Handbook of Statistical Methods for Precision Medicine

The statistical study and development of analytic methodology for individualization of treatments is no longer in its infancy. Many methods of study design, estimation, and inference exist, and the tools available to the analyst are ever growing. This handbook introduces the foundations of modern statistical approaches to precision medicine, bridging key ideas to active lines of current research in precision medicine.

The contributions in this handbook vary in their level of assumed statistical knowledge; all contributions are accessible to a wide readership of statisticians and computer scientists including graduate students and new researchers in the area. Many contributions, particularly those that are more comprehensive reviews, are suitable for epidemiologists and clinical researchers with some statistical training. The handbook is split into three sections: Study Design for Precision Medicine, Estimation of Optimal Treatment Strategies, and Precision Medicine in High Dimensions.

The first focuses on designed experiments, in many instances, building and extending on the notion of sequential multiple assignment randomized trials. Dose finding and simulation-based designs using agent-based modelling are also featured. The second section contains both introductory contributions and more advanced methods, suitable for estimating optimal adaptive treatment strategies from a variety of data sources including non-experimental (observational) studies. The final section turns to estimation in the many-covariate setting, providing approaches suitable to the challenges posed by electronic health records, wearable devices, or any other settings where the number of possible variables (whether confounders, tailoring variables, or other) is high. Together, these three sections bring together some of the foremost leaders in the field of precision medicine, offering new insights and ideas as this field moves towards its third decade.

Chapman & Hall/CRC
Handbooks of Modern Statistical Methods

Series Editor
Garrett Fitzmaurice, *Department of Biostatistics, Harvard School of Public Health, Boston, MA, U.S.A.*

The objective of the series is to provide high-quality volumes covering the state-of-the-art in the theory and applications of statistical methodology. The books in the series are thoroughly edited and present comprehensive, coherent, and unified summaries of specific methodological topics from statistics. The chapters are written by the leading researchers in the field and present a good balance of theory and application through a synthesis of the key methodological developments and examples and case studies using real data.

Published Titles

Handbook of Mixture Analysis
Sylvia Frühwirth-Schnatter, Gilles Celeux, and Christian P. Robert

Handbook of Infectious Disease Data Analysis
Leonhard Held, Niel Hens, Philip O'Neill, and Jacco Walllinga

Handbook of Meta-Analysis
Christopher H. Schmid, Theo Stijnen, and Ian White

Handbook of Forensic Statistics
David L. Banks, Karen Kafadar, David H. Kaye, and Maria Tackett

Handbook of Statistical Methods for Randomized Controlled Trials
KyungMann Kim, Frank Bretz, Ying Kuen K. Cheung, and Lisa Hampson

Handbook of Measurement Error Models
Grace Yi, Aurore Delaigle, and Paul Gustafson

Handbook of Multiple Comparisons
Xinping Cui, Thorsten Dickhaus, Ying Ding, and Jason C. Hsu

Handbook of Bayesian Variable Selection
Mahlet Tadesse and Marina Vannucci

Handbook of Matching and Weighting Adjustments for Causal Inference
José Zubizarreta, Elizabeth A. Stuart, Dylan Small, Paul R. Rosenbaum

Handbook of Bayesian, Fiducial, and Frequentist Inference
James Berger, Xiao-Li Meng, Nancy Reid and Min-ge Xie

Handbook of Sharing Confidential Data: Differential Privacy, Secure Multiparty Computation, and Synthetic Data
Jörg Drechsler, Daniel Kifer, Jerome Reiter and Aleksandra Slavkovic

For more information about this series, please visit: https://www.crcpress.com/Chapman--HallCRC-Handbooks-of-Modern-Statistical-Methods/book-series/CHHANMODSTA

Handbook of Statistical Methods for Precision Medicine

Edited by
Eric Laber
Bibhas Chakraborty
Erica E. M. Moodie
Tianxi Cai
Mark van der Laan

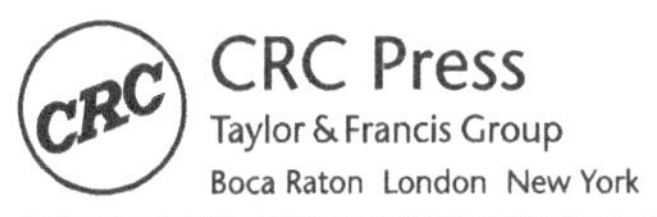

CRC Press is an imprint of the
Taylor & Francis Group, an **informa** business
A CHAPMAN & HALL BOOK

First edition published 2025
by CRC Press
2385 NW Executive Center Drive, Suite 320, Boca Raton FL 33431

and by CRC Press
4 Park Square, Milton Park, Abingdon, Oxon, OX14 4RN

CRC Press is an imprint of Taylor & Francis Group, LLC

Library of Congress Cataloging-in-Publication Data
Names: Laber, Eric B., editor.
Title: Handbook of statistical methods for precision medicine / edited by Eric Laber, Bibhas Chakraborty, Erica E.M. Moodie, Tianxi Cai and Mark van der Laan.
Description: First edition. | Boca Raton, FL : CRC Press, 2025. | Series: Chapman & Hall/CRC handbooks of modern statistical methods | Includes bibliographical references and index.
Identifiers: LCCN 2024015853 (print) | LCCN 2024015854 (ebook) | ISBN 9781032106151 (hardback) | ISBN 9781032106168 (paperback) | ISBN 9781003216223 (ebook)
Subjects: LCSH: Precision medicine--Statistical methods--Handbooks, manuals, etc.
Classification: LCC RM301.3.G45 H365 2025 (print) | LCC RM301.3.G45 (ebook) | DDC 610.2/1--dc23/eng/20240722
LC record available at https://lccn.loc.gov/2024015853
LC ebook record available at https://lccn.loc.gov/2024015854

ISBN: 978-1-032-10615-1 (hbk)
ISBN: 978-1-032-10616-8 (pbk)
ISBN: 978-1-003-21622-3 (ebk)

DOI: 10.1201/9781003216223

Typeset in CMR10 font
by KnowledgeWorks Global Ltd.

Publisher's note: This book has been prepared from camera-ready copy provided by the authors.

Contents

List of Tables

List of Figures

Preface

The statistical study and development of analytic methodology for the individualization of treatments are no longer in their infancy. Many methods of study design, estimation, and inference exist, and the tools available to the analyst are ever growing. This handbook introduces the foundations of modern statistical approaches to precision medicine, bridging seminal ideas to active lines of current research.

The contributions in this handbook vary in their level of assumed statistical knowledge; all contributions are accessible to a wide readership of statisticians and computer scientists including graduate students and new researchers in the area. Many contributions, particularly those that are more comprehensive reviews, are suitable for epidemiologists and clinical researchers with some statistical training. The volume in split into three sections: *Study Design For Precision Medicine*, *Estimation of Optimal Treatment Strategies*, and *Precision Medicine in High Dimensions*. The first focuses on designed experiments, in many instances, building and extending on the notion of sequential multiple assignment randomized trials. Dose finding and simulation-based designs using agent-based modelling are also featured. The second section contains both introductory and more advanced methods, suitable for estimating optimal adaptive treatment strategies from a variety of data sources including non-experimental (observational) studies. The final section considers settings in which the number of covariates (whether confounders, tailoring variables, or other) is large relative to the sample size. Applications include electronic health records, data from wearable devices, and genetics. Together, these three sections bring together some of the foremost leaders in the field of precision medicine, offering new insights and ideas as this field moves towards its third decade.

Acknowledgements

Eric B. Laber is supported by funding from the National Science Foundation and National Institutes of Health. Bibhas Chakraborty is supported by research grants from the Duke-National University of Singapore Medical School and the Ministry of Education, Singapore. Erica E. M. Moodie is supported by a Canada Research Chair in Statistical Methods for Precision Medicine from the Canadian Institutes of Health Research and by a chercheur de mérite career award from the Fonds de recherche du Québec, Santé (FRQS).

We are indebted to our colleagues and collaborators, and the contributors to this diverse volume of insightful reviews and exciting new ideas. We extend sincere thanks to Shomoita Alam and Utek Leong for their assistance in reviewing this work.

Funding for specific works, data statements, and acknowledgements of individual contributors are noted at the end of each chapter.

Durham, USA	*Eric B. Laber*
Singapore	*Bibhas Chakraborty*
Montreal, Canada	*Erica E. M. Moodie*
Boston, USA	*Tianxi Cai*
Berkeley, USA	*Mark van der Laan*

July 2024

Editors

Eric B. Laber is the James B. Duke Distinguished Professor of Statistical Sciences and Biostatistics and Bioinformatics at Duke University. He is a fellow of the American Statistical Association and International Statistical Institute as well as the recipient of the Gottfried E. Noether Award, the Raymond J. Carroll Award, and the American Statistical Association Outstanding Application Award.

Bibhas Chakraborty is an Associate Professor jointly appointed by the Duke-National University of Singapore Medical School (Duke-NUS) and the Department of Statistics and Data Science at the National University of Singapore. He also holds an adjunct faculty position with the Department of Biostatistics and Bioinformatics at Duke University. He is a 2011 recipient of the Calderone Research Prize for Junior Faculty from Columbia University, a 2017 recipient of the Young Statistical Scientist Award from the International Indian Statistical Association and is an Elected Member of the International Statistical Institute (ISI). Along with Dr. Erica E.M. Moodie, he co-authored the first textbook on dynamic treatment regimes (Springer, New York, 2013). Currently he serves as an Associate Editor for Biometrics.

Erica E. M. Moodie is Professor of Biostatistics and Canada Research Chair in Statistical Methods for Precision Medicine at McGill University. She is the 2020 recipient of the CRM-SSC Prize in Statistics, is an Elected Member of the International Statistical Institute, and holds a chercheur de mérite career award from the Fonds de recherche du Québec-Santé. Dr. Moodie is the Co-Editor of Biometrics and a Statistical Editor of Journal of Infectious Diseases.

Tianxi Cai is the John Rock Professor of Population and Translational Data Science at Harvard Chan School of Public Health (HSPH) and a Professor of Biomedical Informatics at Harvard Medical School (HMS). Dr. Cai's research includes statistical learning methods for efficient analysis of multi-institutional electronic health records data, real world evidence, and precision medicine using large scale genomic and phenomic data.

Mark van der Laan is the Jiann-Ping Hsu/Karl E. Peace Professor in Biostatistics and Statistics at the University of California, Berkeley. Mark's research interests include censored data, causal inference, genomics and adaptive designs. Mark has led the development of Targeted Learning, including Super Learning and Targeted maximum likelihood estimation (TMLE). In 2005 Mark was awarded the Committee of Presidents of Statistical Societies (COPSS) Presidential Award. He also received the 2004 Spiegelman Award and 2005 van Dantzig Award. He is co-founder of the international Journal of Biostatistics and Journal of Causal Inference, and has authored various Springer books on Targeted Learning, Censored Data and Multiple Testing.

List of Contributors

Sahir Bhatnagar
McGill University
Montreal, Quebec, USA

Zeyu Bian
University of Miami,
Miami, Florida, USA

Thomas Braun
University of Michigan
Ann Arbor, Michigan, USA

Thomas Burnett
University of Bath
Bath, UK

Nilanjan Chatterjee
John Hopkins
Baltimore, Maryland, USA

Bin Cheng
Columbia University
New York City, New York, USA

Ying Kuen Cheung
Columbia University
New York City, New York, USA

Incheoul Chung
University of Washington
Seattle, Washington, USA

Nadège Costa
University Hospital of Toulouse
Toulouse, France

Romain Demeulemeester
University Hospital of Toulouse
Toulouse, France

Ashkan Ertefaie
University of Rochester
Rochester, New York, USA

Qijia He
University of Washington
Seattle, Washington, USA

Xinyu Hu
Columbia University
New York City, New York, USA

Thomas Jaki
University of Cambridge
Cambridge, UK

Jin Jin
John Hopkins University, University of Pennsylvania
Philadelphia, Pennsylvania, USA

Jeremiah Jones
University of Rochester
Rochester, New York, USA

Edward H Kennedy
Carnegie Mellon University
Pittsburgh, Pennsylvania, USA

Ronald C. Kessler
Harvard Medical School
Boston, Massachusetts, USA

Kelley M Kidwell
University of Michigan
Ann Arbor, Michigan, USA

Michael R. Kosorok
University of North Carolina
Chapel Hill, North Carolina, USA

Sylvie Lambert
McGill University
Montreal, Quebec, USA

Juhee Lee
University of California Santa Cruz
Santa Cruz, California, USA

Alex R. Leudtke
University of Washington
Seattle, Washington, USA

Chen Lu
Massachusetts Institute of Technology
Cambridge, Massachusetts, USA

Yangyi Lu
University of Michigan
Ann Arbor, Michigan, USA

Xinkun Nie
Stanford University
Stanford, California, USA

Min Qian
Columbia University
New York City, New York, USA

David S. Robertson
University of Cambridge
Cambridge, UK

Philippe Saint-Pierre
University of Toulouse
Toulouse, France

Nicolas Savy
University Toulouse III
Toulouse, France

Susan M Shortreed
Kaiser Permenente Washington Health Research Institute
Seattle, Washington, USA

John Sperger
University of North Carolina
Chapel Hill, North Carolina, USA

David A. Stephens
McGill University
Montreal, Quebec, Canada

Robert L. Strawderman
University of Rochester
Rochester, New York, USA

Roy Tamura
University of South Florida
Tampa, Florida, USA

Ambuj Tewari
University of Michigan
Ann Arbor, Michigan, USA

Peter F. Thall
M.D. Anderson Cancer Center
Houston, Texas, USA

Tyler J. Vander
Weele Harvard University
Boston, Massachusetts, USA

Sofia S. Villar
University of Cambridge – MRC Biostatistics Unit
Cambridge, UK

Stefan Wager
Stanford Graduate School of Business
Stanford, California, USA

Michael Wallace
University of Waterloo
Waterloo, Ontario, Canada

Sidi Wang
University of Michigan
Ann Arbor, Michigan, USA

Ziping Xu
University of Michigan
Ann Arbor, Michigan, USA

Ying-Qi Zhao
Fred Hutchinson Cancer Center
Seattle, Washington, USA

Xiaobo Zhong
Bristol Myers Squibb
Englewood Cliffs, New Jersey, USA

Part I

Study Design For Precision Medicine

Chapter 1

Adaptive Designs for Precision Medicine: Fundamental Statistical Considerations

David S. Robertson, Thomas Burnett, Thomas Jaki, Sofia S. Villar

1.1 What are Adaptive Designs?

In a traditional clinical trial, the study design is fixed in advance, the study is carried out and the data are only analyzed after trial completion (Friedman et al., 2010). In contrast, adaptive clinical trial designs pre-plan possible modifications of the study as part of the trial protocol while preserving the validity and integrity of conclusions, with such modifications being made on the basis of the data accumulating over the course of the trial as well as external information (US Department of Health and Human Services Food and Drug Administration, 2019; Dimairo et al., 2020; Pallmann et al., 2018; Burnett et al., 2020). Possible modifications of the trial include changing the sample size, the number of treatments, the study populations or the allocation ratio to different arms. As noted by Burnett et al. (2020), this flexibility is a gateway to potentially more efficient and/or ethical trials where futile treatments may be dropped earlier, more patients can receive a superior treatment, fewer patients may be required overall and/or better conclusions can be reached sooner. The general statistical methodology underpinning the validity of adaptive design has been around for more than 30 years (Bauer et al., 2016). Methods for Group Sequential Designs are even older (Pocock, 1977) and are now well-established and commonly used, while methods for Response-Adaptive Randomization (see Section 1.3.2) date back to the 1930s (Thompson, 1933). Adaptive designs can be used throughout the different phases of the clinical development process, which we now describe.

The clinical development process: phases of clinical trials
Clinical trials are experiments designed to evaluate treatments (e.g., drugs, surgical procedures, digital interventions) on patients and have been typically classified into four phases (Jennison and Turnbull, 1999; Senn, 2021). Phase I trials are usually small experiments conducted to assess the safety of a treatment, the aim being to establish the safety profile across a range of available doses in order to select a dose for further testing. Phase II trials are moderate-sized experiments aimed at early clinical assessment of treatments, to identify if a treatment works well enough to progress for a definitive assessment in the next phase and to assess side effects. Phase III clinical trials imply a full-scale, confirmatory evaluation of the novel treatment option and usually involves many more patients than in phases I or II. Finally, phase IV studies (also known as post-marketing surveillance) are conducted after a treatment has been shown to work in phase III and has been licensed, and aim to find out how well treatments work when used more widely as well as long-term risks and benefits.

How can adaptive designs be used for precision medicine in clinical trials?
The goal of precision medicine is to develop evidence-based treatment options that take into account individual patient characteristics, such as through the identification of

DOI: 10.1201/9781003216223-1

subpopulations that differ in their susceptibility to a disease or response to a treatment (National Research Council, Division on Earth and Life Studies, Board on Life Sciences, Committee on A Framework for Developing a New Taxonomy of Disease, 2011). The possibilities and promise of applying this idea have been dramatically increased by recent developments. Large-scale biologic databases (such as the 1000 genomes project), powerful methods for characterizing patients (such as proteomics, metabolomics, genomics, diverse cellular assays, and mobile health technology) together with computational resources for analyzing large data sets have boosted the interest in precision medicine (Collins and Varmus, 2015). Precision medicine objectives can be relevant to all the phases of clinical trials mentioned above. While we provide some examples for Phase I trials (see Section 1.2.1), our main focus is on Phase II and III trials.

Traditional clinical trials are typically designed to find differences in averages between one experimental treatment and a control, or between doses of the same treatment, and may not easily or efficiently accommodate precision medicine goals. Adaptive designs can offer a framework for delivering precision medicine when needed, and more generally allow multiple treatment options to be efficiently evaluated and tailored to deliver better outcomes for multiple subpopulations of interest. In this chapter, we take a broad look at different classes of adaptive designs and highlight how they can be used with different precision medicine goals in mind.

When using adaptive designs, it is crucial that the adaptive nature of a design does not undermine the trial's integrity and validity (Chow et al., 2005). By integrity of a trial we mean that the trial data and processes have not been compromised while validity requires that the trial appropriately answers the original research questions. Adaptive designs require that the data are collected, analyzed and stored in an appropriate manner at every stage of the trial, with specialized statistical methodology for inference. The primary focus of this chapter is the statistical considerations around the use of adaptive designs; for discussion around practical and logistical issues we refer the interested reader to Pallmann et al. (2018); Quinlan and Krams (2006).

To demonstrate how and when adaptive designs can be useful in the context of precision medicine, we focus on key questions of scientific interest when developing and testing novel treatments: "What is a safe dose to treat a patient group?" (Section 1.2); "Which is the best treatment among multiple options for a patient group?" (Section 1.3); and "Which groups of patients will benefit from a treatment?" (Section 1.4). In each of these Sections, we review the relevant adaptive designs and the corresponding statistical methodology and briefly illustrate their application through real-world examples. First, though we introduce the notation that will be used throughout this chapter.

1.1.1 Notation

In this chapter, we are concerned with evaluating the performance of $K \in \mathbb{Z}^+$ experimental treatments $T_1, ..., T_K$, which (when appropriate) will be compared with a control treatment T_0, which is usually either a standard of care or a placebo. Alternatively, in dose finding studies each T_k can represent a certain dose of a common treatment, and the goal could be to select one of them to carry forward for further evaluation. For simplicity, when presenting notation we shall refer to T_k generically as *arms* to represent either experimental treatments or doses of an identical treatment. In the context of precision medicine, we will typically also be interested in evaluating arms in $L \in \mathbb{Z}^+$ subgroups or subpopulations of patients, which we assume are non-overlapping. In a traditional (non-adaptive) trial design, the number of arms K, subgroups L and total sample size N are assumed to be fixed and known in advance. In contrast, adaptive designs can include the option of modifying K, L and N based on interim trial data. We assume that there are a total of $J - 1$ interim analyses, giving rise to a J-stage trial design (where $J \in \mathbb{Z}^+$). Note that in some adaptive designs,

J need not be fixed but can itself be adapted based on the interim data. In dose finding studies, a stage can represent a cohort of patients.

For what follows, it is useful to define the sample size for each stage. We let $r^{(j)}$ denote the proportion of the total sample size N in stage $j \in \{1, \ldots, J\}$, where $\sum_{j=1}^{J} r^{(j)} = 1$ and $0 < r^{(j)} < 1$. Similarly, we let $r_{k,l}^{(j)}$ denote the proportion of the total sample size N allocated to arm $k \in \{0, 1, \ldots, K\}$ and subgroup $l \in \{1, \ldots, L\}$, where $\sum_{j=1}^{J} \sum_{k=0}^{K} \sum_{l=1}^{L} r_{k,l}^{(j)} = 1$ and $0 \leq r_{k,l}^{(j)} \leq 1$. For example, in the simplest case where equal randomization is used, $r^{(j)} = 1/J$ and $r_{k,l}^{(j)} = 1/(J(K+1)L)$. Note that since N can be a random variable, we may also want to fix a maximum feasible sample size n_{max} for the trial.

When arm k is assigned to patient $i \in \{1, \ldots, N\}$ belonging to subgroup l, this generates a patient outcome $Y_{i,k,l}$. This is a random variable representing the primary outcome measure of the clinical trial. We assume that $Y_{i,k,l}$ depends on the arm and subgroup-specific parameter of interest $\theta_{k,l}$. We also allow $Y_{i,k,l}$ to depend on a vector of $C \in \mathbb{Z}^+$ patient covariates (also known as prognostic factors), denoted $\boldsymbol{X}_{i,l} = (X_{1,i,l}, \ldots, X_{C,i,l})$. For example, with continuous outcomes one could have a linear regression model for patient responses:

$$Y_{i,k,l} = \theta_{k,l} + \boldsymbol{X}_{i,l}^T \boldsymbol{\beta} + \epsilon_i$$

where $\boldsymbol{\beta} = (\beta_1, \ldots, \beta_C)$ and $\epsilon_i \sim \mathcal{N}(0, \sigma^2)$. Equally, one could consider other types of models for alternative outcomes of interest, such as a logistic regression model for binary outcomes.

A final concept we introduce is that of hypothesis testing for the parameters of interest $\theta_{k,l}$. We focus on the case where the null hypotheses are given by $H_{0,k,l} : \theta_{k,l} \leq \theta_{0,l}$ versus one-sided alternative hypotheses $H_{1,k,l} : \theta_{k,l} > \theta_{0,l}$ for $k \in \{1, \ldots, K\}$, assuming a larger value of $\theta_{k,l}$ represents a desirable outcome. Hence we are focusing on superiority trials where an active arm is compared with a placebo; if there is an active control, then two-sided hypothesis testing might be more appropriate (providing symmetry in testing for superiority). In general, the question of whether to use one-sided or two-sided tests in clinical trials is somewhat controversial; see Bland and Bland (1994); Fisher (1991); Knottnerus and Bouter (2001) for examples of different viewpoints.

At the end of stage j of the trial, we can calculate an estimator $\hat{\theta}_{k,l}^{(j)}$ of the parameter of interest, such as the maximum likelihood estimator (MLE). Typically, we can then use this estimator to form a test statistic $\mathcal{T}_{k,l}^{(j)}$ to test the null hypothesis (see Section 1.1.2.1) at stage $j < J$ if the adaptive design calls for this; otherwise, hypothesis testing will only be done at the end of the trial (i.e. stage J).

Formal definition of an adaptive design

Given the notation and concepts introduced above, one can also consider the following more formal definitions of trial designs (i.e., one that determines the sampling strategy or the patient allocation to treatments during the trial) both in the "traditional" and "adaptive" sense. A traditional design of a clinical trial would determine *fixed* values of all the design elements in Table 1.1 in advance of observing any data on $Y_{i,k,l}$ and $\boldsymbol{X}_{i,l}$, based on statistical considerations (e.g., a set of values for the parameter(s) $\theta_{k,l}$, some hypotheses of interest and associated statistical tests). In contrast, an adaptive design would use a (set of) rule(s) to determine the design elements as the accumulating trial data $Y_{i,k,l}$ and $\boldsymbol{X}_{i,l}$ (as well as any trial-external information) are observed. Note that the design elements at stage j can themselves be random until the data at stage $j-1$ is observed, and that the rules themselves can change based on previously observed data. A key property of these rules is that they will preserve the trial's integrity and validity (e.g., for frequentist adaptive designs, preserving error rates associated with the hypotheses of interest is central; see Section 1.1.2.1).

Table 1.1 *Summary of notation used in this chapter. The subscript i refers to patient $i \in \{1, \ldots, N\}$, k refers to treatment $k \in \{0, 1, \ldots, K\}$ and l refers to subgroup $l \in \{1, \ldots, L\}$. The superscript (j) refers to stage $j \in \{1, \ldots, J\}$. When $J = 1$, $K = 1$ or $L = 1$, we drop the corresponding superscript or subscript for notational convenience.*

Symbol	**Meaning**
Design elements	
K	number of arms (treatments or doses)
J	number of stages/cohorts
L	number of subgroups
N	total sample size
n_{max}	maximum sample size
T_k	treatment or dose k
$r_{k,l}^{(j)}$	proportion of patients
Data available	
$Y_{i,k,l}$	patient outcome
$\boldsymbol{X}_{i,l}$	patient covariates
Statistical concepts	
$\theta_{k,l}$	parameter of interest
$\hat{\theta}_{k,l}^{(j)}$	estimator of parameter of interest
$\mathcal{T}_{k,l}^{(j)}$	test statistic of parameter of interest
$H_{0,k,l}$	null hypothesis
$H_{1,k,l}$	alternative hypothesis

1.1.2 Key Statistical Concepts and Trial Metrics

In this subsection, we discuss key statistical issues to consider for adaptive designs for precision medicine, from both a frequentist and a Bayesian perspective. As part of this, we highlight the most commonly reported metrics for adaptive designs.

1.1.2.1 Principles of Error Control

We start by recapping traditional concepts of frequentist type I error control. These concepts are especially important from a regulatory perspective (US Department of Health and Human Services Food and Drug Administration, 2019; Committee for Medicinal Products for Human Use, 2007) for confirmatory adaptive designs. The type I error rate for a single null hypothesis $H_{0,k,l} : \theta_{k,l} \leq \theta_{0,l}$ is defined as $\sup_{\theta_{k,l} \leq \theta_{0,l}} Pr(\text{rejecting } H_{0,k,l} \,|\, \theta_{k,l})$, and for confirmatory trials this is controlled below a pre-specified level $\alpha \in (0,1)$, e.g., 0.05 or 0.025. In many contexts, the type I error rate will be maximized on the boundary of the null parameter space, i.e., when $\theta_{k,l} = \theta_{0,k}$, such as when using a likelihood ratio test with a monotone likelihood function. More generally, when there is repeated testing of $H_{0,k,l}$ at stages $j = 1,\ldots,J$, the overall type I error rate is given by $\sup_{\theta_{k,l}\leq\theta_{0,l}} \sum_{j=1}^{J} Pr(\text{rejecting } H_{0,k,l} \text{ at stage } j \,|\, \theta_{k,l})$; see Sections 1.3.1 for further details in the context of multi-arm multi-stage (MAMS) designs. Note that in what follows, we typically assume that a test statistic $\mathcal{T}$ of the parameter of interest follows a known distribution (at least asymptotically). However, if the trial adaptations are complex, then this is not trivial to achieve and methods for robust inference (e.g., bootstrap methods) may be required instead.

Conditional invariance principle, combination tests and conditional error functions
A general approach to control the type I error rate for confirmatory adaptive designs is known as the *conditional invariance principle* (Brannath et al., 2007). To fix ideas and for simplicity, we focus on trials with $J = 2$ stages (i.e. a single interim analysis) and consider a single null hypothesis (i.e. $K = L = 1$) $H_{0,1,1}$, denoted H_0 for convenience. Generalizations to $J > 2$ stages are relatively straightforward (see references provided below), and later in this subsection, we discuss testing multiple hypotheses.

In our two-stage trial setting, the design characteristics of the second stage are chosen based on the first-stage data (as well as any external information). Let $\mathcal{T}^{(2)}$ denote the test statistic for H_0 calculated using only the second stage data. In general, $\mathcal{T}^{(2)}$ will depend on the first-stage data as this determines the second stage-design characteristics. However, it is often possible to transform $\mathcal{T}^{(2)}$ so that the conditional null distribution of $\mathcal{T}^{(2)}$ given the first-stage data and the second stage design is invariant (i.e., equals a fixed pre-specified distribution). Typically this can be achieved by transforming $\mathcal{T}^{(2)}$ into a p-value p_2 which is conditionally uniformly distributed under the null. This usually implies that p_2 is stochastically independent of the first stage data, see Liu et al. (2002). Hence the joint distribution of p_2 and the first stage data is known and invariant with respect to the adaptation rules, which allows the specification of an invariant rejection region in terms of the first stage data and p_2.

An invariant rejection region can be specified using *combination tests* or *conditional error functions* and we now describe each in turn. Starting with combination tests, let p_1 denote the p-value calculated using only the first stage data. A two-stage combination test (Bauer and Köhne, 1994) is defined using a combination function $C(p_1, p_2)$ that is monotonically increasing in both arguments, boundaries for early stopping α_0, α_1 and a critical value c for the final analysis. At the interim analysis, the trial is stopped early for efficacy (with the rejection of H_0) if $p_1 \leq \alpha_1$ or for futility (otherwise known as lack-of-benefit) if $p_1 > \alpha_0$. If $\alpha_1 < p_1 \leq \alpha_0$, the trial continues to the second stage and H_0 is rejected if $C(p,q) \leq c$, where

$$\alpha_1 + \int_{\alpha_1}^{\alpha_0} \int_0^1 \mathbf{1}[C(x,y) \leq c]\, dy\, dx = \alpha.$$

This procedure defines a level-α test as long as the distribution of p_2 conditioned on p_1 is stochastically larger than or equal to the uniform distribution (Brannath et al., 2002). Examples of combination functions in the context of adaptive designs can be found in Bauer et al. (2016), while the extension of the combination test approach to $J > 2$ stages is described in Brannath et al. (2002).

Turning to the conditional error function approach, let $\mathcal{D}_1$ denote the first stage data and $B(\mathcal{D}_1)$ denote a measurable function (known as the conditional error function) from the first stage sample space to $[0,1]$ such that $E_{H_0}(B) \leq \alpha$. If the trial proceeds to the second stage, H_0 is rejected if $p_2 \leq B(\mathcal{D}_1)$. Note that $B = 0$ corresponds to early stopping for futility while $B = 1$ corresponds to early rejection of H_0. This procedure defines a level-α test as long as the distribution of p_2 conditioned on $\mathcal{D}_1$ is stochastically larger than or equal to the uniform distribution (Bauer et al., 2016). Combination tests and conditional error functions are in fact equivalent, see Posch and Bauer (1999).

Multiple hypotheses and type I error rate control

In our context, when $K > 1$ or $L > 1$ there are multiple hypotheses of interest. Various generalizations of the type I error rate can be considered, the most common in the adaptive trial setting being the familywise error rate (FWER), which is the probability of making at least one type I error. To define this more formally, we first need to define the family $\mathcal{F}$ of hypotheses. Depending on the trial context and goals, the family could include all hypotheses tested in the adaptive design, $\mathcal{F} = \{H_{0,k,l}\}_{k=1,\ldots,K;\, l=1,\ldots,L}$, or only a subset of interest, such as a treatment-specific family $\mathcal{F}_k = \{H_{0,k,l}\}_{l=1,\ldots,L}$. For further discussion on defining families of hypotheses for error control when there are both treatments and patient subgroups within the same trial protocol, see Stallard et al. (2019).

Once a family $\mathcal{F}$ with corresponding index set $\mathcal{I}$ is defined, let Θ denote the parameter space for $\{\theta_{k,l}\}_{(k,l)\in\mathcal{I}}$. We denote the index set of true null hypotheses by $\mathcal{I}_0$ and the number of false rejections by $V = \#\{i \in \mathcal{I}_0 : H_{0,i} \text{ is rejected}\}$. The FWER, given a parameter configuration $\theta \in \Theta$, is defined as $\text{FWER}_\theta = Pr(V \geq 1 \,|\, \theta)$, and this can be controlled in the strong or weak sense. Weak control of the FWER is defined under the global null $\mathcal{H}_0 = \bigcap_{i\in\mathcal{I}} H_{0,i}$, so that $\sup_{\theta\in\Theta_0} \text{FWER}_\theta \leq \alpha$, where Θ_0 is the parameter space under $\mathcal{H}_0$. In contrast, strong control of the FWER guarantees that the FWER is controlled below α regardless of which or how many null hypotheses are true, i.e. $\sup_{\theta\in\Theta} \text{FWER}_\theta \leq \alpha$. In confirmatory adaptive designs, strong FWER control is typically required for the primary family of interest (US Department of Health and Human Services Food and Drug Administration, 2019).

A recent development has been the consideration of the false discovery rate (FDR) for adaptive trials (Wason and Robertson, 2021), in particular for master protocol designs such as platform or umbrella trials (see Sections 1.3.3 and 1.4.2) The FDR is defined as the expected proportion of the hypotheses rejected that are in fact false (i.e. incorrectly rejected). More formally, $\text{FDR} = E[V/R]$, where V is defined as above and R is the total number of rejections made (and by definition, $\text{FDR} = 0$ when $V = R = 0$). The FDR is a more liberal error rate control criterion than the FWER, but this means that FDR-controlling procedures will typically have a greater power. In what follows though, we will mainly focus on the FWER as the error metric of choice.

Closed testing procedures

A powerful and general way to construct multiple testing strategies is to use the closed testing principle (Marcus et al., 1976). Given a family of hypotheses $\mathcal{F}$ with index set $\mathcal{I}$ as above, we define the corresponding closed system of all hypotheses, consisting of all possible intersection hypotheses $\mathcal{H}_\mathcal{J} = \bigcap_{j\in\mathcal{J}} H_j$, $\mathcal{J} \subseteq \mathcal{I}$. Note that this includes all the individual (also known as 'elementary') hypotheses $H_i, i \in \mathcal{I}$. For each possible intersection hypothesis, a suitable level-α test is defined that takes into account the multiplicity – for example, using a Bonferroni test or a Dunnett test (see Section 1.3.1). Given the observed data, we reject an individual hypothesis H_i, $i \in \mathcal{I}$ only if all intersection hypotheses containing H_i are also rejected (each at level α). That is, we globally reject H_i at level α if for all $\mathcal{J} \subseteq \mathcal{I}$ with $i \in \mathcal{J}$, we reject tests of $H_\mathcal{J}$ at level α.

A desirable property of a closed testing procedure is that of *consonance* so that the rejection of an intersection hypothesis $\mathcal{H}_\mathcal{J}$ implies that at least one individual hypothesis $H_j, j \in \mathcal{J}$ is also rejected. Romano et al. (2011) showed that any multiple testing procedure that is not consonant can be replaced by a consonant multiple testing procedure that rejects at least as many hypotheses. More generally, Burnett and Jennison (2021) proved that a procedure strongly controls the FWER if and only if it is a closed testing procedure, i.e. even if not defined as such, any testing procedure that strongly controls the FWER implies a closed testing procedure. Closed testing procedures can be used in conjunction with combination tests or conditional error functions, allowing trial adaptivity while also controlling the FWER. We refer the reader to Bauer and Kieser (1999) and the tutorial of Bretz et al. (2009) for concrete examples.

Power considerations
Aside from type I error rate control, another key frequentist consideration is the type II error rate or (equivalently) the power of an adaptive design. For a single hypothesis $H_{0,k,l} : \theta_{k,l} \leq \theta_{0,l}$ the power is typically defined as $1 - \beta = Pr(\text{rejecting } H_{0,k,l} \,|\, \theta_{k,l} = \theta_{0,l} + \delta_{k,l})$, where $\delta_{k,l} > 0$ is a pre-defined treatment effect of interest (for a review of Bayesian interpretations of 'power' that move away from point alternatives, see Kunzmann et al. (2021)). However, in our context when $K > 1$ or $L > 1$, power can have various definitions (Vickerstaff et al., 2019). Common ones include

- Marginal power: $Pr(\text{rejecting } H_{0,k,l} \,|\, \theta_{k,l} = \theta_{0,l} + \delta_{k,l})$ given k and l
- Disjunctive power: $Pr(\text{rejecting at least one } H_{0,k,l} \,|\, \boldsymbol{\theta})$
- Conjunctive power: $Pr(\text{rejecting all } H_{0,k,l} \,|\, \boldsymbol{\theta})$

where $\boldsymbol{\theta}$ is the vector of $\theta_{k,l}$ for $k = 1, \ldots, K$ and $l = 1, \ldots, L$, with $\theta_{k,l} = \theta_{0,l} + \delta_{k,l}$. The definitions of disjunctive and conjunctive power above can straightforwardly be refined to focus on a particular experimental treatment by keeping k fixed, or a particular subgroup by keeping l fixed. The choice of the $\delta_{k,l}$ depends on the trial context; see Section 1.3.1 for an example of power under the least favorable configuration for MAMS designs.

1.1.2.2 Estimation

While type I error rate control and power considerations are typically paramount for confirmatory adaptive designs, *estimation* of the parameter of interest (such as the treatment effect) is also a key consideration. An issue with adaptive designs in general is that conventional end-of-trial point estimates (e.g. the MLE) are prone to statistical bias (US Department of Health and Human Services Food and Drug Administration, 2019; Marschner, 2021). This is defined as a systematic tendency for the estimate of treatment effect to deviate from its true value. More formally, the mean bias of an estimator $\hat{\theta}_{k,l}$ is defined as $E(\hat{\theta}_{k,l}) - \theta_{k,l}$. An estimator may be biased due to the trial adaptations affecting its sampling distribution, such as the selection of a treatment or subgroup. Apart from bias, it is also important to consider the variance $\text{Var}(\hat{\theta}_{k,l})$ or mean-squared error $E[(\hat{\theta}_{k,l} - \theta_{k,l})^2]$ of an estimator, reflecting the classical bias-variance trade-off. Although the precision of estimators is less often reported in the literature, this can be compared using estimation efficiency measures; see for example Sverdlov and Rosenberger (2013). In order to correct for the bias in point estimators (while ideally maintaining reasonable variance), a variety of unbiased and bias-reduced estimators for different classes of adaptive designs have been proposed; see Robertson et al. (2021) for an up-to-date systematic methodological review.

The construction of confidence intervals (or regions) for the parameter(s) of interest is another important consideration. In a similar way to point estimation, confidence interval estimation can also be affected by trial adaptations so that standard confidence intervals may not achieve their nominal coverage. A number of proposals have been made for constructing a confidence interval for a single parameter of interest $\theta_{k,l}$, see Brannath et al. (2006). One such proposal is the repeated confidence interval approach, where a sequence $\mathcal{C}_j$, $j = 1, \ldots J$ are defined so that $Pr(\theta_{k,l} \in \mathcal{C}_j \text{ for all } j) \geq 1 - \alpha$ for all $\theta_{k,l}$. Repeated confidence intervals can be obtained using the duality of confidence intervals and the hypothesis testing strategy, and are valid even if one does not adhere to the pre-specified stopping rules. Meanwhile, for inference about a parameter vector $\boldsymbol{\theta}$, simultaneous confidence intervals have been proposed for closed testing procedures in adaptive designs (Magirr et al., 2013; Posch et al., 2005).

1.1.2.3 Patient Benefit Metrics

Particularly in the context of precision medicine, different metrics to reflect the "ethical" or patient benefit properties of adaptive designs have been considered. However, these metrics are still not commonly reported or standardized in their definitions, reflecting the priority of inferential and estimation goals. Some relevant examples of possibly useful patient benefit metrics include:

- The number of treatment successes (for binary outcomes) or the total response (for continuous outcomes) in the trial: $\sum_{i=1}^{N} Y_{i,k,l}$. When averaged over trial realizations for binary outcomes, this is referred to as the expected number of successes (ENS). Alternatively, for binary outcomes some authors focus on the number of treatment failures $\sum_{i=1}^{N}(1 - Y_{i,k,l})$ and report the expected number of failures (ENF). These metrics can also be considered focusing on a particular subgroup l.
- The proportion of patients allocated to the best arm for each subgroup l: $\sum_{i=1}^{N} 1\{a_{i,k^*,l} = 1\}/N_l$, where $a_{i,k,l} = 1$ if patient i is allocated to treatment k (and is equal to 0 otherwise), $k^* = \text{argmax}_k\{\theta_{k,l}\}$ and N_l is the number of patients in subgroup l.

Typically the above patient benefit properties refer to patients within the trial only, but these metrics could also be considered including patients outside the trial (but who could potentially benefit from the trial's results). However, if one were to do that, then the corresponding inferential properties of the design (such as power) would also have to take into account future patients (Kaptein, 2019).

1.1.2.4 Bayesian Approaches to Trial Design

The standard statistical approach to designing and analyzing traditional clinical trials is a *frequentist* one. There are many virtues of this traditional approach, including its extreme rigor and narrowness of focus to the experiment at hand, but a side effect of this virtue is inflexibility (Berry, 2006). Frequentist adaptive designs aim to address the latter point, but they usually require either restrictions to the design in terms of adaptations that can be considered, or a specific analysis (or both) in order to preserve the validity of the study. The Bayesian perspective of a clinical trial can allow greater flexibility through the use of prior information that is updated using the accumulating data from the trial (with the possibility of being assessed at any time), and with the possibility of modifying the design of the trial based on this. Bayesian statistical methods are being increasingly used in clinical trial designs, and are naturally well-suited to designing adaptive trials. Computational cost is no longer such a large barrier thanks to increased computing power and efficient algorithms for sampling and describing posterior distributions.

We refer the reader to the books Berry et al. (2010); and Spiegelhalter et al. (2004) for a detailed resource on Bayesian adaptive designs. Section 1.2 of the book by Berry et al. (2010) describes seven key aspects in which a Bayesian and frequentist perspective on trial design differ. Here we briefly mention some concepts that will help the reader follow the discussions presented in the later sections.

- The parameter of interest $\theta_{k,l}$ is considered a random variable rather than an unknown constant as in the frequentist paradigm. Bayesians will associate a prior probability distribution to $\theta_{k,l}$ (i.e., before any data is available) and a posterior one (i.e. once some data is observed).

- Bayes theorem can be used to revise prior probabilities in light of the data collected as follows:
$$p(\theta_{k,l}|Y) = \frac{p(Y|\theta_{k,l})}{p(Y)} \times p(\theta_{k,l}) \tag{1.1}$$
where $p(\theta_{k,l}|Y)$ is the posterior probability of $\theta_{k,l}$ given the observed outcome data Y, $p(Y|\theta_{k,l})$ is the likelihood of the observations Y and $p(\theta_{k,l})$ is the prior distribution of $\theta_{k,l}$. This implies that data can be used continually as accumulated to update this probability (or to derive the posterior probability of the null or alternative hypothesis being true).
- Predictive probabilities can be computed by averaging conditional probabilities (i.e. conditioned on $\theta_{k,l}$ as in a frequentist approach) over all possible values of the unknown parameters. These probabilities are important as they can also be used for decision-making and defining an adaptive design based on them.
- The Bayesian approach is flexible in incorporating wider aspects of decision-making. Traditional frequentist statistics is geared towards the use of observed data $Y_{i,k,l}$ to make inferences around $\theta_{k,l}$. Such inferences are usually made without explicit regard to the decision that will be made based on them. Clinical trials are decision problems, treatment recommendations will be made based on them, and treatment decisions will also be made during the clinical experiment itself. Each possible decision will generate future observations, and each will be associated with different benefits and costs, which can be modeled as a loss function (or a utility function). These different scenarios can be weighted with predictive probabilities.
- Randomization in clinical trials (to allocate patients to treatments) is a defining element of a well-conducted study, ensuring comparability of treatment groups, mitigating selection bias, and providing the basis for statistical inference (Rosenberger and Lachin, 2015). The latter is not defined for a Bayesian analysis which is based on subjective probability.
- In analyzing the results of a clinical trial, the Bayesian approach naturally permits bringing in all available information to bear on the scientific question being addressed and into the decision process. In a frequentist perspective, such potentially important information can be used to inform the interpretation of the statistical results but is usually not formally incorporated into the decision process.

It is worth pointing out that the frequentist perspective is still dominant among regulatory agencies. Therefore, frequentist operating characteristics (such as type I/II errors) are very important to regulators, specially so for confirmatory or later-phase trials. Bayesian ideas for designing adaptive designs are however routinely applied in dose-finding trials and more widely used with an explicit goal to build sequential adaptive designs with good frequentist operating characteristics than to implement a fully Bayesian approach. This makes it difficult to classify an adaptive design as frequentist or Bayesian. This distinction may apply to the inference procedure used for the final analysis and/or to the design of the adaptive trial itself. In our opinion, the inferential classification may not be helpful, since the choice of inference procedure depends on a study's goals and regulators' preferences between these two approaches. Moreover, many innovative trial approaches have Bayesian design aspects but the inference procedure focuses on the frequentist operating characteristics, e.g. Ventz et al. (2017).

Some could argue that the use of a prior (informative) distribution would make an adaptive design Bayesian but we instead follow the definition in Robertson et al. (2023) (for response-adaptive designs) by which we define a Bayesian adaptive design as "a design rule that depends recursively on the posterior probability of the parameters" (Atkinson and Biswas, 2019), where the recursive updating of the allocation probabilities is done via Bayes Theorem. Such adaptive designs are "fully Bayesian" as in Ryan et al. (2016), and allow for the full probabilistic description of all uncertainties, including future outcomes (e.g. through predictive probabilities).

1.2 What is a Safe Dose to Treat a Patient Group?

Phase I trials in many therapeutic areas have the goal of identifying the maximum tolerated dose (MTD), which is the highest dose that is safe in the sense of controlling the risk of unacceptable side effects (NIH, 2014). In practice, this means identifying the dose at which the probability of a dose-limiting toxicity (DLT) is equal to some pre-specified target level, usually around 20–33%. We denote this toxicity target as θ^*. Experiments with a goal of selecting a dose among several ones is a well-established area to apply precision medicine concepts. For example, in many contexts (like oncology), finding a safe dose requires identifying one that gives a suitable compromise between toxicity and efficacy. In that setting, one could account for a potential subgroup effect (i.e., a different safe dose among subgroups) in dose-finding studies (Babb and Rogatko, 2001). However, this can be challenging to achieve and requires careful design considerations, since the exclusion of a subgroup that could in fact benefit from a safe treatment can cause a beneficial effect to be missed (Cotterill and Jaki, 2018; Neuenschwander et al., 2016). An extra challenge in these study designs is how to reduce the potentially large number of covariates (or biomarkers of interest) and covariate-dose interactions to a few of interest that can be efficiently studied in experiments with small sample sizes (Guo and Yuan, 2017).

Since dose-finding studies are usually small and treat consenting patients sequentially at different doses (until too high a proportion of unacceptable side effects are observed, or a suitable dose is identified), adaptive designs are a natural fit to implement these. In this chapter, we do not go into the full details of adaptive designs for dose-finding studies (See the introduction of Chapter 4 for references) but aim to briefly describe one of the currently commonly used model-based (adaptive) approach to dose finding as an introduction to other adaptive designs we will explore later on. Model-based, model assisted and/or curve-free Bayesian approaches have been found to be preferable to algorithmic methods on statistical and practical grounds. Specifically, these approaches exhibit a superior performance in terms of identifying the dose with the desired toxicity rate and allocating a greater expected proportion of patients to doses at, or close to, that dose (Jaki et al., 2013; Paoletti et al., 2015). Additionally, selecting early-phase designs with such statistical properties impact the success prospect of later (confirmatory) studies (Conaway and Petroni, 2019) as well as its efficiency or speed in challenging contexts (Harrington et al., 2013; Riviere et al., 2015). Further personalization of a dose-finding study can be formulated as an appropriate extension of the model described in section 1.2.1. We will discuss some of these extensions, including designs that are aimed at finding a best dose (as in a phase II setting) at the end of this section.

1.2.1 Continual Reassessment Method (CRM)

Suppose a trial will recruit patients in J stages in which $d_j \in \{1, \ldots, K\}$ denotes the dose allocated to all patients in the jth cohort and let $Y_{i,k} \in \{0, 1\}$ be the response of patient i to dose k (where 1 denotes a DLT occurring). Thus, we define a data set at stage j of the trial, after data have been collected from j cohorts, by the sequence of doses and responses $(d_i, Y_{i,k})$ for $i = 1, \ldots, j * b$, where b is the cohort size. Note that b can be as small as 1 and does not even have to have a constant size but in practice, this is usually a small number of patients.

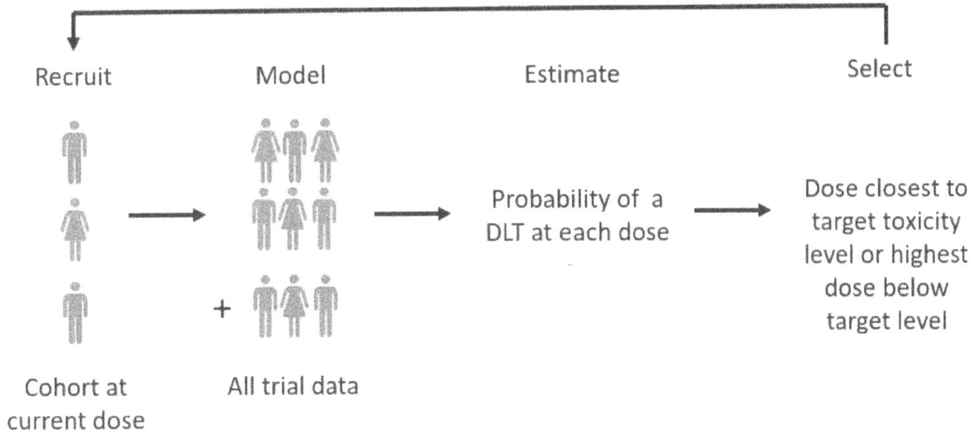

Figure 1.1 *Schematic of a trial using the continual reassessment method (CRM).*

O'Quigley et al. (1990) introduced the CRM model and considered a one-parameter model for the relationship between dose and toxicity such as

$$Pr(Y_{i,k} = 1, d_i = k) = \omega(k, a) = \left(\frac{\tanh(T_k) + 1}{2}\right)^a,$$

where a is the model parameter that is assumed to be negatively related with the chances of a DTL and T_k represents dose level k. One method of deriving these *transformed* doses is to elicit prior estimates of the probability of each dose causing a DLT, and then solve the above equation to obtain the transformed doses for each dose level k. Further details on this can be found in Cheung (2011). In general, *transforming* doses creates dose labels that ensure the model fits well before the trial starts; as discussed in Wheeler et al. (2019), the actual dose scale of the drug does not matter. For an example transformation from drug-specific doses to dose labels see Figure 3 in Wheeler et al. (2019). Common model choices, prior reference values, and resultant dose labels can be found in Table 1 by Wheeler et al. (2019).

The MTD is defined as the dose level k^* that has an associated probability of a DLT closest to some target toxicity level θ^*. In general, the CRM models the relationship between dose and the risk of a patient experiencing a DLT, using an iterative process to make use of all available trial data when choosing the dose for the next patient cohort (O'Quigley et al., 1990; O'Quigley and Shen, 1996). Based on all available data from the trial the relationship between dose and toxicity is modeled to inform the choice of dose for the next cohort. The aim of this experiment is to learn about the parameter a in order to estimate the MTD from the resulting curve. Patients enter the trial sequentially in cohorts and each cohort is allocated the dose level that is the current best estimate of the MTD or the highest available dose below the target level. This process is iterated for each new cohort of patients, ensuring that at all times all available data are used. Figure 1.1 gives a schematic of a trial using the CRM.

The CRM is an example of a Bayesian Adaptive design (as described in 1.1.2.4) and hence requires a prior density function, $\pi(a)$, that represents beliefs about the parameter a before conducting the trial. Note that in general, the parameter a could be a vector of one or more parameters that alters the shape of the dose-toxicity relationship. As in O'Quigley et al. (1990), if $a > 0$ then we can set $\pi(a) = \exp(-a)$. The posterior density function for a, $f(a, \boldsymbol{Y}_k^{(j)})$ is defined via Bayes' theorem at each interim $j > 0$, where $\boldsymbol{Y}_k^{(j)}$ is the set of observed responses from the first j cohorts. We define $\boldsymbol{Y}_k^{(0)}$ as the empty set, so that

$f(a, \mathbf{Y}_k^{(0)}) = \pi(a)$. In the CRM model, the posterior density given the current data $\mathbf{Y}_k^{(j)}$ is updated recursively. This generates an update for the estimates of the probability of a DLT occurring if cohort $j+1$ is allocated to each of the k possible dose levels. These estimated toxicity probabilities can be computed as follows:

$$\hat{\theta}_k^{(j)} = \int \omega(k, a) f(a, \mathbf{Y}_k^{(j)})\, da.$$

Patients in each cohort are allocated the dose level that is the current best estimate of the MTD, defined as the dose level k for which $|\hat{\theta}_k^{(j)} - \theta^*|$ is the smallest.

The application of the CRM design is highly flexible, allowing the investigators to adjust the design to suit the particular trial and trialist (making use of all trial data wherever it is introduced, as is seen in the example to follow). Both the cohort size b and the sample size N of a CRM trial are determined before the trial begins; sample sizes are often planned with practical constraints in mind rather than statistical properties, and simulation may be used to understand statistical operating characteristics (Wheeler et al., 2019). Similarly, the total number of doses K is usually determined before the trial starts.

1.2.1.1 Example: Using the CRM to Find a Tolerable Dose of a Repurposed Cancer Drug

Imatinib is a medicine licensed for some types of cancers. A recently published study (Wilkins et al., 2021) has shown that Imatinib may have beneficial effects in the subgroup of patients with Pulmonary Arterial Hypertension (PAH), a rare condition. However, there have been concerns about its safety and the typical doses used in oncology have been found to not be well tolerated in PAH patients (Hoeper et al., 2013). To improve the investigator's understanding, of the PIPAH study (Wilkins et al., 2021) uses a CRM model to study the best tolerated dose (i.e. a dose which has a 20% probability that a patient will not be able to continue Imatinib for 5 consecutive days) assuming this dose may be much lower than that currently recommended for cancer patients.

1.2.2 Other Adaptive Designs for Finding a Safe Dose

Since the proposal of the CRM 30 years ago, numerous modifications of the design have been proposed. The Escalation with Overdose Control (EWOC) approach (Babb et al., 1998) is one of them and was proposed in response to concerns that the CRM tended to allocate too many subjects to dose levels with an associated probability of DLT corresponding to overdosing. Similarly to the CRM, the EWOC uses all available data to make dose-escalation decisions with a target toxicity level used to choose which dose level the next patient or cohort should receive. However, the EWOC approach assigns the next patient using a skewed allocation criterion to account for the fact that the overdosing of patients is much more undesirable compared to the underdosing. This results in a more conservative patient allocation approach, with fewer patients being exposed to possible overdosing compared to the CRM, while still benefiting from the model attempting to allocate the patients near the MTD (Wheeler et al., 2017; Tighiouart and Rogatko, 2010). Additionally, the same statistical model is re-expressed in a way that allows focus on the clinically relevant parameters, the MTD, and the probability of a DLT at the lowest dose. This means that prior information about the treatment being investigated can easily be incorporated and one can visualise how the distribution of the MTD changes over the course of the trial.

As discussed in Burnett et al. (2020), the model-based approaches above serve as the main framework for other proposed approaches designed for trials with novel drug combinations, endpoints that use time-to-event data and/or efficacy outcomes, or information about the severity of observed toxicities. These designs have found their way into clinical practice in recent years, primarily in oncology for cytotoxic treatments. However, they can be used for novel molecularly targeted anti-cancer therapies (Mandrekar et al., 2007), and in other disease areas altogether: O'Quigley et al. (2001) proposed CRM-type designs for anti-retroviral drugs to treat Human Immunodeficiency Virus (HIV); Lu et al. (2016) conducted a dose-escalation study of quercetin in patients with Hepatitis C; Whitehead et al. (2006) proposed a model-based design for trials in healthy volunteers; and Lyden et al. (2019) used a CRM design in the RHAPSODY trial in stroke patients.

In the CRM (and other dose-finding approaches), a common assumption is that of a monotonic relationship between toxicity probabilities and doses. While this may hold for single-agent trials there are other treatments (e.g., in oncology) in which this will not be the case. In such a setting, alternative designs such as the No Monotonicity Assumption or Partial Ordering Continual Reassessment Method designs should be used (Abbas et al., 2020). Many other types of dose-finding designs have also been proposed, including ones based on optimal design theory (Haines et al., 2003; Azriel, 2014; Haines and Clark, 2014; Liu and Yuan, 2015) and model-free designs (Gasparini and Eisele, 2000; Mander and Sweeting, 2015; Yuan et al., 2016; Mozgunov and Jaki, 2019)

1.2.3 How to Identify the Best Dose

Once a safe range of doses has been found, the next question is how to choose the 'best' or 'optimal' dose, i.e. the lowest safe dose that achieves the highest efficacy (Riviere et al., 2018; Shen et al., 2020). The question of finding the best dose is typically addressed in phase II dose-ranging studies, where patients are randomized to one of a number of doses (including possibly a placebo dose). As stated by Thall (2021), such designs can be seen as a type of enrichment: "Another type of enrichment is done in sequentially adaptive early-phase trials that choose an optimal regime, which may be a dose, dose pair, schedule, or dose-schedule combination, for successive patient cohorts. This repeatedly enriches the regimes seen interimly to have superior outcomes in terms of the optimization criterion that is used." Some of these designs use adaptations that will be described later in the chapter. For example, Riviere et al. (2014) uses response-adaptive randomization (Section 1.3.2) to explore the dose-space.

One approach to finding the best dose could be based on all possible pairwise comparisons among candidate doses. However, this only uses the information from the doses under comparison and typically results in larger sample sizes required in the trial (Xub and Bretz, 2017). The traditional approach instead is to compare many doses to the control using a step-down Dunnett test (Dunnett and Tamhane, 1991). An alternative, two-stage approach, known as multiple comparison procedures and modeling approaches (MCP-Mod) (Bretz et al., 2005; Pinheiro et al., 2014) uses a dose-response model allowing for interpolation between the doses. In the first stage, the possible models for the dose-response relationship are defined. The inclusion of several models addresses the issue of some of the models being misspecified. In the second stage, once data is observed, the MCP step checks whether there is any dose-response signal. This is done through hypothesis tests for each model, adjusting for the fact that there are multiple candidate models. If no models are found to be statistically significant, it is concluded that the dose-response signal cannot be detected given the observed data. If a dose-response signal is established, it could be that a single model is selected or multiple models are selected and an average is made. The selection of models can be based either on tests performed at the MCP step or on some other measures such as information criterion. The chosen model is used to select the best dose. We refer the reader to the works focusing on the step-by-step application of MCP-Mod in practice (Xub and Bretz, 2017; Bornkamp et al., 2009). An alternative approach to finding an optimal dose is to use a framework for constructing step-wise multiple testing procedures based on general contrasts to control the FWER, as proposed by Tamhane et al. (1996); Dunnett and Tamhane (1998).

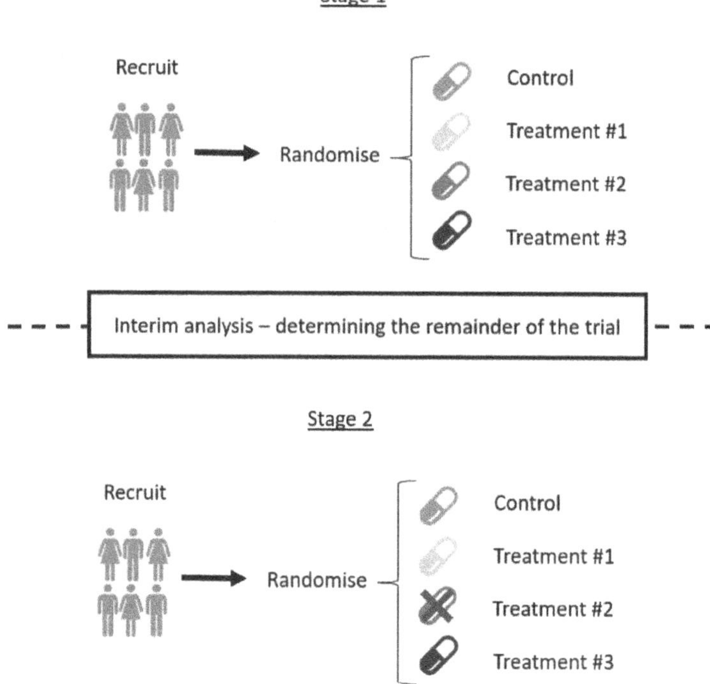

Figure 1.2 *Schematic of a two-stage Multi-arm Multi-stage (MAMS) trial design. At the interim analysis treatment 2 is stopped early for futility. This is Fig. 1 in Burnett et al. (2020), licensed under CC BY 4.0 (https://creativecommons.org/licenses/by/4.0/)*

1.3 Which is the Best Treatment Among Multiple Options for a Patient Group?

We next consider clinical trials that aim to select the best treatment among multiple experimental treatment arms. The methods we explore are typically considered for use in Phase II of the development process, where we wish to select a treatment for further study in Phase III. We explore methods that seek to remove less beneficial treatments from the trial quickly, giving patients a higher chance of receiving an efficacious treatment.

1.3.1 Multi-Arm Multi-Stage Designs

Multi-Arm Multi-Stage (MAMS) designs allow the simultaneous comparison of multiple experimental treatment arms with a single common control (Jaki, 2015). They are conducted over multiple stages, allowing for the early stopping of recruitment for either efficacy or futility (see Subsection 1.3.1.2). For example, if an experimental treatment is found to be performing poorly it may be dropped for futility/lack-of-benefit at a pre-planned interim analysis (if all experimental arms are dropped, the trial is stopped for futility); alternatively, the trial may end early when a treatment is shown to be sufficiently efficacious. MAMS trials are designed using a pre-planned set of adaptation rules to find the best treatment to carry forward for further study (Stallard and Todd, 2003) or carry forward all promising treatments (Magirr et al., 2012). Figure 1.2 gives a schematic of a two-stage MAMS trial with three experimental treatments, and at the interim analysis treatment 2 is stopped early for futility.

The multi-arm nature of such designs reduces the number of patients allocated to the control treatment compared to conducting multiple two-arm trials, while removing treatments during the course of the trial offers a reduction in the expected sample size (at the cost of an increase in the maximum sample size). The drop-the-loser design discussed later in this section gives a guaranteed reduction in sample size without providing as much benefit as a traditional MAMS trial. In a precision medicine setting our chief concern is selecting the best treatment(s) for subpopulations of patients to carry forward for further study, a problem which MAMS designs are well equipped to efficiently answer.

1.3.1.1 Trial Design

Let μ_k be the expected response of a patient to T_k for $k = 0, 1, ..., K$, so that our parameter of interest is the treatment effect for each experimental treatment $\theta_k = \mu_k - \mu_0$ for $k = 1, ..., K$. We define the corresponding null hypotheses $H_{0,k} : \theta_k \leq 0$ versus the alternatives $H_{1,k} : \theta_k > 0$. To compare the K experimental treatments (multi-arm) we plan a J-stage trial (multi-stage). Recruitment for the trial is split into J cohorts of patients, with an analysis conducted after each stage of the design. At the design stage of the trial we fix recruitment proportions $r_k^{(j)}$ for each stage j and treatment k. A notable restriction on these recruitment proportions is that the ratio of patients assigned to each treatment must remain constant throughout the trial, that is

$$\frac{r_0^{(j_1)}}{r_k^{(j_1)}} = \frac{r_0^{(j_2)}}{r_k^{(j_2)}} = r \text{ for all } k = 1, \ldots, K \text{ and } j_1, j_2 = 1, \ldots, J,$$

which is required to ensure the distribution of the test statistics does not depend on any μ_k (Koenig et al., 2008). At the start of the trial we define the maximum possible sample size n_{max}, since treatments maybe removed from the trial at any interim analysis. For example, suppose at analysis j' for treatment k we observe $\hat{\theta}_k^{(j')}$ such that we wish to remove the experimental treatment k from consideration (either for futility or due to efficacy); in this case, we cease recruiting to T_k, that is $r_k^{(j)} = 0$ for all $j > j'$ and no further analysis is conducted regarding θ_k. If all experimental treatments are removed from consideration then the trial is concluded; this is the only scenario in which we drop the control T_0.

To demonstrate in full how such designs are constructed, we consider a scenario with normally distributed outcomes for patients on each treatment. That is, at analysis j for treatment $k \in \{0, 1, .., K\}$ we have observed outcomes $Y_{i,k}$ for $i \in \{1, \ldots, r_k^{(j)} n\}$ that are independent with

$$Y_{i,k} \sim \mathcal{N}(\mu_k, \sigma_k^2).$$

Estimation of the treatment effect follows in the usual way where at stage j for treatment $k \in \{1, \ldots, K\}$

$$\hat{\theta}_k^{(j)} = \frac{\Sigma_{i=1}^{r_k^{(j)} n} Y_{i,k}}{r_k^{(j)} n} - \frac{\Sigma_{i=1}^{r_0^{(j)} n} Y_{i,0}}{r_0^{(j)} n}.$$

For later use, we define the Z-value corresponding to these estimates, at stage j for treatment k we have $Z_k^{(j)} = \hat{\theta}_k^{(j)} (\sigma_k^2 / r_k^{(j)} n)^{-1/2}$ where

$$Z_k^{(j)} \sim \mathcal{N}(\theta_k (\sigma_k^2 / r_k^{(j)} n)^{-1/2}, 1).$$

The common control arm introduces a known correlation structure for the Z-values, $corr(Z_k^{(j)}, Z_k^{(j)}) = 1$ for all $k \in \{1, ..., K\}$ while for $k_1 \neq k_2$ $(k_1, k_2 \in \{1, \ldots, K\})$

$$corr(Z_{k_1}^{(j)}, Z_{k_2}^{(j)}) = \frac{\sigma_0^2/r_0^{(j)}}{\left\{\left(\sigma_{k_1}^2/r_{k_1}^{(j)} + \sigma_0^2/r_0^{(j)}\right)\left(\sigma_{k_2}^2/r_{k_2}^{(j)} + \sigma_0^2/r_0^{(j)}\right)\right\}^{1/2}}.$$

Thus $Z^{(j)} = (Z_1^{(j)}, \ldots, Z_K^{(j)})$ follow a multivariate normal distribution with mean $\Theta = (\theta_1, \ldots, \theta_K)$ and a known correlation matrix $\Sigma^{(j)}$. These designs are not restricted to normally distributed observations. The key is that the test statistics at each stage of the trial follow a known joint distribution under the null hypothesis to allow for the testing procedures to follow to be constructed.

1.3.1.2 Decision Making Using the Generalized Dunnett Test

Magirr et al. (2012) introduce the generalized Dunnett testing procedure for MAMS designs. At the design stage of the trial, we define upper and lower stopping boundaries, $U = (u^{(1)}, \ldots, u^{(j)})$ and $L = (l^{(1)}, \ldots, l^{(j)})$. These boundaries are used to sequentially test each $H_{0,k}$; at analysis j if $Z_k^{(j)} > u^{(j)}$ we reject $H_{0,k}$ and the study is stopped, while if $Z_k^{(j)} < l^{(j)}$ then T_k is dropped from the trial as described in Section 1.3.1.1.

Under such a testing procedure the FWER is maximized under the global null $\mathcal{H}_0$ (that is $\theta_k = 0$ for all $k \in \{1, .., K\}$). Thus we choose U and L such that

$$Pr(\text{rejecting } \mathcal{H}_0 | \Theta = 0) = \alpha.$$

For a given set of design parameters J, K, n and $r_k^{(j)}$ for $j \in \{1, ..., J\}$ and $k \in \{1, ..., K\}$ and distribution assumptions for θ_k and σ_k^2 the choices of U and L are not unique. It is important to note that the choice for U and L will influence the operating characteristics such as the maximum and expected sample size and the probabilities of rejecting combinations of null hypotheses, so when constructing such designs, consideration should be given as to which testing boundaries will be used. Magirr et al. (2012) provide several options for the shape of the boundaries following common group sequential methods (Jennison and Turnbull, 1999).

To compute the required maximum sample size n_{max} we must choose which operating characteristic is key for our design. In this setting, it is typical to consider the power to reject null hypotheses. As discussed in Section 1.1.2.1, in our context with K hypotheses being tested there are several definitions of power that we might consider. In particular, it is common to focus on the disjunctive power for some configuration of Θ,

$$Pr(\text{rejecting at least one } H_{0,k} \,|\, \Theta),$$

which is computationally similar to computing the error rate for given boundaries U and L. That is, for a configuration of Θ we compute a maximum sample size n_{max} to give some target disjunctive power $1 - \beta$.

The Least Favourable Configuration (LFC) (Thall et al., 1988) is a useful tool for planning such designs. Let δ be the treatment effect of interest (upon which we wish to base our power calculation for the trial in the usual way), suppose that we further have $\delta_0 < \delta$ such that if $\theta_k < \delta_0$ (for any $k \in \{1, \ldots, K\}$) we would not wish to investigate T_k any further. If $\delta_0 = 0$ this would imply that we are interested in detecting any positive treatment effect, but in practice, we would expect that some choice of $\delta_0 > 0$ would be more reasonable. Without loss of generality, the LFC is given by $\theta_1 = \delta$ and $\theta_k = \delta_0$ for any $k \in \{2, \ldots, K\}$. This is known as the least favourable configuration since it minimises the probability of rejecting $H_{0,1}$ when compared to all other choices of Θ such that $\theta_1 \geq \delta$ and $\theta_k \leq \delta_0$ (for any $k \in \{2, \ldots, K\}$).

Defining the closed testing procedure
An alternative way to view the generalized Dunnett testing procedure is as a closed testing procedure. Recall from Section 1.1.2.1 that if $\mathcal{I} = \{1, \ldots, K\}$ the global null may be written as $\mathcal{H}_0 = \bigcap_{k \in \mathcal{I}} H_{0,k}$, thus by definition of the testing procedure, for any $\mathcal{J} \subset \mathcal{I}$ we have a test of $H_{\mathcal{J}}$ constructed at level α. Such a testing procedure is implicitly consonant, the consequence being that if we use the same L and U for the test of $H_{\mathcal{J}}$ then $Pr_{\Theta=\Theta_0}(\text{Reject } \mathcal{H}_{\mathcal{J}}) < \alpha$. So if we reject $H_{0,k}$ using the generalized Dunnett procedure we have indeed rejected each $H_{\mathcal{J}}$ for all $\mathcal{J}$ with $k \in \mathcal{J}$ and so have applied a closed testing procedure. Each such test of $H_{\mathcal{J}}$ is conservative by construction. Urach and Posch (2016) propose extending the generalized Dunnett testing procedure by directly defining the group sequential tests for each element of the closed testing procedure. This allows for a potential increase in power, particularly when considering the probability of rejecting multiple hypotheses.

Binding and non-binding futility
The futility boundaries, L may be either binding (they must be strictly adhered to) or non-binding (they need not be strictly adhered to). In the case of binding futility boundaries this is accounted for in the construction of U and thus the binding nature is accounted for in the error rate of the design. In the case of non-binding futility, U is computed with $l^{(j)} = -\infty$ for all $j \in \{1, \ldots, J\}$, although alternative choices for L may be used in the trial itself.

1.3.1.3 Drop the Loser

Drop The Loser (DTL) designs (Thall et al., 1989; Sampson and Sill, 2005) are very closely related to MAMS designs (Wason et al., 2017) as they compare several experimental treatments to a common control over multiple stages. The designs are sufficiently close that we consider how a drop-the-loser design might operate using the same framework for observations as discussed for MAMS in Section 1.3.1.1. The main difference is that for a DTL design a pre-determined number of treatments are dropped at each analysis. As the name suggests we remove the worst performing experimental treatment(s) at each analysis, until one treatment remains to be compared to the control in the final analysis.

Following the construction of Section 1.3.1.1, at each analysis we drop a pre-determined number of arms. As before we consider a trial comparing K experimental treatments with a common control, at each interim analysis $j \in \{1, ..., J-1\}$ we will choose the number of treatments for the next stage of the trial $\kappa^{(j+1)}$. Note that $\kappa^{(j)}$ must be pre-defined and chosen such that $\kappa^{(j)} > \kappa^{(j+1)}$. At each analysis the test statistics $Z^{(j)}_{k_1}, Z^{(j)}_{k_2}, \ldots$ (where $\{k_1, k_2, \ldots\}$ is the set of experimental treatments under consideration at stage j of the trial) are ordered and the top $\kappa^{(j+1)}$ treatments are selected for the next stage of the study (removing all other experimental treatments). At the final analysis the remaining $Z^{(J)}_{k_1}, Z^{(J)}_{k_2}, \ldots$ may be compared with a critical value for the hypothesis test c, rejecting H_{0,k_i} if $Z^{(J)}_{k_i} > c$ for all $k_i \in \{k_1, k_2, \ldots\}$. Wason et al. (2017) describe a version of this design where only one experimental the arm remains at the final analysis, showing how to select the critical value while maintaining strong control of the FWER.

1.3.1.4 Example

The TAILoR trial (Pushpakom et al., 2015) was a Phase II trial of telmisartan in HIV-positive individuals using a two-stage MAMS design. The trial planned recruitment of up to 336 patients over a 48-week period, with a single interim analysis planned after 168 patients had completed 24 weeks on either an intervention or control treatment. Patients were randomized with equal probability to one of four groups: no treatment (control), 20mg telmisartan daily, 40mg telmisartan daily, or 80mg telmisartan daily. In the interim analysis, there were three possible outcomes based on assessment of change in the reduction in insulin resistance from baseline to 24 weeks: if one telmisartan dose was substantially more effective than control, the study would stop and that dose would be recommended for further study; if all telmisartan doses were less effective than control, the study would stop with no dose recommended for further study; if one or more doses were better than the control but none met the first criterion, the study would continue and patients would have been randomized between these remaining dose(s) and control. If a second stage was conducted then a final analysis was be conducted with two possible outcomes: either the best dose is significantly more effective than the control in which case it is recommended for further study; or no dose is significantly better than control the in which case no dose is recommended.

A total of 377 patients were recruited (Pushpakom et al., 2020) (note this difference in sample size was due to higher than expected drop-out). In stage one, 48, 49, 47, and 45 patients were randomized to control and 20, 40, and 80 mg telmisartan, respectively. At the interim analysis, the 20 and 40 mg telmisartan groups performed worse than control on average and so only 80 mg telmisartan was taken forward into stage two. At the end of stage two, 105 patients had been recruited to control and 106 to the 80-mg arm (in total), there was no difference in HOMA-IR (estimated effect, 0.007; SE, 0.106) at 24 weeks between the telmisartan (80 mg) and control arm. If a traditional fixed sample design had been used in place of a MAMS design all experimental arms would have been studied throughout the trial, requiring a further 100 or so patients for arms that ultimately did not demonstrate an effect of the experimental treatment.

1.3.1.5 Summary

MAMS designs are potentially useful when there are multiple promising treatments with no strong belief that one treatment will be more beneficial. Using the methods such as those outlined in this Section allows for several benefits. As we have seen all treatments are directly compared within the same trial, this allows for exploration over which of the treatments may offer the most benefit. Within this comparison, there is no restriction to a hierarchy within the treatments (such as multiple doses of the same treatment). The use of a shared control group considerably reduces the number of patients that need to be recruited compared to separate trials testing each treatment, with a further reduction in expected sample size from the multi-stage nature of a traditional MAMS design, or a guaranteed reduction in sample size from a DTL design.

Removing treatments that are not sufficiently beneficial to patients during the course of the trial is ethically appealing. Further to this, since patients have a higher chance of receiving an experimental treatment compared to a two-arm trial, this may improve recruitment to the study (Dumville et al., 2006; Meurer et al., 2012). Administratively and logistically effort is only required for one trial and thus can substantially speed up the development process (Parmar et al., 2008). As with all adaptive designs, there is a cost for these benefits, in addition to those in common with many other adaptive designs. In the case of MAMS designs the potentially higher maximum sample size can be unappealing, however this is offset by the reduction in the expected sample size. A variable sample size and variation in which treatments may be required can make planning such designs more cumbersome, although the possible pathways are pre-defined; this is more variable than is typical of even other adaptive designs because decisions relate to each treatment individually. From a statistical perspective planning for such designs is more involved, and requires more statistician time. However, open source software is available to assist in the design and analysis of MAMS trials in the form of the "MAMS" package in R (Jaki et al., 2019). Alternatively in STATA there are several modules available such as "nStage" (Royston et al., 2014), "nStagebin" (Bratton, 2014), and "DESMA" (Grayling, 2019).

1.3.2 *Response-Adaptive Randomization (RAR)*

In order to allocate treatments to patients, traditionally clinical trials have used fixed randomization schemes that do not change as a result of patients' responses to treatments. Alternatively, randomization probabilities can be adapted during the trial based on the accrued data on responses, with the aim of achieving experimental objectives while ideally preserving inferential validity. A common motivation for doing so is to allocate more patients to a treatment that is estimated to be more effective during the trial, but RAR can also target other objectives such as increasing the power of a specific treatment comparison. Many different classes of RAR procedures have been proposed for various trial contexts. As stated by Thall (2021), some types of RAR can be considered as "an extreme form of enrichment", with the updated randomization probabilities seen as enriching the arm(s) that have superior performance based on the interim data. RAR can also be used in conjunction with other types of trial adaptations, such as treatment and subgroup selection (see also Section 1.3.2.1). For example, if the allocation probability goes below or rises above a certain value, arms can be dropped for futility or selected in a similar way to a MAMS design (Wason and Trippa, 2014; Lin and Bunn, 2017). For clarity, we first describe the use of RAR without the consideration of patient subgroups or covariates, which we defer to Section 1.3.2.1. A recent review of methodological and practical issues around the use of RAR in clinical trials can be found in Robertson et al. (2023).

A general way to represent treatment allocation rules is to consider the allocation probabilities for each patient. Let $a_{i,k}$ be a binary indicator variable denoting the treatment allocation for patient i, with $a_{i,k} = 1$ if patient i is allocated to treatment T_k and 0 otherwise. Each patient is assumed to be allocated to one treatment only, and hence $\sum_{k=0}^{K} a_{i,k} = 1$. Typically patients enter the trial and are treated sequentially, either individually or in groups. Using our notation, we can consider RAR with J 'stages' or groups corresponding to (potential) updates to the allocation probabilities, where $J = N$ is a fully sequential RAR procedure as is commonly presented in the RAR literature. Let $\pi_{i,k}^{(j)} = P(a_{i,k} = 1)$ denote the probability that patient i in group j is allocated treatment k. Note that we require $\sum_{k=0}^{K} \pi_{k,i}^{(j)} = 1$ and $\pi_{i,k}^{(j)} > 0$ for all i (i.e., our definition excludes non-randomized response-adaptive methods like the Gittins Index (Villar et al., 2015)). As an example, equal randomization has $\pi_{i,k}^{(j)} = 1/(K+1)$ for all i, j, k.

In a RAR procedure, the allocation probabilities are adapted throughout the course of the trial based on past treatment allocations and response data. More formally, let $\boldsymbol{a_i} = (a_{0,i}, a_{1,i}, \ldots, a_{K,i})$ denote the allocation vector for patient i. We also let $\boldsymbol{a}^{(j)} = \{\boldsymbol{a_1}, \ldots, \boldsymbol{a_{N_j}}\}$ and $\boldsymbol{y}^{(j)} = \{y_1, \ldots, y_{N_j}\}$ respectively denote the sequence of allocations and responses observed for the first j groups of patients, where N_j is the number of patients observed in the first j groups, and both $\boldsymbol{a}^{(0)}$ and $\boldsymbol{y}^{(0)}$ are defined as the empty set. RAR defines the allocation probability $\pi_{i,k}^{(j)}$ conditional on $\boldsymbol{a}^{(j-1)}$ and $\boldsymbol{y}^{(j-1)}$, i.e.

$$\pi_{i,k}^{(j)} = Pr\left(a_{i,k} = 1 \,|\, \boldsymbol{a}^{(j-1)}, \boldsymbol{y}^{(j-1)}\right). \tag{1.2}$$

Hence the proportion of patients $r_k^{(j)}$ defined earlier is determined by the allocation probabilities $\pi_{i,k}^{(j)}$.

As a concrete example, we consider Bayesian RAR procedures based on Thompson sampling (Thompson, 1933), which has been popular in the methodological literature. For simplicity, we focus on the case with $K = 1$ experimental treatment. The allocation probabilities are given by

$$\pi_{i,1}^{(j)} = \frac{\left[Pr(\theta_1 > \theta_0 \,|\, \boldsymbol{a}^{j-1}, \boldsymbol{y}^{j-1})\right]^c}{\left[Pr(\theta_1 > \theta_0 \,|\, \boldsymbol{a}^{j-1}, \boldsymbol{y}^{j-1})\right]^c + \left[1 - Pr(\theta_1 > \theta_0 \,|\, \boldsymbol{a}^{j-1}, \boldsymbol{y}^{j-1})\right]^c}$$

and $\pi_{i,0}^{(j)} = 1 - \pi_{i,1}^{(j)}$. Here $Pr(\theta_1 > \theta_0 \mid \boldsymbol{a}^{j-1}, \boldsymbol{y}^{j-1})$ is the posterior probability that the experimental treatment has a larger parameter of interest than the control treatment (given the allocations $\boldsymbol{a}^{j-1}$ and observed responses $\boldsymbol{y}^{j-1}$) from all of the previous $j-1$ blocks. The parameter c controls the variability of the resulting procedure. Setting $c = 0$ gives equal randomization, while setting $c = 1$ gives the original Thompson sampling. Thall and Wathen (2007) propose setting c equal to 1/2 or $N_j/(2N)$. From a Bayesian perspective, the posterior probabilities $Pr(\theta_1 > \theta_0 \mid \boldsymbol{a}^{j-1}, \boldsymbol{y}^{j-1})$ can naturally be used to stop the trial early for futility or efficacy according to pre-defined early stopping thresholds.

1.3.2.1 Covariate-Adjusted Response-Adaptive Randomization (CARA)

RAR can also be used with the objective of identifying and selecting subgroups where treatment could have a differential effect (i.e. a treatment-covariate interaction exists). Let $\tilde{\boldsymbol{x}}^{(j)}$ denote the covariate vector sequence of interest observed for the first j groups of patients. Additionally, based on $\tilde{\boldsymbol{x}}^{(j)}$ one could define pre-specified non-overlapping groups of interest and define l partitions based on the specific value of covariates for patient i. To allow for the RAR procedure to depend on $\tilde{\boldsymbol{x}}^{(j)}$ and let the $r_{k,l}^{(j)}$ be determined accordingly one can extend equation (1.2) as follows

$$\pi_{i,k}^{(j)} = Pr\left(a_{i,k} = 1 \mid \boldsymbol{a}^{(j-1)}, \boldsymbol{y}^{(j-1)}, \tilde{\boldsymbol{x}}^{(j)}\right). \tag{1.3}$$

We note that in precision medicine, the role of covariates is of course crucial in developing targeted therapies for patient subgroups. More generally, covariates (sometimes called prognostic factors) are especially important in clinical trials if there are treatment interactions. However, there are covariates that may be important for other reasons in most clinical trials, e.g., centre/country effects (in multicentre or international studies), demographic subgroups (such as gender, age, and race) and time trends (a drift in patient characteristics over time). These can result in a CARA procedure that aims for balance (as a way to achieve a power constraint) rather than increasing the allocation of patients within a subgroup to a superior treatment. For further discussion of the use of covariates in randomization, we refer the reader to the review paper by Rosenberger and Sverdlov (2008), more recent methodological papers by Atkinson et al. (2011); Baldi Antognini and Zagoraiou (2011); Antognini and Zagoraiou (2012); Metelkina and Pronzato (2017) and the book by Sverdlov (2015). Another useful reference is Zagoraiou (2017), which discusses how to choose a covariate-adaptive randomization procedure in practice.

For precision medicine trials, in those cases in which one expects a treatment-covariate interaction, a CARA algorithm could be applied to each possible stratum according to the pre-specified group of interest. Continuing with the RAR example, we consider a Bayesian CARA procedure based on Thompson sampling (Thompson, 1933), variants of which have been used or influential in the design of trials such as BATTLE (Kim et al., 2011) or I-SPY 2 (Barker et al., 2009). For simplicity, we focus on the case with $K = 1$ experimental treatments. The allocation probabilities for patient i in subgroup l (which we denote by $\tilde{\boldsymbol{x}}^{(j)} \in \boldsymbol{l}$) are given by

$$\begin{aligned}\pi_{i,1,l}^{(j)} = {} & \left[Pr(\theta_{1,l} > \theta_{0,l} \mid \boldsymbol{a}^{(j-1)}, \boldsymbol{y}^{(j-1)}, \tilde{\boldsymbol{x}}^{(j)} \in \boldsymbol{l})\right]^c \\ & \times 1/\left\{ \left[Pr(\theta_{1,l} > \theta_{0,l} \mid \boldsymbol{a}^{(j-1)}, \boldsymbol{y}^{(j-1)}, \tilde{\boldsymbol{x}}^{(j)} \in \boldsymbol{l})\right]^c \right. \\ & \left. + \left[1 - Pr(\theta_{1,l} > \theta_{0,l} \mid \boldsymbol{a}^{(j-1)}, \boldsymbol{y}^{(j-1)}, \tilde{\boldsymbol{x}}^{(j)} \in \boldsymbol{l})\right]^c \right\}\end{aligned}$$

and $\pi_{i,0,l}^{(j)} = 1 - \pi_{i,1,l}^{(j)}$. Here $Pr(\theta_{1,l} > \theta_{0,l} \mid \boldsymbol{a}^{(j-1)}, \boldsymbol{y}^{(j-1)}, \tilde{\boldsymbol{x}}^{(j)} \in \boldsymbol{l})$ is the posterior probability that the experimental treatment has a larger parameter of interest than the control treatment in subgroup l given the allocations $\boldsymbol{a}^{(j-1)}$ and observed responses $\boldsymbol{y}^{(j-1)}$ from all of the previous $j-1$ blocks. Similar to what can be done with RAR, and following a Bayesian perspective, the above posterior probabilities can be used to make decisions such as early stopping of treatments in subgroups (either based on futility or efficacy grounds) and/or to stop the trial altogether.

1.3.2.2 *Summary*

As many different classes of RAR (including CARA) procedures have been proposed, it is challenging to draw conclusions about the disadvantages or advantages of RAR designs as a whole. However, as already noted, the most common motivation for using RAR is to increase the overall proportion of patients enrolled in the trial who benefit from the treatment they receive (while controlling the statistical operating characteristics) (Villar et al., 2018; Robertson et al., 2023). This can mitigate potential ethical conflicts (London, 2018) that can arise when equipoise is disturbed during a trial by the accumulating evidence, and makes the trial more appealing to patients (Meurer et al., 2012) which may improve trial recruitment (Tehranisa and Meurer, 2014). It is also possible to use RAR to optimize other characteristics of the trial such as power (Hu and Rosenberger, 2003). In a multi-armed trial context, RAR can shorten the development time and more efficiently identify responding patient populations (Berry, 2010).

RAR designs have been criticized for a number of reasons (Proschan and Evans, 2020; Robertson et al., 2023) although many of the raised concerns can be addressed or may only apply to a specific class of RAR. Logistics of trial conduct is one obstacle in RAR due to the constantly changing randomization (Korn and Freidlin, 2011). For RAR procedures that are patient-benefit oriented, this may come at the cost of other characteristics; for example, a two-arm RAR trial may require, larger sample sizes than a traditional fixed randomized design to achieve the same power; methods to account for such compromise have been proposed (Villar et al., 2018; Viele et al., 2020). Finally, the question of frequentist hypothesis testing (and statistical inference more generally) becomes more complex for RAR designs; see for example, Robertson and Wason (2019); Barnett et al. (2023); Deliu et al. (2021).

1.3.3 *Platform Trials*

The use of MAMS designs can increase the efficiency of the drug development process through the early stopping of experimental treatment arms and the use of a common control group. However, experimental drugs are often not all in the same stage of development, and hence new treatments can become available for evaluation *during* the course of a MAMS trial. By including these in the trial as they become available within an overarching trial framework, there are benefits in terms of reduced logistical and administrative effort (compared with starting a completely new trial) and allowing direct comparisons of experimental treatments within the same trial. The term *platform trial* (also known as an 'open' or 'perpetual' platform trial) is used to describe MAMS designs which allow the flexibility of adding new treatment arms over time. Figure 1.3 gives a schematic of a typical platform trial, showing how treatment arms enter into the trial as they become available, are evaluated, and then 'dropped' for futility/lack-of-benefit or 'graduated' from the trial once demonstrated as being efficacious. The criteria used to drop or graduate arms can be based on frequentist or Bayesian metrics; for example, the I-SPY2 platform trial was conducted using a Bayesian framework (Barker et al., 2009) whereas the STAMPEDE platform trial (see below) used a frequentist framework (Sydes et al., 2009). Platform trials can also incorporate RAR as part of their design, such as Bayesian RAR as used in the I-SPY2 trial.

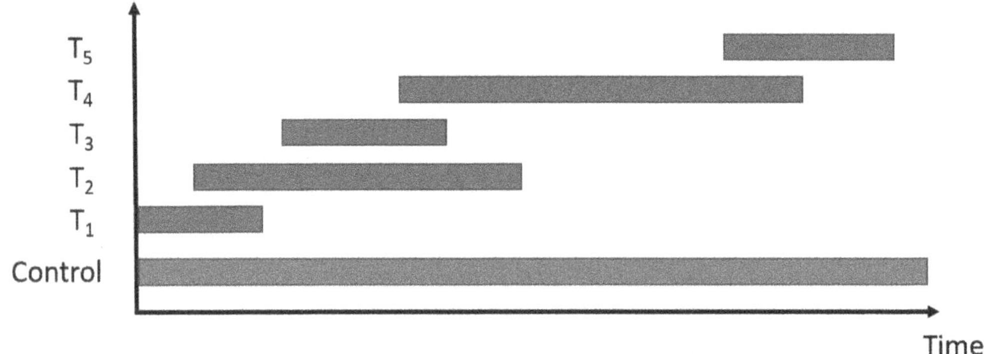

Figure 1.3 *Schematic of a typical platform trial. Treatment arms $T_1, \ldots, T_5$ enter the trial when available, are evaluated against a common control, and can then be dropped from the trial for futility/lack-of-benefit or graduated if efficacious.*

From a statistical perspective, the additional challenge for platform trials compared with standard MAMS designs is allowing the addition of treatment arms while still ensuring appropriate statistical inference. A useful recent review of statistical (and practical) considerations when adding new treatment arms to an ongoing platform trial is given by Lee et al. (2021). They highlight two key considerations when making inference about new treatment comparisons:

1. Analysis approaches: whether to use all of the control data or only concurrent control data.
2. Type I error control: whether adjustment for multiplicity is required, and if so whether FWER (see below) or FDR control (Wason and Robertson, 2021) is more appropriate.

Additional complications in inference will occur if the control arm used in the platform, trial changes over time.

1.3.3.1 Adding Treatment Arms While Maintaining Strong FWER Control

In contexts where strong FWER control is required, different approaches have been proposed (Lee et al., 2021). Here we describe the framework proposed by Burnett et al. (2020) to add experimental treatment arms to a platform trial in progress, using the notation for MAMS designs introduced in Section 1.3.1.

Consider a MAMS trial with J stages and K experimental treatments, where we shall test the null hypotheses $H_{0,k}$ versus alternatives $H_{1,k}$ for $k \in \{1, \ldots, K\}$. Following the construction of Urach and Posch (2016) we define the local tests for each element of the closed testing procedure, that is for all $\mathcal{K} \subseteq \{1, \ldots, K\}$ the intersection hypothesis defined as $H_{0,\mathcal{K}} = \bigcap_{k \in \mathcal{K}} H_{0,k}$ is tested using the pre-defined upper and lower stopping boundaries $U_{\mathcal{K}} = (u_{\mathcal{K}}^{(1)}, \ldots, u_{\mathcal{K}}^{(J)})$ and $L_{\mathcal{K}} = (l_{\mathcal{K}}^{(1)}, \ldots, l_{\mathcal{K}}^{(J)})$ constructed to ensure each test is at some target error rate α.

Suppose this trial is still in progress after analysis $J' \in \{1, \ldots, J-1\}$ (that is, the trial is still recruiting for at least one experimental treatment and the control for the next stage $J'+1$). At analysis $J' \in \{1, \ldots, J-1\}$, say $A \in \mathbb{Z}^+$ new experimental treatments become available and can be added to the trial. Hence there are now up to $K' = K+1+A$ treatments for the trial in total (assuming that the original $K+1$ treatment arms are still in the trial). For the existing $K+1$ treatment arms, suppose we do not alter the recruitment (not a strict requirement but useful for now). For the new treatment arms, there is no recruitment before they are added and hence $r_k^{(j)} = 0$ for $k = K+1, \ldots, K+A$ and $j = 1, \ldots, J'$

with no corresponding Z-values. We then add recruitment $r_k^{(j)}N$ for each new treatment $k = K+1, \dots, K+A$ for the remaining trial stages $j = J'+1, \dots, J$ where this is planned and fixed at the point where the new treatments are added.

To make formal inferences about all treatments now in the trial we wish to incorporate formal testing of the hypotheses $H_{0,k} : \theta_k = 0$ for $k = 1, \dots, K+A$, and thus our requirement for strong control of the FWER now extends across all $K+A$ tests. For each $\mathcal{K} \subseteq \{1, \dots, K\}$, since there is no modification of the design, we continue with the pre-defined test. For $\mathcal{K} \subseteq \{K+1, \dots, K+A\}$, there is no existing information and thus we must choose $U_{\mathcal{K}} = (u_{\mathcal{K}}^{(J'+1)}, \dots, u_{\mathcal{K}}^{(J)})$ and $L_{\mathcal{K}} = (l_{\mathcal{K}}^{(J'+1)}, \dots, l_{\mathcal{K}}^{(J)})$ such that the test is constructed at level α; note these are chosen at the interim analysis where the treatments are added and treated as pre-defined testing boundaries for the remainder of the trial.

The only case that remains is $\mathcal{K} = \mathcal{K}_K \cup \mathcal{K}_A$ where $\mathcal{K}_K \subseteq \{1, \dots, K\}$ and $\mathcal{K}_A \subseteq \{K+1, \dots, K+A\}$ (intersections involving both the original K hypotheses and additional A hypotheses). For any such $H_{0,\mathcal{K}}$ we use the conditional error principle (Proschan and Hunsberger, 1995; Koenig et al., 2008; Hommel, 2001) to include the existing information for all θ_k where $k \in \mathcal{K}_K$. Letting $\boldsymbol{\theta}_{\mathcal{K}_K}^{(J')}$ be the vector of estimates of the treatment effects, the corresponding conditional error is given by

$$B_{\mathcal{K}_k}(\hat{\boldsymbol{\theta}}^{(J')}) = Pr_{\mathcal{K}_k}(R \,|\, \hat{\boldsymbol{\theta}}^{(J')}) \quad \text{for all } \boldsymbol{\theta} = (\theta_1, \dots, \theta_K),$$

where R is the event that we reject one or more true null hypotheses and this probability is computed under $H_{0,\mathcal{K}_k}$. Since $H_{0,\mathcal{K}}$ implies $H_{0,\mathcal{K}_k}$ we have that

$$\int_{\hat{\boldsymbol{\theta}}^{(J')}} f(\hat{\boldsymbol{\theta}}^{(J')}) B_{\mathcal{K}_k}(\hat{\boldsymbol{\theta}}^{(J')}) \, \mathrm{d}\hat{\boldsymbol{\theta}}^{(J')} = \alpha$$

where $f(\cdot)$ denotes the probability density function of the Z-values based on the data up to stage J'. Constructing the test for $H_{0,\mathcal{K}}$ we choose $U_{\mathcal{K}} = (u_{\mathcal{K}}^{(J'+1)}, \dots, u_{\mathcal{K}}^{(J)})$ and $L_{\mathcal{K}} = (l_{\mathcal{K}}^{(J'+1)}, \dots, l_{\mathcal{K}}^{(J)})$ such that the test is constructed at level $B_{\mathcal{K}_k}(\hat{\boldsymbol{\theta}}^{(J')})$. This ensures that for the trial as a whole the test of each such $H_{0,\mathcal{K}_k}$ is constructed at level α. Thus each element of the closed testing procedure is constructed at level α and the FWER is strongly controlled at level α as required.

1.3.3.2 Example: STAMPEDE Trial

STAMPEDE is a platform trial for patients with prostate cancer, which assess the effects of adding different agents (both individually and in combination) to the standard of care, which is the control arm. The trial started in 2005 with five original comparisons (Sydes et al., 2009), but since then the trial has been repeatedly amended to include an additional six comparisons. Statistical power and type I error rates were calculated based on pairwise comparisons with concurrent control, without any adjustment for multiplicity. The initial allocation ratio for the five original experimental treatments was 2:1:1:1:1:1 (i.e. favouring the control arm by 2:1), and for the six additional experimental treatments a 1:1 ratio was used. In STAMPEDE, the decision rules to drop or progress treatment arms are based on the estimated hazard ratio (compared with the concurrent control data) being above or below pre-specified boundaries.

1.4 Which Groups of Patients will Benefit from a Treatment?

An important aspect of precision medicine (and clinical trials in general) is to ensure the right patients receive the treatment (i.e. those who will gain a meaningful benefit). Here, we focus on trials that use clinically relevant biomarkers to identify patients who may be sensitive to a treatment and therefore likely to respond.

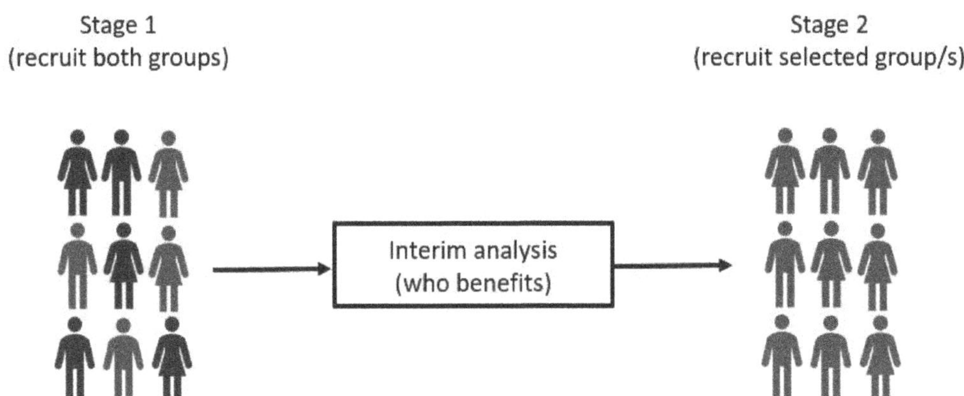

Figure 1.4 *Schematic of a typical adaptive enrichment (AE) trial with two biomarker-defined subgroups of interest. This is Fig. 4 in Burnett et al. Burnett et al. (2020), licensed under CC BY 4.0 (https://creativecommons.org/licenses/by/4.0/)*

1.4.1 Adaptive Enrichment

Adaptive Enrichment (AE) designs (also often referred to as population enrichment designs) make use of biomarker-defined subgroups; importantly, these subgroups must be well defined before the trial commences as they will be incorporated directly into the design of the trial. In such a setting there is often uncertainty about how the treatment might perform in each subgroup, and with the goal of precision medicine in mind we would like to ensure that we understand which subgroup(s) actually receive the real benefit of the treatment. AE designs start by recruiting all patients to the trial, then at an interim analysis allow the modification of recruitment defining how to recruit the remainder of the trial. Usually this involves the removal of subgroups (with numerous decision criteria for how to select which subgroups are kept in the trial). It is also possible, as an alternative strategy, to change the proportion of the recruitment assigned to each subgroup. Such designs make use of flexible hypothesis testing methods (Bretz et al., 2006; Schmidli et al., 2006; Marcus et al., 1976) that preserves the statistical integrity of the trial while allowing freedom in the decision-making process at the interim analysis. This has lead to a rich environment with many different takes on decision-making methodology, with both Bayesian (Brannath et al., 2009; Burnett, 2017; Ondra et al., 2019) and classical techniques being applied (Götte et al., 2015; Magnusson and Turnbull, 2013). Figure 1.4 shows a schematic of a typical AE trial with two biomarker-defined subgroups of interest. At the interim analysis, the green subgroup is determined to benefit from the treatment and so is recruited for the remainder of the trial.

1.4.1.1 Recruitment

AE designs can be defined for several configurations of the trial population. For example, we could consider a population split into disjoint subgroups, subgroups within a larger group, and subgroups where patients are able to be in one or more groups. In this Section we reduce the problem to a configuration where we are concerned with a subgroup of interest $\mathcal{S}_1$ and the full-population $\mathcal{S}_3$, we also define the complement $\mathcal{S}_2$ where $\mathcal{S}_3 = \mathcal{S}_1 \cup \mathcal{S}_2$. Within $\mathcal{S}_1$ and $\mathcal{S}_3$ we compare an experimental treatment T_1 with a control T_0. Let $\mu_{k,l}$ be the expected response of a patient from subgroup $l \in \{1, 2\}$ to T_k for $k \in \{0, 1\}$, and let us define the treatment effect in each subgroup as $\theta_l = \mu_{1,l} - \mu_{1,0}$. Let λ $(0 < \lambda < 1)$ be the proportion of $\mathcal{S}_3$ that are also in $\mathcal{S}_1$, then $\theta_3 = \lambda\theta_1 + (1-\lambda)\theta_2$. In this configuration of populations we wish to conduct formal analyses in $\mathcal{S}_1$ and $\mathcal{S}_3$, that is we test the null hypothesis $\mathcal{H}_{0,l} : \theta_l \leq 0$ versus the alternative $\mathcal{H}_{1,l} : \theta_l > 0$ for $l \in \{1, 3\}$.

AE designs typically split recruitment into two stages. Recruitment in each stage of the trial is split according to the two subgroups, $\mathcal{S}_1$ and $\mathcal{S}_2$, in subgroup $l \in \{1, 2\}$ at stage $j \in \{1, 2\}$ on treatment k we plan to recruit $r_{k,l}^{(j)} n$ patients. In an AE trial the $r_{k,l}^{(j)}$ are chosen at the design stage for all $l \in \{1, 2\}$ and $j \in \{1, 2\}$; however, $r_{k,l}^{(2)}$ may be modified at the interim analysis with the restrictions that $r_{0,l}^{(2)}/r_{1,l}^{(2)}$ and $r_{0,1}^{(2)} + r_{1,1}^{(2)} + r_{0,2}^{(2)} + r_{1,2}^{(2)}$ take the same value before and after the modification. For illustrative purposes we consider a scenario with normally distributed observations from each patient. That is, in subgroup $l \in \{1, 2\}$ at analysis j on treatment k we have observations $Y_{i,k,l}$ that are independent with

$$Y_{i,k,l} \sim N(\mu_{k,l}, \sigma_{k,l}^2).$$

Estimation of the treatment effect in each subgroup follows in the usual way, that is, at stage j in subgroup $l \in \{1, 2\}$ the estimator of interest is

$$\hat{\theta}_l^{(j)} = \frac{\Sigma_{i=1}^{r_{1,l}^{(j)} n} Y_{i,1,l}}{r_{1,l}^{(j)} n} - \frac{\Sigma_{i=1}^{r_{0,l}^{(j)} n} Y_{i,0,l}}{r_{0,l}^{(j)} n},$$

while for $\mathcal{S}_3$ we have

$$\hat{\theta}_3^{(j)} = \lambda \hat{\theta}_1^{(j)} + (1 - \lambda) \hat{\theta}_2^{(j)}.$$

These estimators follow known distributions. For $l \in \{1, 2\}$ let

$$\mathcal{V}_l^{(j)} = \frac{\sigma_{1,l}^2}{r_{1,l}^{(j)} n} + \frac{\sigma_{0,l}^2}{r_{0,l}^{(j)} n},$$

then we have $\hat{\theta}_l^{(j)} \sim N(\theta_l, \mathcal{V}_l^{(j)})$, while for $\mathcal{S}_3$ with $\mathcal{V}_3^{(j)} = \lambda^2 \mathcal{V}_1^{(j)} + (1-\lambda)^2 \mathcal{V}_2^{(j)}$ we have $\hat{\theta}_3^{(j)} \sim N(\theta_3, \mathcal{V}_3^{(j)})$. The joint distribution of $(\hat{\theta}_1^{(j)}, \hat{\theta}_3^{(j)})$ is bivariate normal with $cov(\hat{\theta}_1^{(j)}, \hat{\theta}_3^{(j)}) = \lambda \mathcal{V}_l^{(j)}$.

In order to allow the modification of $r_{k,l}^{(2)}$ During the trial while also testing the hypotheses we make use of a flexible testing methodology (Bretz et al., 2006; Schmidli et al., 2006; Marcus et al., 1976). We follow the approach of Burnett and Jennison (2021) using a combination test to combine the stages of each element of the closed testing procedure. At stage j of the trial for $l \in \{1, 3\}$ we compute Z-values $Z_l^{(j)} = \hat{\theta}_l^{(j)} (\mathcal{V}_l^{(j)})^{-1/2}$ corresponding to $H_{0,1}$ and $H_{0,3}$ respectively; note under the null hypotheses each $Z_l^{(j)} \sim N(0, 1)$. In addition, to complete the closed testing procedure we require a test of $H_{0,\{1,3\}} = H_{0,1} \cap H_{0,3}$, which can be constructed for example using a Dunnett-type method (Dunnett, 1955), taking the test statistic to be

$$\mathcal{T}^{(j)} = \max(Z_1^{(j)}, Z_3^{(j)});$$

(the choice to take the maximum of the Z-values makes the assumption that we wish to evaluate the test statistics on the same scale). Note that the test statistic in each stage does not follow a standard normal distribution under the null hypothesis, but we can transform them into such that this property does hold. Let $\Phi_2(T^{(j)}, \Sigma^{(j)})$ be the cumulative bivariate normal distribution with mean zero and correlation matrix $\Sigma^{(j)}$ corresponding to the correlation matrix of $(Z_1^{(j)}, Z_3^{(j)})$ (which is known), evaluated over a region with a lower limit of $-\infty$ an upper limit of $T^{(j)}$ in each dimension. Then the z-value for $H_{0,\{1,3\}}$ is given by

$$Z_{13}^{(j)} = \Phi^{-1} \left[\Phi_2(T^{(j)}, \Sigma^{(j)}) \right],$$

where $Z_{13}^{(j)} \sim N(0,1)$ under $H_{0,\{1,3\}}$. In this configuration of populations we might consider removing $H_{0,3}$ from consideration in the interim analysis, thus we no longer need to recruit patients to $\mathcal{S}_2$ setting $r_{k,2}^{(2)} = 0$ for $k \in \{0,1\}$. In this case, we do not find $Z_3^{(2)}$ and we set $Z_{13}^{(2)} = Z_1^{(2)}$.

We find the overall test statistics for the trial using the weighted inverse normal (Bauer and Köhne, 1994; Lehmacher and Wassmer, 1999; Hartung, 1999) combination test. Using pre-defined weights $w^{(1)}$ and $w^{(2)}$ chosen such that $(w^{(1)})^2 + (w^{(2)})^2 = 1$, the combined Z-values for $l \in \{1,3,\{1,3\}\}$ for the trial are then given by

$$Z_l = w^{(1)} Z_l^{(1)} + w^{(2)} Z_l^{(2)}.$$

Under the corresponding null hypothesis $Z_l \sim N(0,1)$ and so we reject the local test of $H_{0,l}$ when $Z_l > \Phi^{-1}(1-\alpha)$ for $l \in \{1,3,13\}$. Globally we reject $H_{0,1}$ at level α if we reject the local tests of $H_{0,1}$ and $H_{0,\{1,3\}}$ at level α. Similarly, globally we reject $H_{0,3}$ at level α if we reject the local tests of $H_{0,3}$ and $H_{0,\{1,3\}}$ at level α. Thus we have a closed testing procedure and the FWER is strongly controlled by this procedure since this is true for any valid choice of $r_{k,l}^{(2)}$ for $k \in \{0,1\}$ and $l \in \{1,2\}$.

1.4.1.2 Decision Making

The interim decision-making in AE trials is a crucial element of the adaptive design, as it should ensure the correct populations are targeted and determines the operating characteristics of the trial. We present some of the more common approaches from the literature here. For simplicity we consider a trial where $\lambda = 0.5$, $\sigma_1^2 = \sigma_0^2$ and $r_{k,l}^{(j)}$ is constant for all $l \in \{1,2\}$, $k \in \{0,1\}$ and $j \in \{1,2\}$. That is $\mathcal{S}_1$ makes up half the full population, the interim analysis is conducted after half the trial with equal recruitment to each subgroup and treatment planned throughout the trial. At the interim analysis, we then allow the choice that the trial continues recruiting as planned, denote this by $\mathcal{A} = 1$, or enrich the trial that is $r_{k,2}^{(2)} = 0$ for $k \in \{0,1\}$, denote this by $\mathcal{A} = 2$.

Threshold comparison

The most intuitive approach is a threshold-type approach (Magnusson and Turnbull, 2013). Originally this is defined to keep all subgroups in the trial for which the score statistic $(\hat{\theta}_l^{(j)} \mathcal{V}_l^{(j)})$ exceeds $(\mathcal{V}_l^{(2)} \sqrt{\mathcal{V}_l^{(2)}})^{-1}$. More generally we might consider in our example that for some constant $a \in \mathbb{R}$ we use the modified recruitment for the second stage of the trial if $Z_3^{(1)} < a$. We might define such thresholds for any groups that may remain in the trial.

Promising zone

The promising zone approach of Mehta and Pocock (2011) differs from the threshold type approach, in that the decision about whether to drop a population at the interim analysis is made based on the probability of rejecting the null hypothesis. In our example, if at the interim analysis $Pr(\text{rejecting } H_{0,3} | \hat{\theta}_3^{(1)}) > a$ (for some constant a chosen before the trial), this defines a 'favourable/promising zone' where the trial continues with the originally planned recruitment. On the other hand, if $Pr(\text{rejecting } H_{0,3} | \hat{\theta}_3^{(1)}) < a$, this defines an 'enrichment zone' where $r_{k,2}^{(2)} = 0$ for $k \in \{0,1\}$.

Following this approach, it is possible to allow for more possible decisions at the interim analysis. We may define the following: the favourable zone, where recruitment continues as planned for the remainder of the trial; the promising zone where the sample size is increased; the enrichment zone where the trial is enriched, maintaining the original total sample size but restricting recruitment to a subgroup of interest; the futility zone where the trial is stopped for futility. The definition of additional options increases the flexibility of the design and thus allows the design to be more closely aligned with the goals of the trial.

1.4.1.3 Bayes Optimal Designs

There is a large body of work investigating the use of Bayesian methods in the decision making of AE designs (Brannath et al., 2009; Burnett, 2017; Ondra et al., 2019; Burnett and Jennison, 2021; Ballarini et al., 2021). Following the work of Burnett and Jennison (2021) we demonstrate the construction of Bayes optimal AE designs, using Bayesian decision theory to make optimal decisions during the interim analysis. Let the density function of the prior distribution for the treatment effects be given by $p(\theta_1)$ and $p(\theta_2)$ (it is possible to allow for correlated prior distributions but here it is sufficient to assume these prior distributions are independent). At the interim analysis, we have estimates $\hat{\theta}_1^{(1)}$ and $\hat{\theta}_2^{(1)}$ which have known density functions $f(\hat{\theta}_1^{(1)})$ and $f(\hat{\theta}_2^{(1)})$. Thus at the interim analysis we use Bayes Theorem (equation (1.1)) to find the posterior distribution $p(\theta_1|\hat{\theta}_1^{(1)})$ and $p(\theta_2|\hat{\theta}_2^{(1)})$ giving the current understanding about the treatment effects. Recall here that θ_1 and θ_2 determine θ_3 and so it is sufficient to define everything in terms of θ_1 and θ_2.

For the purpose of interim decision making, we also require the definition of a utility function as discussed in Section 1.1.2.4 based on the outcomes for the trial $\boldsymbol{Y}$. This $\boldsymbol{Y}$ will be made up of all relevant information from the trial, for example, $\hat{\theta}_1^{(1)}$, $\hat{\theta}_2^{(1)}$, $\hat{\theta}_1^{(2)}$, $\hat{\theta}_2^{(2)}$ and the decision at the interim analysis (which of course may depend on $\hat{\theta}_1^{(1)}$, $\hat{\theta}_2^{(1)}$). For example, we might define a simple gain function

$$G(\boldsymbol{\theta}, X) = \lambda\theta_1 \mathbb{1}[\text{Reject } H_{0,1}] + \theta_3 \mathbb{1}[\text{Reject } H_{0,3}],$$

that is, at the end of the trial if we have rejected a null hypothesis we achieve a benefit proportional to the associated sample size and size of the population. For optimization purposes, our goal is to maximize the expected value of the gain. In particular, at the interim analysis, the Bayes optimal decision is given by the choice of action $\mathcal{A}$ that maximizes the expected gain given the posterior distributions

$$\mathbb{E}_{p(\boldsymbol{\theta}|\hat{\boldsymbol{\theta}})}[G(\boldsymbol{\theta}, X)].$$

Such optimal decisions are non-trivial to compute; in the trial itself this is not problematic since the decision will only be made once at the interim analysis. However, at the design stage, it is responsible to compare the operating characteristics of the planned design with those of alternative methods, for example, a trial that maintains the same recruitment throughout either recruiting the full population or only $\mathcal{S}_1$ throughout the trial. Burnett and Jennison (2021) propose an efficient method for the creation of a lookup table allowing the swift computation of the interim decision over the space of possible values of $\hat{\theta}_1^{(1)}$ and $\hat{\theta}_2^{(1)}$. This allows simulation of the design to allow for the comparison of the operating characteristics with other designs. It is clear from our description of the design that the interim decision is not the only design choice that we must make. Ballarini et al. (2021) construct fully optimal AE designs, optimizing recruitment over both stages of the trial using the same Bayesian decision framework ideas.

1.4.1.4 Example: TAPPAS

TAPPAS (Jones et al., 2017; Mehta et al., 2019) is a trial of TRC105 (an antibody) and pazopanib versus pazopanib alone in patients with advanced angiosarcoma. The study identified two subgroups, those with cutaneous advanced angiosarcoma and those with non-cutaneous advanced angiosarcoma. There was an indication of greater tumour sensitivity to

TRC105 in the cutaneous subgroup. The primary endpoint for this study was progression-free survival, with an initial sample size of 124 patients to be followed until 95 events (progression or death) have been observed.

An AE design was used where the data monitoring committee were able to recommend one of three pre-planned actions at the interim analysis: continue as planned with the full population (recruiting 124 patients followed until 95 events in total); continue with the full population and an increase in sample size and progression-free survival events (recruiting 200 patients followed until 170 events in total); continue with only the cutaneous subgroup, thereby enriching the study population (recruiting 170 patients followed until 110 events in total). This decision making the procedure followed the promising zone approach (Mehta and Pocock, 2011), where the choice of which option would be followed is based upon the probability of rejecting the null hypotheses given the data available at the interim analysis.

The study recruited from the full population throughout, as dictated by the data observed at the interim analysis. A total of 128 patients were recruited (close to the targeted recruitment of 124), with 64 patients randomized to each of the experimental treatments and the control. It was concluded that TRC105 did not demonstrate activity when combined with pazopanib.

1.4.1.5 Summary

AE designs recruit fewer patients from subgroups that are demonstrated to not benefit from the treatment based on accumulating trial data. This is particularly helpful when there is uncertainty about which subgroups benefit from the experimental treatment before the trial begins, allowing a compromise over selecting only one of the subgroups before the trial begins. The adaptation allows the direct targeting of the appropriate subgroups while maintaining a fixed overall sample size.

However, this adaptation is not without cost; suppose before the trial we knew which subgroups truly received a benefit, it would be more efficient to conduct a trial only using these subgroups. Take for example a subgroup within a full population; if we knew only the subgroup received a benefit from the outset of the trial we could allocate the full sample size to only that subgroup which would clearly be more efficient. Even in a best case scenario it is rare that the AE design offers an advantage in terms of statistical efficiency, with the benefit coming from equivalent performance to nonadaptive alternatives while accessing the adaptive features.

1.4.2 Umbrella and Basket Trials

The advent of next-generation genomic sequencing has led to an increasing focus on developing treatments that target specific genetic mutations, particularly in oncology. Indeed, the potential promise of precision oncology is that it will be possible to sequence each patient, find the driver mutations and then treat them with a specific inhibitor of that gene (Bui and Kummar, 2018). Two key trial designs have recently evolved to accommodate this approach, namely basket and umbrella trials. These designs typically make use of more detailed biomarker/genetic information than that seen in Section 1.4.1, and can accommodate multiple treatments, disease types and biomarkers. We distinguish each trial design below.

Basket trials

In a basket trial, we examine a single targeted treatment for patients sharing a single biomarker or genomic feature but across multiple diseases or disease subtypes (e.g. tumours in different organs of the body) (Renfro and Mandrekar, 2018; Woodcock and LaVange, 2017). Figure 1.5 gives a schematic of a typical basket trial with a single basket, where all

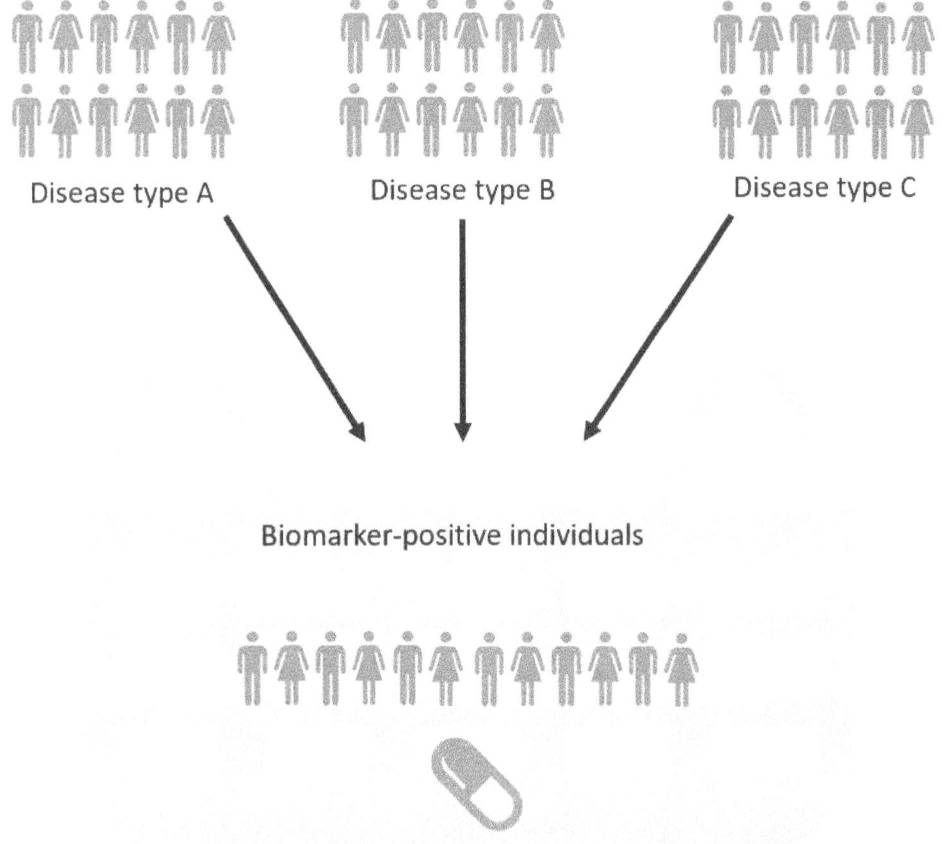

Figure 1.5 *Schematic of a typical basket trial with a single basket. All biomarker-positive patients across the three different disease (sub)types are treated with a single targeted treatment.*

biomarker-positive patients across the different disease types are treated with a targeted therapy. Note that a basket trial may have multiple baskets, where each basket corresponds to a different biomarker.

Basket trials are typically single-arm Phase II trials, where each basket studies a target-response hypothesis (Renfro and Mandrekar, 2018). The number of patients in a basket is typically small, with promising results then leading to a larger randomized Phase III trial for confirmation. The design of a basket trial could incorporate multiple stages with early stopping rules, similar to those discussed in Section 1.4.1.2. A key advantage of basket trials is that they allow the evaluation of targeted therapies for genetic mutations that would be too rare to study within a tumour-specific context (Chu and Yuan, 2018).

Umbrella trials

In an umbrella trial, we consider a single disease or disease type (the overarching "umbrella") and evaluate multiple targeted treatments. More specifically, we identify multiple biomarker-defined subgroups and pair each with a specific treatment. Figure 1.6 gives a schematic of a typical umbrella trial, where the patients with the disease are screened for the presence of biomarkers and then assigned to receive the corresponding targeted therapy. Note that biomarker-negative cohorts can also be included. Umbrella trials can be phase II

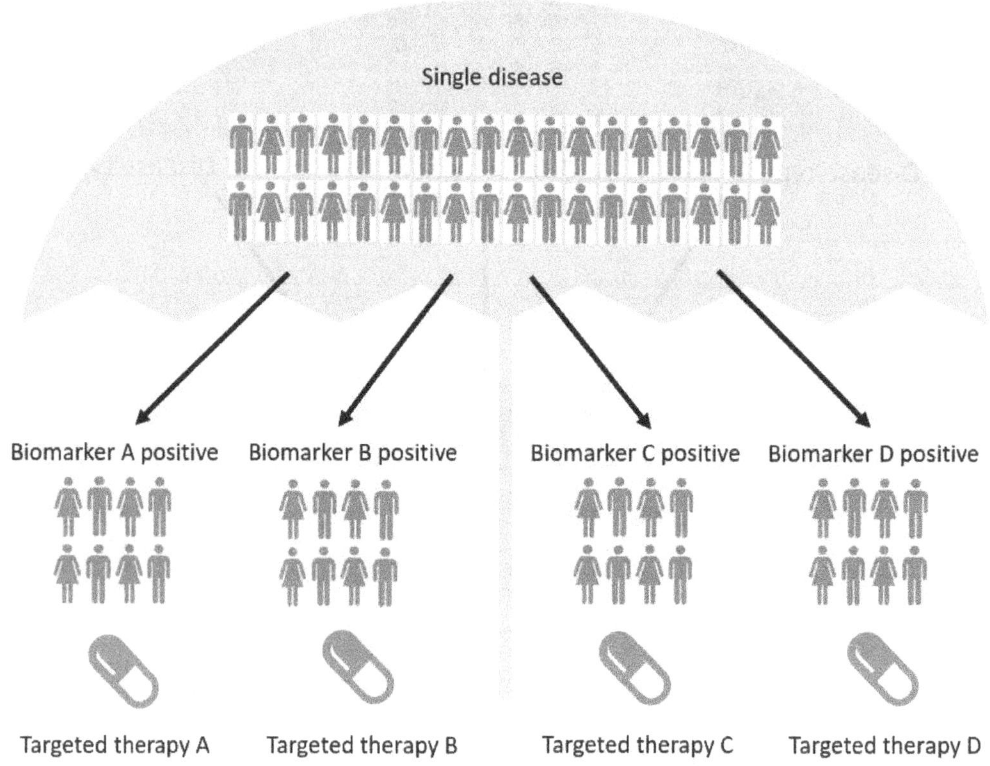

Figure 1.6 *Schematic of a typical umbrella trial. Patients with the disease are screened for the presence of biomarkers and then assigned to receive the corresponding targeted treatment.*

or III trials, where the individual biomarker-specific sub-trials may be single-arm studies, or randomized studies comparing the targeted treatment with control (Renfro and Mandrekar, 2018). Each of these sub-trials may contain adaptive elements such as early stopping or response-adaptive randomization.

1.4.2.1 Statistical Considerations

We can draw some parallels with both MAMS and AE designs of Sections 1.3.1 and 1.4.1, as we may have multiple treatments and subgroups to incorporate into the design. However, the comparison is not so direct as it might first appear. While we may consider conducting analyses following the methods described previously, the emphasis in such designs is often more exploratory with the goal being to understanding the relationship between patient subgroups and the treatment(s). As noted above, this more exploratory emphasis is particularly the case for basket trials.

For both basket and umbrella trials, clearly, it is possible to perform separate statistical analyses: i.e. in a basket trial evaluating the treatment effect in each tumour type separately, and in an umbrella trial separately analyzing the biomarker-specific sub-trials. However, the nature of the designs themselves suggests that there can often be information that can be learned across these 'modules', and hence the borrowing of information from a Bayesian perspective can be a natural choice when it comes to analyzing such trials.

Thall et al. (2003) proposed using a Bayesian hierarchical model (BHM) to adaptively borrow information across subgroups, which was then applied to basket trials by

Berry et al. (2013). These approaches rely on a shrinkage parameter η to control the degree of information borrowing across subgroups. More formally, given L strata, a BHM assumes the outcome data Y_l from subgroup $l = 1, \ldots, L$ follows a distribution F parameterized by a subgroup-specific parameter θ_l: $Y_l|\theta_l \sim F(\theta_l)$, where θ_l itself follows a distribution $\theta_l \sim G(\eta)$. Inference for η can be done in a frequentist or Bayesian manner, with the latter requiring the specification of a (typically non-informative) prior on η.

These methods have since been extended for basket trials in a number of ways. The EXNEX model (Neuenschwander et al., 2016) relaxes the standard exchangeability assumption in order to reduce the risk of too much shrinkage and excessive borrowing for extreme strata, using a robust mixture model. Another proposal is the Bayesian calibrated prior model (Chu and Yuan, 2018), which models η as a function of the measure of homogeneity between the subgroups in order to better control the frequentist type I error rate. Meanwhile, for umbrella trials there has been a recent proposal to also use BHM to allow effect size clustering and information borrowing across multiple biomarker-treatment pairs (Kang et al., 2021).

1.4.2.2 Example: BRAF V600 Basket Trial

This phase II basket trial evaluated the efficacy of the drug vermurafenib in multiple non-melanoma cancers with BRAF V600 mutations (Hyman et al., 2015). The trial used Simon's two-stage design to evaluate the response rate, as measured using the RECIST criteria, in eight tumor-specific cohorts (plus an "all-others" cohort). There were 122 adults enrolled, with the number recruited in the tumor-specific cohorts ranging from 5 to 27. The trial concluded that there were promising signals of activity in three individual tumor types (namely non-small-cell lung cancer, Erdheim-Chester disease and Langerhans'-cell histiocytosis), which could then be further investigated in follow-up phase III trials.

1.4.2.3 Master Protocols

Basket, umbrella as well as platform trials (see Section 1.3.3) are key examples of the wider class of *master protocols*, defined as any top-level or overarching clinical trial protocol that comprises several parallel sub-trials, designed to answer multiple scientific questions (Renfro and Mandrekar, 2018; Woodcock and LaVange, 2017). This may involve multiple treatments, diseases and biomarkers of interest. A master protocol governs centralized processes (e.g. patient enrollment and screening for biomarkers) and standardized design components and operational aspects across its sub-protocols. Master protocols are becoming increasingly popular in practice (Park et al., 2019) as an efficient way to investigate multiple hypotheses of interest. We can consider a "mix and match" approach as well through combining aspects of such trials, e.g. a platform trial with a basket or umbrella structure. Renfro and Mandrekar (2018) give a number of examples of recent or currently ongoing trials that can be considered as both a platform and a basket/umbrella trial.

1.5 Discussion

The adaptive designs we have presented and discussed in this book chapter form a wide class of methods focused on improving the power and participant benefit of clinical trials, all of which may be essential requirements to deliver precision medicine in practice. Despite the many clear benefits of many adaptive designs, these study designs are still far from established as typical practice (Le Tourneau et al., 2009; Jaki, 2013; Chevret, 2012). Many reasons for this have been discussed (Dimairo et al., 2015; Jaki, 2013; Dimairo et al., 2015) and include: lack of expertise and experience (in the application of adaptive designs among clinicians, trialists and trial statisticians); lack of design and analysis software; additional time required for planning and analysis; inadequate funding structure to account for design uncertainty; and the fact that chief investigators may prefer more established methods. Ambiguous terminology and vague definitions also add to this confusion (Dragalin, 2006).

We have not been exhaustive in our presentation of adaptive designs, focusing instead on a few key designs to answer some of the most common clinical questions from a precision medicine perspective. Seamless designs (Bretz et al., 2006; Schmidli et al., 2006; Jennison and Turnbull, 2006), which we have not discussed in detail, use a similar adaptive design methodology to combine phases of clinical development: designs may be inferentially seamless, where data from the earlier stage are incorporated into the overall trial results; operationally seamless, avoiding any break in recruitment between the stages of the development process but excluding data from earlier stages from the final analysis of the latter; or both. There are many motivations for conducting seamless designs (Cuffe et al., 2014), making it an active area of research (Graham et al., 2019).

While we are enthusiastic about adaptive designs and their use in many clinical situations and we also believe they can be highly complementary to a precision medicine goal, we are nevertheless very much aware that they are not always beneficial. The suitability of adaptive methods depends largely on the clinical question being addressed. We have presented some key clinical questions for which adaptive designs may be of use across a wide range of disease areas, study settings and outcome/response variables. In some situations, adaptive designs may provide little efficiency advantage or could be even detrimental to the quality of information provided by the trial. We share the view expressed by Wason et al. (2019) that: "factors that reduce the efficiency of adaptive designs are systematically downplayed or ignored in methodological papers, which may lead researchers into believing they are more beneficial than they actually are". Thus, we advise some caution on the expectations of what adaptive designs may achieve.

Regulatory bodies are increasingly recognising the desire for the use of adaptive designs and accepting their use, although it is recommended that regulators be engaged early in the process whenever using any novel methodology (US Department of Health and Human Services Food and Drug Administration, 2019; Committee for Medicinal Products for Human Use, 2007). Funding bodies are also increasingly comfortable with the use of adaptive designs, the TAILoR trial discussed in Section 1.3.1 appears as a case study on the National Institute for Health Research website (NIHR, NIHR). Additionally new reporting guidance for adaptive designs (Dimairo et al., 2020) have recently been published to facilitate uptake further.

For many years one major obstacle to the use of adaptive designs in practice has been the lack of suitable software to aid both the design and conduct of trials. This issue is increasingly being tackled by those researching the methods, with many open-source packages available for the design and analysis of adaptive methods some of which have been cited in this work. For example, `rpact` (Wassmer and Pahlke, 2019) is an R package that assists in the design and analysis of confirmatory clinical trials. In addition, there is a steep learning curve to the implementation of such designs; training courses are becoming increasingly available to address this.

From a methodological standpoint, there are some practical issues that go beyond the scope of what we have discussed in this book chapter that should be considered when proposing an adaptive design, for example potential information leakage or the introduction of bias (Sanchez-Kam et al., 2014; Chow et al., 2012). The Practical Adaptive and Novel Designs and Analysis (PANDA) toolkit (Dimairo, Pallmann, Jaki, Wheeler, Bradburn, Flight, Cooper, and Marsh, Dimairo et al.) is an online resource that addresses and explains broader issues in the use of adaptive designs.

For each possible adaptive design, there will be advantages and disadvantages. In general, advantages may include: an increase in efficiency of the design in terms of the expected number of patients or a clear benefit in understanding the question of scientific interest; clear ethical advantages to ensuring the right patients are given the best available treatment whenever possible; and the key disadvantage is the additional burden, both in the planning of the trial and the interim analyses.

At the design stage of any clinical trial (adaptive or not), some assumptions must be made. These assumptions influence the overall performance of the trial and inadequate assumptions can lead to a sub-optimal design. With the additional complexity of many adaptive designs, there are more assumptions to be made and it is critical that these are well understood by the trial team to consider the impact of these choices and for the choice to be adequate. Communication and establishing of common practice between the statistical methodology and the trial community will be key in seeing the wider spread application of such methods.

Despite the challenges in the design and analysis of an adaptive trial we believe that under the right circumstance the benefits introduced by the increased flexibility clearly outweighs these issues. The COVID-19 pandemic has led to an unprecedented response in terms of clinical research activity and has opened up a large potential for the use of adaptive designs. The results from this COVID-19 research needed to be obtained as quickly as possible and presented a number of challenges associated with considerable uncertainty (including the nature of the disease, the number and characteristics of patients affected, and the emergence of new potential therapies). These challenges made adaptive designs for clinical trials a particularly attractive option (Stallard et al., 2020) and we expect this is likely to result in an increased uptake of these methods in the near future.

Acknowledgements

This research was supported by the NIHR Cambridge Biomedical Research Centre (BRC-1215-20014). This report is independent research supported by the National Institute for Health Research (T Jaki's Senior Research Fellowship, NIHR-SRF-2015-08-001). The views expressed in this publication are those of the authors and not necessarily those of the NHS, the National Institute for Health Research or the Department of Health and Social Care (DHSC). SS Villar received funding from the UK Medical Research Council (MC_UU_00002/15), T Jaki and DS Robertson received funding from the UK Medical Research Council (MC_UU_00002/14). DS Robertson also received funding from the Biometrika Trust.

Chapter 2

Small Sample, Sequential, Multiple Assignment, Randomized Trial Design and Analysis

Sidi Wang, Thomas Braun, Roy Tamura, Kelley M. Kidwell

2.1 Introduction

With the power of genetic and genomic sequencing, what we previously categorized as common diseases, we now classify as many smaller, distinct diseases. That is, with technology we have the ability to better identify patient heterogeneity. In acknowledging heterogeneity, studying treatment effects in large groups of individuals and averaging over their heterogeneity may not lead to beneficial outcomes for many individuals. Understanding how best to treat small samples of individuals is imperative to the success of precision medicine.

A randomized, controlled clinical trial (RCT) is generally regarded as providing the strongest scientific evidence for treatment efficacy (Grimes and Schulz, 2002). However, clinical trials are difficult to conduct in small samples for a number of reasons, most notably the low number of individuals affected that can be recruited to the study. Further, it may be challenging to meet standard, frequentist operating characteristics like 80% power and two-sided 5% type I error.

Unfortunately, these hindrances have lessened the number and quality of clinical trials in rare diseases. In the United States, a rare disease is defined as a disorder or condition that affects less than 200,000 people (107th Congress, 2002). In total, it is estimated that 25-30 million people in the U.S. (8-12% of the population) are affected by over 7,000 rare diseases (Griggs et al., 2009). However, approved treatments are only developed for approximately 5% of these rare disorders, which leads to substantial unmet medical needs for many patients (Food and Drug Administration, 2015). As best described by Smith, Williamson and Beresford, 'even when adequately powered RCTs may be infeasible, there is a strong argument that some level of randomized evidence is much better than none.' (Smith et al., 2014).

Crossover designs are often used to study treatments in small samples due to the gain in power by having each participant receive each treatment and serve as their own control thereby decreasing confounding and variance of treatment effects. A 2×2 (2 treatments and 2 periods) crossover design randomizes patients to a particular sequence of treatments so that, for example, participants receive treatment A in period 1 followed by treatment B in period 2 or treatment B in period 1 followed by treatment A in period 2. An N-of-1 design is a crossover design within one person such that instead of randomizing a group of participants, one individual receives treatments in a randomized order across several periods. For example, a person may receive treatments A then B then B then A then B then A again across three ordered treatment periods. If individuals and treatments are similar, N-of-1 trials can be aggregated and summarized using meta-analytic, frequentist or Bayesian methods (Zucker et al., 2010).

DOI: 10.1201/9781003216223-2

Both crossover and N-of-1 trials are important designs to identify effective treatments, but both designs have limitations for small sample treatment efficacy or effectiveness studies. Both designs are only appropriate for chronic or incurable conditions where the goal is not to cure, are susceptible to dropouts (especially if a positive response is obtained on the first treatment), require participants to switch treatments, and require rapidly available and measurable responses. Difficulties in conducting and analyzing these designs, as well as the limitations of the designs for conventional two-arm randomized trials noted above, have motivated the need for more innovative small sample, clinical trial designs (Gupta et al., 2011).

In this chapter, we introduce design and methodology for small n, sequential, multiple assignment, randomized trials (snSMARTs) (Tamura et al., 2016) as an alternative approach to study treatments in small samples. snSMART designs address some of the issues that limit the use of crossover and N-of-1 trials by allowing those who respond to treatment to remain on that treatment. The designs and methodology presented here have primarily been motivated by studies of treatments for isolated skin vasculitis, a rare disease characterized by painful lesions. The first trial to implement an snSMART design was A Randomized Multicenter Study for Isolated Skin Vasculitis (ARAMIS, NCT02939573), but the design and methods are applicable beyond ARAMIS and those that formally meet the definition of a rare disease. snSMARTs may be appropriate trial designs in precision medicine for any disease or disorder that affects a small number of individuals and can remain stable over the course of the trial unless treatment is effective.

First, we briefly review the characteristics of traditional SMART designs in Section 2.2. We then describe snSMART designs in contrast to the traditional SMART and in more details via specific variations of snSMART designs in Section 2.3. Current methods for analyses depending on the type of outcome and goal of the trial are presented in Section 2.4. The chapter ends with an illustration of the application of the methods using the R package snSMART and a short discussion of the practical implementation of snSMART design and methods.

2.2 Traditional SMART Designs

Before we more fully describe an snSMART, we introduce the traditional SMART design used in large samples. A SMART is a multi-stage (usually two-stage) trial with the goal of informing the development of dynamic treatment regimens (DTRs) (Lavori and Dawson, 2000; Dawson and Lavori, 2012; Murphy, 2005a) or tailored sequences of treatments. The same group of participants is followed through each stage of the trial. In a traditional SMART, participants are randomized among several treatments in the first stage (Figure 2.1). An intermediate outcome, known as a tailoring variable, is assessed at a specific time or over time. The tailoring variable is often defined as a response to the previous treatment so that responders may receive a different set of treatment options than non-responders. Specifically, in a generic two-stage SMART design, participants are randomized among several treatments $(A_1, A_2, ..., A_n)$ in stage 1. After being followed for a predetermined period, participants are assessed for response. In stage 2, those responding to A_1 may be randomized to a set of treatments $(B_1^1, B_2^1, ..., B_m^1)$, with a similar approach for those responding to each of the other treatments assigned in stage 1, e.g those responding to A_2 are randomized in stage 2 to $(B_1^2, B_2^2, ..., B_m^2)$, etc. However, for practical reasons, instead of randomizing responders among a set of new treatments, another approach is to directly assign responders to receive their stage 1 treatment again in stage 2. A similar randomization approach is used for participants who do not respond to their stage 1 treatment. Specifically, participants not responding to A_1 in stage 1 may be randomized to a set of treatments $(C_1^1, C_2^1, ..., C_k^1)$, again with a similar approach used for those not responding to each of $A2, A3, \ldots A_n$. Again, for practical reasons, non-responders are almost always randomized

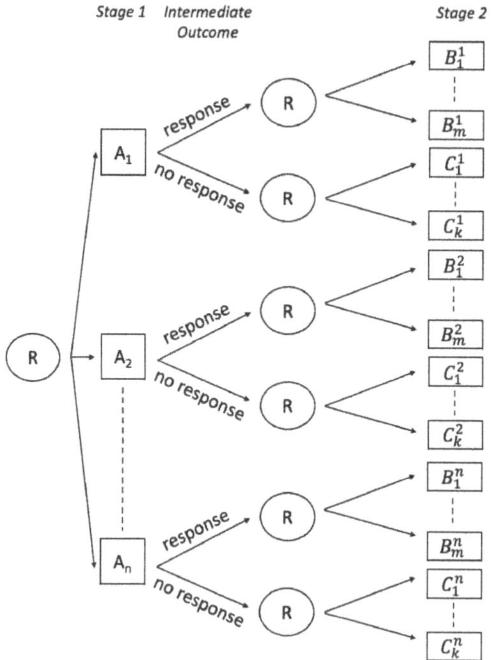

Figure 2.1 *Generic design of SMART.*
A generic two-stage SMART design. Stage 1: participants are randomized among treatments $A_1, A_2, ..., A_n$. Intermediate outcomes are assessed after stage 1 such that responders and non-responders from each stage 1 group are re-randomized among their own corresponding stage 2 treatments. The same participants are followed throughout the study. "R" represents randomization.

to a new treatment, although it is possible to directly augment or change the treatment of non-responders to a specific treatment without randomization.

DTRs are embedded within a SMART design. Each DTR is a guideline for a tailored sequence of treatments including an initial treatment, a subsequent treatment if the patient responds to the initial treatment, and a subsequent treatment if the patient does not respond to the initial treatment. For example, two DTRs embedded in Figure 2.1 are $\{A_1, B_1^1, C_1^1\}$ and $\{A_3, B_2^3, C_1^3\}$. At the end of the trial, the treatment effects of the embedded DTRs can be estimated, and promising DTRs can be further studied in a confirmatory trial against the standard of care. Other chapters in this book are dedicated to the estimation of these tailored sequences of treatments either from a SMART or observational data. Instead, we present the traditional SMART design and analytic goals so that we can compare it to those of an snSMART which we describe in more detail in the following section.

2.3 Variations on snSMART Designs

As with a traditional SMART, an snSMART is a multi-stage trial where for a two-stage design, randomization in the second stage depends on the outcome to first-stage treatment (see Figure 2.2). However, there are additional requirements for an snSMART design not found in traditional SMARTs. Often in a traditional SMART, the intermediate outcome or tailoring variable differs from the second-stage outcome (e.g. the tailoring variable may be a binary response variable and the second-stage endpoint may be continuous) and the first stage is shorter than the second stage. Instead, an snSMART design requires that the same outcome is measured at the end of the first stage and at the end of the second stage.

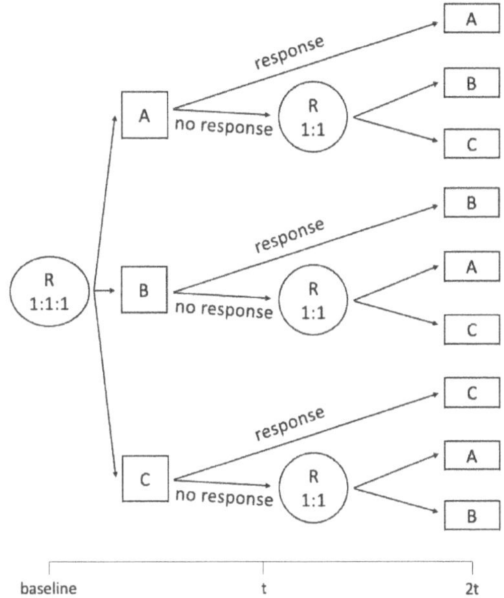

Figure 2.2 *Study design of an snSMART.*
Participants are randomized to one of the three treatment arms in stage 1 with equal probability. After being followed for time t, participants are assessed on their response to initial treatment. The responders continue the same treatment in stage 2, while the non-responders are re-randomized to one of the remaining treatments in stage 2.

The "tailoring variable" used in an snSMART design is not an early indication of treatment success or failure, but rather, the outcome of interest which requires the treatment be administered long enough to be effective. Thus, an snSMART has the specific feature that the length of time of both stages must be the same.

Beyond differences in design, an snSMART and traditional SMART also differ with respect to their primary goal. Specifically, snSMARTs are motivated to identify the superior first-stage treatment (or dosage level) using both stages of data, whereas SMARTs are motivated to identify effective two-stage treatment sequences or DTRs that define a personalized treatment plan (Robins, 1986; Murphy, 2003). Data are shared across the two stages of the snSMART design to more efficiently estimate the first-stage treatment effects. In order to share the data across stages, treatments are repeated from the first-stage to the second stage of an snSMART design and in order to circumvent some of the pitfalls of crossover designs, responders to first-stage treatment remain on that treatment. Thus, there is less flexibility (i.e. fewer variations) in snSMART designs compared to the many variations of SMART designs, such that snSMARTs have fewer types and numbers of treatments at the first and second stages. Because the inferential goals differ and snSMART designs will likely have a much smaller sample size than classic SMART designs, most of the existing methods for analyzing data from a classic SMART do not apply in the snSMART setting.

2.3.1 snSMART with Three Active Treatments and a Binary Outcome

The snSMART design shown in Figure 2.2 is a generalized version of the design used for the ARAMIS (Micheletti et al., 2020) trial. In the snSMART design, participants are equally randomized between three active treatments in the first stage which we denote as A, B, and C. Each stage is set to the same period of time in which the treatment could have a full effect, e.g. each stage in ARAMIS is six months. At the end of each stage, treatment response is assessed. In ARAMIS, response was defined via a composite physician and patient-reported set of outcomes, but this outcome can be any binary or dichotomized variable of scientific interest. Unlike a crossover trial, where all participants crossover to another treatment in the second stage (period), in an snSMART, responders to the initial treatment continue to receive their initial treatment. Non-responders to initial treatment are equally re-randomized to one of the other two treatments that they did not initially receive. At the end of the second stage, the same outcome, e.g. response, is measured on all participants.

2.3.1.1 Group Sequential snSMART

The snSMART design with three active treatments can include adaptive components such that an inferior treatment arm can be removed at an interim point during the trial (Chao et al., 2020). Adaptive designs have been recommended for studying rare diseases by many (Gupta et al., 2011; Chow and Chang, 2019) and are often used in earlier phase designs with smaller samples (Cheung, 2011). Group sequential designs are a type of adaptive design where interim analyses are planned prior to the start of the trial so that decisions can be made based on accumulated data to modify aspects of the trial in a predetermined way (e.g. to remove a treatment arm or stop a trial early due to futility or efficacy). Dropping a treatment arm or ending the trial early allows the potential of: i) more participants receiving better-performing treatments, or ii) a smaller expected sample size of the trial. The first feature may improve the engagement and recruitment of participants because participants are less likely to be treated with an inferior treatment if it is removed during the trial, while the latter feature may be desirable for investigators and sponsors of the trial due to restricted resources. The group sequential snSMART allows for the removal of an inferior treatment arm (Chao et al., 2020).

The group sequential snSMART design includes several predetermined interim analysis points (or looks) $l = 1, 2, ..., L$, where L is the maximum number of interim analyses performed during a trial. Here 'stage' and 'look' are two different concepts. 'Stage' refers to a period of time that is specific to when each participant is followed for a response (i.e. there are two stages of equal length in an snSMART), whereas 'look' refers to a period of time that is specific to the entire study when the accrued data are analyzed in an interim analysis (Chao et al., 2020).

A group sequential snSMART begins as a standard snSMART with three active treatments. At each interim point, treatment effects are estimated and the preset decision rules are used to determine if a treatment can be dropped. If an interim analysis suggests there is an inferior treatment, then that treatment is removed. Stage 1 non-responders to this inferior treatment have equal chances of being assigned to the other two treatments in stage 2, and responders to this inferior treatment will keep receiving this treatment in stage 2 even if it has been removed after the interim analysis. Stage 1 non-responders to each of the non-inferior treatments are switched deterministically to the other non-inferior treatment in stage 2 (Figure 2.3). At most, one treatment arm is removed and two active treatments remain until the end of the trial. If none of the treatments is statistically inferior to the others at a particular interim point, all treatments are kept in the trial.

2.3.2 snSMART with Three Active Treatments and a Continuous Outcome

The snSMART design in Figure 2.2 and the group sequential design in Figure 2.3 assume a binary outcome measured at the end of the first and second stages. Dichotomization of a continuous outcome may not be feasible based on insufficient prior knowledge or the outcome of interest may inherently be continuous. An extension to the snSMART design

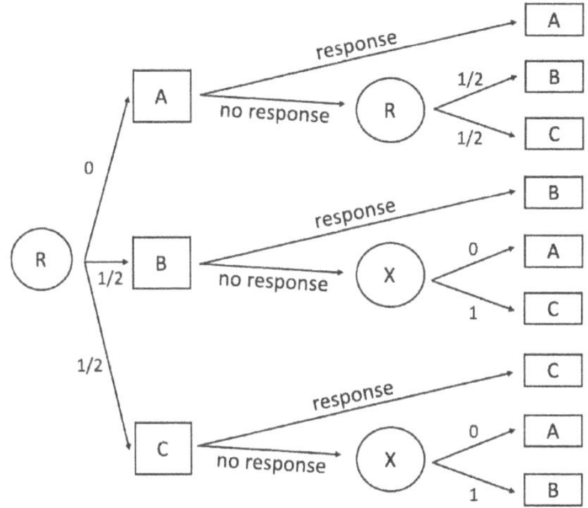

Figure 2.3 *Study design of a group sequential snSMART after treatment A has been removed. R denotes randomization to the following treatment; X denotes deterministic assignment to the following treatment. Numbers on the plot denote the probability of being assigned to the following treatments.*

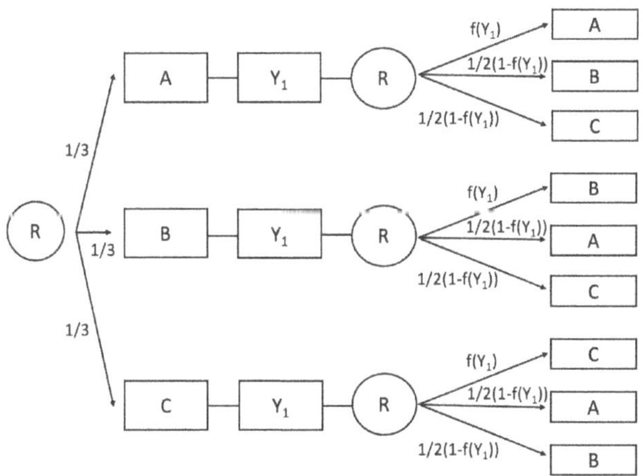

Figure 2.4 *Study design of an snSMART with a mapping function. R denotes randomization to the following treatment; A, B, and C are treatments, and $f(Y_1)$ is the mapping function. Expressions on the arrows denote the probability of being assigned to the following treatments. Each stage is the same length of time.*

presented in Figure 2.2 allows for a continuous outcome measured at the end of both stages (Hartman et al., 2021). The first stage of this design (shown in Figure 2.4) mimics the standard design where all participants are equally randomized to one of the three first-stage treatments. Participants are followed for a predetermined period of time before their continuous outcome Y_1 is recorded at the end of stage 1. There are no 'responders' or 'non-responders'; instead, the probability of staying on the same treatment for any participant is a function of their continuous outcome $f(Y_1)$. We call this function a mapping function. Given that the output of a mapping function is a probability, the range of the mapping

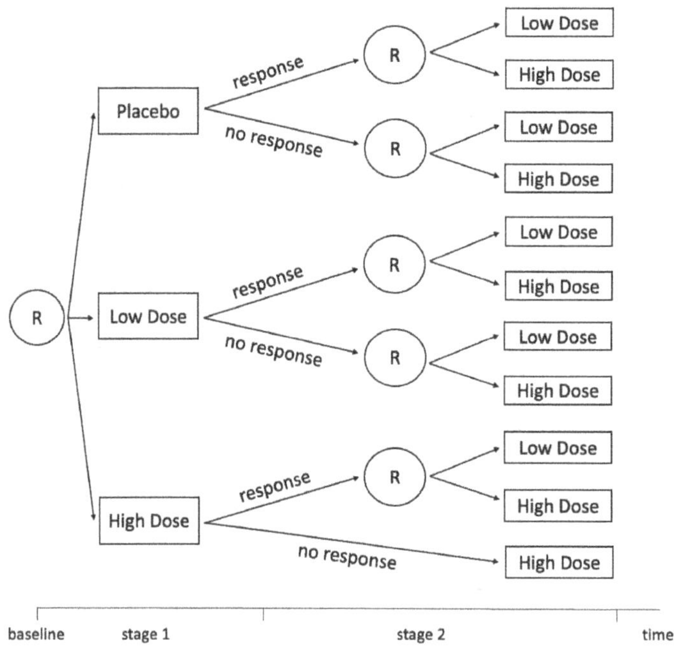

Figure 2.5 *Study design of a snSMART with two dose levels and a placebo. Participants are randomized among placebo, low dose and high dose equally in stage 1. After being followed for a predetermined period of time, participants are assessed on their response to the initial treatment. The stage 2 dosage assignment for each patient is based on their dosage group and response status to the initial treatment. Outcomes are collected at the end of both stage 1 and stage 2.*

function is between 0 and 1. We include more details on the choice of the mapping function in Section 2.4.2. Participants have probability $f(Y_1)$ of receiving the same treatment and probability $[1 - f(Y_1)]/2$ of receiving either of the two remaining treatments. At the end of stage 2, the continuous outcome is measured again.

2.3.3 snSMART with Two Dose Levels and a Placebo and a Binary Outcome

The snSMART design in Figure 2.2 was motivated by ARAMIS where there were several active treatments in use for isolated skin vasculitis. Very often, however, the purpose of a clinical trial is to find the optimal dose of a drug of interest, determine the efficacy of that dose and register the drug and dosage with the Food and Drug Administration (FDA). Thus, a variation of the snSMART design that focuses on a single drug and placebo was proposed by Fang et al. (2021). This variation alters the snSMART design in Figure 2.2 by replacing three active drugs with two dose levels of one drug and a placebo (see Figure 2.5). This snSMART design enables all participants to receive at least one dosage level of the drug and the estimation of the differences in the probability of response to treatment between the two dose levels and placebo. All participants receive an active treatment by the end of the study which aids in the recruitment of participants. In addition, more than one dosage level of a drug can be compared in the same trial making it possible to demonstrate if a lower, less toxic dose is as efficacious as a high dose.

In this design, participants have an equal chance of being randomized to receive a placebo, low dose, and high dose in stage 1. After receiving the initial assignment for a pre-specified period of time, participants in the study are assessed for binary response.

Based on their stage 1 treatment and response to that treatment, participants are assigned to either the same or a different dose of treatment in stage 2. Participants who received a placebo or low dose in stage 1 are re-randomized to either low or high dose in stage 2, so that every participant receives some dose of the drug in the trial. Non-responders to the stage 1 high dose remain on the high dose in stage 2, and responders to the stage 1 high dose are re-randomized equally to either low or high dose in stage 2 (Figure 2.5). This re-randomization of high-dose responders allows for all participants to receive an active dose with additional data on low dose and to explore if the same treatment effect from stage 1 on a high dose can be seen in stage 2 on a low dose with potentially better tolerability.

2.4 Analytic Methods for snSMART Designs

Here, we present both Bayesian and frequentist methods to analyze data from the snSMART designs presented in Section 2.3. First, in Section 2.4.1 we present a Bayesian Joint Stage Model (BJSM) for the binary outcome snSMART design seen in Figure 2.2. We compare this BJSM to a frequentist log-linear Poisson joint stage model that does not incorporate prior information and does not make the same assumptions on some of the model parameters. We show how the BJSM is used in the group sequential design from Figure 2.3 in Section 2.4.1.3. In Section 2.4.2, we present another version of the BJSM that estimates first-stage treatment effects when the outcome of interest is continuous and the mapping function is used for re-randomization. Finally, in Section 2.4.3, we modify the BJSM to analyze data from an snSMART design that considers dose levels and placebo.

2.4.1 Analysis of snSMART with Three Active Treatments and a Binary Outcome

2.4.1.1 Bayesian Joint Stage Model (BJSM)

In this design (Figure 2.2), the primary goal of the trial is to estimate the first-stage response rate of each treatment and to provide estimates of the pairwise treatment differences with their corresponding credible intervals. To estimate the first-stage response rate of each treatment, a Bayesian approach that borrows information across the first and second stages was proposed by Wei et al. (2018) for a two-stage snSMART design. Parameters are used to link the stage 1 and stage 2 treatment response rates.

Notation is as follows:

- participants in the trial: $i = 1, ..., N$, N is the total sample size,
- stage of the trial: $j = 1, 2$,
- treatment: $m = A, B, C$,
- linkage parameter that connects first-stage response to second-stage response for first-stage non-responders: β_0,
- linkage parameter that connects first-stage response to second-stage response for first-stage responders: β_1,
- observed response outcome for patient i in stage j on treatment m: Y_{ijm},
- first-stage response rate: π_m for treatment m,
- second-stage response rate for first-stage responders: $\beta_1 \pi_m$, and
- second-stage response rate for non-responders to treatment m in the first stage who receive treatment m' in the second stage: $\beta_0 \pi_{m'}$.

The proposed BJSM model is

$$\begin{aligned} Y_{i1m}|\pi_m &\sim Bernoulli(\pi_m) \\ Y_{i2m'}|Y_{i1m},\pi_m &\sim Bernoulli((\beta_1\pi_m)^{Y_{i1m}}(\beta_0\pi_{m'})^{1-Y_{i1m}}). \end{aligned} \tag{2.1}$$

To facilitate a parsimonious model and constrain the estimation space for the linkage parameters, we assume the following:

1. the linkage parameters β_0 and β_1 do not depend on the initial treatment m,
2. $\beta_0 < 1$: the response rate in stage 2 for treatment m is less than the response rate for treatment m in stage 1 for non-responders, and
3. $\beta_1 > 1$: the response rate in stage 2 for treatment m is higher than the response rate for treatment m in stage 1 for responders.

These assumptions were appropriate when designing ARAMIS and enabled the use of specific prior distributions. However, all model assumptions should be specific to the disease and treatments being studied. The BJSM does not require these specific assumptions and can be made more flexible by eliminating these assumptions. For example, the linkage parameters can depend on first-stage treatment such that there may be six linkage parameters β_{0m} and β_{1m}. Additionally, the linkage parameters need not be constrained and can be estimated across the real line.

Prior distributions for the treatment response rates, π_m and the linkage parameters β_0 and β_1 must also be specified. Suggested priors for the parameters in the BJSM that satisfy the assumptions listed previously are i) $\pi_m \sim Beta(\zeta_m, \eta_m)$, ii) $\beta_0 \sim Beta(\zeta_0, \eta_0)$, and iii) $\beta_1 \sim Pareto(1, \phi)$. The Beta distribution is a conjugate prior for a binary outcome and has properties such that the mean of the distribution is $\zeta_m/(\zeta_m + \eta_m)$ and the prior sample size is the sum of the two hyperparameters $\zeta_m + \eta_m$. As a reasonable prior setting in the ARAMIS study, $\zeta_m = 0.4$ and $\eta_m = 1.6$ since investigators believed an ineffective treatment would have an average response rate of 0.2. Separate priors for each treatment were not specified, but the model can accommodate this. Furthermore, the sum of the hyperparameters specified for ARAMIS suggested that the prior estimate of an ineffective treatment was based on a prior sample of two individuals. Two individuals are small in comparison to the expected total sample size of 90 for the trial, so the influence of the prior is small at the end of the study. Since Wei et al. (2018) assumed the linkage parameter for the non-responders ranged from 0 to 1 a uniform distribution or a Beta distribution with $\zeta_0 = 1$ and $\eta_0 = 1$ was suggested. For the linkage parameter for responders, a Pareto distribution allows for values greater than or equal to 1, but has most of its mass between 1 to 3. This was chosen for ARAMIS since it was believed that on average the response rate would be 1.5 times greater in stage 2 than in stage 1 for responders to stage 1 treatment. With the prior distributions specified, the joint stage model, and the observed data from the trial, response rates for each treatment are estimated from the posterior distribution of π_m using Markov Chain Monte Carlo sampling.

While the primary goal of an snSMART is to estimate the first-stage treatment effects, DTR effects can also be estimated from an snSMART. If DTRs are of interest, then the BJSM model should consider 6 linkage parameters, (β_{0m}, β_{1m}), so that the linkage parameters can depend on first-stage treatment. This parameterization takes advantage of any differences that may occur in each treatment-specific pathway and will allow more unique treatment effect estimates for each DTR. The restriction on the prior distribution of β_{1m} can be loosened so that β_{1m} ranges from 0 to infinity as opposed to 1 to infinity. For this, we recommend a Gamma(ζ_1, η_1) prior, where for example, $\zeta_1 = \eta_1 = 2$.

Then, posterior draws can be computed for each DTR $\pi_{mmm'}$ using the posterior draws of β_{0m}, β_{1m} and π_m where $\pi_{mmm'} = \pi_m(\pi_m\beta_{1m}) + (1 - \pi_m)(\pi_{m'}\beta_{0m})$. Using the BJSM to estimate DTR effects takes advantage of all outcomes collected at the end of the first and second stages, as opposed to weighted and replicated regression (Nahum-Shani et al., 2012; Kidwell et al., 2018) used to estimate DTR effects from traditional SMART designs that only use the second-stage outcome. The BJSM method may result in slightly higher bias but is more efficient than using the weighted and replicated regression method; this bias-variance tradeoff is not uncommon in rare disease treatment estimation.

2.4.1.2 Log-linear Poisson Joint Stage Modeling (LPJSM) for a Binary Outcome

The LPJSM is a frequentist approach of modeling data from two stages that parallels the BJSM. The mean of the outcome is modeled using a log link and the variance is modeled by the Poisson family due to the potential convergence issues when using the binomial family variance in small samples (Williamson et al., 2013).

We extend the notation from the section above for the LPJSM such that:

- $\mathbb{1}\{\cdot\}$: indicator function,
- α_m, γ_1 and γ_0: the logged values of π_m, β_1 and β_0 from the BJSM model, respectively,
- $\boldsymbol{Y}_i = (Y_{i1m}, Y_{i2m'})^T, \boldsymbol{\mu}_i = (\mu_{i1m}, \mu_{i2m'})^T$,
- $\boldsymbol{\theta} = (\alpha_A, \alpha_B, \alpha_C, \gamma_1, \gamma_0)^T$, and
- $\boldsymbol{V}_i$ is the working covariance matrix of $\boldsymbol{Y}_i$ with $\boldsymbol{V}_i = \boldsymbol{A}_i^{1/2}\boldsymbol{A}_i^{1/2}$, and $\boldsymbol{A}_i^{1/2}$ is a diagonal matrix with elements being the square root of $Var(Y_{ijm})$, which is modeled with a Poisson family variance structure, i.e. $Var(Y_{ijm}) = \mu_{ijm}$.

The LPJSM is specified as:

$$\begin{aligned}\log(E(Y_{i1m})) = \log(\mu_{i1m}) = \alpha_A \mathbb{1}\{m = A\} + \alpha_B \mathbb{1}\{m = B\} \\ + \alpha_C \mathbb{1}\{m = C\}\end{aligned} \tag{2.2}$$

$$\begin{aligned}\log(E(Y_{i2m'})) = \log(\mu_{i2m'}) = \alpha_A \mathbb{1}\{m' = A\} + \alpha_B \mathbb{1}\{m' = B\} \\ + \alpha_C \mathbb{1}\{m' = C\} + \gamma_1 Y_{i1m} + \gamma_0(1 - Y_{i1m})\end{aligned} \tag{2.3}$$

The parameters are estimated via generalized estimating equations (GEE):

$$\sum_{i=1}^{N} \frac{\partial \boldsymbol{\mu}_i^T}{\partial \boldsymbol{\theta}} \boldsymbol{V}_i^{-1}(\boldsymbol{Y}_i - \boldsymbol{\mu}_i) = 0. \tag{2.4}$$

The robust "sandwich" covariance estimator $(\sum_0^{-1} \sum_1 \sum_0^{-1})$ is used to estimate the variance of $\hat{\boldsymbol{\theta}}$.

Simulation studies conducted by Wei et al. (2018) illustrated that the root-mean-square error (which considers both bias and efficiency) and the width of the 95% credible intervals of the BJSM estimators are smaller than the LPJSM approach in realistic settings. If the BJSM model assumptions about the linkage parameters are violated, the estimator generated by the BJSM is more likely to be biased but is still more efficient than estimators from the LPJSM.

2.4.1.3 Two Step Dropping Rule for a Group Sequential snSMART

Sequential design is often used in clinical trials where accumulated data can be used to make a decision regarding the treatments under study before reaching full accrual. Here, we present how the BJSM can be used to include interim decision-making to drop an inferior treatment arm. We present methods from Chao et al. (2020) that incorporate a two-step dropping rule into the snSMART design based on the posterior distributions of the response rates at each interim look. This group sequential design is applicable to rare diseases or small sample trials where the rate of accrual is slow in comparison to the timing of the outcome measurements so that the interim decisions can impact future patient treatment assignment.

We extend the notation from the BJSM from Section 2.4.1 to facilitate interim analysis. At each interim look l, we use all of the available outcome data Y_{i1m} and $Y_{i2m'}$ for all $m, m' \equiv A, B, C$ and implement the BJSM to provide the posterior distribution of the response rates of all treatments even though stage 2 outcomes may be missing for some participants. Hence, the patients who have the stage 2 outcome $Y_{i2m'}$ at look l are a subset of the patients who provide their stage 1 outcome Y_{i1m}. Additionally, at interim analysis look l, we denote

- N_l is the sample size at each look,
- $P_{m,l}$ is the interim posterior probability that treatment m has the greatest response rate given the data up to look l,
- $Q_{m,l}$ is the interim posterior probability that treatment m has the smallest response rate given the data up to look l, and
- τ_l and ψ_l are tuning parameters used in the decision rules to maintain desired operating characteristics of the trial.

The two-step decision rule defines a process that allows us to decide if we should drop a treatment arm at look l. The first step of the decision rule is based on $P_{m,l}$ such that we drop the inferior treatment arm when there is one inferior treatment. The second step is based on $Q_{m,l}$ such that we can drop the worst-performing arm when there is one superior treatment. Chao et al. (2020) suggest at most two looks due to the small sample size, and if a treatment is dropped at the first look, the second look is not performed. The Bayesian decision rule is as follows:

1. Calculate $P_{m,l}$ for each treatment m and compare with a prespecified cut-off τ_l.
2. If $P_{m,l} > \tau_l$ for any m, then compute $Q_{m',l}$ for treatments $m' \neq m$ and remove the treatment with higher $Q_{m',l}$.
3. If $P_{m,l} \leq \tau_l$ for all m, then compute $Q_{m,l}$ for all m and compare the posterior probability $Q_{m,l}$ with the prespecified cut-off ψ_l. If $Q_{m,l} > \psi_l$ for any m then treatment m will be removed. Otherwise, all treatments are kept in the trial.

The tuning parameters τ_l and ψ_l are selected through simulation over a grid of values to control the probability of incorrectly removing an effective treatment, a quantity similar to type I error. The operating characteristics of a group sequential snSMART are robust to small differences in these tuning parameters.

This group sequential design allows one treatment to be dropped at an interim analysis if it is clearly inferior to the others or if one treatment is clearly better than the other two treatments. In the case of one superior treatment then one of the lower performing of the two treatments could be removed based on the point estimates of the response or investigators could choose to continue the trial without removing an arm.

The group sequential snSMART design differs from the standard snSMART design in that treatment assignment can become deterministic after an interim analysis for some stage 1 non-responders. Chao et al. (2020) proved that the BJSM still provides unbiased estimates of the response rates even if an arm is removed during the trial. The treatment effect estimates using the BJSM continue to be more efficient than a standard, parallel trial with only 1 stage and on average, more patients are treated with the better-performing treatments than an snSMART without interim analyses.

2.4.2 Analysis of snSMART with Three Active Treatments and a Continuous Outcome

The previous methods assumed a binary outcome measured at the end of stages 1 and 2. Some trials, however, may measure a continuous endpoint such as patient-reported outcomes or utilities that consider both efficacy and tolerability. Thus, the extension of the snSMART design to consider continuous endpoints at the end of stage 1 and stage 2 using a mapping function is shown in Figure 2.4. We elaborate here on the choice of the mapping function to facilitate re-randomization in the second stage and then present a version of the BJSM that considers continuous outcomes.

2.4.2.1 Mapping Function

The mapping function (MF) maps the stage 1 outcome Y_{i1} to [0,1], which is the probability of staying on the same treatment. A probability closer to 1 indicates a better outcome for the patient on that treatment so that they have a higher chance of staying on the same treatment. The mapping function may be formulated as:

$$f(Y_{i1}) = \left(\frac{Y_{i1} - Y_{min}}{Y_{max} - Y_{min}}\right)^s,$$

but any monotonic function that maps Y_{i1} to [0,1] can be used. We consider three specific versions of this MF. The first MF or linear MF (s=1) may be used when little information is known about the distribution of Y_1, but minimum and maximum values are known. If there are extreme values within the possible range of Y_1, we can select a more practical minimum and maximum of Y_1 and truncate the MF at 0 and 1. The second MF (when $Y_{min} = 0$ and $Y_{max} = 1$ reduces to $f(Y_{i1}) = Y_{i1}^s$, $0 < s < 1$) may be used when there is a high proportion of patients who are expected to stay on the same treatment through both stages or when the outcome may be right skewed. The third MF (when $Y_{min} = 0$ and $Y_{max} = 1$ reduces to $f(Y_{i1}) = Y_{i1}^s$, $s > 1$) is appropriate when a high proportion of patients are expected to switch treatments or the outcome is left skewed.
Additional notation for the BJSM considering continuous outcomes is as follows.

- outcome of each stage: Y_{ij}, a continuous outcome,
- treatment for patient i in stage j: M_{ij}, where $j = 1, 2$ for a two-stage design,
- mean outcome for stage 1: μ_1, a function of only the stage 1 treatment,
- mean outcome for stage 2: μ_2, a function of both the stage 1 and stage 2 treatments, a weighted average of the treatment effects from stage 1 and stage 2 with an additional effect if the patient stays on the same treatment,
- expected effect of treatment $m, m = A, B, C$ in the first stage: ξ_m, where the primary goal of the snSMART is to estimate ξ_m and identify the best treatment in stage 1, and
- effects of how treatments differ from stage 1 to stage 2: ϕ_1, ϕ_2, ϕ_3, where a detailed definition is provided below.

We assume the data from the snSMART design with a mapping function has a multivariate normal likelihood where the covariance matrix is a function of the sequence of treatments the participant received:

$$F(x) = \begin{bmatrix} Y_{i1} \\ Y_{i2} \end{bmatrix} |M_{i1}, M_{i2} \sim MVN\left(\begin{bmatrix} \mu_1(M_{i1}) \\ \mu_2(M_{i1}, M_{i2}) \end{bmatrix}, \boldsymbol{V}(M_{i1}, M_{i2})\right).$$

Then the proposed BJSM for an snSMART with a mapping function jointly models the first-stage and second-stage mean treatment effects as such:

$$\mu_1(M_{i1}) = \textstyle\sum_{m=A}^{C} \xi_m I(M_{i1} = m),$$
$$\mu_2(M_{i1}, M_{i2}) = \phi_1 \textstyle\sum_{m=A}^{C} \xi_m I(M_{i1} = m) + \phi_2 \sum_{m'=A}^{C} \xi_{m'} I(M_{i2} = m') + \phi_3 I(M_{i1} = M_{i2}).$$

For patients who switch treatments in the second stage, the mean model for the stage 2 outcome is a combination of some lingering effect of the first treatment (ϕ_1) and some additional effect of the second treatment (ϕ_2), where $\phi_1, \phi_2 > 0$. If the patient stays on the same treatment in both stages, the mean treatment effect in the second stage is the first-stage treatment effect plus an additional effect from staying on the treatment longer. These ϕ_1 and ϕ_2 terms are similar to the β_0 and β_1 linkage parameters for the standard snSMART. Our interest here for the snSMART with an MF is in the ξ_k parameters to estimate the first-stage treatment means.

The covariance between first and second-stage outcomes is modeled so that $\boldsymbol{V}(M_{i1}, M_{i2}) = V_1 I(M_{i1} = M_{i2}) + V_2 I(M_{i1} \neq M_{i2})$ where V_1 and V_2 are both 2×2 variance-covariance matrices. This specification allows those who stay on the same treatment to have a different correlation between stage 1 and stage 2 outcomes than those who switch treatments.

Hartman et al. (2021) proposed the following constraints for the ϕ_m parameters to help facilitate a parsimonious model:

- $\phi_2 = 1 - \phi_1$, $\phi_1, \phi_2 > 0$,
- $\phi_2 > \phi_1$, so that the stage 2 treatment has a larger effect on the stage 2 outcome than the stage 1 treatment
- $\phi_3 \geq 0$, so that staying on the same treatment has either no effect or a positive effect on the expected stage 2 outcome.

The priors were specified as such:

- $\pi_m \sim N(\mu, \sigma)$ for all m, where Hartman et al. implemented $\mu_m = 50$ and $\sigma_m = 50$ for all m,
- $\phi_1 \sim Unif(0, 0.5)$, in this way we have $\phi_2 > \phi_1$ based on the constraints above,
- $\phi_3 \sim FM(mean = 0, sd = \zeta)$, given that ϕ_3 is non-negative.where Hartman et al. suggested $\zeta = 20$, and
- $V_1, V_2 \sim IW_2\left(\begin{bmatrix} 1 & 0 \\ 0 & 1 \end{bmatrix}, 2\right)$ since Inverse Wishart (IW) distributions are conjugate priors for multivariate normal covariances. The low degrees of freedom (2) make the prior relatively uninformative.

Through simulation, Hartman et al. show that the two-stage snSMART design with an MF outperforms one-stage designs in estimating and correctly identifying the best first-stage treatment regardless of the MF used Hartman et al. (2021). In addition, modeling the continuous outcome with an MF provided higher efficiency and less bias than dichotomizing the continuous outcome and treating it as a binary variable at the end of the first and second stages.

2.4.3 Analysis of an snSMART with Dose Levels and Placebo and a Binary Outcome

The BJSM method for snSMART with dose levels and placebo (Fang et al., 2021) is very similar to that of the snSMART with three active treatments. The design, however, differs and therefore so do some of the model assumptions and prior distributions for parameters. Since both responders and non-responders are re-randomized in the second stage and two dose levels are considered, the model allows for a dose-response relationship between low and high doses. We use the same notation as the standard BJSM used in Section 2.4.1.1, but here $m = P, L, H$. The proposed BJSM model is the same as proposed for the three active treatment snSMART found in equation 2.4.
However, we adapt different prior distributions as follows:

- $\pi_P \sim Beta(\zeta_m, \eta_m)$

Fang et al. selected $\zeta_m = 3$ and $\eta_m = 17$ which is equivalent to a (spontaneous) response rate of 15%, but these parameters would be tailored to the disease considered.

- $\log(\pi_L/\pi_P) \sim N(\mu, \sigma^2)$ and $\log(\pi_H/\pi_P) \sim N(\mu, \sigma^2)$
  Fang et al. selected $\mu = 0.2$ and $\sigma^2 = 100$ to allow for a weak tendency for the drug response rates to be greater than the effect of the placebo.
- $\beta_0, \beta_1 \sim Gamma(\alpha, \beta)$
  Fang et al. selected $\alpha = 2$ and $\beta = 2$ for the prior of both linkage parameters, which allows $\beta_{1m}\pi_{m'}$ and $\beta_{0m}\pi_{m*}$ to be greater than 1. This choice is based on:
  (a) simplicity,
  (b) most of the values range between 0 and 3, which serves as a restriction to the prior distributions of the linkage parameters, and
  (c) $Gamma(2, 2)$ is centered at 1 with variance equal to 0.5, which makes it possible to have linkage parameters that are below or above 1.

Through simulation, Fang et al. compared bias, root-mean-square error (rMSE), coverage rates, and widths of the 95% confidence/credible intervals (CIs) between their proposed BJSM method and the frequentist method LPJSM. They concluded that BJSM could provide reasonable estimates of π_P, π_L and π_H when the true response rates were low, while LPJSM method was likely to have convergence issues under this scenario. Even though LPJSM outperformed BJSM in estimating each individual response rate when the true response rate and sample size were large, the BJSM, in general, provided more accurate estimations of the difference between the response rates of different dosage levels. In addition, the BJSM method was robust to different prior distributions.

2.5 Hypothetical Data Analysis in R

An R package **snSMART** (available at `https://github.com/sidiwang/snSMART`) incorporates many statistical methods to design and analyze snSMART data. This package provides functions for simulating trial data of various snSMART designs, calculating the required sample size for an snSMART with three active treatments and a binary outcome, and analyzing trial data via both Bayesian and frequentist approaches. Here we illustrate two of the functions given an snSMART with three active treatments, no interim analyses, and a binary outcome.

2.5.1 Sample Size Calculation

A sample size calculation specific to the BJSM using the average coverage criterion (Adcock, 1988) was developed by Wei et al. (2020). This calculation determines the minimum number of individuals to enroll in an snSMART more quickly than through a simulation-based, trial and error approach. The sample size calculation assumes three active treatments with one unique, best treatment and finds the sample size per arm such that the credible interval of the difference between the two best treatments rules out zero with a specified probability. The treatment with the highest posterior mean is compared to the treatment with the second highest posterior means based on the user input information and the BJSM.

To calculate the sample size for an snSMART as shown in Figure 2.2, we need to specify the expected response rates of treatments (π_m, ranges between 0 and 1), means of the linkage parameters (β_0 and β_1) where β_1 ranges between 1 to 1/largest response rate and β_0 ranges from 0 to 1, the desired coverage rate for the posterior difference of the best two treatments which can be considered as $1 - \alpha$ where α is similar to the desired type I error, the probability that the credible interval of the difference of the best two treatments excludes zero (similar to power), the prior means for each response rate (which will likely equal the expected response rates, but may be more conservative), and prior effective sample size for each response rate. In the `sample_size()` function shown below, we set $\pi_A = 0.6, \pi_B = 0.3, \pi_C = 0.3, \beta_0 = 0.5, \beta_1 = 1.4$, coverage rate $= 0.9$, power $= 0.8$. The prior means for treatment A, B, C are set to their expected response rates of 0.6, 0.3 and 0.3, respectively, and the prior sample size for treatment A, B, C are set as 4, 2 and 3.

```
N = sample_size(pi = c(0.6, 0.3, 0.3), beta1 = 1.5,
beta0 = 0.5, coverage = 0.9, power = 0.8,
mu = c(0.6, 0.3, 0.3), n = c(4, 2, 3))
```

R output:

```
With given settings, the estimated sample size per
arm for an snSMART is: 17
This implies that for an snSMART with sample size
of 17 per arm (51 in total for three agents): The
probability of successfully identifying the best
treatment is 0.8 when the difference of response
rates between the best and second best treatment
is at least 0.3, and the response rate of the best
treatment is 0.6
```

Thus, we require 17 participants on each treatment arm to distinguish the best treatment from the second-best treatment using the BJSM and the specified trial characteristics.

2.5.2 Data Analysis via BJSM

We assume that we have an snSMART design with 18 participants per arm in stage 1, and 5 patients dropped out before the second stage re-randomization. Data from an snSMART can be described via two 3x3 tables. Table 2.1 describes the number of individuals who receive each treatment sequence such that the first-stage response rate can be inferred by the number of individuals on the diagonals divided by the number of individuals randomized to each first-stage treatment. Table 2.2 describes the number of individuals who respond at the end of the second stage for each treatment sequence.

Table 2.1 *Describes the number of participants who received each treatment sequence in an snSMART with three active treatments*

First stage	Second stage treatment			
treatment	A	B	C	N/A
A	13	2	2	1
B	6	3	7	2
C	6	6	4	2

Table 2.2 *Describes the number of participants who responded to each treatment sequence in an snSMART with three active treatments*

First stage	Second stage treatment		
treatment	A	B	C
A	11	0	0
B	4	2	3
C	1	0	3

Given this trial data, we can create a dataframe using the package via the function `trial_dataset()`.

```
trial_data = trial_dataset(trt = c(18, 18, 18),
resp = c(13, 3, 4), trt_same_II = c(13, 3, 4),
resp_same_II = c(11, 2, 3), trt_negA = c(2, 2),
trt_negB = c(5, 6), trt_negc = c(6, 6),
resp_negA = c(0, 0), resp_negB = c(4, 3),
resp_negC = c(1, 0))
```

The first 18 lines of the generated dataset is shown below:

```
   treatment_stageI response_stageI treatment_stageII response_stageII
1                 1               1                 1                1
2                 1               1                 1                1
3                 1               1                 1                1
4                 1               1                 1                1
5                 1               1                 1                1
6                 1               1                 1                1
7                 1               1                 1                1
8                 1               1                 1                1
9                 1               1                 1                1
10                1               1                 1                1
11                1               1                 1                1
12                1               1                 1                0
13                1               1                 1                0
14                1               0                 2                0
15                1               0                 2                0
16                1               0                 3                0
17                1               0                 3                0
18                1               0                NA               NA
```

Next, we use the `BJSM_binary()` function to analyze the generated trial dataset. To run this function, we need to specify the prior distributions for both treatment response rates and linkage parameters, the details of MCMC simulations, and the number of linkage parameters (two or six) used in the BJSM model. This function creates an object of class 'BJSM_binary' that contains a list of components: posterior samples of linkage parameters and treatment response rates; estimates of linkage parameters, estimates of treatment response rates, estimated pairwise response rate differences of all treatments; and expected response rate of DTRs.

```
BJSM_result = BJSM_binary(data = trial_data,
prior_dist = c("beta", "beta", "pareto"),
pi_prior.a = c(0.4, 0.4, 0.4),
pi_prior.b = c(1.6, 1.6, 1.6),
beta0_prior = c(1.6, 0.4),
beta1_prior = c(3, 1), n_MCMC_chain = 1,
BURN.IN = 10000, MCMC_SAMPLE = 60000,
ci = 0.95, six = TRUE, DTR = TRUE)
```

Here, `data = trial_data` is the trial data generated in the previous step. `prior_dist = c("beta", "beta", "pareto")` specifies the prior distributions for π, β_0 and β_1 respectively. `pi_prior.a = c(0.4, 0.4, 0.4)`, `pi_prior.b = c(1.6, 1.6, 1.6)` input the parameter a and parameter b of the prior distribution for each π_m. Similarly, `beta0_prior = c(1.6, 0.4)`, `beta1_prior = c(3, 1)` input the parameters of the prior distrubtions for β_0 and β_1. `n_MCMC_chain = 1` shows that 1 MCMC chain is generated. `BURN.IN = 10000` shows that the number of burn-in iterations for MCMC is set to 10,000. `MCMC_SAMPLE =`

60000 says that 60,000 iterations is included in the MCMC. `ci = 0.95` shows that the coverage probability for credible intervals is set to 0.95. `six = TRUE` is to specify that the six linkage parameters model is fitted. `DTR = TRUE` shows that the expected response rate of DTR is also included in the function output.

Function output is shown below:

```
Treatment Effects Estimate:
Estimate Std. Error C.I.  CI low CI high
trtA  0.66487   0.084265 0.95 0.49931 0.82529
trtB  0.18914   0.074060 0.95 0.05509 0.33309
trtC  0.30428   0.079656 0.95 0.15169 0.45945
Differences between Treatments:
Estimate Std.Error C.I.   CI low CI high
diffAB  0.47573   0.10996 0.95  0.25485 0.68262
diffBC -0.11514   0.10848 0.95 -0.32464 0.10276
diffAC  0.36059   0.11608 0.95  0.12827 0.58227
Linkage Parameter Estimate:
Estimate Std. Error C.I.  CI low CI high
beta0A  0.72691     0.26962 0.95 0.18840  1.0000
beta0B  0.92185     0.10022 0.95 0.70758  1.0000
beta0C  0.47192     0.24345 0.95 0.12678  1.0000
beta1A  1.21674     0.17276 0.95 1.00000  1.5479
beta1B  1.77648     0.90879 0.95 1.00000  3.5465
beta1C  1.65666     0.62715 0.95 1.00000  2.8851

Expected Response Rate of Dynamic Treatment
Regimens (DTR):
result
rep_AB 0.58003
rep_AC 0.60808
rep_BA 0.56321
rep_BC 0.29409
rep_CA 0.36821
rep_CB 0.21398
```

The result shows that the response rates for treatment A, treatment B and treatment C are estimated to be 0.665 (95% credible intervals (CI): 0.499 - 0.825), 0.189 (95% CI: 0.055 - 0.333), and 0.304 (95% CI: 0.152, 0.459) respectively. The treatment response rates between A and B, A and C are statistically significant. Treatment A is identified as the best treatment.

2.6 Discussion

In this chapter, we introduced snSMART designs and methods as an alternative approach to study treatments in small samples which are common in precision medicine. Variations of the snSMART design and corresponding BJSM are available to analyze the data adapting to the type of treatments being tested in the trial as well as the type of outcome considered. The design and methods can be extended to consider more treatments or stages, but three treatments and two stages are likely to be used most commonly due to small sample size, timing, and logistics.

We focused on applying the Bayesian framework to analyze data from the snSMART variations, but data may also be analyzed under the frequentist framework. The Bayesian approach formally incorporates expert opinion, registry data, or other prior knowledge into the prior distributions of the parameters, and provides intuitive interpretations of treatment effect estimates. Across simulations, the Bayesian framework provided more efficient treatment effect estimators than similar frequentist estimators. Often the Bayesian estimates were slightly more biased, but the bias was negligible. A sensitivity analysis of snSMART data via the frequentist approach is recommended to verify any assumptions made by the Bayesian analysis. The efficiency gains from two stages versus one via the design and implementing a Bayesian approach versus a frequentist approach via the analysis make the snSMART and BJSM desirable in small samples.

The presented methods and corresponding R package can handle missingness and continue to provide treatment effect estimates, but more research is needed to fully understand the impact of missingness with respect to the proportion missing and type of missingness. In implementation, clinical trials often have missing data from discontinuation of participants due to severe adverse events, low efficacy of the treatment, or the inconvenience of participation (Little et al., 2012). In addition, current snSMART methods estimate the average treatment effect for all patients and do not include covariates in the analyses. Incorporating covariates, e.g. patients' characteristics, into the model, can further personalize the treatment with the goal of precision medicine. This additional level of personalization needs to be balanced with the small sample size and heterogeneity of participants.

The snSMART design is not appropriate for all small sample trials, but can result in efficiency gains where the disease setting is relatively stable over the trial period and carry-over effects are minimal or can be eliminated with a short wash-out period. The snSMART design is an alternative to a crossover design and may increase participation and retention due to allowing individuals who respond to remain on that treatment. In addition, if placebo is required in the trial, an snSMART allows the estimation of a concurrent placebo arm, while also allowing each individual who first receives placebo to receive an active (dose of) treatment. The multi-stage design requires a longer time period to conduct the trial than a single stage design, but this increase in time is balanced via increased observations from individuals leading to increased efficiency in treatment effect estimates. As precision medicine divides diseases into smaller and smaller subsets, the snSMART and BJSM may be powerful tools to identify effective treatments that may otherwise not be studied in these small samples.

Chapter 3

Sequential Multiple Assignment Randomized Trials with Adaptive Randomization (SMART-AR) for Mobile Health Devices

Xiaobo Zhong, Bibhas Chakraborty, Ying Kuen Cheung

3.1 Introduction

In this chapter, we introduce a design that uses an adaptive randomization (AR) scheme within the sequential multiple assignment randomized trial (SMART), with the dual goals of learning about the effectiveness of selecting different dynamic treatment regimens (DTRs) and improving the quality of care for patients who participate in the trial. DTR is a multistage treatment program consisting of a sequence of decision-making rules, one per treatment decision, that allows for selecting a treatment based on the clinical information collected by each decision-making time point (Kosorok and Laber, 2019). DTR is alternatively called adaptive treatment strategy (Murphy, 2005a), treatment policy (Lunceford et al., 2002), or adaptive intervention (Collins et al., 2004; Zhong et al., 2019). Compared to a traditional intervention, under which a patient receives a fixed treatment throughout the entire course, the treatment level and type under a DTR can be repeatedly adjusted according to the individual's needs and thus provide opportunities to optimize the treatment selection as a function of time-dependent clinical information (Chakraborty and Murphy, 2014). DTR is particularly effective for managing chronic conditions, such as substance abuse disorder, depression management, and cancer.

We will illustrate the method in the context of a platform of smartphone apps for managing depression. While depression is a common mental health problem, only a small segment of the population with related symptoms can access standard one-on-one treatment. Behavioral intervention technologies, which harness smartphone apps to deliver psychological therapies, are increasingly argued to be a solution for extending psychological therapies to more people with depression and anxiety (Karyotaki et al., 2017). Firth et al. (2017) reported that smartphone apps could effectively reduce symptoms of depression and anxiety. However, mental health apps pose new design challenges, partly due to how people use their smartphones. People typically turn to their phones in spare moments and engage in a brief burst of activities to accomplish specific tasks due to resource competition (Vaish et al., 2014). Research indicates that people tend to use their smartphone apps in brief interactions. Specifically, 70% of the interactions occurred in less than 60 seconds (Andrews et al., 2015). As such, smartphone apps that require more than a minute or two to use, or require complex navigation, are unlikely to be used repeatedly. Meanwhile, there are various psychological strategies such as goal setting, cognitive restructuring, behavior activation, and positive psychological interventions that can be useful for people with common mental health problems. Apps can also differ in terms of interactional elements, such as text versus photographic entry, daily tasks versus as-needed tasks, etc.

Cheung et al. (2018) reported a mobile app recommendation system, IntelliCare, which consisted of a suite of apps for depression management. IntelliCare was based on the notion

DOI: 10.1201/9781003216223-3

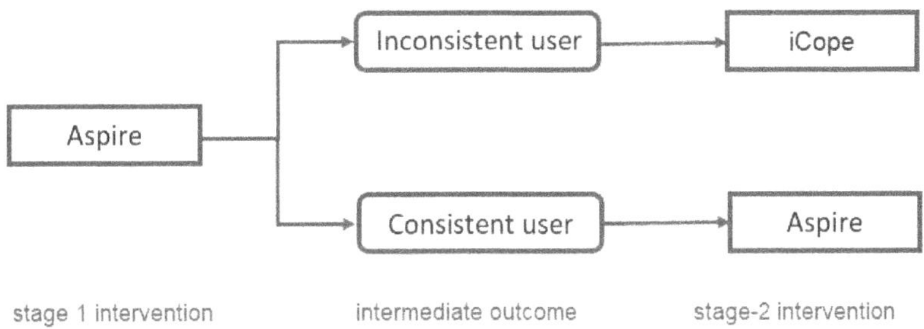

Figure 3.1 *Example of 2-stage DTR for depression management using two smartphone apps, Aspire and iCope.*

that people would be better served by a collection of simple apps, each with a specific goal, psychological strategy, and simple interactional element. It was designed as a prototype for such a platform that provides users with 12 apps that would instantiate different psychological strategies to support acquiring a set of depression management skills. For example, Aspire is an app designed to help a user identify the values that guide one's life and the actions (or "paths") that one takes to live these values. It helps keep track of these actions throughout the day and supports the users in living a purpose-driven and satisfying life. Another example app is iCope, which allows the user to send oneself inspirational messages and reassuring statements, written in their own words, to help the user get through tough spots or challenging situations. However, although numerous apps are available, depression management for these patients remains poor due to suboptimal treatment administration (Thombs et al., 2008). As the management of depression may involve multiple treatment components given over a relatively long period, a successful intervention is likely a direct result of administering a single component or a combination in an optimal treatment sequence, possibly based on intermediate outcomes, with an objective to maximize the eventual health outcome. Thus, the optimal intervention is potentially a DTR. Figure 3.1 is an example of a two-stage DTR consisting of two apps (i.e., Aspire and iCope). Under the example DTR, a patient will download and use the app Aspire initially for four weeks at stage 1, followed by using the same app for another six months at stage 2 if the user engagement data show that Aspire has been used consistently during stage 1, or switching to download and use iCope at stage 2 otherwise.

An efficient design for comparing multiple DTRs to improve the care of patients with depression is SMART, wherein a patient is first randomized to a treatment component and then re-randomized at a subsequent stage based on the intermediate outcome (Thall et al., 2000). Figure 3.2 shows a SMART for comparing different 2-stage depression management DTRs based on two apps (i.e., Aspire and iCope) in IntelliCare, in which a patient is first recommended to download and use an app for four weeks at stage 1 via a Hub, according to the result of initial randomization. Note that the Hub itself does not play any role as a treatment component. Instead, it sends out notifications to recommend particular intervention apps, and then provides links for downloading these apps within the platform such that users do not need to find these apps separately in other app marketplaces. At the end of stage 1, an intermediate evaluation is given to assess the user engagement for recommended apps, and patients are classified as consistent users or inconsistent users. Then, a new recommendation is sent to each patient based on the results of the second randomization, according to different histories of stage-1 treatment and intermediate outcomes. The final primary outcome is the reduction of depression symptoms, measured by the Beck Depression Inventory (BDI), six months after the second randomization. For more details on

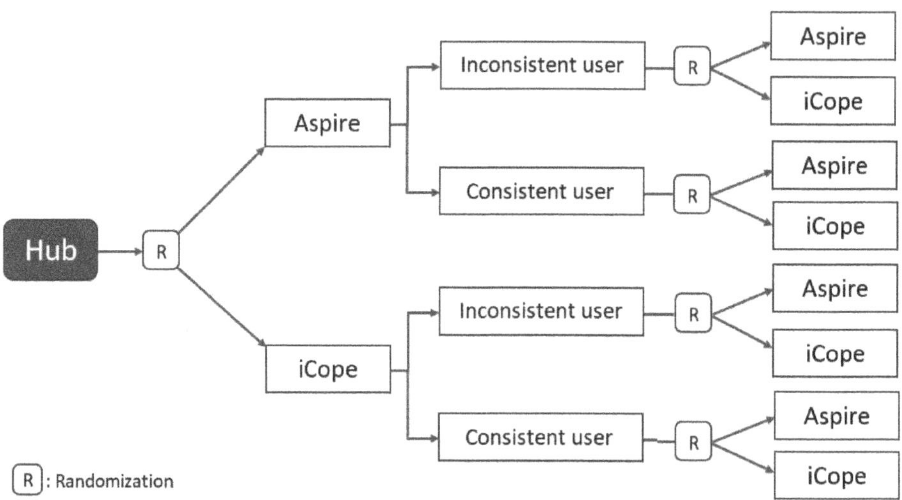

Figure 3.2 *A SMART based on apps for depression management.*

this design, see Section 3.2. By virtue of randomization, the assumption of ignorable treatment, which asserts that the assignment of treatment is independent of the future potential outcomes, conditioning on the subject's clinical history, can consistently hold (Rubin, 1974; Robins, 1997). Therefore, we can conduct causal inference for comparing multiple DTRs based on the data collected from a SMART.

It is common to conduct implementation studies to facilitate the uptake of new interventions, particularly in behavioral interventions for chronic conditions. An implementation study aims to adapt existing treatments in a care setting or treatment program to improve the quality of care for patients enrolled in the program while producing knowledge about the treatment (Cheung and Duan, 2014). A regular SMART design randomizes subjects to available treatment options according to pre-specified probabilities, often without regard to the likely benefits of the treatment. In particular, a typical strategy aims to achieve equal sample sizes across possible treatment sequences Murphy (2005a), but it does not go well with the objective of an implementation study. In addition, to cover all possible branches of the treatment sequence, a SMART design may suffer from the "curse of dimensionality". In drug trials such as the CATIE for schizophrenia (Schneider et al., 2001), the curse of dimensionality can be alleviated by restricting intervention options that are ethically and scientifically feasible, thus reducing the number of possible interventions to be evaluated. For example, it is quite common to use the play-the-winner strategy (Zhong et al., 2019), whereby a patient with a positive intermediate outcome will stay on the same treatment. In giving cancer therapy, the frontline treatment is typically continued upon a response or stable disease (Thall et al., 2000). In the above illustration example, however, although it is reasonable to suggest continuing the same app that is consistently used in stage 1, playing the winner is unnecessary for the ethical or optimal approach in behavioral intervention apps.

Motivated by these practical considerations, Cheung et al. (2015) proposed the sequential multiple-assignment randomized trial with adaptive randomization (SMART-AR) design for implementation research. This design addresses three main concerns of an implementation study: it allows incorporation of historical data or opinions for study design; it includes randomization for learning purposes; it aims to improve patients' care by adapting the treatment selection based on the ongoing trial information throughout the program. The idea of AR is to use the outcome data from patients treated previously in an ongoing study to unbalance the randomization probabilities in favor of the empirically superior treatments for the subsequent patients who enroll in the same study later. This idea is appealing for quality improvement in a care program. Here, the term "adaptive" in AR refers to the fact that treatment decisions are adapted between-patient rather than within-patient. We will discuss the method in more detail in the following sections.

3.2 Q-Learning: Review and Notation

A non-adaptive SMART allows the evaluation of DTRs that adapt treatments within patients but do not adapt treatments between patients. Lee et al. (2014) proposed to apply ε-greedy randomization in a dose-finding trial to adapt dose assignment based on the posterior expectation of Q-function-type utilities. Similarly, the AR strategy in SMART-AR is also based on Q-function in Q-learning. In this section, we first review the notations and method of Q-learning in a two-stage SMART setting.

We define a stage as a time interval during which a patient receives a particular treatment. Let t be the indicator of stage and thus $t = 1, 2$ in a 2-stage SMART. Let $i = 1, \ldots, N$ be the patient indicator, where N is the total number of patients enrolled in the trial. Let A_{ti} denote the treatment given to the ith patient at stage t, and S_t denote the set of treatment options at stage t so that $A_{ti} \in S_t$. Let J_t be the number of treatment options at stage t. The objective of Q-learning is to identify the optimal decision $d_t^*(h_t) \in S_t$ for the stage-t intervention given the patient's history $H_{ti} = h_{ti}$ prior to the decision-making point at the beginning of stage t, for maximizing the expected final outcome Y_i. For illustration purposes, we will focus on identifying optimal two-stage DTR based on the Q-learning approach, by which we define Q-functions as

$$Q_2(h_2, a_2) = E(Y_i | H_{2i} = h_2, A_{2i} = a_2) \tag{3.1}$$

for stage 2 and

$$Q_1(h_1, a_1) = E(\max_{a_2 \in S_2} Q_2(h_{2i}, a_2) | H_{1i} - h_1, A_{1i} = a_1) \tag{3.2}$$

for stage 1. In settings where the stage-1 treatment selection is not adapted to any baseline information, that is $H_{1i} = \phi$, the value of Q_1 only depends on the choice of stage-1 treatment option a_1, and thus (3.1) reduces to $Q_1(h_1, a_1) = E(max_{a_2 \in S_2} Q_2(h_{2i}, a_2) | A_{1i} = a_1)$. If the Q-functions were known, we could use backward induction to evaluate the optimal DTR that maximizes the expected value of the eventual outcome for patient i as

$$d_t^*(h_{ti}) = \arg\max_{a_t \in S_t} Q_t(h_{ti}, a_t)$$

for $t = 1, 2$. However, in practice, the true Q-functions are never known a priori and need to be estimated from the data. Q-learning postulates the conceptual model for stage-t Q-function using linear regression for a continuous eventual outcome:

$$Q_t(h_t, a_t; \theta_t) = \theta_0 + \theta_{t1}^T a_t + \theta_{t2}^T h_t + \theta_{t3}^T h_t a_t,$$

where the design matrix comprises of clinical history h_t and treatment selection a_t that can be properly coded as continuous or dummy variables. For stage 2, the regression coefficients θ_2 can be estimated by the least square method such that

$$\widehat{\theta}_2 = \arg\min_{\theta_2} \sum_{i=1}^{n} \{Y_i - Q_2(H_{2i}, A_{2i}; \theta_2)\}^2. \tag{3.3}$$

For stage 1, we define for patient i a pseudo-outcome

$$\widehat{Y}_i = \max_{a_2 \in S_2} Q_2(H_{2i}, a_2; \widehat{\theta}_2) \tag{3.4}$$

as a proxy for the quantity under expectation in the definition of $Q_1(h_1, a_1)$, and then estimate θ_1 using least squares based on the pseudo-outcomes:

$$\widehat{\theta}_1 = \arg\min_{\theta_1} \sum_{i=1}^{n} \{\widehat{Y}_i - Q_1(H_{1i}, A_{1i}; \theta_1)\}^2. \tag{3.5}$$

With the model-based estimates of the Q-functions, we can apply backward induction to obtain an estimate of the optimal DTR as

$$\widehat{d}_t^*(h_{ti}) = \arg\max_{a_t \in S_t} Q_t(h_{ti}, a_t; \widehat{\theta}_t)$$

for $t = 2$ and 1.

Algorithm 3.1: General approach to identify optimal 2-stage DTR using Q-learning method

1 Define Q-functions as in Equations (3.1) and (3.2).
2 Estimate coefficients θ_2 for stage-2 Q-function by (3.3).
3 Calculate the pseudo maximum value $\widehat{Y}_i$ for patient i, where $i = 1, \ldots, N$, by (3.4).
4 Estimate coefficients θ_1 for stage-1 Q-function by (3.5).
5 Estimate the optimal decision for stage 1.
6 Estimate the optimal decisions $(\widehat{d}_{20}^*, \widehat{d}_{21}^*)$ for stage 2 based on estimated $\widehat{d}_1^*$, where

$$\widehat{d}_{20}^* = \arg\max_{a_2 \in S_2} Q_2(A_1 = \widehat{d}_1^*, r = 0, A_2 = a_2; \widehat{\theta}_2)$$

$$\widehat{d}_{21}^* = \arg\max_{a_2 \in S_2} Q_2(A_1 = \widehat{d}_1^*, r = 1, A_2 = a_2; \widehat{\theta}_2).$$

Algorithm 3.1 summarizes the standard approach to estimate the optimal two-stage DTR by the Q-learning method, which can be further generalized to SMART design with more than two stages. In this case, the result of intermediate evaluation is summarized as a binary outcome and patients are classified as either responders (i.e., $r = 1$) or non-responders (i.e., $r = 0$) at the end of stage 1. In the depression management apps example, we consider two options of mobile apps that are to be recommended by the Hub for a user at the time of initial sign-in and possibly modified after four weeks of the first download. Let A_{ti} be the apps recommended to patient i at stage-t for $t = 1, 2$; that is, $S_{ti} = 0, 1$ for $t = 1, 2$, with 0 representing Aspire and 1 for iCope. At the end of stage 1, an intermediate evaluation will be given to each patient based on the user engagement data. And then, patients will be classified as high-engagement or low-engagement users. The number of sessions of an app that a user launched in a week will be counted, and the weekly counts measuring the "loyalty" of the user to the app will be summarized across the 4-week period. The concept of loyalty index was first developed for web analytics and later adapted for smartphone apps to measure user engagement. In this case, the loyalty index can be calculated by

$$\begin{aligned}\text{Loyalty index} &= 1 - \frac{1}{\text{number of sessions during the observed period}} \\ &= 1 - \frac{1}{\sum_{i=1}^{4} \text{weekly counts}}\end{aligned}$$

Table 3.1 *Treatment sequences and the results of Q-learning for smartphone apps data* ($N = 400$)

Sequence indicator	Stage-1 treatment	Intermediate outcome	Stage-2 treatment	N of patients	$\widehat{Q}_2$	Pseudo outcome	$\widehat{Q}_1$
1	Aspire	Low user engagement	Aspire	51	0.86	10.53	11.00
2	Aspire	Low user engagement	iCope	56	10.53	10.53	
3	Aspire	High user engagement	Aspire	51	11.53	11.53	
4	Aspire	High user engagement	iCope	43	6.04	11.53	
5	iCope	Low user engagement	Aspire	53	7.77	7.77	14.51
6	iCope	Low user engagement	iCope	49	4.25	7.77	
7	iCope	High user engagement	Aspire	52	21.60	21.60	
8	iCope	High user engagement	iCope	45	11.73	21.60	

Suppose a patient only launches the app when it is downloaded but never uses it afterwards; the number of sessions launched will be 1 for the first week and 0s for the rest 3 weeks. Therefore, the number of sessions during the 4-week observed period will be 1 and then the loyalty index will be 0. In contrast, if a patient accesses the app once a day for five days per week across the 4-week period, the loyalty index will be 0.95. A high-engagement user, in this case, is defined as a patient with a loyalty index of at least 0.95. Let R_i denote the binary intermediate outcome for patient i measured at the end of stage 1, coded as 1 for high engagement users and 0 for low engagement users. Also, let Y_i be the eventual outcome of BDI reduction six months after the second randomization. As a result, the longitudinal trajectory of patient i is given by $\{A_{1i}, R_i, A_{2i}, Y_i\}$. The two stage-specific recommendations made by the Hub for patient i are A_{1i} with history $H_{1i} = \phi$ and A_{2i} with history $H_{2i} = \{A_{1i}, R_i\}$. We define the Q-functions as the stage-specific saturated linear regression models as

$$Q_2(h_{2i}, a_{2i}|\theta_2) = \beta_0 + \beta_1 a_{1i} + \beta_2 r_i + \beta_3 a_{2i} + \beta_4 a_{1i} r_i + \beta_5 a_{2i} r_i \\ + \beta_6 a_{1i} a_{2i} + \beta_7 a_{1i} r_i a_{2i}$$

for stage 2 with the linear parameters $\theta_2 = (\beta_0, \beta_1, \beta_2, \beta_3, \beta_4, \beta_5, \beta_6, \beta_7)$, and

$$Q_1(h_{1i}, a_{1i}|\theta_1) = Q_1(a_{1i}|\theta_1) = \gamma_0 + \gamma_1 a_{1i}$$

for stage 1 with the linear parameters $\theta_1 = (\gamma_0, \gamma_1)$.

Suppose we conducted a preliminary pilot study under the design of Figure 3.2 and collected data from all 400 patients with the complete intermediate outcomes (i.e., consistent or inconsistent use of the app initially downloaded in stage 1) and the final primary outcomes (i.e., six-month reduction of BDI after the second randomization). Table 3.1 summarize all possible sequences of (A_1, r, A_2) embedded in the SMART and the sample size corresponding to each sequence is as follows.

We define the Q function for stage 2 as the saturated linear regression model as

$$Q_2(a_{1i}, r_i, a_{2i}|\theta_2) = \beta_0 + \beta_1 a_{1i} + \beta_2 r_i + \beta_3 a_{2i} + \beta_4 a_{1i} r_i + \beta_5 a_{2i} r_i \\ + \beta_6 a_{1i} a_{2i} + \beta_7 a_{1i} r_i a_{2i},$$

where the linear parameters $\theta_2 = (\beta_0, \beta_1, \beta_2, \beta_3, \beta_4, \beta_5, \beta_6, \beta_7)$ can be estimated based on the observed data using the least squares method:

$$\widehat{\theta}_2 = \arg\min_{\theta_2} \sum_{i=1}^{n} \{Y_i - Q_2(a_{1i}, r_i, a_{2i}; \theta_2)\}^2.$$

Consequently, we obtained the estimated parameters as

$$\widehat{\theta}_2 = (0.86, 6.90, 10.66, 9.67, 3.17, -13.18, -15.15, 8.79).$$

For each observed sequence in Table 3.1, we can calculate the estimated value of Q_2 according to the corresponding values of (a_{1i}, r_i, a_{2i}) and $\widehat{\theta}_2$, as shown in Column 6 of Table 3.1. Similarly, we can define a linear Q function for stage 1. Assuming that the selection of stage-1 apps does not depend on baseline information, we have

$$Q_1(h_{1i}, a_{1i}|\theta_1) = Q_1(a_{1i}|\theta_1) = \gamma_0 + \gamma_1 a_{1i}$$

To estimate θ_1, we define for patient i a pseudo-outcome

$$\widehat{Y}_i = \max_{a_2 \in s_2} Q_2(a_{1i}, r_i, a_2; \widehat{\theta}_2), \tag{3.6}$$

as a proxy for the quantity under the expectation in the definition of $Q_1(h_1, a_1)$, and thus $\theta_1 = (\gamma_0, \gamma_1)$ can be estimated by using least squares based on the pseudo-outcomes:

$$\widehat{\theta}_1 = \arg\min_{\theta_1} \sum_{i=1}^{n} \{\widehat{Y}_i - Q_1(a_{1i}; \theta_1)\}^2.$$

Column 7 of Table 3.1 provides the pseudo-outcomes defined by (3.6) for estimating θ_1 given the history up to a_2. As result, we can obtain the estimated regression parameters for the stage-1 Q function as

$$\widehat{\theta}_1 = (11.00, 3.51).$$

Column 8 of Table 3.1 is the estimated Q_1 given $A_1 = 0$ (i.e., Aspire) and $A_1 = 1$ (i.e., iCope). Based on these results, we conclude that the optimal stage-1 decision is iCope. Meanwhile, the optimal stage-2 decision given that a patient downloads iCope but fails to use it consistently at stage 1 is Aspire. On the other hand, for a patient who consistently uses iCope at stage 1, the best decision for stage 2 is still Aspire. Thus, the estimated best DTR uses iCope for four weeks in stage 1 and then switches to Aspire in stage 2 regardless of the user engagement during stage 1. This DTR leads to an expected BDI reduction at six months of 14.51.

We provide the R codes that helped conduct the above calculations, including those to estimate the Q-functions and those to identify the optimal DTR based on the Q-learning method. The illustrated data was simulated based on the characteristics of smartphone apps usage data collected from IntelliCare apps in Google Play Store (Cheung et al., 2018). For details of the data generative model, see Section 3.3. The data and all the R program codes related to the results in this chapter are available for download from GitHub at `https://github.com/tonizhong/SMARTAR_sample_code`.

3.3 SMARTs with Adaptive Randomization (SMART-AR)

If the true optimal DTR d^* were known for the target population served by a treatment program, it would be natural to treat every patient with d^*. However, in most situations, we will need to learn about d^* using the data from patients in the program. Hence, some randomization of the treatment sequences is needed. In a classic non-adaptive SMART design, the ith patient who enrolled in the trial is assigned to a stage-t intervention a_t with randomization probability $\pi_t(a_t|h_{ti})$, where the function $\pi_t(a_t|h_t)$ is pre-specified such that $\sum_{a_t \in S_t} \pi_t(a_t|h_t) = 1$ for each given h_t. For example, by setting $\pi_t(a_t|h_t) = 1/J_t$ for all $a_t \in S_t$, we aim to apply balanced randomization, under which a patient has an equal opportunity of being assigned to any treatment option at a decision-making point given the history of h_t.

The idea of AR is to determine the function $\pi_t(a_t|h_t)$ using the data collected from the ongoing study. The AR criterion here is based on the fact that Q-learning aims to maximize $Q_t(h_t, a_t|\widehat{\theta}_t)$ for a given h_t. Precisely, let $n(i)$ denote the number of patients who have completed the trial with the final outcome evaluated just prior to the enrollment of patient i. It is likely that $n(i) < i - 1$ as patients are enrolled in a staggered fashion. For patient i, we randomly assign a treatment based on an initial set of probabilities $\{\pi_t^0(a|h_{ti})\}$ if $n(i) < N_{\min}$ for a pre-specified $N_{\min}$. The set π_t^0 may be chosen based on the data from previous studies and thus be viewed as historical randomization probabilities. Once there are at least $N_{\min}$ patients with complete data, that is $n(i) \geq N_{\min}$, we start updating the randomization probabilities using the data of the first $n(i)$ patients. Specifically, for patient i at stage t, define treatment a_t

$$\widehat{\rho}_t(a_t|h_{ti}) = \exp\left\{\frac{Q_t(h_{ti}, a_t|\widehat{\theta}_t)}{\widehat{\sigma}_t}\log b\right\} \tag{3.7}$$

for some pre-specific base $b \geq 1$, the least squares estimate $\widehat{\theta}_t$ in (3.7) evaluated using the data in the first $n(i)$ patients who have completed the trial, and $\widehat{\sigma}_t^2$ is the mean square error due to $\widehat{\theta}_t$, such that

$$\widehat{\sigma}_1^2 = \frac{\sum_{k=1}^{n(i)}\{Y_k - Q_1(H_{1k}, A_{1k}; \widehat{\theta}_1)\}^2}{n(i) - \dim(\widehat{\theta}_1)} \quad \text{and}$$
$$\widehat{\sigma}_2^2 = \frac{\sum_{k=1}^{n(i)}\{Y_k - Q_2(H_{2k}, A_{2k}; \widehat{\theta}_2)\}^2}{n(i) - \dim(\widehat{\theta}_2)},$$

where $\dim(\theta)$ denotes the dimension of the vector θ. The empirical randomization probability for treatment a is then calculated by normalizing $\widehat{\rho}_t$, that is,

$$\widehat{\pi}_t(a_t|h_{ti}) = \frac{\widehat{\rho}_t(a_t|h_{ti})}{\sum_{a_t \in S_t}\widehat{\rho}_t(a_t|h_{ti})} = \frac{\exp\{\widehat{\Delta}_{ti}(a_t)\log b\}}{\sum_{a_t \in S_t}\exp\{\widehat{\Delta}_{ti}(a_t)\log b\}}, \tag{3.8}$$

where $\widehat{\Delta}_{ti}(a_t) = \{Q_t(h_{ti}, a_t; \widehat{\theta}_t) - Q_t(h_{ti}, a_{ti}^w; \widehat{\theta}_t)\}/\widehat{\sigma}_t$ and $\widehat{a}_{ti}^w$ is the estimated worst action given h_{ti}. To allow input from historical data or perspective, we can use a weighted average of the historical and empirical randomization probabilities on the logarithm scale, defined as

$$\widetilde{\rho}_t(a|h_{ti}) = \exp\{\lambda_n^{b-1}\log\pi_t^0(a|h_{ti}) + (1 - \lambda_n^{b-1}) log\widehat{\pi}_t(a|h_{ti})\} \tag{3.9}$$

where λ_n typically takes a value from 0 to 1 and goes to zero as $n = n(i)$ grows. For example, Cheung et al. (2015) suggested considering $\lambda_n = \tau^{1/(b-1)}N_{\min}/n$ for $b > 1$ for $\tau \in [0, 1]$. The randomization probabilities to treatment a at stage t given h_{ti} are given by normalizing $\widetilde{\rho}_t(a|h_{ti})$:

$$\tilde{\pi}_t(a_t|h_{ti}) = \frac{\widetilde{\rho}_t(a_t|h_{ti})}{\sum_{a_t \in S_t}\widetilde{\rho}_t(a_t|h_{ti})}. \tag{3.10}$$

Thus, under (3.9), the historical randomization probability π_t^0 influences the randomization probabilities even after AR is in effect, although its contribution gradually decreases and eventually goes to zero as n increases when $b > 1$. Algorithm 3.2 provides a general guide to calculate the adaptive randomization probabilities in SMART-AR.

Figure 3.3 shows the trend of stage-1 and stage-2 randomization probabilities in a simulated SMART-AR trial for identifying the optimal DTR for smartphone apps in depression management. The historical SMART data was simulated based on a balanced randomization scheme. Specifically, the randomization probabilities were set to be $P(A_1 = 1) = 0.5$ at stage 1 and $P(A_2 = 1|H_2 = h_2) = 0.5$ given any possible treatment history and intermediate response at stage 2. The intermediate response rate was set as $P(R = 1|A_1 = 0) = 0.45$

Algorithm 3.2: Standard approach to calculate the adaptive randomization probabilities for SMART

Specify three design parameters $N_{\min}$, b, and τ.
Calculate the initial randomization probabilities $\pi_t^0(a|h_{ti})$ for the first $N_{\min}$ patients.
Start from patient i, where $i = N_{\min} + 1$, calculate $\widehat{\rho}_t(a|h_{ti})$ by (3.7).
Calculate the empirical randomization probabilities $\widehat{\pi}_t(a_t|h_{ti})$ by (3.8).
Combine the information of initial and empirical randomization probabilities as $\widetilde{\rho}_t(a|h_{ti})$ by (3.9).
Update the final adaptive randomization probabilities $\widetilde{\rho}_t(a_t|h_{ti})$ by (3.10).

and $P(R = 1|A_1 = 1) = 0.50$. Given the ith patient's treatment history and intermediate response, (A_{1i}, R_i, A_{2i}), the primary outcome Y_i, was randomly generated from a normal distribution with mean

$$E(Y|A_1, R, A_2) = (1.32, 10.50, 10.88, 5.20, 7.80, 5.16, 22.00, 10.88)$$

and variance $\sigma^2 = 25$ for $A_1 \in (0,1), R \in (0,1)$ and $A_2 \in (0,1)$. Under the illustrative SMART-AR design, we used historical SMART data to generate the initial stage-1 randomization probabilities for the first 100 patients who enrolled in the trial ($N_{\min} = 100$) given a total sample size of 400. Meanwhile, the initial randomization probabilities of stage-2 randomization were set to 0.5. Starting from the 101st patient, we updated the randomization probabilities for patient i based on the results of all the previous patients who enrolled in the trial, assuming $n(i) = i - 1$. Figure 3.3(A) shows that the stage-1 randomization

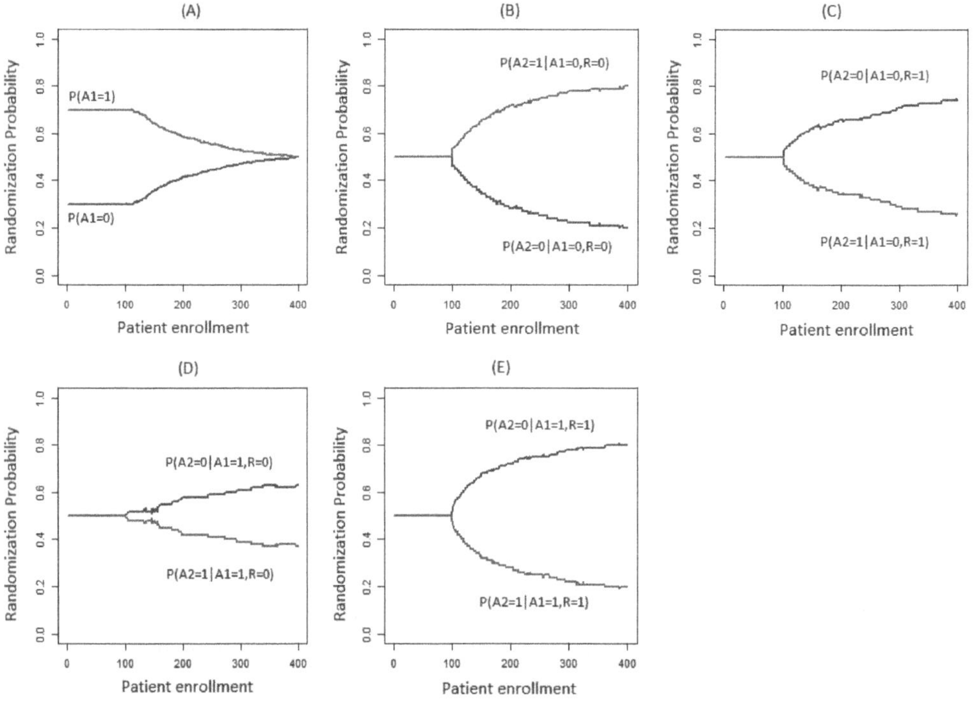

Figure 3.3 *Change of stage-1 and -2 randomization probabilities in a simulated trial ($N = 400$) for comparing 8 DTRs of smartphone apps for depression management ($N_{\min} = 100, b = 10, \tau = 0.9$).*

probabilities for the first 100 patients are $\pi_1^0(a_1 = 0) = 0.3$ and $\pi_1^0(a_1 = 1) = 0.7$, respectively. As the number of patients enrolled and evaluated increased, the stage-1 randomization probability corresponding to Aspire gradually increased to $\pi_1^0(a_1 = 0) = 0.5$ for the last patient (i.e., i=400). Figures 3.3(B) to 3.3(D) are stage-2 randomization probabilities given different histories of stage-1 treatments and intermediate responses.

3.4 Design Parameters

In addition to $\{\pi_t^0\}$, a SMART-AR design requires specifying three parameters: b, $N_{\min}$, and $\{\lambda_n\}$. The base b indicates how "greedy" the AR scheme is. When $b = 1$, the trial reduces to a non-adaptive SMART design with fixed randomization probabilities π_t^0 for allocation. When $b > 1$, the allocation tends to favor the options with larger $Q_t(h_{ti}, a_t|\widehat{\theta}_t)$. As the value of b increases, the weight related to empirical randomization probability $\widehat{\pi}_t$ increases, and thus the ongoing trial information has more impact on the allocation for those patients later enrolled in the trial. Cheung et al. (2015) recommend set the value of b from 2 to 100 to span a reasonably wide range of "greediness" for a moderate effect size $\widehat{\Delta}_{ti}(a)$, defined as

$$\widehat{\Delta}_{ti}(a) = \{Q_t(h_{ti}, a_t|\widehat{\theta}_t) - Q_t(h_{ti}, \widehat{a}_t^w|\widehat{\theta}_t)\},$$

where $\widehat{a}_t^w$ is the estimated worst action given a history of h_{ti}. Typically, the randomization probabilities move quicker as the value of b increases.

The minimum sample size $N_{\min}$ indicates how early AR comes into effect. The choice of $N_{\min}$ depends on the dimension of Q-function $\dim(\theta_t)$ so that the Q-functions can be reliably estimated. Based on the experience with linear regression models, Cheung et al. (2015)) suggests setting $N_{\min} \geq 3 \times \max_t\{\dim(\theta_t)\}$.

While there are many possible choices of λ_n for (3.9), it is common to take the value of

$$\lambda_n = \tau^{1/(b-1)} \frac{N_{\min}}{n},$$

where $\tau \in [0, 1]$ and $n = n(i)$. The value of parameter τ attenuates the greediness of AR via the weight given to initial randomization probability π_t^0, which equals τ when AR first comes into effect. Generally, a larger value of τ leads to more attenuation, whereas $\tau = 0$ implies no attenuation so that the SMART-AR uses the empirical randomization probabilities for allocation, that is, $\widetilde{\pi}_t = \widehat{\pi}_t$. Together with b and $N_{\min}$, the attenuation τ allows a wide range of specifications of a SMART-AR design. Cheung et al. (2015) discussed the design calibration of SMART-AR based on the general calibration approach proposed by Lee and Cheung (2009). Overall, the average patient outcome in SMART-AR increases with a large b, small $N_{\min}$, and small τ, and the optimal SMART-AR design should account for both the efficiency of identifying the best DTR and the quality improvement of patient care. Readers who are interested in it can see more details in Cheung et al. (2015). In practice, we suggest that designers use a similar approach to determine the SMART-AR design parameters $(b, N_{\min}, \tau)$ that show satisfactory operating characteristics in simulation studies.

3.5 Discussion

In this chapter, we have introduced a synthesis of Q-learning and adaptive randomization for designing a SMART-AR. In the example trial, we defined the binary intermediate outcome based on the user engagement data. Specifically, the intermediate response was defined as a loyalty index $\geq$ 95% across the 4-week period. One could also classify a response into three (or more) categories, for example, the inactive user (loyalty index < 50%), the medium active user (loyalty index 50%–95%), and the active user (loyalty index $\geq$ 95%), depending on the interest of the study. Such design enrichment needs to be coupled with a larger model for the Q-function. Generally, with C response categories in a two-stage DTR, $\dim(\theta_2)$ is of the order $J_1 \times C \times J_2$: the actual number of parameters depends on how many interaction terms are postulated, while it is important to include interactions in the search for optimal DTR. Therefore, when a program starts and data are limited, it is necessary to consider "simple" designs with fewer interactions. As the enrollment grows, one can enrich the design to account for more information by incorporating interaction effects with patient covariates, e.g., refining and increasing treatment options such as different types of smartphone apps, redefining the intermediate response categories, and adopting more than two stages of treatments. The proposed AR scheme accommodates such enrichment to the extent that Q-learning is feasible given the sample size. The use of AR improves the performance and robustness of Q-learning by allocating patients away from treatment sequences that are not promising. In the context of DTRs, due to the curse of dimensionality, the advantage offered by AR is potentially enormous.

Since the weighted average (3.9) combines the historical and the empirical inputs on the probability scale, it can be easily applied with other empirical randomization schemes. For example, the empirical component (3.8) may be replaced with an ε-optimal criterion as in Lee et al. (2015), who adopt a Bayesian approach and estimate the Q-function using full likelihood. The method introduced in this chapter, while less formal than a fully Bayesian approach, offers flexibility. It can be easily extended to deal with a broader set of problems, such as when the outcome is binary (e.g., Moodie et al. (2014)). However, to use either approach, it is critical to properly calibrate the design parameters $(b, N_{\min}, \tau)$ in this method, and an ε-sequence and the prior distribution for the Bayesian model in Lee et al. (2015).

As in any sequential method, the advantages of AR diminish with fast patient accrual. Specifically, a SMART-AR converges to a non-adaptive SMART, as more patients are enrolled before adaptation begins. The non-adaptive SMART can thus be used to provide a lower bound of performance for SMART-AR. This fact underlines the crucial role of historical input π_t^0. This point should be read in light of the nature of implementation research, in which the SMART-AR is used as a dissemination tool to deploy existing treatments to a community. Thus, a historical perspective is often available and useful, and may prove more beneficial than applying balanced randomization initially.

Chapter 4

Bayesian Dose-Finding in Two Treatment Cycles based on Efficacy and Toxicity

Peter F. Thall, Juhee Lee

4.1 Introduction

Practicing physicians routinely use DTRs to make multi-cycle decisions for their patients. Most clinical trial designs ignore the actual DTRs being used, and instead only evaluate the treatments given initially, as if each patient's clinical outcomes were due to the first treatment alone. A common example in oncology arises when salvage therapy is given after disease progression following an initial front-line treatment. While the two-stage DTR is (front-line, salvage), with the possible outcomes in each stage determined by the times to progression, death, or administrative censoring, most designs and data analyses evaluate the front-line treatments and ignore salvage therapy. A flawed rationale for this dysfunctional convention is that effects of different salvage therapies on patients' times from progression to death will somehow "average out." A detailed description of this pervasive practice, and its consequences, is given in Chapter 12 of Thall (2020). This problem also is very common in early-phase dose-finding trial designs, nearly all of which are myopic in that they focus on the dose or dose combination given initially while ignoring treatments and doses given in cycles of therapy after the first. Consequently, the nominally "optimal" dose chosen by such a design actually pertains only to the first cycle of therapy. The design described in this chapter was motivated by the desire to provide an alternative to this convention.

There is an extensive literature on adaptive dose-finding designs for phase I clinical trials, which are based on toxicity, and phase I-II clinical trials, which are based on both efficacy and toxicity. Reviews have been given by Chevret (2006); Zohar and Chevret (2007); Yin (2012); Yan et al. (2018); and Gauthier et al. (2019), among many others. Detailed discussions of phase I-II designs are given in the book by Yuan et al. (2016).

The first early phase design accounting for the administration schedule was given by Braun et al. (2005). They proposed a phase I design to optimize the administration schedule, with a fixed per-administration dose, using between-patient adaptive rules based on time-to-toxicity. Braun et al. (2007) extended this by allowing both schedule and per-administration dose to vary, and jointly optimizing the (dose, schedule) regime using a criterion similar to that of the time-to-event continual reassessment method (Cheung and Chappell, 2000). Li et al. (2008) proposed a phase I-II design to optimize (dose, schedule) for two nested schedules and bivariate binary outcomes. Zhang and Braun (2013) proposed a design to optimize (dose, schedule) while accounting for multiple within-patient administrations.

This chapter reviews a Bayesian phase I-II dose-finding design proposed by Lee et al. (2015) that treats the actions taken in a two-cycle therapeutic regime as a DTR. Possible actions are to choose a dose, or not treat the patient due to the absence of any acceptable dose. For a given experimental agent, the design adaptively optimizes the action taken for each patient in each of two treatment cycles using an objective function computed from elicited joint utilities of binary (efficacy, toxicity) outcomes in each cycle. The design is called DTM2, an acronym for "decision theoretic two-cycle method." While a more general

DOI: 10.1201/9781003216223-4

version of DTM2 that accommodates two ordinal outcomes is given by Lee et al. (2016), this chapter will review the binary outcome case in order to focus on the main ideas and the dose-outcome model's structure.

DTM2 relies on a Bayesian hierarchical multivariate probit regression model that includes Gaussian latent outcome variables used to define the observed binary outcomes and random patient effects on the latent outcome variables that induce association. An objective function is defined using elicited numerical utilities that quantify risk-benefit trade-offs of the possible (efficacy, toxicity) pairs; this objective function is structurally similar to that used in Q-learning (Watkins, 1989; Murphy, 2003; Zhao et al., 2011) and related methods in reinforcement learning (Sutton and Barto, 2018). The DTM2 design chooses an optimal action in each cycle by maximizing the posterior expected mean of the objective function. This is done by applying a recursive Bellman equation (Bellman, 1957) and assuming when making the decision in cycle 1, that the optimal action will be taken in cycle 2. At the end of the trial, the method provides an optimal two-stage DTR consisting of two actions, $\mathbf{a} = (a_1, a_2)$. Either a_1 says to not treat any patient because no dose is acceptable, or a_1 = a cycle 1 dose, and a_2 = a function of the patient's cycle 1 dose and (efficacy, toxicity) outcomes that either chooses a cycle 2 dose or says to not treat the patient in cycle 2. Because all decisions are based on posterior quantities computed using all patients' data, the method is adaptive both within and between patients. This is very different from simply choosing two nominally "optimal" doses, one for each cycle, where the "optimal" cycle 2 dose is chosen for all patients while ignoring each patient's observed cycle 1 data.

4.2 Dose-Outcome Model

The Bayesian model used by DTM2 is an extension of the multivariate probit model (Ashford and Sowden, 1970; Chib and Greenberg, 1998). A vector of unobserved, correlated latent multivariate normal variables is used to define each observed toxicity and efficacy variable as the indicator that its corresponding latent variable is greater than 0. Correlation between the latent normal variables thus induces association between the observed binary variables. The DTM2 model extends a standard multivariate probit model by including a Bayesian hierarchical structure and accounting for two cycles. Posteriors are computed by applying Markov chain Monte Carlo (MCMC) methods (see, for example, Robert and Casella, 2004) for latent variable models, with posterior computation done via Gibbs sampling (Albert and Chib, 1993; Chib and Greenberg, 1998).

Let N be a pre-specified maximum sample size and $n \leq N$ the number of patients accrued and given at least one cycle of treatment up to a trial time when an adaptive decision must be made. Index patients by $i = 1, \ldots, n$. The dose-outcome model does not depend on numerical dose values, and m increasing doses are identified by the integers $\{1, \ldots, m\}$. For treatment cycle c =1 or 2, denote the ith patient's dose by $d_{i,c}$, outcome indicators $Y_{i,c} \in \{0,1\}$ for toxicity and $Z_{i,c} \in \{0,1\}$ for efficacy, and the 2-cycle vectors $\mathbf{d}_i = (d_{i,1}, d_{i,2})$, $\mathbf{Y}_i = (Y_{i,1}, Y_{i,2})$, and $\mathbf{Z}_i = (Z_{i,1}, Z_{i,2})$. Denote the current observed data from all patients by $\mathcal{D} = \{(\mathbf{Y}_i, \mathbf{Z}_i, \mathbf{d}_i) : i = 1, \ldots, n\}$.

A tractable joint distribution for $[\mathbf{Y}_i, \mathbf{Z}_i \mid \mathbf{d}_i]$ is constructed by defining the binary outcomes in terms of four real-valued latent outcome variables, $\boldsymbol{\xi}_i = (\xi_{i,1}, \xi_{i,2})$ for $\mathbf{Y}_i$ and $\boldsymbol{\eta}_i = (\eta_{i,1}, \eta_{i,2})$ for $\mathbf{Z}_i$, with $(\boldsymbol{\xi}_i, \boldsymbol{\eta}_i)$ assumed to follow a four-dimensional normal distribution having random means that vary with $\mathbf{d}_i$. Denoting the indicator function of event A by $\mathrm{I}(A)$, the observed outcomes are defined as $Y_{i,c} = \mathrm{I}(\xi_{i,c} > 0)$ and $Z_{i,c} = \mathrm{I}(\eta_{i,c} > 0)$, so the distribution of $[\mathbf{Y}_i, \mathbf{Z}_i \mid \mathbf{d}_i]$ is induced by that of $[\boldsymbol{\xi}_i, \boldsymbol{\eta}_i \mid \mathbf{d}_i]$. The dose-outcome structure of the following Bayesian hierarchical model for two cycles is similar to the non-hierarchical model for multiple toxicities in one cycle of therapy used by Bekele and Thall (2004). The DTM2 model is based on a conditional likelihood for the cycle-specific latent variable pairs $[\xi_{i,c}, \eta_{i,c} \mid d_{i,c}]$, for $c = 1, 2$, using patient-specific random effects (u_i, v_i) that account for association of the two outcomes between and within cycles for the ith patient. Denote the univariate normal distribution with mean μ and variance σ^2 by $N(\mu, \sigma^2)$, with pdf $\phi(\cdot \mid \mu, \sigma^2)$, and the k-variate normal distribution with mean vector $\boldsymbol{\mu}$ and variance-covariance matrix Σ by $\text{MVN}_k(\boldsymbol{\mu}, \Sigma)$.

The Bayesian model includes the following Level 1 and Level 2 priors:

Level 1 Priors on the Latent Variables. For patient i given dose $d_{i,c} = d$ in cycle c,

$$\begin{aligned} \xi_{i,c} \mid u_i, \bar{\xi}_{c,d}, \sigma_\xi^2 &\sim \text{N}(\bar{\xi}_{c,d} + u_i, \sigma_\xi^2) \quad \text{and} \\ \eta_{i,c} \mid v_i, \bar{\eta}_{c,d}, \sigma_\eta^2 &\sim \text{N}(\bar{\eta}_{c,d} + v_i, \sigma_\eta^2), \end{aligned} \tag{4.1}$$

assuming that $\boldsymbol{\xi}_i$ and $\boldsymbol{\eta}_i$ are conditionally independent given (u_i, v_i). The variances, σ_ξ^2 and σ_η^2 are fixed hyperparameters, but the patient effects, (u_i, v_i), and the mean cycle-specific dose effects, $(\bar{\xi}_{c,d}, \bar{\eta}_{c,d})$, are random. The patient effects are assumed to follow the following Level 2 priors:

Level 2 Priors on the Random Patient Effects. For patient i,

$$u_i, v_i \mid \rho, \tau^2 \overset{iid}{\sim} \text{MVN}_2(\mathbf{0}_2, \Sigma_{u,v}), \quad i = 1, \cdots, n, \tag{4.2}$$

where $\mathbf{0}_2 = (0, 0)$ and $\Sigma_{u,v}$ is the 2×2 matrix with diagonal elements τ^2 and off-diagonal elements $\rho\tau^2$. The hyperparameters, $\rho \in (-1, 1)$ and τ^2 are fixed. This Level 2 prior induces association, parameterized by (ρ, τ^2), among $(\xi_{i,1}, \eta_{i,1}, \xi_{i,2}, \eta_{i,2})$ via the latent variable model (4.1) and thus, in turn, induces association among the observed toxicity and efficacy outcomes in two cycles, $(Y_{i,1}, Z_{i,1}, Y_{i,2}, Z_{i,2})$.

Denote the mean vectors $\bar{\boldsymbol{\xi}}_c = (\bar{\xi}_{c,1}, \ldots, \bar{\xi}_{c,m})$ and $\bar{\boldsymbol{\eta}}_c = (\bar{\eta}_{c,1}, \ldots, \bar{\eta}_{c,m})$. For each dose d, the following level 2 priors are assumed:

Level 2 Priors on the Means of the Gaussian Latent Variables. Let $\bar{\xi}_{c,1} \overset{indep}{\sim} \text{N}(\xi_{c,0}, \sigma^2_{\xi_{c,0}})$ and $\bar{\eta}_{c,1} \overset{indep}{\sim} \text{N}(\eta_{c,0}, \sigma^2_{\eta_{c,0}})$. For $d = 2, \ldots, m$,

$$\begin{aligned} p(\bar{\xi}_{c,d} \mid \bar{\xi}_{c,1}, \ldots, \bar{\xi}_{c,d-1}) &\propto \phi(\bar{\xi}_{c,d} \mid \xi_{c,0}, \sigma^2_{\xi_{c,0}}) 1(\bar{\xi}_{c,d-1} < \bar{\xi}_{c,d}) \\ p(\bar{\eta}_{c,d} \mid \bar{\eta}_{c,1} \ldots, \bar{\eta}_{c,d-1}) &\propto \phi(\bar{\eta}_{c,d} \mid \eta_{c,0}, \sigma^2_{\eta_{c,0}}) 1(\bar{\eta}_{c,d-1} < \bar{\eta}_{c,d}). \end{aligned} \tag{4.3}$$

These priors induce association among the elements of the Level 1 prior means $\bar{\boldsymbol{\xi}}_{c,d}$ and $\bar{\boldsymbol{\eta}}_{c,d}$. The order constraints imposed on the mean dose effects in (4.3) ensure that $\xi_{i,c}$ and $\eta_{i,c}$ each increase stochastically in dose, hence that the probabilities of toxicity and efficacy both increase with dose in each cycle. In clinical settings where this assumption is not appropriate, such as trials of biological agents where either efficacy or toxicity may not be monotone increasing in dose (see Lee et al. (2019)), one or both of the above constraints may be dropped.

Collecting terms from (4.1), (4.2), and (4.3), the 12 fixed parameters that determine all Level 1 and Level 2 priors are $\tilde{\boldsymbol{\theta}} = (\boldsymbol{\xi}_0, \boldsymbol{\eta}_0, \boldsymbol{\sigma}^2_{\xi_0}, \boldsymbol{\sigma}^2_{\eta_0}, \sigma^2_\xi, \sigma^2_\eta, \tau^2, \rho)$, where $\boldsymbol{\xi}_0 = (\xi_{1,0}, \xi_{2,0})$, $\boldsymbol{\eta}_0 = (\eta_{1,0}, \eta_{2,0})$, $\boldsymbol{\sigma}^2_{\xi_0} = (\sigma^2_{\xi_{1,0}}, \sigma^2_{\xi_{2,0}})$, and $\boldsymbol{\sigma}^2_{\eta_0} = (\sigma^2_{\eta_{1,0}}, \sigma^2_{\eta_{2,0}})$. Denoting $\bar{\boldsymbol{\xi}} = (\bar{\boldsymbol{\xi}}_1, \bar{\boldsymbol{\xi}}_2)$, $\bar{\boldsymbol{\eta}} = (\bar{\boldsymbol{\eta}}_1, \bar{\boldsymbol{\eta}}_2)$, $\boldsymbol{\mu}_{\mathbf{d}_i} = (\bar{\xi}_{1,d_{i,1}}, \bar{\xi}_{2,d_{i,2}}, \bar{\eta}_{1,d_{i,1}}, \bar{\eta}_{2,d_{i,2}})$, and the covariance matrix

$$\Sigma_{\xi,\eta} = \begin{bmatrix} \sigma_\xi^2 + \tau^2 & \tau^2 & \rho\tau^2 & \rho\tau^2 \\ & \sigma_\xi^2 + \tau^2 & \rho\tau^2 & \rho\tau^2 \\ & & \sigma_\eta^2 + \tau^2 & \tau^2 \\ & & & \sigma_\eta^2 + \tau^2 \end{bmatrix},$$

and integrating over (u_i, v_i), the joint distribution of the four Gaussian latent variables is

$$\boldsymbol{\xi}_i, \boldsymbol{\eta}_i \mid \mathbf{d}_i, \bar{\boldsymbol{\xi}}, \bar{\boldsymbol{\eta}}, \tilde{\boldsymbol{\theta}} \overset{iid}{\sim} \text{MVN}_4(\boldsymbol{\mu}_{\mathbf{d}_i}, \Sigma_{\xi,\eta}), \quad i = 1, \cdots, n. \tag{4.4}$$

The mean vector $\boldsymbol{\mu}_{\mathbf{d}}$ is a function of the dose levels and, as noted earlier, does not depend on numerical dose values. The hyperparameters τ^2 and ρ quantify associations between cycle 1 and cycle 2 and between efficacy outcomes and toxicity outcomes. If $-1 < \rho < 0$, then efficacy and toxicity are negatively associated, so higher toxicity is associated with lower efficacy. If $0 < \rho < 1$, then efficacy and toxicity are positively associated, so lower toxicity is associated with lower efficacy.

Denote $\boldsymbol{\theta} = (\bar{\boldsymbol{\xi}}, \bar{\boldsymbol{\eta}})$, and temporarily suppress $\tilde{\boldsymbol{\theta}}$ and the patient index i. Integrating over the latent patent effects (u, v) and the latent outcome variables $(\boldsymbol{\xi}, \boldsymbol{\eta})$ gives the joint likelihood for the four observable outcomes $(\mathbf{y}, \mathbf{z})$ of a given patient,

$$\begin{aligned} p(\mathbf{y}, \mathbf{z} \mid \mathbf{d}, \boldsymbol{\theta}) &= \Pr(Y_1 = y_1, Y_2 = y_2, Z_1 = z_1, Z_2 = z_2 \mid \mathbf{d}, \boldsymbol{\theta}) \\ &= \Pr(\gamma_{1,y_1} \leq \xi_1 < \gamma_{1,y_1+1}, \gamma_{1,y_2} \leq \xi_2 < \gamma_{1,y_2+1}, \\ &\qquad \gamma_{2,z_1} \leq \eta_1 < \gamma_{2,z_1+1}, \gamma_{2,y_2} \leq \eta_2 < \gamma_{2,z_2+1} | \mathbf{d}, \boldsymbol{\theta}) \\ &= \int_{\gamma_{1,y_1}}^{\gamma_{1,y_1+1}} \int_{\gamma_{1,y_2}}^{\gamma_{1,y_2+1}} \int_{\gamma_{2,z_1}}^{\gamma_{2,z_1+1}} \int_{\gamma_{2,z_2}}^{\gamma_{2,z_2+1}} \phi(\boldsymbol{\xi}, \boldsymbol{\eta} | \boldsymbol{\mu}_{\mathbf{d}}, \Sigma_{\xi,\eta}) \\ &\qquad d\eta_2 d\eta_1 d\xi_2 d\xi_1, \end{aligned}$$

where the cutoff vectors $(\gamma_{10}, \gamma_{11}, \gamma_{12})$ for Y_c and $(\gamma_{20}, \gamma_{21}, \gamma_{22})$ for Z_c both equal $(-\infty, 0, \infty)$, for $c = 1, 2$. The conditional distribution of the observed cycle 2 outcomes (Y_2, Z_2) given the observed cycle 1 outcomes $(Y_1 = y_1, Z_1 = z_1)$ is

$$\begin{aligned} p(y_2, z_2 \mid y_1, z_1, \mathbf{d}, \boldsymbol{\theta}) &= \Pr(Y_2 = y_2, Z_2 = z_2 \mid Y_1 = y_1, Z_1 = z_1, \mathbf{d}) \\ &= \Pr(\gamma_{1y_2} \leq \xi_2 < \gamma_{1,y_2+1}, \gamma_{2z_2} \leq \eta_2 < \gamma_{2,z_2+1} \\ &\qquad \mid \gamma_{1y_1} \leq \xi_1 < \gamma_{1,y_1+1}, \gamma_{2,z_1} \leq \eta_{i1} < \gamma_{2,z_1+1}, \mathbf{d}) \\ &= \frac{p(\mathbf{y}, \mathbf{z} \mid \mathbf{d}, \boldsymbol{\theta})}{p(y_1, z_1 \mid d_1, \boldsymbol{\theta})}. \end{aligned} \tag{4.5}$$

The bivariate marginal for the cycle 1 outcomes is

$$p(y_1, z_1 \mid d_1, \boldsymbol{\theta}) = \int_{\gamma_{1y_1}}^{\gamma_{1,y_1+1}} \int_{\gamma_{2z_1}}^{\gamma_{2,z_1+1}} \phi([\xi_1, \eta_1] | \boldsymbol{\mu}_{d_1}^1, \Sigma_{\xi,\eta}^1) d\eta_1 d\xi_1 \tag{4.6}$$

where

$$\boldsymbol{\mu}_{d_1}^1 = \begin{bmatrix} \bar{\xi}_{1,d_1} \\ \bar{\eta}_{1,d_1} \end{bmatrix} \text{ and } \Sigma_{\xi,\eta}^1 = \begin{bmatrix} \sigma_\xi^2 + \tau^2 & \rho\tau^2 \\ \rho\tau^2 & \sigma_\eta^2 + \tau^2 \end{bmatrix}.$$

4.3 Decision Criteria

To define the design's decision rules, it is important to distinguish between choosing doses and taking action. The possible actions must allow a given patient's therapy to be terminated early, e.g. if the patient has unacceptable toxicity in cycle 1 (cf. Wang et al. (2012)). To accommodate this, the possible actions in cycle c may be either a dose in $\{1, \cdots, m\}$, or the decision to give no treatment, indexed by 0. The possible actions in each cycle thus are $\mathcal{A} = \{0, 1, \cdots, m\}$. The cycle 1 action, $a_1 \in \mathcal{A}$, allows the optimal action to be $a_1 = 0$ (do not treat) for any patient at any point in the trial, and if this occurs then the trial is terminated with the conclusion no dose is acceptable in cycle 1. Otherwise, if a_1 is a dose

d_1, the patient receives $a_2 \in \mathcal{A}$ for cycle 2, which is a function of the patient's cycle 1 dose and outcomes, (d_1, Y_1, Z_1), and the current data $\mathcal{D}$ from all patients.

As an example, suppose that the cycle 1 dose $a_1 = d_1$ produces toxicity, $Y_1 = 1$. Then, provided that $d_1 > 1$, the possible cycle 2 actions might vary with Z_1, as follows:

- $a_2(d_1, 1, 1, \mathcal{D}) = d_1 - 1$. This says that if there was toxicity, $Y_1 = 1$, and a response, $Z_1 = 1$, at d_1, then give a dose one level lower than d_1 in cycle 2.

- $a_2(d_1, 1, 0, \mathcal{D}) = 0$. This says that if there was toxicity, $Y_1 = 1$, and a no response, $Z_1 = 0$, at d_1, then do not treat the patient in cycle 2.

If $a_1 = d_1 = 1$, the lowest dose level, and $Y_1 = 1$ is observed then, depending on the numerical utilities and possibly additional safety rules, it may be that $d_2(d_1, 1, Z_1, \mathcal{D}) = 0$ regardless of whether $Z_1 = 0$ or 1. If, instead, a two-cycle regime (a_1, a_2) ignores the patient's cycle 1 dose and outcomes, $(a_1 = d_1, Y_1, Z_1)$, it is unlikely to be optimal, and it may be considered unethical. In the 2-cycle DTR, (d_1, Y_1, Z_1) are tailoring variables used by a_2, and optimizing $\boldsymbol{a} = (a_1, a_2)$ in terms of a well-defined objective function is the scientific goal of the design.

4.3.1 Objective Function

The objective function is constructed from a numerical utility function, $U(y, z)$, that quantifies the desirability of each outcome $(Y_c, Z_c) = (y, z)$ in each cycle $c = 1$ or 2. In practice, it is convenient to first fix $U(0,1) = 100$ and $U(1,0) = 0$, since these are the respective utilities of the best and worst possible outcomes, and then elicit the intermediate values $U(0,0)$ and $U(1,1)$ from the physicians planning the trial. The domain [0, 100] facilitates elicitation, but any finite interval will work. A necessary admissibility requirement is that $U(1,0) < U(1,1), U(0,0) < U(0,1)$. These inequalities say that (no toxicity and response) must be more desirable than (toxicity and response), and that (no toxicity and no response) must be more desirable than (toxicity and no response). Otherwise, U would not make sense. In the simulations given below, the design is based on the numerical utilities $U(1,0) = 0$, $U(0,0) = 35$, $U(1,1) = 65$, $U(0,1) = 100$. Since the design is based on one utility, in practice, if two or more physicians disagree about $U(0,0)$ and $U(1,1)$, this may be resolved by simulating the design under their respective utilities, showing them the results, and asking that they reach a consensus.

In the language of Q-learning, for each cycle $c = 1, 2$, a_c is the "action", $U(Y_c, Z_c)$ is the "reward", and $(a_1, Y_1, Z_1) = (d_1, Y_1, Z_1)$ is the "state" prior to taking action a_2 in cycle 2. More generally, a vector $\boldsymbol{X}$ including baseline covariates such as age, disease severity, or biomarker values for a targeted agent might be used to characterize the patient's initial state. In this more general setting, $\boldsymbol{X}$ would be the tailoring variables for a_1 and $(\boldsymbol{X}, d_1, Y_1, Z_1)$ would be the tailoring variables for a_2. Since the final optimal actions (a_1, a_2) then would be a function of $\boldsymbol{X}$, the rules would be called "personalized medicine". While this generalization is attractive, in practice, even in the single-cycle setting choosing covariate-specific doses can be quite complicated (cf. Thall et al. (2008); Chapple and Thall (2018); Lin et al. (2021). Two important practical considerations are that it would be necessary to quickly evaluate any biomarkers in $\boldsymbol{X}$, to avoid delaying any patient's therapy in order to apply an adaptive rule, and that the cost of evaluating the biomarkers cannot be prohibitively expensive.

The objective function for a two-cycle regime uses the idea of Bellman (1957), by starting in cycle 2 and working backwards. Recall that a cycle 2 action is taken only if a_1 is a dose $d_1 \in \{1, \cdots, d_m\}$, since if $a_1 = 0$ then the trial has ended. Given a patient's cycle 1 data

$(a_1 = d_1, Y_1, Z_1)$, the mean utility of action a_2 in cycle 2 is

$$Q_2(a_2, a_1, Y_1, Z_1, \boldsymbol{\theta}) = E\{U(Y_2, Z_2) \mid a_2, a_1, Y_1, Z_1, \boldsymbol{\theta}\} \\ = \sum_{y_2=0}^{1} \sum_{z_2=0}^{1} U(y_2, z_2) p(y_2, z_2 \mid a_2, a_1, Y_1, Z_1, \boldsymbol{\theta}). \quad (4.7)$$

The cycle 2 objective function is then defined as the posterior mean,

$$q_2(a_2, a_1, Y_1, Z_1, \mathcal{D}) = E\{Q_2(a_2, a_1, Y_1, Z_1, \boldsymbol{\theta}) \mid a_2, a_1, Y_1, Z_1, \mathcal{D}\}. \quad (4.8)$$

When $a_2 = 0$, that is, the patient is not treated in cycle 2,

$$p(Y_2 = 0, Z_2 = 0 \mid a_2 = 0, a_1, Y_1, Z_1, \boldsymbol{\theta}) = 1$$

and $q_2(a_2 = 0, a_1, Y_1, Z_1, \mathcal{D}) = U(0,0)$, which is the utility of having neither toxicity nor efficacy. If $a_2 \neq 0$, so that a dose is given in cycle 2, then $q_2(a_2, a_1, Y_1, Z_1, \mathcal{D})$ is the posterior mean utility of giving dose $a_2 = d_2$ in cycle 2 given the cycle 1 data $(a_1 = d_1, Y_1, Z_1)$. This shows the importance of the admissibility requirement $U(0,0) > U(1,0)$, that it must be more desirable to have [no toxicity and no efficacy] than to have [toxicity and no efficacy]. Given $(a_1 = d_1, Y_1, Z_1)$ and current data $\mathcal{D}$, the optimal cycle 2 action is

$$a_2^{opt}(a_1 = d_1, Y_1, Z_1, \mathcal{D}) = \underset{a_2}{\text{argmax}}\ q_2(a_2, a_1, Y_1, Z_1, \mathcal{D}),$$

subject to additional dose acceptability rules that will be presented below.

The decision algorithm next moves backwards to the cycle 1 optimization. Following Bellman (1957), it is assumed that, for any current data $\mathcal{D}$, the optimal action will be taken in cycle 2, and the payoff $q_2(a_2^{opt}, a_1 = d_1, Y_1, Z_1, \mathcal{D})$ for the optimal cycle 2 action is known for all possible cycle 1 histories (d_1, Y_1, Z_1). The expected utility of giving dose d_1 in cycle 1 given $\boldsymbol{\theta}$ is

$$Q_1(d_1, \boldsymbol{\theta}) = E\{U(Y_1, Z_1) \mid d_1, \boldsymbol{\theta}\} = \sum_{y_1=0}^{1} \sum_{z_1=0}^{1} U(y_1, z_1) p(y_1, z_1 | d_1, \boldsymbol{\theta}).$$

To define an overall objective function over both cycles, as usually done in Q-learning the cycle 2 payoff is discounted by using a fixed parameter, $0 < \lambda < 1$. The expected total payoff of giving dose d_1 in cycle 1, assuming that the optimal action a_2^{opt} will be taken in cycle 2, is defined to be

$$\begin{aligned} q_1(d_1, \mathcal{D}) &= E\,[E\{U(Y_1, Z_1) \\ &\qquad + \lambda q_2(a_2^{opt}(d_1, Y_1, Z_1, \mathcal{D}), d_1, Y_1, Z_1, \mathcal{D}) | \boldsymbol{\theta}, d_1\} | d_1, \mathcal{D}] \\ &= E\{Q_1(d_1, \boldsymbol{\theta}) | d_1, \mathcal{D}\} \\ &\qquad + \lambda \sum_{y_1=0}^{1} \sum_{z_1=0}^{1} q_2(a_2^{opt}(d_1, y_1, z_1, \mathcal{D}), d_1, y_1, z_1, \mathcal{D}) \\ &\qquad\qquad p(y_1, z_1 | d_1, \mathcal{D}), \end{aligned} \quad (4.9)$$

where $p(y_1, z_1 | d_1, \mathcal{D})$ is the posterior probability distribution of (y_1, z_1) given d_1 and $\mathcal{D}$. The optimal cycle 1 action, $a_1^{opt} = d_1^{opt}$, maximizes this quantity over the doses $\{1, \ldots, m\}$, while defining $a_1^{opt} = 0$ when $q_1(d_1, \mathcal{D}) < (1 + \lambda) U(0,0)$ for all $d_1 \in \{1, \cdots, m\}$. Maximizing q_1 and q_2 yields the optimal action pair $\boldsymbol{a}^{opt} = (a_1^{opt}, a_2^{opt})$. To summarize,

1) each a_c^{opt} is either a dose or 0 (do not treat the patient),

2) a_2^{opt} is computed only when $a_1^{opt} \neq 0$, i.e. a_1^{opt} is a dose, and

3) both a_1^{opt} and a_2^{opt} are functions of $\mathcal{D}$.

As a logistical issue, additional data from other patients may be obtained between administration of dose $a_1^{opt} = d_1$ and optimization of a_2, due to the fact that $\mathcal{D}$ has changed because additional outcome data were observed on other patients while waiting to evaluate a given patient's cycle 1 outcomes (Y_1, Z_1). In this case, the posterior and hence the patient's optimal cycle 2 action a_2^{opt} might change since more information has become available.

4.3.2 Dose Acceptability

In addition to the formal utility-based optimization criteria, the DTM2 design also includes dose acceptability criteria that are commonly used in dose-finding trials. This is motivated by ethical considerations because maximizing a posterior utility-based objective function is not enough to allow a dose to be administered in practice. Although an optimal policy under a given utility function is mathematically well-defined, it is an indirect solution based on an optimization done in terms of expected values computed under an assumed model. Because a clinical trial's first purpose is to treat the patients enrolled in the trial, essentially, the acceptability rules act as gatekeepers to protect patient safety. An important case arises when it has been determined from interim data that no dose is both safe and efficacious in either cycle. In this case, it is no longer ethical to treat any patient with any dose, and the trial must be stopped. Additionally, in some applications, a decision-theoretic solution might turn out to have undesirable features that were not anticipated when specifying the outcomes, model, and utility function.

The DTM2 design mitigates these concerns by adding three additional dose acceptability criteria that restrict the set of acceptable solutions when maximizing (4.8) and (4.9). The first constraint is very simple, that an untried dose level may not be skipped when escalating. To formalize this, let d_1^M denote the highest dose level among those that have been tried in cycle 1, and let $d_{1,2}^M$ denote the highest dose level among those that have been tried in either cycle 1 or cycle 2. The search for optimal actions is constrained so that $1 \leq d_1 \leq \min(d_1^M + 1, m)$ and $1 \leq d_2 \leq \min(d_{1,2}^M + 1, m)$. The second constraint also is very simple. It does not allow a patient's dose level in cycle 2 to be escalated to a higher level if toxicity was observed in cycle 1, $Y_1 = 1$. These two restrictions are based on the assumption that the probability of toxicity increases with dose. If this assumption is not valid, for example in a study of a biologic agent or cellular therapy, as in Lee et al. (2019), then these restrictions should be dropped. The third constraint is probabilistic, defined in terms of expected utility, and is imposed to avoid giving undesirable dose pairs. For cycle 2, *dose d_2 is unacceptable* if it (1) violates the do-not-skip rule, (2) escalates after $Y_1 = 1$, or (3) satisfies the inequality

$$q_2(d_2, d_1, Y_1, Z_1, \mathcal{D}) < U(0, 0). \tag{4.10}$$

The inequality (4.10) says that the posterior expected utility of treating the patient with dose d_2 given (d_1, Y_1, Z_1) is smaller than that obtained by not giving a cycle 2 treatment to the patient. The set of acceptable cycle 2 doses for a patient with cycle 1 data (d_1, Y_1, Z_1) is denoted by $\mathcal{A}_2(d_1, Y_1, Z_1, \mathcal{D})$. The importance of using each patient's cycle 1 data to choose their cycle 2 dose is shown by the fact that, for given data $\mathcal{D}$, a cycle 2 dose d_2 may be acceptable for some patients' cycle 1 data (d_1, Y_1, Z_1) but not acceptable for others. That is, cycle 2 dose acceptability depends on each patient's previous history.

Table 4.3 illustrates the true expected cycle 2 utilities of d_2 conditional on (d_1, Y_1, Z_1) under simulation scenario 4, which will be described below. Assume that the true parameter values $\boldsymbol{\theta}^{true}$ and $\tilde{\boldsymbol{\theta}}^{true}$ are known, and suppress $\tilde{\boldsymbol{\theta}}^{true}$ for brevity. The table gives values of

$q_1(d_1, \boldsymbol{\theta}^{true})$ and, in the block under d_2, values of

$$E\{U(Y_1, Z_1) + \lambda Q_2(d_2^{opt}(d_1, Y_1, Z_1, \boldsymbol{\theta}^{true}), d_1, Y_1, Z_1, \boldsymbol{\theta}^{true})|\boldsymbol{\theta}^{true}, d_1\}.$$

The function $Q_2(d_2, d_1, Y_1, Z_1, \boldsymbol{\theta}^{true})$ in Table 4.3 is similar to (4.7). For example, the values of $Q_2(a_2, d_1 = 3, Y_1 = 0, Z_1 = 0, \boldsymbol{\theta}^{true})$ given in the first row of the third box from the top are (35.98, 39.49, 39.70, 36.30, 27.17) for d_2 =(1, 2, 3, 4, 5), respectively. Since $Q_2(5, 3, 0, 0, \boldsymbol{\theta}^{true}) < U(0, 0)$, it follows that $d_2 = 5$ is not acceptable due to the requirement (4.10). Since the other four dose levels are acceptable, $\mathcal{A}_2(3, 0, 0, \boldsymbol{\theta}^{true}) = \{1, 2, 3, 4\}$, with $d_2^{opt}(d_1 = 3, Y_1 = 0, Z_1 = 0, \boldsymbol{\theta}^{true}) = 3$. When $(d_1, Y_1, Z_1) = (3, 1, 0)$, it follows that no $d_2 \in \{1, \cdots, m\}$ produces an expected utility $> U(0, 0)$, and $d_2 = 3, 4, 5$ are not acceptable due to the no-escalation-after toxicity rule. Thus, $\mathcal{A}_2(3, 0, 0, \boldsymbol{\theta}^{true}) = \{0\}$, so $d_2^{opt}(d_1 = 3, Y_1 = 1, Z_1 = 0, \boldsymbol{\theta}^{true}) = 0$. The last column of the table lists $d_2^{opt}(d_1, Y_1, Z_1, \boldsymbol{\theta}^{true})$ for all combinations of (d_1, Y_1, Z_1).

To identify acceptable cycle 1 doses, assume that $d_2^{opt}(d_1, Y_1, Z_1, \mathcal{D})$ is chosen from the set $\mathcal{A}_2(d_1, Y_1, Z_1, \mathcal{D})$, that is, it satisfies the three acceptability rules. For cycle 1, *action* d_1 *is unacceptable* if it violates the do-not-skip rule or satisfies the utility-based criterion

$$q_1(d_1, \mathcal{D}) < (1 + \lambda)U(0, 0). \tag{4.11}$$

Looking at the form of q_1 in (4.9), this is simply a formalization of the requirement that d_1 is unacceptable in cycle 1 if it gives a smaller posterior expected payoff than not treating the patient at all. Denote the set of acceptable cycle 1 doses by $\mathcal{A}_1 \subset \mathcal{A}$. While $\mathcal{A}_1(\mathcal{D})$ is adaptive between patients since it is a function of other patients' data, $\mathcal{A}_2(d_1, Y_1, Z_1, \mathcal{D})$ is adaptive both between and within patients.

4.3.3 Adaptive Randomization to Reduce Stickiness

While, on average, the pair $\mathbf{d}^{opt}$ yields the best clinical outcomes, the reliability of the decision-making process over the entire trial can be improved by including adaptive randomization (AR) among $\mathbf{d}$ giving values of the objective function near the maximum at $\mathbf{d}^{opt}$. This is done to address the problem that a "greedy" search algorithm that always takes the optimal action by maximizing an objective function may have a non-trivial probability of getting stuck at an action that is locally optimal but globally suboptimal. Because the suboptimal action where the algorithm is stuck is taken repeatedly, little or no data are obtained for other actions (here, doses) that may, in fact, be globally optimal. This sometimes is called the "exploitation versus exploration" problem, or "stickiness", and it has been well-known for many years in the sequential analysis and optimization literature (cf. Sutton and Barto (2018); Tokic (2010)).

A practical solution for stickiness is to introduce some additional randomness into the search process. This can be done in a dose-finding setting by using AR which, if carefully implemented, can decrease the probability of getting stuck at a suboptimal $\mathbf{d}$. Perhaps counter-intuitively, AR also leads to more patients being treated at doses with larger utilities, on average. This is because AR spreads the sample of patients more widely over the set of doses being studied, compared to a greedy algorithm (Bartroff and Lai (2010); Azriel et al. (2011); Thall and Nguyen (2012); Braun et al. (2016); Lin et al. (2020)). In the more general setting of a phase I-II-III design that allows dose re-optimization after the first stage of phase III based on mean survival time following phase I-II dose-finding based on early efficacy and toxicity, proposed by Chapple and Thall (2019), using AR in phase I-II substantially increases the generalized power of the overall design.

AR is implemented in DTM2 by first defining a function ϵ_i that decreases in patient index i. Denote $\boldsymbol{\epsilon} = (\epsilon_1, \cdots, \epsilon_n)$. The set of ϵ*-optimal doses in cycle 1* is defined to be

$$\mathcal{A}_{\epsilon,1}(\mathcal{D}) = \{d_1 : |q_1(d_{i,1}^{opt}, \mathcal{D}) - q_1(d_1, \mathcal{D})| < \epsilon_i,\ d_1 \in \mathcal{A}_1(\mathcal{D})\}.$$

Thus, the set $\mathcal{A}_{\epsilon,1}(\mathcal{D})$ contains all $d_1 \in \mathcal{A}_1(\mathcal{D})$ having posterior mean utility within ϵ_i of the maximum posterior mean utility. That is, it contains cycle 1 doses that are at least nearly optimal, based on the current data. Using the same idea, the set of *ϵ-optimal doses for cycle 2 given* $(d_{i,1}, Y_{i,1}, Z_{i,1})$ is defined to be

$$\begin{aligned}\mathcal{A}_{\epsilon,2}(d_{i,1}, Y_{i,1}, Z_{i,1}, \mathcal{D}) = \{d_2 :& |q_2(d_{i,2}^{opt}(d_{i,1}, Y_{i,1}, Z_{i,1}, \mathcal{D}), Y_{i,1}, Z_{i,1}, d_{i,1}, \mathcal{D}) \\ & - q_2(d_2, d_{i,1}, Y_{i,1}, Z_{i,1}, \mathcal{D})| < \epsilon_i/2, \\ & d_2 \in \mathcal{A}_2(d_{i,1}, Y_{i,1}, Z_{i,1}, \mathcal{D})\}.\end{aligned}$$

In cycle 2, the upper limit $\epsilon_i/2$ is used rather than ϵ_i because $q_2(d_2, d_1, Y_1, Z_1, \mathcal{D})$ is the posterior expected utility for cycle 2 only. Given this structure for defining what is meant by a dose being "close to optimal" as the sample accumulates, DTM2 randomizes patients fairly among the doses in $\mathcal{A}_{\epsilon,1}$ for cycle 1 and fairly among doses in $\mathcal{A}_{\epsilon,2}$ for cycle 2. This procedure will be called AR($\boldsymbol{\epsilon}$). In practice, the numerical values of ϵ_i depend on the numerical values of $U(y, z)$, and they must be determined by conducting preliminary trial simulations.

4.3.4 Trial Design

The DTM2 design and simulations are based on an illustrative trial constructed to be a prototypical phase I-II trial with five dose levels, but accounting for two cycles of therapy rather than only one. The maximum sample size is $n = 60$ with a cohort size of 2. Based on preliminary simulations using the utility function given earlier, with $U(0, 0) = 35$ and $U(1, 1) = 65$, the DTM2 design's AR parameters were set to $\epsilon_i = 20$ for the first 10 patients, $\epsilon_i = 15$ for patients 11 to 20, and $\epsilon_i = 10$ for the remaining 40 patients. While this choice of AR parameters is *ad hoc*, in this setting it gives a design with good properties.

To start, the first cohort of 2 patients, $i = 1, 2$, are treated at the lowest dose level $d = 1$ in cycle 1, their cycle 1 outcomes $(Y_{i,1}, Z_{i,1})$ are observed, the first posterior of $\boldsymbol{\theta}$ is computed, and cycle 2 actions are taken for each patient. If $\mathcal{A}_{i,2} = \{0\}$ then patient i does not receive a second cycle of treatment. If $\mathcal{A}_{i,2} \neq \{0\}$, then AR($\boldsymbol{\epsilon}$) is used to choose an action for cycle 2 from $\mathcal{A}_{\epsilon,2}$. When $(Y_{i,2}, Z_{i,2})$ are observed in cycle 2, the posterior of $\boldsymbol{\theta}$ is updated.

The second cohort is enrolled after both patients in the first cohort have been evaluated for cycle 1. For all cohorts after the first, the posterior is updated after the outcomes of all previous cohorts have been observed, and the posterior expected utility, $q_{i,1}(d_1, \mathcal{D})$, is computed using $\lambda = 0.8$. For all $i > 2$, if $\mathcal{A}_{i,1}(\mathcal{D}) = \{0\}$ for any interim $\mathcal{D}$, then $d_{i,1}(\mathcal{D}) = 0$, and the trial is terminated. If $\mathcal{A}_{i,1}(\mathcal{D}) \neq \{0\}$, then a cycle 1 dose is chosen from $\mathcal{A}_{\epsilon,1}$ using AR($\boldsymbol{\epsilon}$). Once the outcomes in cycle 1 are observed, the posterior is updated. Using $(d_{i,1}, Y_{i,1}, Z_{i,1}, \mathcal{D})$ and ϵ_i, $\mathcal{A}_{\epsilon,2}$ is searched. If $\mathcal{A}_{\epsilon,2} = \{0\}$, then $d_{i,2} = 0$ and a cycle 2 dose is not given to patient i. Otherwise, $d_{i,2}$ is selected from $\mathcal{A}_{\epsilon,2}(d_{i,1}, Y_{i,1}, Z_{i,1}, \mathcal{D})$ using AR($\boldsymbol{\epsilon}$). When $(Y_{i,2}, Z_{i,2})$ are observed from cycle 2, the posterior of $\boldsymbol{\theta}$ is updated. These steps are repeated until either the trial has been stopped early or the maximum sample size $N = 60$ has been reached, and in this case, a final optimal two-cycle regime $\mathbf{d}_{select}$ is chosen. The goal is to determine the best pair of actions a_1^{opt} and $a_2^{opt}(d_1^{opt}, y_1, z_1) \in \mathcal{A}$, provided that there is an acceptable starting dose $a_1^{opt} = d_1^{opt} \in \{1, \cdots, m\}$.

4.3.5 Comparator Designs

To evaluate the DTM2 design, it was compared to four other designs. In order to obtain reasonably fair comparisons, each comparator was constructed as a 2-cycle extension of an existing 1-cycle dose-finding design. These 1-cycle designs were 3+3 algorithms, the continual reassessment method (CRM, O'Quigley et al. (1990)), and a Bayesian design using toxicity and efficacy odds ratios (TEOR, Yin et al. (2006)). Two versions of the (3+3) method were considered, one that implicitly targets a dose with $P(Y_1 = 1) \leq 0.17$, called (3+3)A, and another that implicitly targets a dose with $P(Y_1 = 1) \leq 0.33$, called (3+3)B. Both (3+3)A and (3+3)B were extended to account for a second cycle by using the following deterministic algorithm to choose a cycle 2 dose level. If toxicity is observed in cycle 1, then the dose is lowered by one level, $d_2 = d_1 - 1$ for cycle 2, and if no toxicity is observed, then the cycle dose is repeated, $d_2 = d_1$. The (3+3)A method, coupled with this deterministic rule for cycle 2, is one of the most commonly used methods in phase I clinical trials. These two-cycle dose-finding algorithms will be denoted by (3+3)A2 and (3+3)B2.

The extended 2-cycle version of the CRM, called CRM2, was defined as follows. For cycle 1, dose selection was based on the commonly assumed model $\Pr(Y_1 = 1 \mid d_1) = p_{d_1}^{\exp(\alpha)}$ where $\alpha \sim N(0, 2)$, and the five fixed probabilities $(p_1, \cdots, p_5)$, often called this CRM model's "skeleton," were assumed to be monotone increasing, $0 < p_1 < \cdots < p_5 < 1$. The skeleton was calibrated using the "getprior" subroutine in the package "dfcrm", setting the fixed target toxicity probability to be 0.30, the prior guess of maximum tolerated dose to be 4, and the desired halfwidth of the indifference intervals to be 0.05 (see Cheung (2011)). The resulting skeleton was $(p_1, \ldots, p_5) = (0.063, 0.123, 0.204, 0.300, 0.402)$. Using this model, each patient's cycle 1 dose was chosen to have posterior mean toxicity probability closest to 0.30. That is, the usual CRM toxicity-based algorithm with target .30 was used. This was implemented using the R function, "crm" in dfcrm, while also imposing the do-not-skip an untried dose rule in cycle 1. To determine a cycle 2 dose, the same deterministic rule was used as that for the extended (3+3) methods, with one more safety requirement. For CRM2, a cycle 2 dose was not given if $\Pr\{\Pr(Y_1 = 1 \text{ or } Y_2 = 1 \mid \alpha) > 0.5 \mid \mathcal{D}, \mathbf{d}\} > 0.9$, assuming conditional independence of $P(Y_1 = 1 \mid \alpha)$ and $P(Y_2 = 1 \mid \alpha)$ for simplicity. For example, following the deterministic rule, a patient treated in cycle 1 at d_1 may be treated at $d_2 \in \{d_1 - 1, d_1\}$, depending on the cycle 1 toxicity outcome. In particular, $d_2 = d_1$ if $Y_1 = 0$. If (d_1, d_1) does not satisfy the safety requirement, however, then a cycle 2 treatment is not given to a patient with d_1 and $Y_1 = 0$. If no cycle 2 dose is allowed for any d_1 regardless of Y_1, that is, if no (d_1, d_2) with $d_2 \in \{d_1 - 1, d_1\}$ satisfies the safety rule, then d_1 is lowered until a cycle 2 value is safe for either $Y_1 = 0$ or $Y_1 = 1$.

Denoting $\pi(a, b \mid d) = \Pr(Y = a, Z = b \mid d)$ for $a, b \in \{0, 1\}$, the TEOR design chooses doses based on the odds ratios

$$OR(d) = \frac{\pi(0,0 \mid d)\, \pi(1,1 \mid d)}{\pi(1,0 \mid d)\, \pi(0,1 \mid d)}$$

for the doses $d = 1, \cdots, m$, and additional dose acceptability criteria. The TEOR design was extended to a 2-cycle version similar to the way that CRM2 was constructed. This 2-cycle extension, named TEOR2, used the following cycle 2 dose acceptability criteria. A dose was not given in cycle 2 if

$$\Pr\{\Pr(Y_1 = 1 \ \text{ or } \ Y_2 = 1) > 0.6 \mid \mathcal{D}, \mathbf{d}\} \ > \ 0.90$$

or

$$\Pr\{\Pr(Z_1 = 0 \text{ and } Z_2 = 1) > 0.8 \mid \mathcal{D}, \mathbf{d}\} \ > \ 0.90,$$

assuming independence of the two cycles for simplicity. In addition, the priors of Yin et al. (2006) were calibrated using the idea of prior effective sample size (ESS) given by Morita et al. (2010), which gave the hyperparameter values $\sigma_\phi^2 = 20$, $\sigma_\psi^2 = 5$ and $\sigma_\theta^2 = 10$. The other TEOR design parameters were set to $\bar{\pi}_T = 0.35$, $\underline{\pi}_E = 0.5$, $p^{escl} = 0.5$, $p^\star = 0.25$ and $q^\star = 0.1$, and $\omega_d^{(3)}$ was used to select a cycle 1 dose for the next patient.

4.4 Simulation Study

The DTM2 design was compared by simulation to (3+3)A2, (3+3)B2, CRM2, and TEOR2, under each of the eight scenarios. To specify simulation scenarios for two cycles, one must

Table 4.1 *Assumed true marginal probabilities of toxicity and efficacy,* $(p_{T,1}, p_{E,1})^{\text{true}}$ *for cycle 1 and* $(p_{T,2}, p_{E,2})^{\text{true}}$ *for cycle 2, under each of scenarios 1 – 7.*

Scenario	Cycles	Doses				
		1	2	3	4	5
1	1	(0.10, 0.02)	(0.15, 0.03)	(0.30, 0.05)	(0.45, 0.08)	(0.55, 0.10)
	2	(0.13, 0.01)	(0.18, 0.02)	(0.33, 0.04)	(0.48, 0.07)	(0.58, 0.09)
2	1	(0.30, 0.50)	(0.32, 0.60)	(0.35, 0.70)	(0.38, 0.80)	(0.40, 0.90)
	2	(0.33, 0.45)	(0.35, 0.55)	(0.38, 0.65)	(0.41, 0.75)	(0.43, 0.85)
3	1	(0.05, 0.10)	(0.18, 0.13)	(0.20, 0.25)	(0.40, 0.26)	(0.50, 0.27)
	2	(0.30, 0.20)	(0.31, 0.35)	(0.32, 0.45)	(0.45, 0.65)	(0.65, 0.70)
4	1	(0.13, 0.06)	(0.15, 0.18)	(0.25, 0.35)	(0.55, 0.38)	(0.75, 0.40)
	2	(0.20, 0.14)	(0.25, 0.23)	(0.35, 0.29)	(0.50, 0.32)	(0.80, 0.35)
5	1	(0.52, 0.01)	(0.61, 0.15)	(0.71, 0.20)	(0.82, 0.25)	(0.90, 0.30)
	2	(0.53, 0.04)	(0.55, 0.20)	(0.62, 0.25)	(0.85, 0.27)	(0.95, 0.33)
6	1	(0.25, 0.10)	(0.28, 0.13)	(0.30, 0.25)	(0.40, 0.35)	(0.50, 0.45)
	2	(0.30, 0.20)	(0.31, 0.35)	(0.32, 0.45)	(0.43, 0.65)	(0.56, 0.70)
7	1	(0.25, 0.10)	(0.28, 0.13)	(0.30, 0.25)	(0.40, 0.38)	(0.65, 0.40)
	2	(0.30, 0.20)	(0.31, 0.35)	(0.32, 0.45)	(0.43, 0.65)	(0.66, 0.67)

specify true joint distributions of $[Y_1, Z_1 \mid d_1]$ and $[Y_2, Z_2 \mid d_1, d_2, Y_1, Z_1]$. Marginal probabilities of toxicity and efficacy in each of the two cycles were simulated using the 4-variate normal distribution given in expression (4.4), with assumed values $\sigma_\xi^{2,\text{true}} = \sigma_\eta^{2,\text{true}} = 0.5^2$, $\tau^{2,\text{true}} = 0.3^2$ and $\rho^{\text{true}} = -0.2$ in all scenarios. The true marginal toxicity and efficacy probabilities for each of the two cycles in each of the first seven scenarios are given in Table 4.1.

For each of scenarios 1 – 7, $\boldsymbol{\xi}^{\text{true}}$ and $\bar{\boldsymbol{\eta}}^{\text{true}}$ were determined by matching $\Pr(Y_c < 0) = \Phi(0 \mid \bar{\xi}_{d_c}^{\text{true}}, \sigma_\xi^{2,true} + \tau^{2,true})$ and $\Pr(Z_c < 0) = \Phi(0 \mid \bar{\eta}_{d_c}^{\text{true}}, \sigma_\eta^{2,\text{true}} + \tau^{2,\text{true}})$ with the assumed true marginal probabilities at each d_c given in Table 4.1. The values $(\bar{\boldsymbol{\xi}}^{\text{true}}, \bar{\boldsymbol{\eta}}^{\text{true}})$ then were used with the assumed nuisance parameter values to simulate $(\mathbf{Y}, \mathbf{Z})$. First, values of (Y_1, Z_1) were simulated from (4.6), with the assumed true values of σ_ξ^2, σ_η^2, τ^2, ρ, and (4.5) then used to generate (Y_2, Z_2) conditional on (Y_1, Z_1).

Scenario 8 was constructed to evaluate robustness, and was based on the following logistic regression model. The fixed marginal cycle 1 toxicity and efficacy probabilities $(p_T(d_1), p_E(d_1))$ of scenario 5 were used to generate outcomes with the following probabilities:

$$\begin{aligned}
\Pr(Y_1 = 1 \mid d_1) &= p_T(d_1), \\
\Pr(Z_1 = 1 \mid d_1, Y_1) &= \text{logit}^{-1}\{\text{logit}(p_E(d_1)) - 0.34(Y_1 - 0.5)\}, \\
\Pr(Y_2 = 1 \mid d_1, d_2, Y_1, Z_1) &= \text{logit}^{-1}\{\text{logit}(p_T(d_1)) + 0.33 d_2 \\
&\quad + 0.4(Y_1 - 0.5) - 0.3(Z_1 - 0.5)\}, \\
\Pr(Z_2 = 1 \mid d_1, d_2, Y_1, Z_1, Y_2) &= \text{logit}^{-1}\{\text{logit}(p_E(d_1)) + 0.76 d_2 \\
&\quad - 0.22(Y_1 - 0.5) + 2.4(Z_1 - 0.5) \\
&\quad - 1.8(Y_2 - 0.5)\}.
\end{aligned}$$

A total of $M = 1{,}000$ trials were simulated under each scenario using each design.

To apply DTM2, the hyperparameters, $\tilde{\boldsymbol{\theta}}$, were calibrated using prior ESS. Values of $\tilde{\boldsymbol{\theta}}$ were determined to give priors with $0.5 \leq \text{ESS} \leq 2$ and used to determine the prior for all simulations. For each scenario, 1,000 pseudo samples of $\boldsymbol{\theta}$ were simulated, setting $\sigma_{\xi_{c0}}^2 =$

Table 4.2 *Optimal treatment sequences for the four possible values of the cycle 1 outcomes* (Z_1, Y_1), *under each of the eight simulation scenarios.*

Scenario	a_1^{opt}	a_2^{opt}			
		(0,0)	(0, 1)	(1,0)	(1,1)
1	0	0	0	0	0
2	5	5	5	4	4
3	3	4	4	2	2
4	3	3	3	0	0
5	0	0	0	0	0
6	5	4	4	4	4
7	4	4	4	3	3
8	5	5	3	4	4

Table 4.3 *True expected utilities in scenario 4 and* $q_1(d_1, \boldsymbol{\theta}^{true})$ = *true expected payoff from giving* d_1 *in cycle 1 assuming that the optimal action will be taken in cycle 2. utility. Entries in the columns under* d_2 *are the true expected cycle 2 utilities,* $q_2(d_2, \boldsymbol{\theta}^{true})$. *The expected utilities in grey are for* d_2 *that violates the no-escalation-after-*$Y_1 = 1$ *rule. Expected utilities in italics are for unacceptable* d_2 *under the utility-based criterion.*

d_1	$q_1(d_1, \boldsymbol{\theta}^{true})$	(Y_1, Z_1)	d_2					a_2^{true}
			1	2	3	4	5	
1	66.19	(0,0)	37.32	41.40	41.85	38.54	*29.66*	3
		(0,1)	48.18	55.07	56.80	54.00	45.04	3
		(1,0)	30.60	33.58	33.07	29.57	23.27	0
		(1,1)	41.20	47.16	47.96	44.80	38.23	0
2	73.38	(0,0)	36.53	40.33	40.66	37.30	*28.38*	3
		(0,1)	45.06	51.39	52.92	50.08	41.15	3
		(1,0)	*30.13*	32.88	32.26	28.70	22.28	0
		(1,1)	38.36	43.71	44.31	41.12	34.54	1
3	80.61	(0,0)	35.98	39.49	39.70	36.30	*27.17*	3
		(0,1)	43.31	49.20	50.62	47.73	38.69	3
		(1,0)	*30.29*	*32.82*	32.12	28.43	21.53	0
		(1,1)	37.34	42.27	42.75	39.46	32.48	2
4	69.71	(0,0)	37.17	40.90	41.40	38.19	*28.65*	3
		(0,1)	44.37	50.46	52.14	49.47	40.09	3
		(1,0)	*32.13*	*34.89*	*34.39*	30.68	22.91	0
		(1,1)	39.17	44.32	45.02	41.74	33.91	3
5	68.16	(0,0)	38.08	42.02	42.80	39.83	*30.06*	3
		(0,1)	45.26	51.52	53.46	51.04	41.51	3
		(1,0)	*33.00*	35.88	35.52	*31.85*	23.69	2
		(1,1)	40.05	45.32	46.16	42.95	34.75	3

$\sigma^2_{\eta c0} = 6^2$, computing probabilities of interest, such as $P(Y_c = 0 \mid d_c)$ and $P(Z_c = 0 \mid d_c)$, based on the pseudo samples, setting $\sigma_\xi^2 = \sigma_\eta^2 = 2^2$, $\tau^2 = 1$ and $\rho = -0.5$.

Table 4.2 shows the optimal actions, d_1^{opt} and $d_2^{opt}(d_1^{opt}, Y_1, Z_1)$, over two cycles under each scenario. For example, in Scenario 3, the optimal cycle 1 action for DTM2 is to give dose 3, and the optimal cycle 2 action is to treat patients with $Y_1 = 0$ at $d_2 = 4$, and those with $Y_1 = 1$ at $d_2 = 2$, regardless of Z_1. To illustrate how the scenario probabilities translate into decision criteria, Table 4.3 gives $q_1(d_1, \boldsymbol{\theta}^{true})$, the true expected total payoff from giving d_1 in cycle 1 assuming that the optimal action will be taken in cycle 2, and the true expected utility for each combination of (d_1, Y_1, Z_1, d_2).

4.4.1 Evaluation Criteria

The following summary statistics were used to evaluate each design's performance. Denote the outcomes of the n patients in a given trial who received at least one cycle of therapy by $\{(Y_{i,1}, Z_{i,1}), (Y_{i,2}, Z_{i,2}), i = 1, ..., n\}$, where $n < 60$ if the trial was stopped early. The empirical mean total utility over both cycles for n patients is $\bar{U} = \sum_{i=1}^{n}\{U(Y_{i,1}, Z_{i,1}) + U(Y_{i,2}, Z_{i,2})\}/n$, with $U(Y_{i,2}, Z_{i,2}) = U(0,0)$ for patients who did not receive a second cycle of therapy. Indexing the M simulated replications of the trial by $m = 1, ..., M$, the empirical mean total payoff for all patents in the trial is

$$\bar{U}_M = \frac{1}{M}\sum_{r=1}^{M}\bar{U}^{(m)}.$$

One may regard $\bar{U}_M$ as a quantification of the ethical desirability of the design for the patients enrolled in the trial, for the assumed utility function $U(y, z)$.

Abusing notation slightly by referring to doses and actions interchangeably, recall that DTM2 selects an optimal dose $d_{1,select}$ for cycle 1, and an optimal function $d_{2,select}$ for use in cycle 2 assuming that $d_{1,select}$ is given, with $d_{2,select}$ not defined if $d_{1,select} = 0$. To evaluate performance in terms of future patient benefit, let $\boldsymbol{\theta}^{true}$ be the true parameter vector assumed for a simulation scenario. Under $\boldsymbol{\theta}^{true}$, the expected payoff in cycle 1 of giving action $d_{1,select}$ to a future patient is

$$Q_{1,select}(d_{1,select}) = E\{U(Y_1, Z_1) \mid d_{1,select}, \boldsymbol{\theta}^{true}\},$$

for $d_{1,select} \neq 0$. This expectation is computed under the distribution of (Y_1, Z_1) conditional on $d_{1,select}$ and $\boldsymbol{\theta}^{true}$, so it may be written more generally as $E^{true}\{U(Y_1, Z_1) \mid d_{1,select}\}$. If the rule $d_{2,select}$ is used, the expected payoff in cycle 2 is

$$\begin{aligned} Q_{2,select}(d_{2,select}) = \sum_{(y_1,z_1)\in\{0,1\}^2} & E\{U(Y_2, Z_2) \\ & \mid d_{1,select}, d_{2,select}(y_1, z_1), y_1, z_1, \boldsymbol{\theta}^{true}\} \\ & \times p(y_1, z_1 \mid d_{1,select}, \boldsymbol{\theta}^{true}), \end{aligned}$$

using the value $E\{U(Y_2, Z_2) \mid d_{1,select}, d_{2,select}(y_1, z_1), y_1, z_1, \boldsymbol{\theta}^{true}\} = U(0,0)$ if $d_{2,select}(y_1, z_1) = 0$. The total expected payoff to a future patient treated using the selected optimal two-cycle regime $\mathbf{d}_{select} = (d_{1,select}, d_{2,select})$ is defined to be

$$Q_{select}(d_{select}) = Q_{1,select}(d_{1,select}) + \lambda\, Q_{2,select}(d_{2,select}).$$

Denote $\delta_{i,2} = 1$ if patient i was treated in cycle 2. For each simulated trial using each design, for the patients who received at least one cycle of therapy, empirical toxicity and efficacy probabilities were computed as

$$\hat{p}(\text{Tox}) = \frac{1}{n}\sum_{i=1}^{n}\frac{1(Y_{i,1} = 1) + \delta_{i,2}1(Y_{i,2} = 1)}{1 + \delta_{i,2}}$$

and

$$\hat{p}(\text{Eff}) = \frac{1}{n}\sum_{i=1}^{n}\frac{1(Z_{i,1} = 1) + \delta_{i,2}1(Z_{i,2} = 1)}{1 + \delta_{i,2}}.$$

Given these empirical per-cycle probability estimates, for each scenario and method, the averages of these values was computed over the replicated trials.

Table 4.4 *Simulation results for DTM2 and four two-cycle comparators.* $\bar{U}_M$ *= mean total payoff for all patients in the trial.* Q_{select} *= total expected payoff to a future patient.* $\hat{p}(Tox)$ *and* $\hat{p}(Eff)$ *are empirical toxicity and efficacy probabilities for patients who received at least 1 cycle of treatment.*

Scenarios	Criterion	DTM2	(3+3)A2	(3+3)B2	CRM2	TEOR2
	$\bar{U}_M$	66.48	59.27	58.81	56.56	61.90
	Q_{select}	57.77	54.36	52.30	51.75	52.43
1	$\hat{p}$(Tox)	0.25	0.22	0.23	0.27	0.25
	$\hat{p}$(Eff)	0.07	0.03	0.03	0.05	0.07
	% completed trials	2.3	88.6	96.5	99.6	4.4
	$\bar{U}_M$	136.35	124.36	118.32	115.86	122.13
	Q_{select}	135.76	103.85	104.48	102.43	108.47
2	$\hat{p}$(Tox)	0.39	0.30	0.33	0.36	0.35
	$\hat{p}$(Eff)	0.72	0.58	0.55	0.56	0.60
	% completed trials	99.4	39.2	64.7	95.6	78.2
	$\bar{U}_M$	94.23	85.95	85.75	89.93	88.04
	Q_{select}	84.39	77.98	80.14	78.43	78.47
3	$\hat{p}$(Tox)	0.38	0.27	0.27	0.30	0.26
	$\hat{p}$(Eff)	0.38	0.27	0.27	0.33	0.28
	% completed trials	79.4	96.6	99.2	100.0	78.50
	$\bar{U}_M$	75.84	81.81	80.12	85.40	84.94
	Q_{select}	69.49	74.92	75.76	78.67	78.87
4	$\hat{p}$(Tox)	0.51	0.25	0.26	0.29	0.28
	$\hat{p}$(Eff)	0.29	0.22	0.21	0.29	0.27
	% completed trials	96.7	83.2	94.7	99.4	81.7
	$\bar{U}_M$	66.65	52.87	52.72	50.41	NA
	Q_{select}	50.64	40.66	40.70	40.61	NA
5	$\hat{p}$(Tox)	0.84	0.43	0.44	0.53	NA
	$\hat{p}$(Eff)	0.35	0.08	0.04	0.03	NA
	% completed trials	0.4	6.8	20.0	9.0	0.0
	$\bar{U}_M$	96.43	82.82	79.27	81.50	86.14
	Q_{select}	92.78	70.30	71.28	71.29	76.24
6	$\hat{p}$(Tox)	0.45	0.28	0.32	0.32	0.32
	$\hat{p}$(Eff)	0.41	0.24	0.23	0.25	0.29
	% completed trials	90.9	51.5	74.7	97.6	58.3
	$\bar{U}_M$	91.88	82.66	79.31	80.99	86.32
	Q_{select}	84.91	70.28	71.27	71.16	76.34
7	$\hat{p}$(Tox)	0.47	0.28	0.32	0.32	0.32
	$\hat{p}$(Eff)	0.38	0.24	0.22	0.25	0.29
	% completed trials	90.3	51.4	73.6	97.5	58.7
	$\bar{U}_M$	95.92	80.24	76.09	79.83	80.75
	Q_{select}	93.22	68.23	69.26	69.28	70.73
8	$\hat{p}$(Tox)	0.54	0.34	0.36	0.37	0.34
	$\hat{p}$(Eff)	0.45	0.25	0.22	0.27	0.27
	% completed trials	84.7	49.4	73.2	97.6	57.9

4.4.2 Simulation Results

The simulation results are summarized in Table 4.4 in terms of $\bar{U}_M$, Q_{select}, the empirical per-cycle toxicity and efficacy probabilities and the percent of trials completed with $d_1 \in \{1, \ldots, m\}$ out of 1,000 simulated trials.

In Scenario 1, Table 4.1 shows that doses d = 1, 2, and 3, are safe, d = 4 and 5 are overly toxic, and all doses have very low efficacy. Thus, in this Scenario there is little or no benefit from any dose. The value $\bar{U}_M$ = 66.48 for DTM2 in Table 4.4 is very close to the utility $U(0,0) + 0.8U(0,0) = 66$ of $(d_1 = 0, d_2 = 0)$, that is, of not treating the patient, and DTM2 correctly terminates the trial 97.7% of the time in this scenario. This is because the utility-based stopping rule of DTM2 recognizes the low utilities. Similarly, TEOR2 terminates 95.6% of the trials before reaching the maximum number of patients due to the low efficacy rates. In contrast, the 2-cycle extensions of the (3+3) algorithm and the CRM are very likely to run the trial to completion, essentially because they ignore efficacy. This is a very useful illustration of the fact that there is little benefit in exploring the safety of an agent if it is inefficacious, and methods that ignore efficacy are very likely to make this mistake. This has little to do with the 2-cycle structure, and it also can be seen when comparing one-cycle phase I-II (efficacy and toxicity-based) designs to phase I (toxicity only) design. To summarize, in Scenario 1, (3+3)A2, (3+3)B2, and CRM2 all have very poor performance, DTM2 and TEOR2 are the only reasonable designs, and DTM2 is superior to TEOR2 in terms of both $\bar{U}_M$ and Q_{select}.

In Scenario 2, Table 4.1 shows that the toxicity probabilities increase with dose from 0.30 to 0.40 in cycle 1 and from 0.33 to 0.43 in cycle 2, while the efficacy probabilities are quite high in both cycles, increasing with dose from 0.50 to 0.90 in cycle 1 and from 0.45 to 0.85 in cycle 2. Thus, if one considers toxicity probabilities around 0.40 to be acceptable trade-offs for these very high efficacy rates, then there is a substantial payoff for escalating to higher doses. The utility function reflects this, with the optimal action $d_1^{opt} = 5$ and $d_2^{opt}(5, Y_1, Z_1) = 4$ or 5 in (Table 4.2). DTM2 obtains larger values of $\bar{U}_M$ and Q_{select} due to much larger $\hat{p}(\text{Eff})$ and slightly larger $\hat{p}(\text{Tox})$, compared to all of the four other designs (Table 4.4). To summarize, in Scenario 2, (3+3)A2 and (3+3)B2 are likely to stop the trial very early, and DTM2 is greatly superior to all four comparators.

In Scenario 3, $d_1^{opt} = 3$, with $d_2^{opt} = 4$ if $Y_1 = 0$ in cycle 1 and $d_2^{opt} = 2$ if $Y_1 = 1$ (Table 4.2). This illustrates the within-patient adaptation of DTM2. The (3+3)A2, (3+3)B2, and CRM2 designs all select $d_1^{opt} = 3$ often because the toxicity probability of $d_1 = 3$ is close to 0.30, but they never select $d_2^{opt} = 2$ for patients with $(d_1, Y_1) = (3, 0)$ because they all ignore Z_1 and do not allow escalation of dose levels for cycle 2 even with $Y_1 = 0$. DTM2 again achieves the largest values of $\bar{U}_M$, Q_{select}, and $\hat{p}(\text{Eff})$, with slightly larger $\hat{p}(\text{Tox})$. To summarize, in Scenario 3, DTM2 is greatly superior to all four comparators.

Scenario 4 is a very challenging case for DTM2, and is favorable for the other three designs. In Scenario 4, $d_1^{opt} = 3$ since its true toxicity probability 0.25 is closest to 0.30. In addition, $d_2^{opt}(d_1^{opt}, Y_1, Z_1)$ is the same as the cycle 2 dose levels chosen by the deterministic rules of (3+3)A2, (3+3)B2 and CRM2, except for $(Y_1, Z_1) = (0, 1)$, which only occurs about 5% of the time. From Table 4.3, the true expected utility of $d_2 = 2$ given $(d_1, Y_1, Z_1) = (3, 0, 1)$ is 32.82, which is very close to $U(0, 0)$. Thus, the three methods, (3+3)A2, (3+3)B2 and CRM2, are likely to select d_1^{opt} by considering only toxicity outcomes and select d_2^{opt} following their deterministic rules. CRM selects $d_1^{opt} = 3$ most of the time, leading to the largest $\bar{U}_M$ and Q_{select}. Similar performance is observed for TEOR2 because d_1^{opt} is considered optimal by TEOR2 and it uses the same deterministic rule for cycle 2. Another way to put this is that a stopped clock is correct twice a day. The smaller values of $\bar{U}_M$ and Q_{select} for DTM2 are due to the fact that it does a stochastic search to determine the optimal actions, using much more general criteria than the other designs. Table 4.3 shows that, for $(d_1, Y_1) = (3, 1)$, the expected cycle 2 utilities are smaller than or very close to $U(0, 0)$ for all the cycle 2 doses, so all cycle 2 doses are barely acceptable or not acceptable. However, $d_1 = 5$ is acceptable and, given $d_1 = 5$, many cycle 2 doses are acceptable, and DTM2 often explores higher doses in cycle 1 than d_1^{opt}. This may be regarded as an illustration of the price that must be paid for using more of the available information to explore the dose domain more extensively based on an efficacy-toxicity utility-based objective function. To summarize, in Scenario 4, all four comparators are superior to DTM2, essentially because this is a case where they all get lucky.

In Scenario 5, the lowest dose is too toxic and therefore even $d_1 = 1$ is unacceptable. All of the designs are very likely to terminate the trial early most of the time. DTM2 stops trials due to the low posterior expected utilities caused by the high toxicity rate at the initial dose, and indirectly through low posterior expected utilities.

Scenarios 6 and 7 have identical true toxicity and efficacy probabilities that are identical for doses 1, 2 and 3. For doses 4 and 5, Scenario 7 has higher toxicity probabilities and lower efficacy probabilities, so a_1^{opt} is a dose lower than a_1^{opt} in Scenario 6. Since dose 3

Table 4.5 *Optimal treatment sequences under scenarios 3, 6 and 7, assuming either high associations or no association between outcomes, for each combination of cycle 1 outcomes* (Y_1, Z_1).

Scenario	Assoc		a_2^{opt}			
		a_1^{opt}	(0,0)	(0, 1)	(1,0)	(1,1)
3	High	3	4	3	0	2
3	None	3	4	4	2	2
6	High	5	5	4	0	3
6	None	5	4	4	4	4
7	High	4	4	4	0	3
7	None	4	4	4	3	3

has a toxicity probability closest to 0.30 in both Scenarios 6 and 7, the other four methods perform very similarly in these two scenarios. DTM2 again has much higher $\bar{U}_M$ and Q_{select} values compared to all of the other designs in these scenarios.

The results for Scenario 8 show that DTM2 is quite robust since the outcome probabilities were generated from a model very different from the DTM2 model. In this scenario, compared to all of the other designs, DTM2 has higher empirical rates of both efficacy and toxicity, $\hat{p}(Eff) = .45$ and $\hat{p}(Tox) = .54$, but also much larger payoffs $\bar{U}_M = 96$ compared to values in the range 76–81, and $Q_{select} = 93$, compared to values in the range 68–71. This underscores the fact that DTM2 is based on a utility that quantifies the risk-benefit trade-off between efficacy and toxicity, while the phase I designs ignore efficacy and TEOR2 uses an odds ratio, which is measure of association, to make decisions. To summarize, in Scenarios 6, 7, and 8, DTM2 is greatly superior to all four comparators.

Additional simulations were conducted to assess the sensitivity of the designs to different assumptions regarding the association between the outcomes, in Scenarios 3, 6 and 7. This was done by setting $(\sigma_\xi^{2,true}, \sigma_\eta^{2,true}\tau^{2,true}, \rho^{true})$ to be either $(0.2, 0.05, 1, -0.5)$ or $(0.5^2, 0.5^2, 0, 0)$. The first set of values induces a high association between outcomes both within each cycle and between cycles, while the second set of values induces no association between outcomes. The changes in these assumed true values lead to different expected utilities in the two cycles, which in turn lead to different optimal decisions. The scenarios are given in Table 4.5, and the simulation results are summarized in Table 4.6. The values of both $\bar{U}_M$ and Q_{select} were larger for all methods in the high-association cases. While the performances of the designs change depending on the assumed true values, regardless of association their comparative performances were approximately the same in all six cases, with DTM2 again by far the best design in terms of both $\bar{U}_M$ and Q_{select}.

4.5 Discussion

It has been well established that doing dose-finding using any phase I design based on toxicity while ignoring efficacy is logically, scientifically, and ethically flawed. Examples and explanations are given by Yuan et al. (2016), Yan et al. (2018), and Thall (2020). These all are based on the simple fact that the first purpose of treatment is to achieve an anti-disease effect, and it never is a good idea to ignore important data. In this chapter, the 2-cycle design deals with this issue from the start by basing decisions in each cycle on both efficacy and toxicity. Since three of the four comparators used in the simulation study are 2-cycle extensions of phase I dose-finding designs, the comparisons of DTM2 to the 2-cycle extensions of these phase I designs may be regarded as unfair. However, in their usual 1-cycle forms, these phase I designs are used very commonly in practice. Moreover, the simulations showed that, in most scenarios, DTM2 is greatly superior to the 2-cycle phase I-II odds ratio-based comparator TEOR2.

Table 4.6 *Simulation results under three selected scenarios, 3, 6 and 7, assuming different values for* $(\sigma_{\xi}^{2,true}, \sigma_{\eta}^{2,true}\tau^{2,true}, \rho^{true})$ *to induce either high association or no association between outcomes.*

Scenario	Criterion	DTM2	(3+3)A2	(3+3)B2	CRM2	TEOR2
	$\bar{U}_M$	97.06	85.68	85.24	88.56	89.85
3	Q_{select}	86.18	78.53	80.53	76.58	79.27
	$\hat{p}$(Tox)	0.37	0.27	0.28	0.31	0.26
	$\hat{p}$(Eff)	0.38	0.26	0.26	0.33	0.29
High Assoc	% completed trials	97.7	96.6	99.2	99.9	77.5
	$\bar{U}_M$	92.05	85.96	85.44	90.06	87.88
3	Q_{select}	82.22	77.83	80.04	79.35	78.75
	$\hat{p}$(Tox)	0.41	0.27	0.27	0.30	0.26
	$\hat{p}$(Eff)	0.36	0.26	0.26	0.33	0.28
No Assoc	% completed trials	98.2	96.6	99.2	99.9	77.5
	$\bar{U}_M$	101.37	85.54	81.74	83.20	89.87
6	Q_{select}	95.18	72.43	73.35	71.40	77.67
	$\hat{p}$(Tox)	0.42	0.26	0.29	0.31	0.31
	$\hat{p}$(Eff)	0.43	0.25	0.22	0.26	0.31
High Assoc	% completed trials	91.1	51.5	74.7	97.5	59.9
	$\bar{U}_M$	94.63	82.45	78.73	81.51	85.11
6	Q_{select}	90.85	69.76	70.75	71.53	76.11
	$\hat{p}$(Tox)	0.46	0.29	0.32	0.33	0.32
	$\hat{p}$(Eff)	0.40	0.24	0.22	0.26	0.28
No Assoc	% completed trials	91.6	51.5	74.7	98.2	57.0
	$\bar{U}_M$	96.67	85.40	81.63	82.94	90.00
7	Q_{select}	87.63	72.44	73.35	71.28	77.84
	$\hat{p}$(Tox)	0.44	0.26	0.29	0.31	0.31
	$\hat{p}$(Eff)	0.41	0.25	0.22	0.26	0.31
High Assoc	% completed trials	90.7	51.4	73.6	97.9	60.2
	$\bar{U}_M$	89.91	82.25	78.64	81.34	85.29
7	Q_{select}	82.89	69.74	70.74	71.23	76.20
	$\hat{p}$(Tox)	0.48	0.29	0.32	0.32	0.32
	$\hat{p}$(Eff)	0.37	0.24	0.22	0.25	0.28
No Assoc	% completed trials	90.8	51.4	73.6	97.5	57.3

While the evaluations of DTM2 showed that it is greatly superior to all four comparators, there still remains substantial room for improvement. One obvious, albeit difficult, way to do this would be to account for more than two cycles in settings where a patient may receive three or more cycles of therapy and the dose of an agent is modified adaptively. A very common example is the long-term use of an immunosuppressive drug in organ or stem cell transplant recipients, to reduce the chance of organ rejection or graft-versus-host disease, but long-term use of the immunosuppressant may have severe adverse effects. Physicians use a wide variety of *ad hoc* adaptive rules to do dose adjustments in such settings, and here the use of sound statistical methods, similar to but more general than the design described here, potentially could be very beneficial. A second type of extension would account for more complex but more realistic outcomes, such as combinations of ordinal variables for disease status and toxicity severity (see Lee et al. (2016)), or time-to-event variables. This would require more complex regression models and utility functions. A third extension, mentioned earlier, would account for patient heterogeneity due to prognostic covariates or specific biomarkers targeted by adoptive cell therapies or biological agents, such as tyrosine kinase inhibitors, immune checkpoint inhibitors, or vascular endothelial growth factor receptor inhibitors. This would require constructing covariate-specific or subgroup-specific decision rules, and the resulting designs would account for both patient heterogeneity and multiple treatment cycles. Finally, incorporating any of these phase I-II multi-cycle designs into the phase I-II-III paradigm of Chapple and Thall (2019), with suitable modifications of the model, decision criteria, and group sequential monitoring rules, would lead to what may be regarded as an ideal family of "all in one" designs for deriving optimal decision rules for precision medicine.

Acknowledgments

This research was supported by NIH/NCI grant 5 P30 CA016672 44.

Chapter 5

Agent-Based Modeling in Medical Research—Example in Health Economics

Philippe Saint-Pierre, Romain Demeulemeester, Nadège Costa, Nicolas Savy

5.1 Introduction

"Simulation is nowadays considered to be the third pillar of science, a peer alongside theory and experimentation" (Siegfried, 2014). This is because simulation provides a valuable method for analyzing complex systems, and sometimes it is the only way to do so. In the field of life sciences, simulation is also crucial, although the challenges are greater due to the vast variability and interdependence of the factors involved. A wide range of questions can be explored through simulation, including PK-PD concerns, translational medicine challenges, trial design optimization, sensitivity analysis, and purely simulation-based issues such as Digital Twin and Simulated Placebo arm.

When using a simulation approach, the initial step is often to define virtual patients using a compartmental model. This involves breaking down the human body into submodels of organs and molecules, creating a top-down approach. For instance, the HumMod project utilizes over 1500 equations and 6500 variables to model body fluids, circulation, electrolytes, hormones, metabolism, and skin temperature, among others (`http://hummod.org/`). However, managing such complex models can be challenging and even with a vast number of variables involved, they may still be too simplistic. This is because the strong dependence structure between variables, which is a fundamental aspect of life's diversity, is often difficult to consider.

On the other hand, agent-based models (ABMs), which are based on numerical simulation, can provide a viable alternative (Cuadros et al., 2014; Bilge and Saka, 2006; Nshimyumukiza et al., 2013). ABMs have a wide range of applications in various fields (Railsback and Grimm, 2019). Notably, a standard protocol for describing an ABM has been published in Grimm et al. (2006). While ABMs have been applied extensively in biology (An et al., 2009) and economics (Tesfatsion and Judd, 2006), their applications in medical research are less common. Some examples include drug development (Pombo-Romero et al., 2013) and public health (Maglio and Mabry, 2011). The simulation process for ABMs can be divided into two phases. Firstly, a group of patients, either real or virtual, is considered. Secondly, the outcomes of each patient are simulated over time under predefined scenarios using predictive models, typically referred to as execution models (Holford et al., 2010). Constructing execution models for outcome modeling involves technical work such as modeling techniques, calibration databases, and expert medical knowledge for selecting variables and modeling disease evolution. The agent-based approach provides results in the form of a distribution of outcomes, making it easy to derive prediction intervals at a given risk, while the population-based approach yields a single prediction of the outcome. In Section 5.2, we will describe agent-based models in the context of clinical trials.

Introducing simulation techniques into clinical research is likely one of the most effective ways to improve clinical trials in various stages, such as design optimization, drug development, clinical operations optimization, and monitoring. The In Silico Clinical Trials (ISCT)

DOI: 10.1201/9781003216223-5

strategy, which involves using simulations (in silico) to identify design weaknesses and measure trial performance in a predefined setting while reducing logistical barriers, aims to make the most rational decisions possible regarding clinical development (see Savy et al. (2019) and references). In Section 5.3, we introduce the challenge of In Silico Clinical Trials, which is an application of agent-based models to drug development.

To develop an agent-based model, two key steps must be considered. The first step is to define the patient cohort to be followed, and the second step is to define the execution models involved. The Baseline Data cohort comprises the baseline values of a patient cohort and is realized as a set of covariates. There are two ways to construct this cohort: by using an existing patient cohort or by generating virtual patients. Our focus is on the generation of virtual patients. In this context, several virtual baseline generators have been developed, which involve Monte-Carlo generations of covariate vectors. These generators include the discrete method, continuous method (see Tannenbaum et al. (2006) and references therein), and copulas method (Bedford and Cooke, 2002). In Section 5.4, we present and compare these methods.

The ultimate goal of using exogenous datasets is to learn and calibrate execution models, which are then used to drive an agent-based model towards one or more pre-defined outcomes of interest. An execution model is essentially an Input/Output model, designed to simulate various aspects of the virtual clinical study. A wide range of candidate models can be used as an execution model, including parametric models such as Markov Process, Cox Process, regression models, Bayesian networks, and non-parametric models such as machine learning techniques like Random Forest, XGBoost, Decision Trees, Support Vector Machines (SVM), and deep learning. However, developing an execution model is a research question in its own right, and the issue of prediction error is of paramount importance. The execution model's purpose is to produce simulated data, not just predicted data, which means that the accuracy of the execution model is crucial. We will delve deeper into this issue in Section 5.5. The case study in Section 5.6 provides examples of execution models in the context of health economics.

The paper is structured as follows: In Section 5.2, we discuss the construction of agent-based models in the context of clinical research. Section 5.3 outlines the properties of agent-based modeling for drug development. In Section 5.4, we present several strategies for generating virtual patient cohorts and compare them using a toy example. The issue of prediction errors in execution models is discussed in Section 5.5, and the importance of accounting for these errors is investigated in the same toy example. Section 5.6 presents a study (Demeulemeester et al., 2021) on HIV treatment switching to generics involving an ABM. Finally, in Section 5.7, we draw some conclusions and make recommendations on the use of agent-based modeling in medical research.

5.2 Agent-Based Models in Medical Research

5.2.1 General Schema of an ABM

Agent-based modeling, in the context of medical research, involves mimicking the behavior of a cohort of patients (agents) in virtual medical research using predefined scenarios. Therefore, an agent-based model typically includes the following:

- The "Baseline Cohort" refers to a group of patients whose values are measured at the start of a study. This cohort can either be actual data from an existing group of patients, or it can be simulated using a "Virtual Baseline Generator" (VBG) model. This model aims to generate a set of virtual patient covariates stochastically. The VBG model must adhere to two main constraints: first, it must be consistent with the research protocol being investigated, and second, it must strike a balance between model complexity and realism of the virtual patients. Specifically, the VBG must generate virtual patient data in

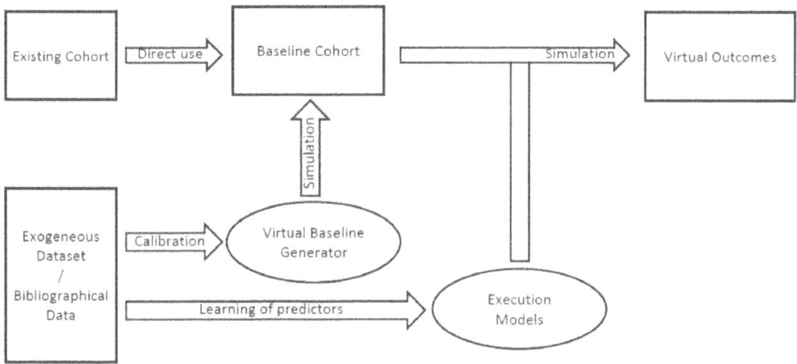

Figure 5.1 *Example of the schema of the simulation design of an ABM for medical research.*

a way that ensures the marginal distributions are consistent with those of the population of interest, and that the correlation structure between covariates is consistent with those of the population of interest. Refer to Section 5.2.3 for more information.

- To enhance and/or enrich a cohort, "Execution Models" are utilized. These models facilitate the evolution through time and completion of the cohort by manipulating the virtual clinical dataset. Execution Models are input/output models which aim to complete or modify the dataset. Several execution models can be implemented, but it's important to consider that they are simulation models rather than solely prediction models. Therefore, it's crucial to account for prediction errors. Further details regarding this point will be discussed in Section 5.2.4.

Agent-based models employ exogenous data to define the VBG and to calibrate or learn the execution models. A generic schema is shown in Figure 5.1.

5.2.2 *What is Agent-Based Modeling for?*

5.2.2.1 *Perform Sensitivity Analyses*

The ABM is a valuable tool for conducting sensitivity analyses of clinical research endpoints. This can be achieved by assessing the performance of a study as a function of various parameters, including patient features, design parameters, and parameters of the execution models. Specifically, the following can be done:

- Modifying patient features by adjusting the marginal distributions of the baseline covariates in the virtual baseline generator.
- Specifying different scenarios for experimental design parameters by defining various parameter sets in the execution models and evaluating trial performance accordingly.
- Assessing the impact of slight modifications to the execution model parameters on trial performance.
- Exploring trial performance for untested execution model parameter values, such as the consequences on trial performance in which a patient is followed for one year but the trial is extended for two years.

5.2.2.2 *Perform Performance Analyses of Predefined Scenarios*

To demonstrate that the difference observed between exposed and unexposed patients is attributable to an intervention, such as a treatment, a common approach is to evaluate a quantity known as the Average Treatment Effect (ATE), which is defined as follows:

$$\text{ATE} = \mathbb{E}\left[Y(1) - Y(0)\right]. \tag{5.1}$$

where for patient i, $Y_i(1)$ is the outcome for patient i exposed and $Y_i(0)$ is the outcome for patient i unexposed. $Y_i(1)$ and $Y_i(0)$ are potential outcomes (Rubin, 1978) and in practice, both of these values cannot be observed simultaneously and ATE cannot be estimated properly. The Average Treatment Effect is usually estimated by

$$\hat{\text{ATE}} = \frac{1}{n_A}\sum_{i=1}^{n_A} Y_i^A - \frac{1}{n_B}\sum_{i=1}^{n_B} Y_i^B$$

where $(Y_i^A, i = 1, \ldots, n_A)$ and $(Y_i^B, i = 1, \ldots, n_B)$ are samples of patients exposed and unexposed, respectively. In the setting of a randomized trial, the quality of this estimation is generally high provided that there are no unmeasured confounders.

In an agent-based model, virtual patients can be assigned to various arms, and in the context of a "digital twin," real patients can be assigned to an additional arm. As a result, the performance of the predefined trial can be accurately evaluated, as the ATE can be directly estimated from (5.1) by:

$$\hat{\text{ATE}} = \frac{1}{n}\sum_{i=1}^{n}(Y_i(1) - Y_i(0)).$$

5.2.3 Baseline Cohort

The initial step in constructing an ABM is to establish a cohort of patients for use in virtual research. There are two primary approaches to achieve this: utilizing an existing cohort of patients or simulating a virtual cohort of patients using a Virtual Baseline Generator. Each approach has its advantages and disadvantages, as previously discussed.

5.2.3.1 Use of an Existing Cohort

The primary advantage of utilizing an existing cohort is that it is realistic and there is no inherent bias in the construction of the cohort. However, it is not possible to modify the population of interest, such as extending the population or specifying a subgroup, without decreasing the sample size. This approach is particularly useful for "digital twin" studies, where the patients from the existing cohort are utilized in virtual research.

5.2.3.2 Use of a Virtual Baseline Generator (VBG)

Using a virtual cohort generated by a Virtual Baseline Generator (VBG) has several advantages and disadvantages compared to using an existing cohort. It allows for easy modifications such as increasing the sample size, specifying a subpopulation or extending the population. However, the quality and realism of the virtual cohort are dependent on the performance of the VBG.

The Virtual Baseline Generator (VBG) involves Monte Carlo generation of a vector of covariates, as detailed in Robert and Casella (2004) and Robert and Casella (2010). However, issues linked to VBG are typical of Monte Carlo generation for multivariate distributions, as discussed in Johnson (1987). Finding a balance between the level of detail for virtual patients and the complexity of the model used to generate them can be challenging, especially since the distributions involved may mix categorical and quantitative variables. The VBG model must satisfy two constraints: the marginal distributions must be consistent with those of the population of interest, and the correlation structure between covariates must also be

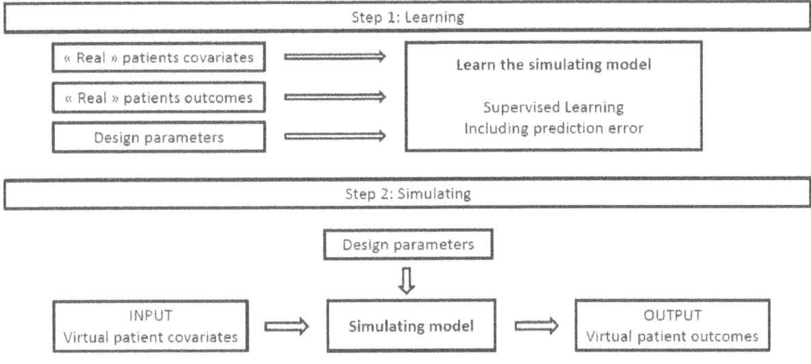

Figure 5.2 *General steps of an execution model.*

consistent. The literature outlines three main approaches: the discrete method (Tannenbaum et al., 2006; Savy et al., 2019), the continuous method (Tannenbaum et al., 2006; Savy et al., 2019), and the Copula method (Bedford and Cooke, 2002). Section 5.4 provides a detailed description of these methods, along with illustrations of their use.

5.2.4 Virtual Outcomes

An execution model is an Input/Output model designed to simulate the course of a virtual clinical trial, as previously discussed. The building process can be divided into two steps. Firstly, a learning step involves a set of real patients' covariates and their outcomes of interest (a learning database). A predictive model of the outcome of interest is calibrated using this learning database. The second step involves simulating the outcome from the patients of interest, whether they are virtual or real, using the model learned in step 1. Figure 5.2 provides a general illustration of an execution model.

There are many different execution models that can be used for simulating virtual clinical trials, ranging from linear regression to machine learning to Markov processes. In order to ensure that the construction of an ABM is versatile, each of these models can be improved separately. This property is known as modularity, and it is a key aspect of building and improving ABMs. It is important to note that these models rely on parameters, which can be categorized into three groups: patient-related parameters, model-related tuning parameters, and design-related parameters. These parameters can be specified as deterministic values or as distributions in a Bayesian framework. The user can choose to fix certain parameters using a Human Machine Interface, which defines the scenario under which the trial is conducted. Alternatively, calibration parameters can be estimated from databases and then fixed during the simulation.

5.3 ABM and Drug Development: In Silico Clinical Trials (ISCT) Challenge

Simulation techniques have been utilized in drug development for approximately three decades. In 2009, Brindley and Dunn demonstrated the benefits of simulation techniques in their study cited in Brindley and Dunn (2009). These benefits include an increased likelihood of achieving study objectives, improved patient safety, reduced study duration, decreased risk of protocol deviations, and prevention of inconclusive outcomes. Although the integration of simulation in clinical research appears to be a logical step, the existing literature does not support this notion. Prior to 2000, as described in Holford et al. (2000) and confirmed by reviews conducted between 2000 and 2010 (Holford et al., 2010) and 2010-2015 (Savy et al., 2018), there was little impact or usage of simulation techniques. This paradox may be attributed to reporting bias, as pharmaceutical companies may conduct investigations that are not published due to confidentiality reasons.

It is worth noting that regulatory agencies are actively promoting the use of simulation in drug development, as cited in Nuventra (2018). For instance, in 2011, the FDA released a strategic plan on Advancing Regulatory Science, which included modeling and simulation as important aspects of their strategy in four out of eight science priority areas (`https://www.fda.gov/media/81109/download`). In a presentation given by Dr. Tina Morrison, Chair of FDA's Agency-wide Modeling and Simulation Working Group and Regulatory Advisor of Computational Modeling for FDA's Office of Device Evaluation, on August 9, 2018 (`https://collaboration.fda.gov/p4r7q3qweuv/`), she provided an overview of current modeling and simulation methodologies and discussed the potential of in silico clinical trials. Similarly, over the past decade, the European Medicines Agency (EMA) has organized several workshops on modeling and simulation, aiming to integrate these techniques in the development and regulatory assessment of medicines. In the 2011 EMA-EFPIA (European Federation of Pharmaceutical Industries and Associations) Workshop on Modelling and Simulation, European regulators agreed to harmonize good modeling and simulation practices and maintain open communication across all parties. To achieve this, the EMA established the Modelling and Simulation Working Group (MSWG) and published the MID3 (Model-Informed Drug Discovery and Development) good practices paper in 2016 (Marshall et al., 2016; Manolis et al., 2017).

Agent-based modeling has led to the development of In Silico Clinical Trials (ISCT), which involve the use of virtual or real patients to simulate their behavior in a virtual clinical trial to evaluate the feasibility and success probability of a clinical trial. This is achieved by using the vast amount of information available on patients, the drug of interest, and trial design in order to build a stochastic model mimicking the course of a clinical trial. In the context of In Silico Clinical Trials (ISCT), virtual patients are represented by a set of covariates that reflect the clinical design (including the criteria for inclusion and exclusion) and the factors known to be associated with the clinical outcomes of interest. Regardless of the study's objective, the general approach is to use exogeneous datasets to train or calibrate a predictive model, which is then applied to an agent-based model to simulate one or more specific outcomes of interest. Examples of execution models include the evolution of Baseline's parameters over time, as demonstrated in Demeulemeester et al. (2021) and Section 5.6, as well as the virtual outcome generator, disease progression model (Cook and Bies, 2016), side effect model, drop-out model, and patients recruitment model (Mijoule et al., 2012; Minois et al., 2017). A wide range of candidate execution models is available, including parametric models such as Markov processes, Cox processes, regression models, and Bayesian networks, as well as non-parametric models such as machine learning techniques like random forests, XGBoost, decision trees, support vector machines (SVM), and deep learning. Developing an execution model is a research question in itself. Figure 5.3 provides an example of a simulation schema for an ISCT involving an execution model that completes the dataset with virtual outcomes at different times and an execution model that introduces adverse events to the dataset.

ISCT enables the performance of sensitivity analyses of clinical trial endpoints by evaluating trial performance as a function of various parameters, including patient features, design parameters, and parameters of the execution models.

- Modifying patient features involves challenging the inclusion/exclusion criteria of a trial.
- Specifying design parameters can include determining the duration of patients' follow-up or the number of centers involved.
- Assessing the impact of small changes in execution model parameters, such as quantifying the effect of a given variation in patients' recruitment rate on trial duration, is also important.

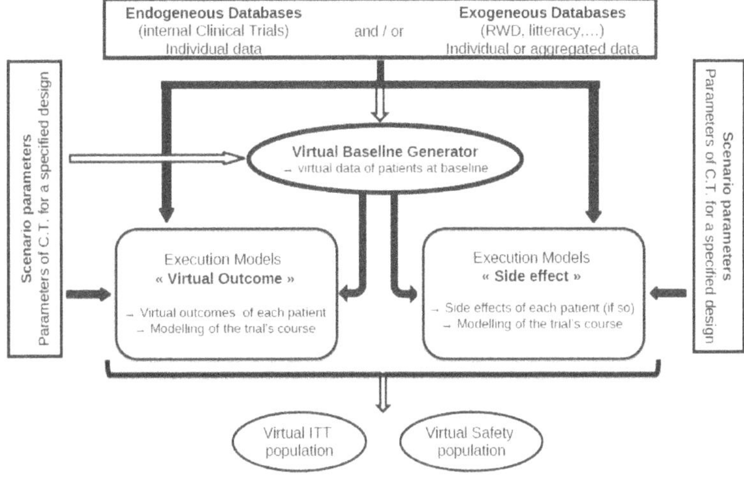

Figure 5.3 *Example of an schema of simulation design of an ISCT.*

- Exploring trial performances for untested values of execution model parameters is another strategy.

It is important to note that these two last strategies are much easier to investigate using parametric execution models than non-parametric ones.

5.4 Virtual Baseline Generator

If one knows the joint distribution of the covariates, denoted as $f_{(C^1,\ldots,C^K)}$ for simplicity, then generating data is simply a matter of Monte Carlo simulation. However, the generation of meaningful data relies on available information about the covariates. This information can be obtained from bibliographical data or from an existing historical database. When dealing with bibliographical data, the parameters of the covariate distribution are considered to be population parameters, while in historical data, these parameters are estimations of population parameters. Although bibliographical data are more relevant, only marginal distributions or summaries of marginal distributions can often be obtained. Assuming covariates are independent is typically the best we can do, which is unsatisfactory. From a historical database, the correlation structure may be estimated, but the question of how to estimate parameters with sufficient precision arises. The reconstruction of a database refers to generating a database with marginal distributions and correlation structures similar to the original ones.

In the following discussion, the k-th covariate is denoted as C^k (where k ranges from 1 to K), and the values of this covariate for the i-th patient are denoted as c_i^k (where i ranges from 1 to n). For simplicity, we use $\vec{c}_i$ to refer to the vector of covariate values for patient i. Covariate C can be either continuous (represented as ${}^cC$) or categorical (represented as ${}^dC$). In this section, we assume that continuous covariates follow a normal distribution, but they can follow any other distribution with a change of variable.

5.4.1 Discrete Method

The discrete method involves splitting the joint distribution of continuous and discrete variables by conditioning. To simplify notation, we can write this as:

$$f_{(C^1,\ldots,C^K)} = f_{(({}^cC^1,\ldots,{}^cC^L)|({}^dC^{L+1},\ldots,{}^dC^K))} \times f_{({}^dC^{L+1},\ldots,{}^dC^K)}$$

5.4.1.1 *Calibrating Method*

The calibration of the model involves two steps:

- First, we fit the distribution of the discrete variables $({}^dC^{L+1}, \ldots, {}^dC^K)$ by estimating the proportion of each modality.
- Second, we fit the conditional distribution of the continuous variables $({}^cC^1, \ldots, {}^cC^L)$ given the categorical variables, by estimating the mean vector and variance-covariance matrix for each configuration of the categorical variables.

5.4.1.2 *Generating Dataset*

To simulate a database of size n, we perform the following algorithm n times:

- Draw a configuration with the probabilities estimated in step 1.
- Given this configuration, draw the remaining values from the multivariate normal distribution estimated in step 2.

It is worth noting that this problem can be split into groups of independent covariates, which can be calibrated and simulated separately. However, when the parameters of the distributions are estimated from data, the discrete method is less efficient, especially when there are a large number of covariates that mix continuous and categorical variables. This is because the technique requires many parameter estimations, and when there are many categorical covariates, the estimation of the parameters of the continuous covariates may be poor due to a small number of data for several modalities.

5.4.2 *Continuous Method*

The continuous Method is an approach introduced in Tannenbaum et al. (2006) to generate databases directly from the population parameters. This method assumes that all covariates follow a normal distribution.

5.4.2.1 *Learning/Calibrating Method*

The calibration step in the continuous Method involves fitting a multivariate normal distribution for all the covariates, regardless of their type. For categorical variables, a recoding of the variable may be used to convert it into numerical data.

5.4.2.2 *Generating Dataset*

To simulate a database of size n, the process involves drawing n sets of values $(u_i^1, \ldots, u_i^K)_{i=1,\ldots,n}$ from a multivariate normal distribution $N(\vec{\mu}, \Sigma)$, which was estimated during the learning step.

- For a continuous covariate, we simply set ${}^cc^k = u^k$ for $k = 1, \ldots, L$.
- For a categorical covariate with M modalities, denoted ${}^dC^k$, we use critical values to generate values. The critical values are defined as follows:

$$\begin{cases} CrV_m^k = \mu_k + \Sigma_{k,k}\phi^{-1}(\sum_{i=1}^m p_i), & 1 \le m \le M-1 \\ CrV_M^k = +\infty \\ CrV_0^k = -\infty \end{cases}$$

  where $(p_i;\ 1 \le i \le M)$ are the proportions of each modality of the categorical covariate, μ_k and $\Sigma_{k,k}$ are the parameters of the normal distribution, ϕ denotes the cumulative function of standard normal distribution.
  Finally, we define ${}^dc^k$ as follows: ${}^dc^k = m$ if and only if $CrV_{m-1}^k < u_i^k \le CrV_m^k$.

The continuous method is an attractive alternative, even though the assumption of multivariate Gaussian distribution may be too restrictive, particularly for capturing multi-modal distributions. The comparison between the discrete and continuous methods, using bibliographic data, has been investigated in Tannenbaum et al. (2006), assuming normally distributed continuous covariates. In this context, the calibration step is not necessary. In Savy et al. (2018, 2019), attention is focused on the performance of these techniques in a setting closer to practical scenarios, where a historical database is available. The objective of the approach is to generate a realistic copy of the historical database, where the marginal distributions are identical, and the correlation structure between the covariates is preserved.

5.4.3 Copula Method

5.4.3.1 Copula

The Copula approach is a practical and powerful tool for constructing multivariate distributions. Copulas aim to describe the dependence structure between a group of random variables, and their specification can be done independently of the marginal distributions. Formally, a copula is a multidimensional cumulative distribution function (CDF) that links the margins of a vector of random variables $\mathbf{X} = (X_1, \ldots, X_d) \in \mathbb{R}^d$ to its joint distribution. Let $F_i(x_i) = \mathbb{P}[X_i \leq x_i]$ be the continuous CDF of X_i for $i = 1, \ldots, d$. According to Sklar's Theorem (Sklar, 1996), every multivariate distribution F_θ can be written as

$$F_\theta(\mathbf{x}) = \mathcal{C}_\theta\left(F_1(x_1), \ldots, F_d(x_d)\right), \tag{5.2}$$

for some appropriate d-dimensional copula $\mathcal{C}_\theta$ with parameter $\theta \in \Theta$. If all marginal distributions are continuous functions, then there exists a unique copula satisfying

$$\mathcal{C}_\theta\left(u_1, \ldots, u_d\right) = F_\theta\left(F_1^{-1}(u_1), \ldots, F_d^{-1}(u_d)\right)$$

where $u_j = F_j(x_j)$. For F_θ absolutely continuous with strictly increasing marginal distributions, one can derive the joint density of $\mathbf{X}$ from (5.2):

$$f_\theta(\mathbf{x}) = \left[\prod_{i=1}^{d} f_k(x_k)\right] c_\theta\left(F_1(x_1), \ldots, F_d(x_d)\right),$$

where c_θ denotes the copula density and $f_i(x_i)$, $i = 1, ..., d$ correspond to the marginal densities.

Many parametric copula families are available and are based on different dependence structures (Nelsen, 2007). However, most of these families are limited to bi-dimensional dependencies, although some can be extended to higher dimensions. A first and naive approach for modeling the dependence structure is assuming a Gaussian copula. In this case, the problem is reduced to determining the input correlation matrix. Such multivariate Gaussian assumption is however very restrictive. Multivariate Archimedean copulas can also be used to describe asymmetric tail dependencies. However, the same copula family describes the dependence among all the pairs, which is not flexible enough. Since the choice of copula has a strong impact on the output distribution, we will consider a flexible approach setting by modeling the input distribution using regular vine copulas (R-vines). R-vine copulas (Joe, 1994) can overcome the constraint of bi-dimensionality and the lack of flexibility of multidimensional copulas by describing multidimensional dependencies by combining multiple pair-copulas.

5.4.3.2 R-vine Copula

In high-dimensional settings, representing multi-dimensional dependence structures is a difficult task. However, a probabilistic method for constructing multivariate distribution functions using pair-copulas has been developed by Joe (1996), providing a flexible approach for high-dimensional copula construction, though not unique. To efficiently describe all possible constructions, Bedford and Cooke (2001) introduced regular vines (R-vines), a graphical tool based on a sequence of trees that decomposes the multivariate probability distribution in a specific way.

For the following definition, we omit the use of θ in f_θ, F_θ and c_θ for the sake of simplicity. The Sklar's theorem states that a copula C is unique and admits a density c if the margins $F_1, \ldots, F_d$ are continuous. Using the chain rule, the joint density f associated with the random vector $\mathbf{X} = (X_1, \ldots, X_d)$ can be written as

$$f(x_1, \ldots, x_d) = c(F_1(x_1), \ldots, F_d(x_d)) \times \prod_{i=1}^{d} f_i(x_i), \tag{5.3}$$

where $f_i(x_i)$, $i = 1, ..., d$, correspond to the marginal densities. By recursive conditioning, the joint density can also be written as

$$\begin{aligned} f(x_1, \ldots, x_d) = {} & f_d(x_d) \times f_{d-1/d}(x_{d-1}|x_d) \times f_{d-2/d-1,d}(x_{d-2}|x_{d-1}, x_d) \\ & \times \cdots \times f_{1/2,\ldots,d}(x_1|x_2, \ldots, x_d), \end{aligned} \tag{5.4}$$

which is unique, up to a re-labelling of the variables.

For example, in a case of three variables, one possible decomposition of the joint density can be written as

$$f(x_1, x_2, x_3) = f_1(x_1) \times f_{2/1}(x_2|x_1) \times f_{3/2,1}(x_3|x_2, x_1) \tag{5.5}$$

The conditional densities can be rewritten using Bayes formula

$$\begin{aligned} f_{3/1,2}(x_3|x_1, x_2) &= \frac{f_{3,1/2}(x_3, x_1|x_2)}{f_{1/2}(x_1|x_2)} \\ &= \frac{1}{f_{1/2}(x_1|x_2)} \times c_{1,3|2}(F_{1/2}(x_1|x_2), F_{3/2}(x_3|x_2)) \\ &\qquad \times f_{1/2}(x_1|x_2) \times f_{3/2}(x_3|x_2) \\ &= c_{1,3|2}(F_{1/2}(x_1|x_2), F_{3/2}(x_3|x_2)) \times f_{3/2}(x_3|x_2) \end{aligned} \tag{5.6}$$

where the second equality comes from Sklar's theorem. By developing $f(x_3|x_2)$ in (5.6) in the same way, we find that

$$\begin{aligned} f_{3/1,2}(x_3|x_1, x_2) = {} & c_{1,3|2}(F_{1/2}(x_1|x_2), F_{3/2}(x_3|x_2)) \\ & \times c_{2,3}(F_2(x_2), F_3(x_3)) \\ & \times f_3(x_3) \end{aligned} \tag{5.7}$$

By doing the same procedure for $f(x_2|x_1)$ in (5.5), one can derive a pair-copula decomposition for the joint density

$$\begin{aligned} f(x_1, x_2, x_3) = {} & f_1(x_1) \times f_2(x_2) \times f_3(x_3) \\ & \times c_{1,2}(F_1(x_1), F_2(x_2)) \times c_{2,3}(F_2(x_2), F_3(x_3)) \\ & \times c_{1,3/2}(F_{1/2}(x_1/x_2), F_{3/2}(x_3/x_2)) \end{aligned} \tag{5.8}$$

Such representation of the joint density in terms of pair-copulas and marginal density is called the pair-copula construction (PCC). The resulting decomposition offers a very flexible way to construct high-dimensional copulas and to model flexible dependence structures

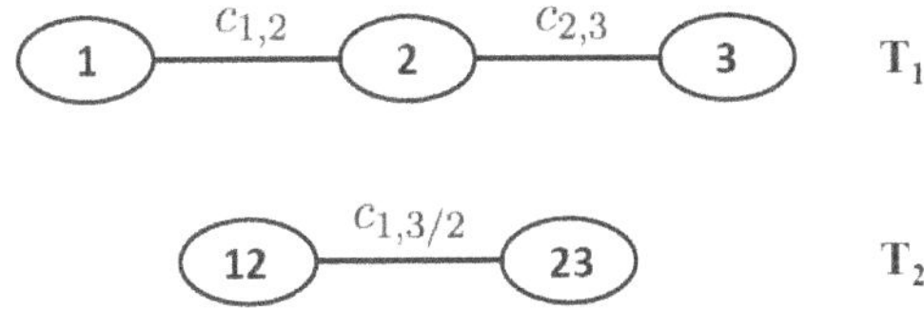

Figure 5.4 *R-vine structure of a dimension $d = 5$ problem.*

using only bivariate copulas. However, the decomposition is not unique. Indeed, (5.3) has numerous decomposition forms and it increases significantly with d.

To help organize them, a graphical model called regular vine (R-vine) was introduced in Bedford and Cooke (2001, 2002) and detailed in Kurowicka and Cooke (2006). Each of these sequences of trees gives a specific way of decomposing the density. A R-vine describes a d-dimensional PCC is a sequence of linked trees where the nodes and edges correspond to the $d(d-1)/2$ pair-copulas. According to Definition 8 in Bedford and Cooke (2001), an R-vine consists of $d-1$ trees $T_1, \ldots, T_{d-1}$ with several constraints. Each tree T_i is composed of $d-i+1$ nodes which are linked by $d-i$ edges for $i = 1, \ldots, d-1$. A node in a tree T_i must be an edge in the tree T_{i-1}, for $i = 2, \ldots, d-1$. Two nodes in a tree T_i can be joined if their respective edges in tree T_{i-1} share a common node, for $i = 2, \ldots, d-1$. The pair copula in the first tree characterizes pairwise unconditional dependencies, while the pair copula in higher-order trees model the conditional dependency between two variables given a set of variables. The number of conditioning variables grows with the tree order. Figure 5.4 illustrates a specific R-vine associated to a density decomposition in dimension 5. Note that a PCC where all trees have a path-like structure defines the D-vine subclass while the star-like structures correspond to the C-vine subclass (Bedford and Cooke, 2001).

5.4.3.3 Discrete Variables and Mixed Case

In practice, the covariates are of mixed nature with discrete and continuous variables. The extension of the PCC to the discrete case has been studied by Panagiotelis et al. (2012). Finally, in the discrete case, the calculations are the same as in the continuous case using probabilities instead of densities. In this case, techniques based on discrete differentiation should be used instead of derivatives. The analogue of conditional densities is pointwise conditional probabilities. The amplitude of the jumps must be evaluated at all considered values. The mixed case with discrete and continuous variables has been studied in Stöber et al. (2015). The results in the continuous and in the discrete case can be combined to derive the pairwise decomposition in the mixed case.

5.4.3.4 Learning/Calibrating Method

The calibration of an R-vine to a multivariate distribution consists of the following steps:

- selecting the tree structure,
- selecting a copula family for each pair-copula in the decomposition,
- estimating the parameter for each pair copula.

In Aas et al. (2009), an approach for selecting an R-vine model based on maximum likelihood estimation is proposed. Other approaches, such as sequential estimation (Kurowicka, 2011; Dissmann et al., 2013), truncation (Aas et al., 2012), and Bayesian estimation (Gruber and Czado, 2015), have also been proposed to select R-vines. Most recent developments, particularly those concerning the extension to the mixed case (discrete and continuous variables), are implemented in the library *vinecopulib* available in R and Python. The R package *rvinecopulib* (Nagler and Vatter, 2019) was used to calibrate the R-vine copula, with maximum likelihood estimation and AIC selection criterion considered.

5.4.3.5 Generating Dataset

Simulating a database of K covariates of size n involves generating n values $(u_i^1, ..., u_i^K)_{i=1,...,n}$ from independent uniform distributions. These uniform marginals are then transformed into the copula sample using the R-vine model. The resulting $n \times K$ matrix of simulated data from the R-vine copula model represents uniform variables, which must be transformed back to their original scales. To do this, the empirical distributions of the original data and their pseudo-inverse are used to transform the uniform variables to their original scales.

5.4.4 A Toy Example

5.4.4.1 Pima Indians Diabetes Dataset

As an illustrative example, consider an extract of the "Pima Indians Diabetes Dataset" which involves predicting the onset of diabetes within 5 years in Pima Indians based on their medical details. It is a binary (2-class) classification problem where the outcome of interest is the binary (Yes - No) variable "Diabetes". For this example, we consider a random subset of 392 patients from the dataset. The covariates in this subset include both qualitative and quantitative variables:

- Have you ever been pregnant? (Yes - No).
- Body mass index (≤ 25, $]25;35]$, > 35).
- Plasma glucose concentration 2 hours after an oral glucose tolerance test.
- Diastolic blood pressure (mm Hg).
- Triceps skinfold thickness (mm).
- 2-Hour serum insulin (mu U/ml).
- Diabetes pedigree function.
- Age (year).

5.4.4.2 Virtual Patients Simulations

The effectiveness of the three simulation approaches can be visually evaluated by comparing the marginal distributions of the simulated variables with those of the original data. Additionally, the pairwise correlation between variables and their correlation with the prognosis can also be compared to that of the original data. Figures 5.5 and 5.6 illustrate the marginal distributions and correlations for the variables *Glucose* and *Skin thickness*, and the variables *Blood pressure* and *Age*, respectively.

According to the findings from Figure 5.5, it appears that the discrete approach is inadequate in capturing the true marginal distribution and the strong correlation between *Glucose* and *Skin thickness*. In contrast, the continuous approach yields consistent results, indicating that the Gaussian assumption is reasonable for this particular analysis. Additionally, the Copula approach appears to be the most efficient method in terms of both marginal distribution and correlation.

Figure 5.6 confirms the conclusion derived from Figure 5.5. Although the continuous method yields better correlation recovery, the original data's marginal distribution and scatter plot are more significant. Surprisingly, the discrete approach does not perform well. Gaussian parameter estimation may suffer when a covariate is poorly balanced.

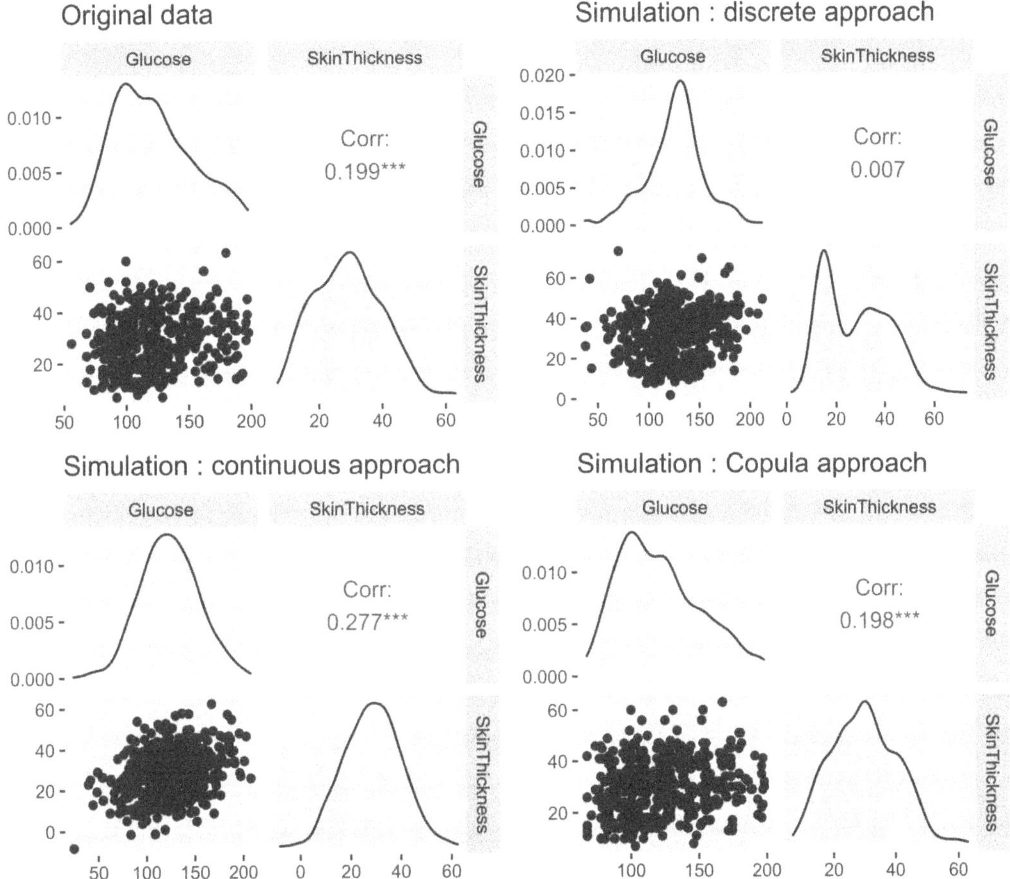

Figure 5.5 *Marginal distribution, correlation and scatter plot of variables Glucose and Skin thickness for the original data and simulated data using the discrete, the continuous and the Copula approaches.*

5.5 Virtual Outcomes

5.5.1 Discussion on the Data

There is a wide range of models available for executing models, including parametric models such as Markov, Cox, linear, logistic, and non-parametric models such as machine learning. The primary difference between these two approaches is that parametric models are calibrated based on data and assumptions, while non-parametric models are entirely data-driven. There are numerous sources of data that can be used, such as completed clinical trials, ongoing clinical trials, and real-world databases with varying levels of quality and accuracy. The quality of the execution model can vary significantly depending on the database used for calibration.

Parametric models face a primary challenge in the estimation of parameters using the available data. The results are more reliable with larger databases, as the inference is better. However, if there is an insufficient amount of data available, it is still possible to make stronger assumptions on the model to simplify it. Another advantage of parametric models is the ability to incorporate data from existing literature or expert knowledge, as well as to fix a value and perform sensitivity analysis.

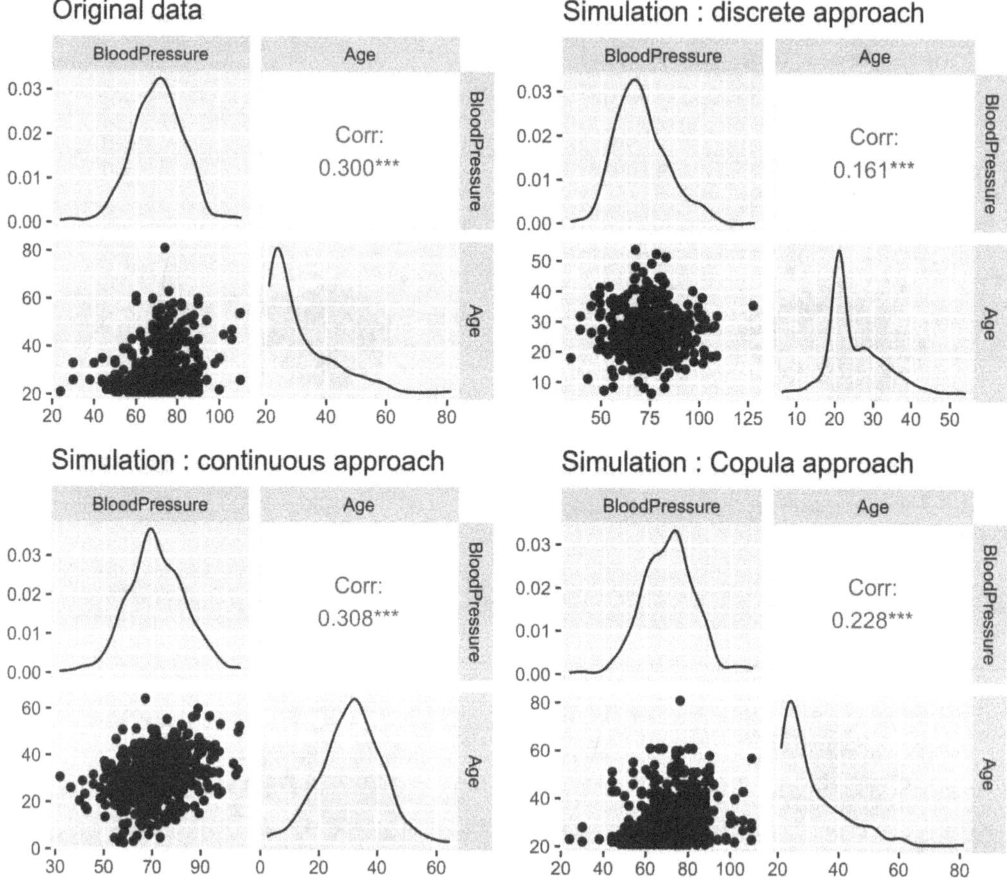

Figure 5.6 *Marginal distribution, correlation and scatter plot of variables Blood pressure and Age for the original data and simulated data using the discrete, the continuous and the Copula approaches. Simulations are executed by either adding or not adding an error in the prediction of the Prognostic variable.*

Non-parametric models face the primary challenge of relying solely on the data-driven approach. Without data, it is not possible to consider a model, and with data, the model is highly sensitive to the quantity and structure of the database. The quality of prediction is linked to the structure of the database, as the model learns from the explored data. If the database does not explore certain values, the prediction associated with those values will be poor or not available. For example, if there is no information on young people (< 30 years old) in the learning database, the predictor will not make any predictions for young people.

Regardless of the model's nature, a common question is the portability of the data. Is it realistic to learn a model (parametric or non-parametric) from a dataset involving patients who are completely different from the patients to be included in the agent-based model, for example, learning from American patients for a European study? To overcome this issue, various algorithms such as the OT-algorithm (Garès et al., 2020) may be of interest.

5.5.2 Discussion on the Generators

The output of an execution model is obtained through a Monte Carlo simulation that considers the chosen model and the values of all the involved parameters. It is crucial to keep in mind that the aim of an execution model is to simulate an outcome and not just to predict it. This is an important point because the model assumptions for simulation are typically stronger than those for prediction. It requires a model not only with good predictive performance but also a model for the error of prediction. It is important to note that confusion between prediction and simulation can lead to an underestimation of the error, making it easier for a factor's effect to be significant.

5.5.3 *Back to the Toy Example*

5.5.3.1 *Virtual Outcome Simulations*

The outcome of interest in the original data is a binary variable, "Diabetes" (yes or no). We can consider subgroups of participants who satisfy "Diabetes = Yes" and "Diabetes = No" separately, and a model can be estimated from the original data to explain the outcome. This model can then be used to simulate the outcome of interest for virtual patients. In this case, a Random Forest algorithm is learned from the original data.

To generate virtual patients, three simulation methods are used, and a set of 500 virtual patients are randomly generated. The corresponding outcome is predicted using the Random Forest algorithm, with and without accounting for the error of prediction. To take the prediction error into account, the predicted value is generated using the confusion matrix of the Random Forest prediction on the original data. For each simulation approach, 100 datasets are simulated together with their *Prognostic* variables (the outcome).

5.5.3.2 *Comparison of Simulation Approaches*

It is possible to evaluate the different simulation approaches by comparing the p-values of the association test between one variable and the prognosis variable in the original dataset and in the simulated dataset. For each simulation approach, the p-values of the association test were evaluated for each dataset (Chi-2 test for categorical variables and Student's t-test for quantitative variables). Figures 5.7, 5.8 and 5.9 provide boxplot and jitter plot of the p-values according to the three simulation approaches for variables *Pregnancy*, *Blood pressure* and *Insulin* respectively. Results are provided in two cases depending on whether the prediction error (or noise) has been added to the simulated *Prognostic* variable.

The p-value obtained for the Chi-2 test between *Pregnancy* and *Prognostic* in the original dataset is approximately 1, indicating the absence of any relationship (Figure 5.7). While the continuous and copula approaches provide consistent results, the discrete method is less reliable as the median p-value is the weakest and significant when simulating data without adding noise. Additionally, there is a considerable variation in the p-values obtained for each simulation run for each approach. In some cases, p-values are significant even when there is no apparent relationship in the original dataset. Therefore, it is crucial to simulate multiple datasets and carefully select the most appropriate one.

Figure 5.8 shows a situation where there is a significant relationship between *Blood pressure* and *Prognostic* ($p = 0.00021$), which is accurately identified and recovered by all three simulation approaches. However, although the median p-value is significant ($p < 0.05$) for all three approaches, around 20% of the simulation runs yield non-significant p-values.

Figure 5.9 presents p-values in the case of a very strong association between *Insulin* and *Prognosis* in the original data. Continuous and Copula methods performed well since there are almost no p-values greater than 0.05. However, in this case, the discrete method fails to recover the association since the median of the p-values is not significant.

After comparing the three simulation approaches, it appears that the discrete method may not be suitable for this application, possibly due to the unbalanced situation. Although the continuous method relies on the strict Gaussian assumption, its results are still acceptable in this case, perhaps due to the unimodal distribution of the marginal distribution. However, the Copula approach appears to provide the most promising and relevant results.

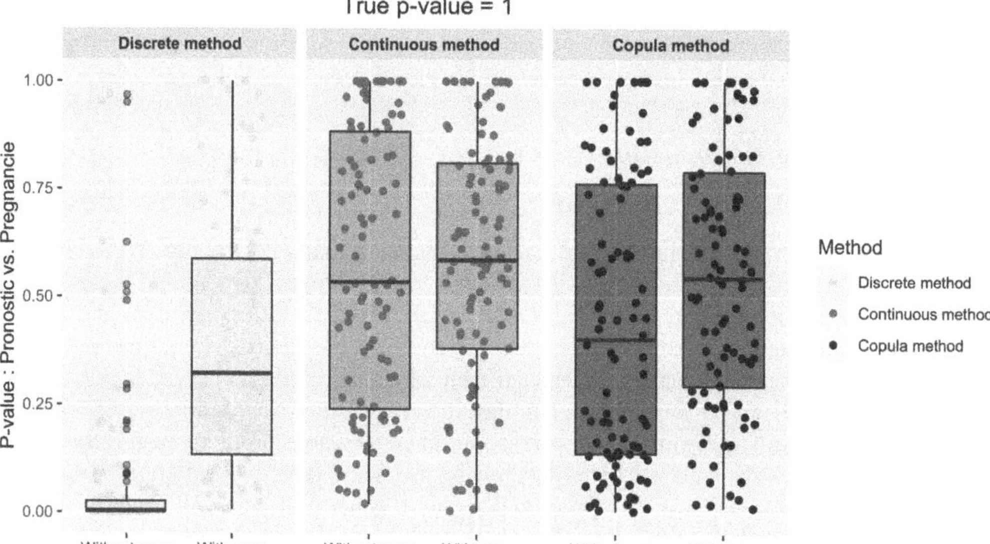

Figure 5.7 *Simulation of* 100 *datasets of* 500 *observations each were performed using the discrete, the continuous and the Copula approaches. For each dataset, the p-value using Chi-2 test between Prognosis variable and Pregnancy were computed and reported using boxplot and jitter plot. The p-value observed in the original data is given in the title. Simulations are performed by either adding or not adding an error in the prediction of the Prognostic variable.*

It is worth noting that the discrepancies between the original data and the simulated data could be due to errors in simulating the virtual patients as well as errors in simulating the outcome, which is the same across all three methods.

5.6 Example in Health Economics

5.6.1 *Context*

In 2014, it was estimated that there were 6,600 new cases of Human Immunodeficiency Virus (HIV) and 156,600 people living with HIV in France, of whom 77% were receiving AntiRetroViral treatment (ARV) (Supervie and Ekouevi, 2014). As ARV therapies became more effective, HIV became a chronic and expensive disease. In 2009, the French Health Insurance (FHI) estimated the direct costs of HIV to be 1.1 billion euros under the Long Term Disease (LTD) scheme, which covers a large portion of disease-related costs (Trapero-Bertran and Oliva-Moreno, 2014). This amounts to 13,000 euros per patient per year, with ARV treatments accounting for 71% of these costs (Caisse Nationale d'Assurance Maladie, 2009). Currently, generic pharmaceutical products account for more than half of the total volume of pharmaceutical products used worldwide, but only 18% of the total pharmaceutical market value (Sheppard, 2018). In France, the proportion of generics sold in the total medicines market was just over 30% in 2014 (Statistica, 2018). From 2012 to 2016, only four ARV generics were available, but in 2017, three new combo generics were launched and are more commonly used. The upcoming years will provide an opportunity to improve efficiency in the allocation of constrained resources as new ARV generics become available and patents for other molecules expire.

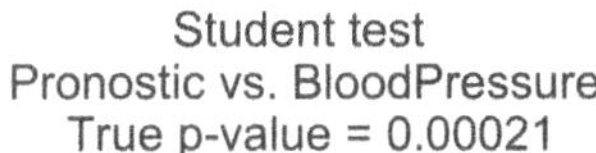

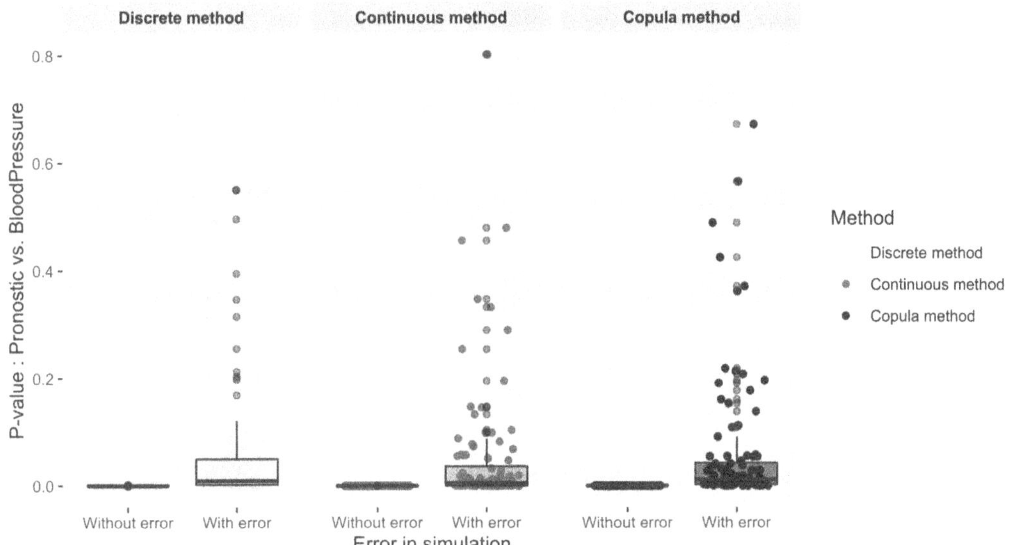

Figure 5.8 *Simulation of* 100 *datasets of* 500 *observations, each were performed using the discrete, the continuous and the Copula approaches. For each dataset, the p-value using Student's t-test between Prognosis variable and Blood pressure were computed and reported using boxplot and jitter plot. The p-value observed in the original data is presented in the title. Simulations are performed by either adding or not adding an error in the prediction of the Prognostic variable.*

Previous studies have conducted limited evaluations of the economic impact of generic drug arrivals (Hill et al., 2014; Restelli et al., 2015). Most of these studies have utilized population-based approaches to predict cost variations in budget impact analyses, which assume average patient behavior and do not consider the inter-patient variability of the different parameters influencing the model. Consequently, such approaches yield punctual predictions of cost variations arising from switching to generics. In Demeulemeester et al. (2021), which is summarized in Section 5.6, the authors developed an ABM to investigate the economic impact of switching to generic HIV medications. Each patient is represented as a vector of covariates that includes information on demographics, medical status, and treatments. Given these covariates, the behavior of each individual over time is simulated using execution models that involve various Markov models mimicking the update of covariates over time, the update of treatments, and the patient's comorbidity status. Each model uses two types of parameters: fixed parameters according to a predefined scenario and calibration parameters estimated from the data (execution model parameters). By simulating individual life trajectories, treatment costs are evaluated under two scenarios: conversion to generics (according to a predefined scheme) and no conversion to generics, enabling the evaluation of differential costs. To ensure the simulation's relevance, scenarios must be set based on fixed parameters, especially the mode of conversion to generics (i.e., marketing authorization date of the generics, penetration rate, tariffs, etc.).

This ABM is based on observational data from the real world, ensuring that the outcomes are relevant to the context of the French investigation. This approach allows for the construction of predictive intervals and for sensitivity analyses of outcomes of interest to the models' parameters. The full results, along with their health economic interpretation, are discussed in Demeulemeester et al. (2021). However, to illustrate the relevance of this

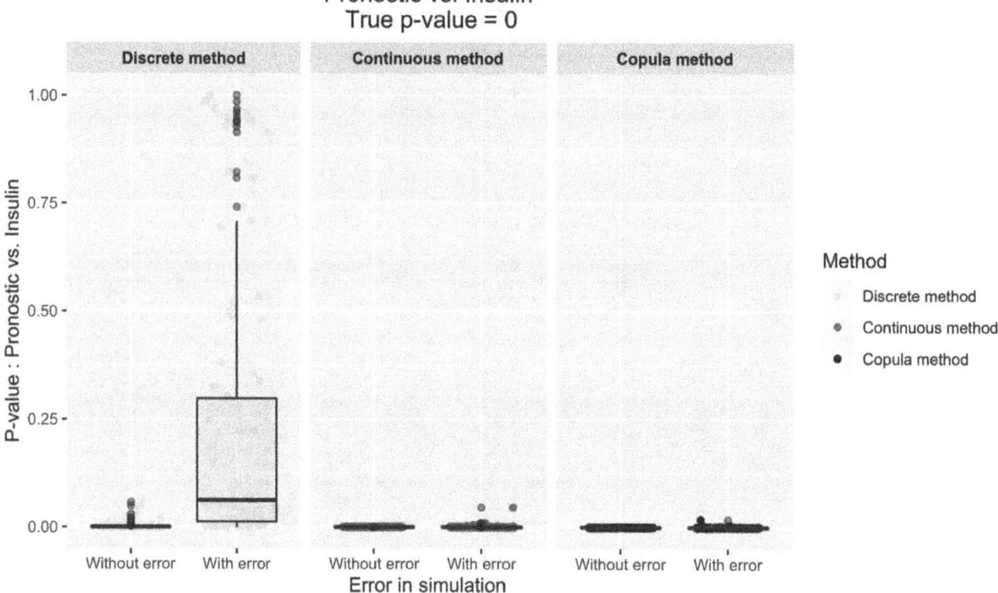

Figure 5.9 *Simulation of* 100 *datasets of* 500 *observations, each were performed using the discrete, the continuous and the Copula approaches. For each dataset, the p-value using Student's t-test between Prognosis variable and Insulin were computed and reported using boxplot and jitter plot. The p-value observed in the original data is presented in the title.*

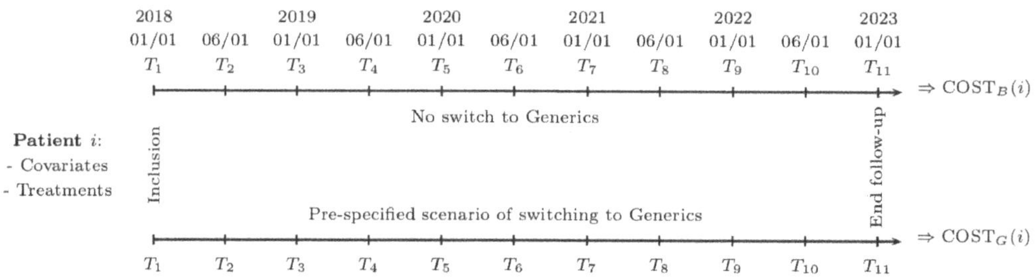

Figure 5.10 *Illustration of the patient's follow-up.*

approach, the impact of the penetration rate on the differential costs is presented in Section 5.6.6.

5.6.2 General Statement of the Agent-Based Model

Let us examine groups of patients who are monitored at six-month intervals over a period of five years, as is standard medical practice. The follow-up period is represented by the set $\{T_u : u = 1, \ldots, 11\}$, and a visual depiction of this timeline can be seen in Figure 5.10.

We can represent the data for patient i at times T_u as a vector $(\texttt{PATIENT}(u, i), \texttt{TREAT}(u, i))$, where $\texttt{PATIENT}(u, i)$ represents the patient-specific covariates at time T_u and $\texttt{TREAT}(u, i)$ represents the treatment-related covariates at time T_u. This splitting between patients covariates and treatments covariates is only motivated by notational convenience.

Notice that ($\texttt{PATIENT}(1,i), \texttt{TREAT}(1,i)$) contains patient i's baseline data and serves as the initial values for the execution models used to simulate the patient's trajectory.

To simulate the trajectory of each patient i, execution models are used to update the patient's characteristics and treatment. Two trajectories are followed for patient i: one trajectory assumes no switch to generic drugs, resulting in a cost denoted as $\text{COST}_B(i)$, while the other trajectory assumes a pre-specified scenario of switching to generic drugs, resulting in a cost denoted as $\text{COST}_G(i)$. In order to estimate the differential cost, for each time T_u, $u \geq 2$, the algorithm is split into four main steps:

Step 1: Update the patient-specific covariates: $\texttt{PATIENT}(u,i)$ is updated based on $\texttt{PATIENT}(u-1,i)$.

Step 2: Update the patient's treatment: $\texttt{TREAT}(u,i)$ is updated based on $\texttt{PATIENT}(u,i)$, the patient's covariates at time T_u.

Step 3: Update the patient's status, considering the possibility of the patient's death.

Step 4: Assess the costs for each scenario during the period $[T_u, T_{u+1}[$, resulting in $\text{COST}_B(u,i)$ and $\text{COST}_G(u,i)$.

Differential costs and their prediction intervals can then be easily derived from the individual costs per period of time. A detailed illustration of the algorithm in given by Figure 5.11. Each step of the algorithm is modeled by an execution model and is specified in Section 5.6.5.

5.6.3 Database Used

In order to specify the characteristics of the patients of interest and to calibrate the execution models, several databases are used or constructed.

NADIS® (Fedialis Medica, Marly le Roi, France) is an Electronic Medical Record (EMR) for HIV, hepatitis B virus (HBV) or hepatitis C virus (HCV) infected adults seeking care in French public hospitals (Pugliese et al., 2003). NADIS® is currently used in 132 French hospital centers. Technical staff and secretaries collect retrospective data during the first months of use of the EMR to ensure completeness of the patient's records. Physicians prospectively provide information on patient's records during each consultation or hospitalization. The resulting database, called NADIS for a sake of simplicity, contains the following information for 27,341 patients.

- Civil status of the patient,
- Social record,
- HIV/Hepatitis clinical record,
- Pathological and therapeutic history,
- Clinical examinations,
- Biological results,
- Antiretroviral genotypes and dosings,
- Medicinal prescriptions,
- Examinations and checkup prescriptions,
- Consultation and diagnosis motivations.

The MEDICATION database is constructed from the NADIS and involves 31 of the main medications used for HIV management. For each medication, the following information are collected:

- `NAMEM`: The name of the medication,
- `REFO`: The amount refunded by Health Insurance,

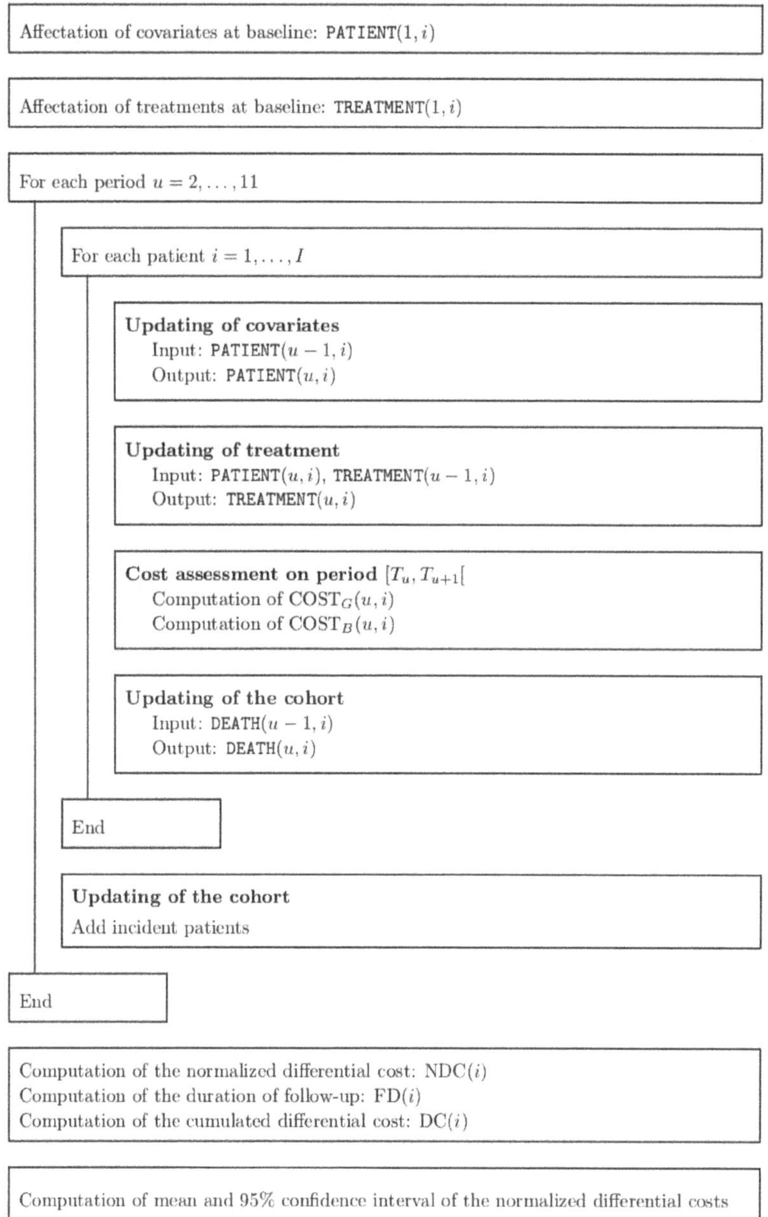

Figure 5.11 *Illustration of the algorithm.*

- `AMMT`: The marketing authorization date.

The database is also enriched with further information on the generic version of the treatment if it exists. This information is governed by parameters related to the simulation scenarios:

- `AMMGM`: The marketing authorization date of the generic version of the medication. For HIV drugs, on average, the difference between the marketing authorization of the drug and its generic version is 13 years.
- `PENRATE`: The maximal penetration rate of the generic version of the medication defined as the proportion of the population that consumes the generic version of a medication.

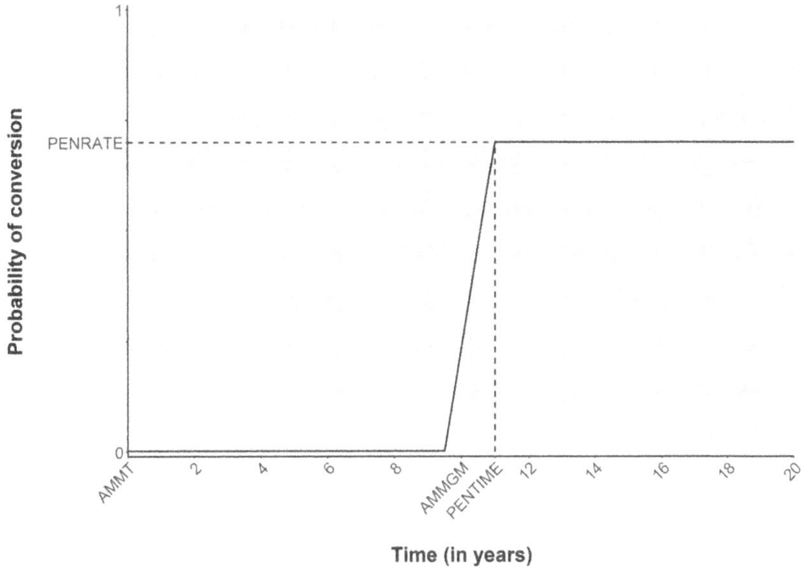

Figure 5.12 *Evolution of the probability of conversion through time, with the assumption that the marketing authorization date for the generic drug is fixed at 10 years after the marketing authorization date of the branded drug.*

In 2012 the penetration rate of generics (all domains combined) reached 69.6% and the maximal rate is 80% (Pugliese et al., 2003).

- `PENTIME`: The penetration time of the generic version of the medication defined as the time at which `PENRATE` is reached. The probability of conversion to generic version (`PROBCONV`) is assumed to increase linearly between `AMMGM` and `PENTIME`. Figure 5.12 in page 103 illustrates the probability of conversion as a function of time.

The TREATMENT database is constructed from the MEDICATION database. In fact, a treatment is a combination of medications due to multi-therapy. This yields a total of more than 800 different treatments in the database. TREATMENT database is composed of,

- `NAMET`: The name of the treatment which is a combination of medications.
- `MEDCOSTB`: The baseline cost for the branded version of the treatment.
- `MEDCOSTG`: The cost for the generic version of the treatment. The cost of the generic version of a drug is observed to be between 30% and 50% of the cost of the branded.

The drug prices are listed on the VIDAL website (`https://www.vidal.fr`), and the tables are organized by time steps to reflect the changing costs. When a generic drug is released, it is priced at 40% of the original tariff at that same date, as required by the current state-pharmaceutical industry framework agreement. Additionally, the tariff for the branded drug decreases by 20% when credits are released. Both branded and generic drugs also see an annual decrease in tariffs of 3.4%, according to INSEE values.

It is important to point that a scenario of evolution will be parameterized by the choice of (`AMMGM`, `PENRATE`, `PENTIME`) and the values of the treatment costs (`MEDCOSTB` and `MEDCOSTG`).

5.6.4 Baseline Cohort

The covariates involved in `PATIENT` are the ones that may have an impact on the evolution of the disease, the side effects, the comorbidities, the evolution of other covariates and the choice of the medication. These covariates can be classified into three categories:

- Demographic covariates,
- Covariates linked to the pathology and its history,
- Covariates linked to the comorbidities,

and are specified in Section 5.6.4.1. Covariates linked to the treatment `TREAT` integrates parameters which allow to investigate different scenarios and are specified in Section 5.6.4.2.

5.6.4.1 Description of Patients Covariates

The patient cohort for this study includes all patients who were being followed in NADIS as of December 31st, 2015. From this cohort, covariates are selected that may have an impact on medication choice or the evolution of other covariates. Baseline values for these covariates can be directly captured in NADIS or derived from other covariates available in NADIS. The covariates are classified into three categories:

Demographic covariates. The first category of covariates is demographic, which includes the main characteristics of the patients. These covariates include `SEX`, which indicates the sex of the patient (0 for male and 1 for female), `AGE`, which indicates the age of the patient in months, and `BC`, which specifies the country of birth and distinguishes patients born in France (modality 1) from those born elsewhere (modality 0). The values of $\texttt{SEX}(T_1)$, $\texttt{AGE}(T_1)$, and $\texttt{BC}(T_1)$ are directly available in the NADIS database.

Covariates linked to the pathology and its history. The second category of covariates includes `CONTA`, which indicates the way the patient was contaminated (1 for homosexual relationship and 0 for not), and `VIHS`, which indicates the status of the infection (1 for AIDS and 0 for not). The duration of the HIV infection (in months), denoted as `VIHD`, is potentially important because initial treatment aims to reduce the number of copies of the virus in the patient's organism. Once this number falls below a certain threshold, the patient can receive a lighter treatment to stabilize the state of the infection. The duration of the last treatment, denoted as `TREATD` (in months), is also crucial, as longer treatment duration reduces the probability of switching to another medication. Finally, the viral load, denoted as `ARN`, is an indicator of the disease's progression and cannot be omitted in this study. The values of $\texttt{CONTA}(T_1)$, $\texttt{VIHS}(T_1)$, $\texttt{VIHD}(T_1)$, and $\texttt{TREATD}(T_1)$ are directly available in the NADIS database. $\texttt{ARN}(T_1)$ is not available in NADIS and is estimated from a quantitative measurement of the viral load (denoted as `ARNVIH`) that exists in the database. This parameter is discretized into three categories (0 for Low, 1 for Medium, and 2 for High) according to the thresholds recommended in Bursaux (1996).

$$\texttt{ARN}(T_1) = \begin{cases} 0 & \text{if } 0 \leq \texttt{ARNVIH}(T_1) < 50 \\ 1 & \text{if } 50 \leq \texttt{ARNVIH}(T_1) < 10,000 \\ 2 & \text{if } \texttt{ARNVIH}(T_1) \geq 10,000 \end{cases}$$

Covariates linked to the comorbidities. Cardiovascular illnesses denoted as `HEART` (1 for Yes and 0 for No), Diabetes, denoted as `DIAB` (1 for Yes and 0 for No) and Renal failure, denoted as `IR` (1 for Yes and 0 for No). The values of $\texttt{HEART}(T_1)$ and $\texttt{DIAB}(T_1)$ are directly available in the NADIS database. `IR` is constructed as

$$\texttt{IR}(T_1) = \begin{cases} 1 & \text{if } \texttt{CREA}(T_1) = 1 \text{ or } \texttt{CREA}(T_1) = 2 \\ 0 & \text{if } \texttt{CREA}(T_1) = 3. \end{cases}$$

where CREA (standing for Creatinine clearance) is a categorical variable with three modalities (0 for Low, 1 for Medium and 2 for High). CREA is constructed using the calculated glomerular filtration flow CGFF that exists in the database:

$$\texttt{CREA}(T_1) = \begin{cases} 1 & \text{if } \texttt{CGFF}(T_1) > 89 \\ 2 & \text{if } 29 < \texttt{CGFF}(T_1) \leq 89 \\ 3 & \text{if } \texttt{CGFF}(T_1) \leq 29 \end{cases}$$

The thresholds used are the ones recommended in Haute Autorité de Santé (2012).
The variable DEATH indicates whether a patient is alive (1 for alive and 0 for dead) and is obviously initiated to 1.

Finally, the vector of patient covariates at baseline PATIENT(1, .) consists of the values at T_1 of the different covariates introduced below.

5.6.4.2 Description of Treatment Variables

The vector of patients treatment at baseline TREAT(1, .) is directly collected from NADIS database and is enriched by the data related to the scenarios involved as described in Section 5.6.3.

5.6.5 The Execution Models

Execution models are parts of the main algorithm in charge of mimicking the behavior of patients at each time step. Each baseline characteristic is then updated according to specific execution models to derive the values of PATIENT(u, .) and TREAT(u, .) for $u = 2, ..., 10$.

5.6.5.1 Step 1: Updating of Patient Covariates

Different models are utilized to update the patient's covariates at each time, and the selection of the model depends on the nature of the covariates and the desired level of precision in the simulations.

Covariates fixed in time. For $u = 2, \dots, 10$, we have $\texttt{SEX}(T_u) = \texttt{SEX}(T_1)$, $\texttt{CONTA}(T_u) = \texttt{CONTA}(T_1)$, $\texttt{BC}(T_u) = \texttt{BC}(T_1)$.

Covariates with deterministic dependence on time. The covariates AGE and VIHD change during the patient's follow-up period as time progresses, since they represent the duration. The change in these covariates is simply an increment of six months. Specifically, for $u = 2, \dots, 10$, we update the covariates as follows: $\texttt{AGE}(T_u) = \texttt{AGE}(T_{u-1}) + 6$ and $\texttt{VIHD}(T_u) = \texttt{VIHD}(T_{u-1}) + 6$. The TREATD covariate also changes in the same manner but needs to be reset to 0 if there is a change in treatment. For $u = 2, \dots, 10$, we update TREATD as follows:

$$\texttt{TREATD}(T_u) = \begin{cases} \texttt{TREATD}(T_{u-1}) + 6, & \text{if there is no switch of treatment,} \\ 0, & \text{if there is a change of treatment at time } T_u. \end{cases}$$

Covariates with random dependence in time. Covariates HEART, DIAB, VIHS and DEATH may change during the patient's follow-up. These changes can lead to a modification of patient treatment. The evolution of these covariates is directed by Markov chains where the transition matrices, denoted $M_{\texttt{HEART}}$, $M_{\texttt{DIAB}}$, $M_{\texttt{VIHS}}$ and $M_{\texttt{DEATH}}$ are chosen to be constant.

Table 5.1 *List of covariates involved together with the associated modalities and execution models. LIN refers to LINear model, C to Constructed model, LBP to Linear By Part model, MC to Markov Chain and MCRT to Markov Chain with Random Transitions.*

Covariate	Name	Modalities	Execution
Age	`AGE`	N/A	LIN
Cardiovascular illnesses	`HEART`	YES / NO	MC
Country of birth (France)	`BC`	YES / NO	N/A
Creatinine clearance	`CREA`	Low / Medium / High	MCRT
Death	`DEATH`	YES / NO	MC
Diabetes	`DIAB`	YES / NO	MC
Duration of the last treatment	`TREATD`	N/A	LBP
Duration of the VIH infection	`VIHD`	N/A	LIN
Renal failure	`IR`	YES / NO	C
Sex	`SEX`	Male / Female	N/A
Status of VIH infection (SIDA)	`VIHS`	YES / NO	MC
Viral load	`ARN`	Low / Medium / High	MCRT
Way of contamination (Hom. Rel.)	`CONTA`	YES / NO	N/A

Covariates with random dependence in time and randomness depending on covariates. For `ARN` and `CREA`, the transition matrices, denoted $M_{\texttt{ARN}}$ and $M_{\texttt{CREA}}$ cannot be assumed to be constant because these transitions depend on the patient's covariates. For these models, the probabilities of transition are modeled by a logistic or a polytomic regression. The covariates involved in the model are selected by a backward stepwise strategy. For $\texttt{ARN}(T_u)$, those are $\texttt{ARN}(T_{u-1})$, $\texttt{IR}(T_{u-1})$, $\texttt{CONTA}(T_{u-1})$, $\texttt{HEART}(T_{u-1})$, $\texttt{VIHS}(T_{u-1})$, $\texttt{AGE}(T_{u-1})$, $\texttt{SEX}(T_{u-1})$, $\texttt{VIHD}(T_{u-1})$ and $\texttt{TREATD}(T_{u-1})$ and for $\texttt{CREA}(T_u)$ the covariates are $\texttt{CREA}(T_{u-1})$, $\texttt{SEX}(T_{u-1})$, $\texttt{ARN}(T_u)$, $\texttt{AGE}(T_{u-1})$, $\texttt{HEART}(T_{u-1})$, $\texttt{TREATD}(T_{u-1})$, $\texttt{VIHS}(T_{u-1})$ and $\texttt{VIHD}(T_{u-1})$.

Calibration of the execution models. The calibration of the models which means the estimation of the coefficients of $M_{\texttt{HEART}}$, $M_{\texttt{DIAB}}$, $M_{\texttt{VIHS}}$ and $M_{\texttt{DEATH}}$ as well as the estimation of the parameters of the logistic (polytomic) regressions involved in the coefficients of $M_{\texttt{ARN}}$ and $M_{\texttt{CREA}}$ are derived from NADIS database.

A summary of the covariates considered in this simulation plan and their related execution models is presented in Table 5.1.

5.6.5.2 Step 2: Updating the Treatment

The update of the treatment at time T_u, as represented by column $\texttt{TREAT}(u, .)$, is governed by four rules:

Rule 1: The patient can continue with their current treatment.

Rule 2: The patient can switch to a different treatment.

Rule 3: The patient can switch to the generic version of their current treatment.

Rule 4: Once a patient switches to the generic version of their treatment, they cannot switch back to the branded version unless they change their treatment altogether.

The execution models, accounting for these rules, are defined as:

- The switching of patients from one treatment to another is modeled using a Markov chain based on transition probabilities estimated from the NADIS database. For transitions observed in a large number of patients, a logistic regression model is fitted to capture the dependence of transition probabilities on selected covariates, which are determined using a backward stepwise approach on a case-by-case basis. When transitions are rare (i.e., observed in fewer than 100 patients), their probabilities are treated as constant.

- The probability of patients switching to the generic version of their treatment depends on time t and is represented by Figure 5.12. The probability is defined as follows:

$$\texttt{PROBCONV(t)} = \begin{cases} 0 & \text{if } t < \texttt{AMMGM}, \\ \texttt{PENRATE}\frac{t-\texttt{AMMGM}}{\texttt{PENTIME}-\texttt{AMMGM}} & \text{if } \texttt{AMMGM} \leq t < \texttt{PENTIME}, \\ \texttt{PENRATE} & \text{if } t > \texttt{PENTIME}. \end{cases}$$

5.6.5.3 *Step 3: Updating of the Cohort*

On one hand, 455 incident cases are included in the cohort at each time step T_u, consistent with the results of literacy studies (Lot et al., 2019) and what is found in the NADIS database. These cases are randomly selected from the $\texttt{PATIENT}(1,.)$ vector, and each case's treatment is randomly selected from the updated treatment variable at time u, $\texttt{TREAT}(u,.)$, to reflect changes in prescription patterns and prices over time.

On the other hand, if a patient i dies during the period $[T_{u-1}, T_u[$, i.e., if $\texttt{DEATH}(u-1,i) = 1$ and $\texttt{DEATH}(u,i) = 0$, they are not removed from the cohort, but their future costs are set to zero.

Finally, let $\text{FD}(i)$ denote the follow-up duration (in semesters) for patient i.

5.6.5.4 *Step 4 : Computation of the Differential Cost*

The differential cost DC for patient i is defined by:

$$\text{DC}(i) = \text{COST}_B(i) - \text{COST}_G(i) = \sum_{u=1}^{10} \left(\text{COST}_B(u,i) - \text{COST}_G(u,i)\right),$$

where $\text{COST}_B(i)$ represents the cost for patient i considering no switch to generics and $\text{COST}_G(i)$ represents the cost assuming a pre-specified scenario of switching to generics. The main indicator of interest is the total differential cost on five years for the French population defined as the sum over patients of the individual differential cost $\text{DC}(i)$ divided by 22.8%, which is an approximation of the fraction of the French HIV population integrated in NADIS. Notice that if a patient i died during the period $[T_u, T_{u+1}[$ his future costs are fixed to zero, this means $\text{COST}_B(v,i) = \text{COST}_G(v,i) = 0$ for any $v \geq u+1$.

The normalized differential cost should be defined by taking into account the possibility of patients dying before the end of the follow-up period and the occurrence of incident cases. The differential cost should be normalized according to the follow-up duration to define the normalized differential cost:

$$\text{NDC}(i) = \frac{\text{DC}(i)}{\text{FD}(i)}.$$

Another metric of interest is the average differential cost per patient per semester, which is calculated as the mean of the normalized differential costs $\text{NDC}(i)$ over all patients in the study.

5.6.6 *Example of Results*

To demonstrate the effectiveness of this approach, this paper presents results on the impact of penetration rate on the differential cost, which is of significant importance in this context. However, the complete results of this study are beyond the scope of this paper, which focuses on the methodological aspects of the agent-based simulation approach from a statistical perspective, with an emphasis on the issue of variability. The full results, along with their health economic interpretation, are presented in Demeulemeester et al. (2021), which includes sensitivity analyses on the marketing authorization date and tariff reductions, among other factors.

5.6.6.1 Scenarios Investigated

The scenarios investigated are as follows, for each treatment k:

- `AMMGM(k)`: is fixed to 13 years after `AMMT`, irrespective of the value of k.
- `PENTIME(k)`: is fixed to one year after `AMMGM`, irrespective of the value of k.
- `PENRATE(k)`: five different penetration rates (10%, 25%, 40%, 55%, and 70%) are considered for each treatment k.
- `MEDCOSTB`: the cost of treatment at baseline is the cost refunded by Health Insurance in the first semester of 2018.
- `MEDCOSTG`: is fixed to 40% of the branded cost at `AMMGM`, irrespective of the value of k.

In order to get an idea of the relevance of the predictions, 100 simulation runs are performed (note that a higher number of simulation runs does not change the results) yielding the empirical distribution of each parameter from which it is easy to derive 90% (or 80%) prediction intervals considering the 5th and 95th (or 10th and 90th) values of the sorted distribution.

5.6.6.2 Results

The results obtained are as follows. It is important to notice that such results cannot be obtained without agent-based modeling.

- The estimate of the total differential cost for five years for the French population together with their 90% and 80% prediction intervals are illustrated by means of boxplots in Figure 5.13.

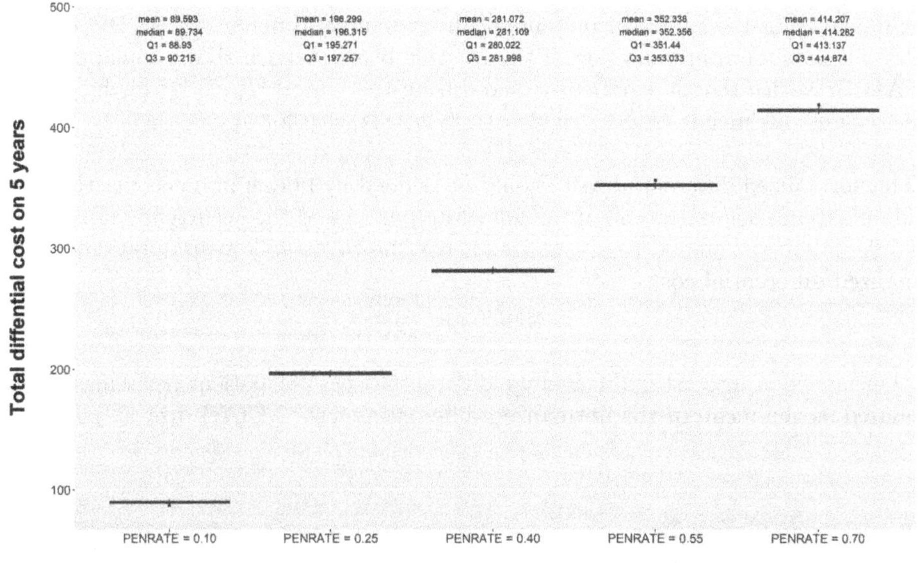

Figure 5.13 *Boxplot of the total differential cost on five years for the French population as a function of the penetration rate (from* 100 *simulation runs, in millions on euros).*

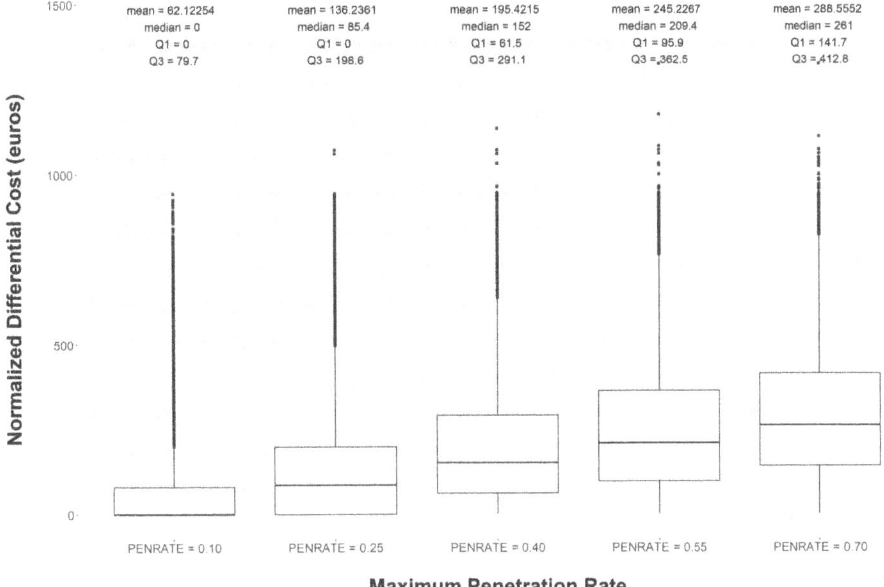

Figure 5.14 *Boxplot of the normalized differential costs per patient per year as a function of scenarios defined by penetration rate (from* 100 *simulation runs, in euros).*

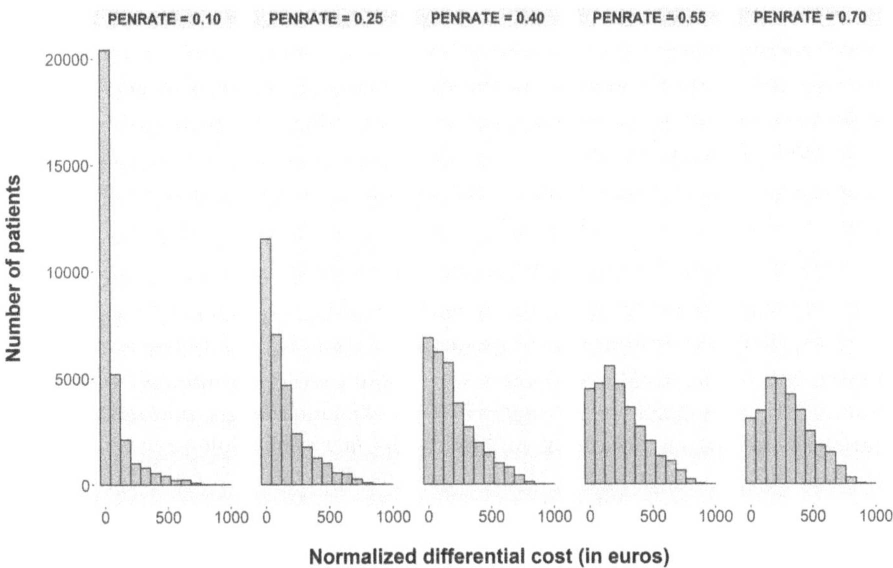

Figure 5.15 *Distribution of the normalized differential costs per patient as a function of scenarios defined by penetration rates (from* 100 *simulation runs, in euros).*

- The estimate of the normalized differential cost per patient per year together with their 90% and 80% prediction intervals are illustrated by means of boxplots in Figure 5.14. These results are enriched by Figure 5.15 which represents, for each scenario, the distributions of the normalized differential cost per patient obtained after 100 simulation

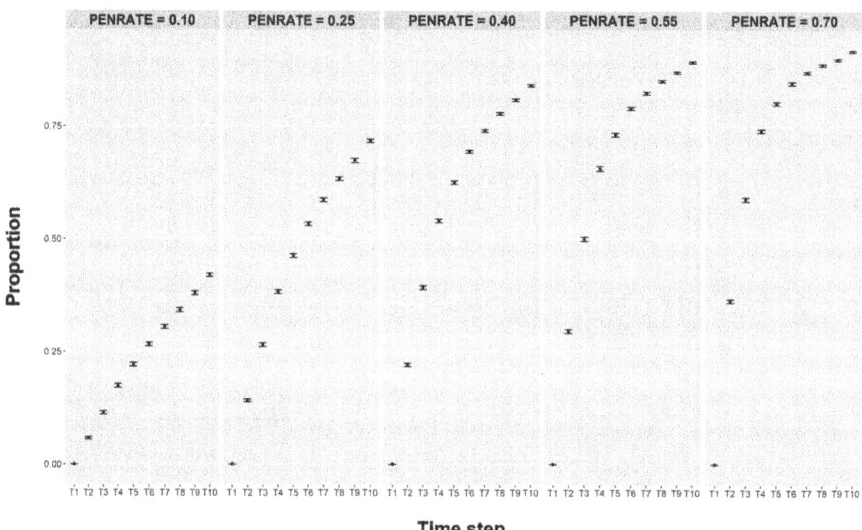

Figure 5.16 *Boxplots of the proportion of patients who were prescribed a generic at least once during the follow up together with their prediction intervals (from* 100 *simulation runs). 80% prediction intervals.*

runs. These plots give us a preview of the distribution of that value in the population for a given simulation run.

- The estimate of the proportion of patients who were prescribed generic at least once during the follow-up together with their 80% prediction intervals are illustrated by means of boxplots in Figure 5.16.

To begin with, it is worth noting that the differential costs increase naturally with the penetration rate, but this increase is not linear. It is also important to note that the precision of the prediction, as measured by the standard deviation of predicted values, increases only slowly as the penetration rate increases. The main finding of this study is the comparison of results for total differential costs, which is a parameter related to the population (as illustrated in Figure 5.13), and per-patient differential cost (as illustrated in Figure 5.14). Results for total differential cost show a very small prediction interval, whereas results for individual patients (as shown in Figure 5.15) yield much larger prediction intervals. This comparison is important because it highlights the fact that while predictions may be quite accurate at the population level, there is a large amount of variability at the individual level. In other words, the differential cost only becomes noticeable at a high penetration rate, which cannot be observed with a population-based approach. The same is true for total differential costs, as very small prediction intervals are observed (as shown in Figure 5.16), and there is no difference between the 90% and 80% confidence intervals.

Finally, it is important to observe the patterns of how the proportion of patients who switch to generics is modified by the maximum penetration rate. It is also noteworthy that 0 is contained in all prediction intervals, except for time T10 at a penetration rate of 70%. This observation is highly correlated with the proportion of patients who switch to generics, as seen in Figure 5.16, where the only proportion that exceeds 90% is the one obtained at time T10 with a penetration rate of 70%.

5.6.7 *Discussion and Conclusions*

The proposed agent-based method in the context of health economics research has four major advantages, as follows:

- Firstly, the method allows for the integration of a greater number of parameters, including individual parameters and their correlation structures, in the prediction of differential costs. This enhances the realism of the predictions.
- Secondly, the method enables the study of time effects through the use of longitudinal models.
- Thirdly, the method incorporates randomness in the system dynamics to assess the precision of the predictions. This can be evaluated through prediction intervals obtained from the distribution of predictions generated by multiple simulation runs. It is a valuable tool for identifying the main sources of randomness and comparing results.
- Fourthly, the method facilitates investigation of individual patient behavior, allowing for both population and individual-level conclusions. The system dynamics incorporate randomness from two sources:
  - Firstly, variability in patient behavior across multiple simulation runs, which can potentially differ greatly from one run to another.
  - Secondly, the dynamic nature of the patient's trajectory, which is simulated via execution models for a given simulation run.

The relevance of the first point may be diminished when dealing with total cost since the prediction involves the aggregation of costs across the entire population.

The primary limitation of the proposed method is a common one in modeling, which stems from the selection of models and the effectiveness of model calibration. The selection of models is based on clinical input on the disease and the available data. In this study, we received substantial support from the NADIS scientific committee, which consists of experts in the management of HIV-infected patients.

The results presented in this study are based on the assumptions underlying the execution models, which are detailed in the corresponding section. It is important to note that we did not consider the ability of some patients to break their medication combination (i.e., switching from a one-pill combination of several medications to several pills). This decision was made to prevent a significant increase in algorithm complexity. However, it is worth noting that this assumption may result in an underestimation of cost savings. By not allowing patients to break their medication combinations, we ensure that when a generic version of a medication that is part of a combination becomes available, patients are not incentivized to break the combination to take the generic, which would lead to further cost savings.

It is widely accepted that the agent-based approach involves finding a balance between the complexity of the model, which ensures its relevance, and its practical use. The more complex a model is, the more challenging it is to calibrate, and the more sensitive the results are to the model. However, the execution models used in this study can be easily adapted and made more complex to account for the specificities of the disease and treatments. For instance, time-dependent covariate logistic regressions or Markov models could be considered. These models could then be modified and applied to other chronic diseases to simulate potential cost savings resulting from switching to generics or modifying treatment costs. These savings could be used to fund preventive care or innovative care that provides better health outcomes for the population in terms of both quantity and quality.

5.7 Conclusion, Recommendations and Take Home Message

The fundamental components of an ABM are the virtual baseline generator and the execution models. Each of these components has its own set of limitations. The virtual baseline generator is responsible for simulating data with realistic correlation structures and marginal distributions. On the other hand, the execution models must generate virtual outcomes that account for prediction errors.

Developing an ABM requires careful consideration of the data used to build the model. This includes selecting appropriate variables, ensuring data availability, assessing the volume of data, and understanding the origin of the data (e.g., real-world data, clinical trials, cohorts). These data considerations inform the choice of execution models that can be implemented. For instance, implementing machine learning algorithms typically requires a minimum volume of data.

The order in which execution models are applied is an important consideration in building an ABM. The sequence of execution models can have a significant impact on the results of simulations.

To achieve reliable results in ABMs, it is essential to consider the sources of variability that arise from both the generation of baseline data (if applicable) and the prediction errors of the execution models. These errors can accumulate and result in highly variable outcomes. Therefore, it is crucial to run simulations multiple times and report results in terms of parameters derived from the empirical distribution obtained from various runs (such as median, prediction interval, and box plot) to ensure consistency.

Building ABMs requires a strong interdisciplinary approach that involves statisticians for building models, health data specialists for identifying and locating databases, and clinicians for identifying the variables of interest and defining the execution models to be considered.

One can observe that the ABMs presented in this study can be expanded to multi-agent models, particularly in an epidemic scenario where agents are not independent. However, the implementation of such models can be more complicated. There are specialized tools, such as the *NetLogo* software, that can be utilized to develop an ABM. Afterwards, it can be incorporated into the R software through the *RNetLogo* package (Thiele, 2017).

Chapter 6

Thompson Sampling for mHealth and Precision Health Applications

John Sperger, Eric B. Laber, Michael R. Kosorok

6.1 Introduction

Technological advancements in mobile-health (mHealth) have made it possible to deliver personalized healthcare at scale. Mobile devices, such as smart phones, allow patients to receive care if, where, and when it is needed, while wearables, such as continuous glucose monitors and accelerometers, allow for efficient collection of rich patient-level data which can be used to tailor and refine treatment decisions. Recent mHealth studies cover a wide range of diseases and disorders including addiction (Carpenter et al., 2020), diet and exercise planning for persons with type I diabetes (Luckett et al., 2020), supportive care for cancer pain (Fisher et al., 2021), and HIV/STI prevention (Mustanski et al., 2022).

However, while it is increasingly recognized that mHealth holds immense potential for scaling and democratizing healthcare (Hernández-Neuta et al., 2019), clinical trials targeting the evaluation and optimization of personalized mHealth-based interventions largely remains in the purview of a small number of specialists. A primary goal of this chapter is to provide an accessible introduction to Thompson Sampling (TS, Thompson, 1933; Russo et al., 2017) as a framework for adaptive randomization in sequential decision problems with a long or indefinite horizon when the goal is to maximize cumulative utility (e.g., patient benefit in mHealth). TS is general and extensible. It applies with continuous, categorical, or time-to-event data with censoring, under a Bayesian or frequentist paradigm, and with parametric, semi-parametric, or non-parametric models. Thus, we believe TS makes an excellent starting point for researchers designing an adaptive trial in mHealth and other settings with many decision points.

We present TS from the perspective of precision medicine and clinical trial design though, as anticipated by its generality, it is applicable much more broadly (see Russo et al. (2017), Lattimore and Szepesvári (2020), and Slivkins et al. (2019)). TS was first proposed by Thompson (1933) nearly a century ago for adaptive treatment allocation with binary treatments. This seminal paper was the antecedent to long and fruitful lines of work on multi-arm bandits (Robbins, 1956), sequential designs (Wald, 1947; Robbins et al., 1952; Chernoff, 1959), and adaptive trials (Armitage, 1960). Furthermore, TS has been a central idea of Bayesian adaptive design for decades (Berry and Fristedt, 1985) and has been applied in multiple cancer clinical trials (see Trippa et al., 2012; Thall and Wathen, 2005, and references therein). Nevertheless, rigorous theoretical and empirical study of TS in realistic environments occurred only in the past 15 years or so. (Chapelle and Li, 2011; Agrawal and Goyal, 2012, 2013b). Distributional approximations and inferential procedures have been developed even more recently (Zhang et al., 2020; Hadad et al., 2021; Bibaut et al., 2021; Wager and Xu, 2021; Zhang et al., 2022). These recent innovations have been instrumental in driving more widespread adoption of TS in sequential decision problems.

The remainder of this chapter is organized as follows. In Section 2, as means of building intuition, we introduce TS using a simple adaptive trial with two treatments. In Section 3,

DOI: 10.1201/9781003216223-6

we present a general version of TS. In Section 4, we discuss some of the statistical properties of TS including regret, power, inference and prior sensitivity. In Section 5, we discuss some practical considerations with modern applications of TS. We close with a summary and brief discussion of future research directions in Section 6.

6.2 Thompson Sampling in the simplest case

To introduce Thompson Sampling (TS), we begin with the original scenario considered by Thompson (1933) in which a set of patients (all with the same ailment) arrive at the clinic one-by-one and, upon arriving, are assigned one of two treatments the result of which is either a success or a failure. In this simple setting, the outcome of the present patient is observed before the next one arrives. Thus, the clinician has available the treatment and outcome history of all prior patients to inform each treatment decision. The goal is to allocate treatments in such a way that the expected number of successes (ENS) is maximized. It can be seen that traditional one-to-one randomization only maximizes ENS if there is no difference in the success rate of the two treatments (in which case, any allocation of the treatments is equally good). Conversely, greedy selection, i.e., always selecting the treatment with the highest estimated probability of success (say, after a burn-in period of equal allocation), need not optimize ENS as it can become stuck allocating the inferior treatment by chance. An ENS-maximizing allocation strategy must balance optimization based on current information with experimentation (choosing the estimated suboptimal treatment). The need to strike this balance is known as the 'exploration-exploitation' dilemma, and is at the heart of sequential decision-making (Sutton and Barto, 2018). Intuitively, as evidence accumulates that a given treatment is optimal, an optimal adaptive treatment allocation strategy should become more likely to recommend that treatment. TS operationalizes this intuition by setting the probability of treatment assignment at each time step equal to the posterior probability that the treatment is optimal; for this reason, TS is sometimes called posterior probability matching. Under TS, as the posterior becomes increasingly concentrated on the true parameter values, the probability of assigning an optimal treatment will increase to one.

To make these ideas concrete, consider a trial which will enroll a total of n subjects. Each subject, $t = 1, \ldots, n$, will be assigned a treatment $A_t \in \mathcal{A} = \{0, 1\}$ and their outcome, success or failure, subsequently observed. The 'complete' set of outcomes are $\{(Y_t^0, Y_t^1)\}_{t=1}^n$ which comprise n i.i.d. copies of (Y^0, Y^1), where Y^a is the potential outcome under treatment $a \in \mathcal{A}$. The observed outcome for subject t is $Y_t = A_t Y_t^1 + (1 - A_t) Y_t^0$, i.e., the observed outcome is the potential outcome under the treatment actually given.

Let $\mu_a = P(Y^a = 1)$ be the success probability under treatment a and let N_a denote the (random) number of subjects assigned to treatment a at the completion of the trial so that $n = N_0 + N_1$. The ENS is thus $\mathcal{E}_n = \mathbb{E}(N_0)\mu_0 + \mathbb{E}(N_1)\mu_1$. Application of classic, aka Bayesian, TS requires a prior $p_0(\mu_0, \mu_1)$ over the success probabilities. A natural choice is to specify independent beta distributions for the success probabilities, i.e., $p(\mu_0, \mu_1) = \rho(\mu_0; \alpha_{0,0}, \beta_{0,0})\rho(\mu_1; \alpha_{1,0}, \beta_{1,0})$ with

$$\rho(\mu_a; \alpha_{a,0}, \beta_{a,0}) = \frac{1}{B(\alpha_{a,0}, \beta_{a,0})} \mu_a^{\alpha_{a,0}-1}(1 - \mu_a)^{\beta_{a,0}-1},$$

for $\mu_a \in [0, 1]$, where $B(\alpha_{a,0}, \beta_{a,0}) = \Gamma(\alpha_{a,0})\Gamma(\beta_{a,0})/\Gamma(\alpha_{a,0}, \beta_{a,0})$ and $\alpha_{a,0}, \beta_{a,0} \geq 0$ are hyper-parameters.

Under this model, the posterior for μ_a after processing the outcome for the tth subject follows a beta distribution with parameters

$$\alpha_{a,t} = \alpha_{a,t-1} + Y_t 1_{A_t = a}$$

$$\beta_{a,t} = \beta_{a,t-1} + (1 - Y_t)1_{A_t=a},$$

where 1_u is an indicator that the clause u is true. Use an overline to denote history so that $\overline{\mathbf{A}}_t = (A_1, \ldots, A_t)$ and $\overline{\mathbf{Y}}_t = (Y_1, \ldots, Y_t)$. Thus, when the tth subject enters the trial, the information available to the clinician is $\mathcal{H}_{t-1}^b = (\overline{\mathbf{A}}_{t-1}, \overline{\mathbf{Y}}_{t-1})$, where $\mathcal{H}_0^b = \emptyset$ (the superscript 'b' is a mnemonic for bandit). Under TS, when the tth subject enters the trial, they are assigned treatment a with probability $P(\mu_a \geq \mu_{1-a}|\mathcal{H}_{t-1}^b)$ (we assume the posterior probability that $\mu_a = \mu_{1-a}$ is zero, if not, one can use random tie-breaking). Thus, one could compute $\theta_{0,t} = P(\mu_0 \geq \mu_1|\mathcal{H}_{t-1}^b)$ and then draw $A_t \sim \text{Bernoulli}(1 - \theta_{0,t})$. An implementation that is simpler, especially in more complex settings, is to draw a sample from the posterior, say $\widetilde{\mu}_{a,t} \sim \rho(\mu_a; \alpha_{a,t-1}, \beta_{a,t-1})$ for each $a \in \mathcal{A}$, and then to select treatment so as to optimize the mean outcome if the sampled parameters were correct, e.g., $A_t = \arg\max_a \widetilde{\mu}_{a,t}$. Algorithm 6.1 provides a schematic for using TS in an adaptive trial with n subjects.

Algorithm 6.1: Beta-Bernoulli TS adaptive trial with two treatments

Input: Hyperparameters $(\alpha_{0,0}, \beta_{0,0}, \alpha_{1,0}, \beta_{1,0})$, trial size n

for Subjects $t = 1, \ldots, n$ **do**
- **for** Treatments $a = 0, 1$ **do**
  - Sample $\tilde{\mu}_{a,t} \sim \rho(\mu_a; \alpha_{a,t-1}, \beta_{a,t-1})$
- Assign treatment $A_t = \arg\max_a \tilde{\mu}_{a,t}$
- Observe outcome Y_t
- Update posterior parameters
  - $\alpha_{a,t} = \alpha_{a,t-1} + Y_t 1_{A_t=a}$
  - $\beta_{a,t} = \beta_{a,t-1} + (1 - Y_t)1_{A_t=a}$

6.2.1 *Simple TS with clipping*

The preceding version of TS does not place guardrails on the treatment assignment probabilities, i.e., the probability of assigning one treatment may converge to zero or one. In clinical settings in which there are a multiple secondary analyses of interest, this behavior may not be desirable as we might not have sufficient power for these analyses. A common remedy is to truncate (i.e., clip) the probabilities to the interval $[c_0, c_1]$ where $0 < c_0 < c_1 < 1$ (Zhang et al., 2020). Clipped-TS will select action a with probability

$$P(A_t = a|\mathcal{H}_{t-1}^b) = \max\left[c_0, \min\left\{c_1, P\left(a = \arg\max_{a'} \mu_{a'}|\mathcal{H}_{t-1}^b\right)\right\}\right].$$

Thus, under clipped-TS, the expected number of subjects assigned to treatment a is bounded below by $c_0 n$ and above by $c_1 n$.

Because Clipped-TS, as described, requires explicitly computing the probabilities of each action, rather than simply computing a draw from the posterior, it can be burdensome to execute in more complex settings. One sampling-based approach that ensures each treatment is selected with some minimal probability is ϵ-TS (Li et al., 2022). In ϵ-TS, for a pre-specified value $\epsilon \in (0, 1)$, when subject t enters the trial they are assigned treatment according to TS with probability $(1 - \epsilon)$ and they are assigned treatment uniformly at random with probability ϵ. Thus, under ϵ-TS with two treatments, the probability of assigning treatment a at time t is always bounded below by $\epsilon/2$. This strategy of mixing uniform random treatment assignment with TS can be applied much more broadly, e.g., with continuous treatments or treatment sets which depend on the decision context (see Section 3).

6.2.2 Simple TS in basket trials

To illustrate how TS can be easily extended to more complex trial designs, we consider a hypothetical basket trial of cancer therapeutic agents. This hypothetical trial begins with two agents, say $\mathcal{A}_0 = \{0, 1\}$, but after (say) the 76th subject is processed, a new agent becomes available so that our set of allowable agents becomes $\mathcal{A}_1 = \{0, 1, 2\}$. Further, suppose that at the time the new agent is introduced, there have been 39 successes and 9 failures under agent 0, and 17 successes and 11 failures under agent 1. Assuming uniform priors for all three agents, the posterior distributions for the success probabilities, μ_0, μ_1, μ_2, are Beta$(40, 10)$, Beta$(18, 10)$, and Beta$(1, 1)$ respectively. When the 77th subject enters the trial, the treatment assignment probabilities for each arm are approximately 78%, 2%, and 20% for treatments 0,1, and 2 respectively. The estimated mean for treatment 1 is 0.6 while the estimated mean for treatment 2 is 0.5, yet treatment 3 is ten times more likely to be selected. This illustrates the dependence of Thompson Sampling on both the estimated mean *and* uncertainty around this estimated mean.

6.3 Beyond the simplest case: contextual bandits

In the preceding section, we considered a one-size-fits-all approach to treatment selection, i.e., the goal was to identify a single treatment which was best (on average) for the entire population. We now consider the setting in which treatment is tailored to individual patient characteristics. As in the preceding section, we consider a trial in which a total of n subjects will be enrolled. However, we now assume that the data generated by the trial will be of the form $\{(\mathbf{X}_t, A_t, Y_t)\}_{t=1}^n$, where $\mathbf{X}_t \in \mathcal{X} \subseteq \mathbb{R}^p$ are characteristics for the tth subject, $A_t \in \mathcal{A} = \{0, 1\}$ is their assigned intervention, and $Y_t \in \mathbb{R}$ is their outcome, coded so that higher values are preferred.

Let Y_t^a denote the potential outcome for the tth subject under treatment $a \in \mathcal{A}$. Under the contextual bandit model, the set of contexts and all potential outcomes $\{(\mathbf{X}_t, Y_t^0, Y_t^1)\}_{t=1}^n$ are assumed to be independent copies of $(\mathbf{X}, Y^0, Y^1)$. We assume the following standard causal conditions hold: (i) no unmeasured confounders, $(Y^0, Y^1) \perp A|\mathbf{X}$; (ii) consistency, $Y = Y^A$; and (iii) positivity, there exists $\epsilon > 0$ such that $P(A = a|\mathbf{X} = \mathbf{x}) \geq \epsilon$ for all $a \in \mathcal{A}$ and $\mathbf{x} \in \mathcal{X}$. In addition, we assume there is no interference nor are there multiple versions of treatment (Hernán and Robins, 2020).

For simplicity, we assume that subjects enroll one-by-one so that the outcome for one subject is observed before the next one is assigned their treatment. As previously, use an overline to denote history so that $\overline{\mathbf{X}}_t = (\mathbf{X}_1, \ldots, \mathbf{X}_t)$, $\overline{\mathbf{A}}_t = (A_1, \ldots, A_t)$, and $\overline{\mathbf{Y}}_t = (Y_1, \ldots, Y_t)$. Define $\mathcal{H}_{t-1}^c = (\overline{\mathbf{X}}_{t-1}, \overline{\mathbf{A}}_{t-1}, \overline{\mathbf{Y}}_{t-1})$ to be the information collected through the first $(t-1)$ subjects with $\mathcal{H}_0^c = \emptyset$ (the superscript 'c' is a mnemonic for contextual bandit). The information available to a clinician in selecting treatment for the tth subject is thus $\mathcal{H}_t^{c-} = (\mathcal{H}_{t-1}^c, \mathbf{X}_t)$.

To illustrate TS in this setting, we assume a linear model for the outcome of the form

$$Y_t = \psi(\mathbf{X}_t, A_t)^{\intercal}\gamma + \epsilon_t,$$

where $\psi(\mathbf{X}_t, A_t) \in \mathbb{R}^q$ is a feature vector constructed from $\mathbf{X}_t$ and A_t, $\gamma \in \mathbf{\Gamma} \subseteq \mathbb{R}^q$ is a vector of unknown coefficients, and ϵ_t is an independent error term with mean zero and finite variance. We assume that $\epsilon_1, \ldots, \epsilon_n$ are drawn *i.i.d.* from a distribution with density $f(\epsilon; \boldsymbol{\eta})$ which is indexed by unknown parameters $\boldsymbol{\eta} \in \mathcal{N} \subseteq \mathbb{R}^d$. Set $\boldsymbol{\theta} = (\gamma^{\intercal}, \boldsymbol{\eta}^{\intercal})^{\intercal} \in \mathbf{\Theta} = \mathbf{\Gamma} \times \mathcal{N}$. To apply TS, we specify a prior $\rho(\boldsymbol{\theta})$ over $\mathbf{\Theta}$. When the tth subject arrives, presenting with context $\mathbf{X}_t$, treatment a is selected with probability

$$P(A_t = a|\mathcal{H}_t^{c-}) = P\left\{a = \arg\max_{a'} \psi(\mathbf{X}_t, a')^{\intercal}\boldsymbol{\theta}|\mathcal{H}_t^{c-}\right\}.$$

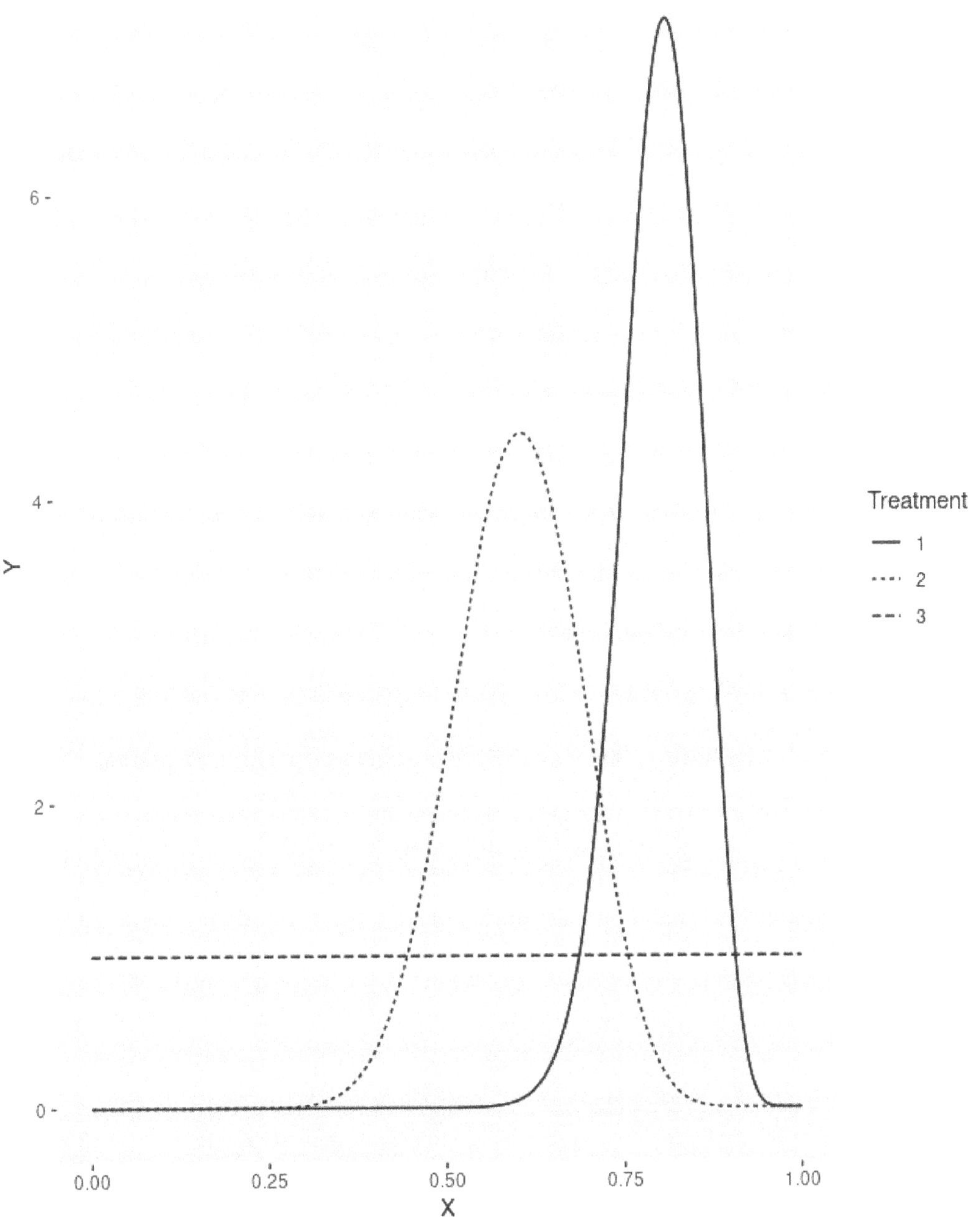

Figure 6.1 *Beta distribution densities for hypothetical basket trial.*

For example, we might assume normal errors so that $\epsilon_t \sim \text{Normal}(0, \tau^{-1})$ and assume an improper prior of the form $\rho(\boldsymbol{\theta}) \propto \tau^{-1}$. In this case, the posterior distribution for $\boldsymbol{\gamma}$ given $\mathcal{H}_t^{c-}$ follows a multivarite t-distribution with $t-1-q$ degrees of freedom, centered at the OLS estimator

$$\widehat{\boldsymbol{\gamma}}_{t-1} = \left\{ \sum_{v=1}^{t-1} \psi(\mathbf{X}_v, A_v)\psi(\mathbf{X}_v, A_v)^{\intercal} \right\}^{-1} \sum_{v=1}^{t-1} \psi(\mathbf{X}_v, A_v) Y_v, \tag{6.1}$$

and with variance equal to

$$\widehat{\Sigma}_{t-1} = \widehat{\sigma}^2_{t-1}\left\{\sum_{v=1}^{t-1}\psi(\mathbf{X}_v, A_v)\psi(\mathbf{X}_v, A_v)^{\mathrm{T}}\right\}^{-1},$$

where $\widehat{\sigma}^2_{t-1} = (t-1-q)^{-1}\sum_{v=1}^{t-1}\left\{Y_v - \psi(\mathbf{X}_v, A_v)^{\mathrm{T}}\widehat{\boldsymbol{\theta}}_{t-1}\right\}^2$, is the usual estimator of the residual variance.

In practice, under the above prior, γ does not have a proper posterior distribution until sufficient data have been collected. Thus, in the early stages of the trial, one may follow simple 1:1 randomization or some other (possibly stratified) randomization scheme. If at time t the posterior distribution of γ is proper, one can compute the TS treatment assignment by first drawing $\widetilde{\gamma}_t \sim \text{Multivariate} - \text{t}\left(\widehat{\gamma}_{t-1}, \widehat{\boldsymbol{\Sigma}}_{t-1}, t-1-q\right)$ and then setting $A_t = \arg\max_{a\in\mathcal{A}} \psi(\mathbf{X}_t, a)^{\mathrm{T}}\widetilde{\gamma}_t$.

6.3.1 Frequentist TS for contextual bandits

The fully Bayesian approach to TS for contextual bandits requires significant modeling and can become computationally burdensome if one does not use conjugate priors. As an alternative, one can use the (estimated) sampling distribution in place of the posterior to obtain a frequentist version of TS that requires fewer modeling assumptions and is often much more computationally tractable.

Consider again the linear model $Y_t = \psi(\mathbf{X}_t, A_t)^{\mathrm{T}}\gamma + \epsilon_t$, where $\gamma \in \boldsymbol{\Gamma}$ is an unknown parameter vector and the error ϵ_t satisfies $\mathbb{E}(\epsilon_t|\mathcal{H}_t^{c-}) = 0$ and $\text{Var}(\epsilon_t|\mathcal{H}_t^{c-}) = \sigma_t^2$ where $0 < \sigma_t^2 < C$ for some constant C and all t. The ordinary least squares estimator $\widehat{\gamma}_{t-1}$ of γ based on $\mathcal{H}_t^{c-}$ is given in (6.1). Of course, $\widehat{\gamma}_{t-1}$ also solves the normal equations

$$\sum_{v=1}^{t-1}\left\{Y_v - \psi(\mathbf{X}_v, A_v)^{\mathrm{T}}\gamma\right\}\psi(\mathbf{X}_v, A_v) = 0.$$

We can approximate the sampling distribution of $\widehat{\gamma}_{t-1}$ using a normal approximation (e.g., Heyde, 1997, see); however, we prefer to use a generalized bootstrap instead as it is trivial to implement and avoids cumbersome derivations (Chatterjee and Bose, 2005). For each t, let $\lambda_{t,1}, \ldots, \lambda_{t,t} \sim_{\text{i.i.d.}} \text{Exp}(1)$ and let $\widehat{\gamma}^{(b)}_{t-1}$ denote the solution to the bootstrap normal equations

$$\sum_{v=1}^{t-1}\lambda_{t,v}\left\{Y_v - \psi(\mathbf{X}_v, A_v)^{\mathrm{T}}\gamma\right\}\psi(\mathbf{X}_v, A_v) = 0, \tag{6.2}$$

then $\widehat{\gamma}^{(b)}_{t-1}$ is a draw from the generalized bootstrap estimator of the sampling distribution of $\widehat{\gamma}_{t-1}$. Under bootstrap TS, the action at time t is $A_t = \arg\max_a \psi(\mathbf{X}_t, a)^{\mathrm{T}}\widehat{\gamma}^{(b)}_{t-1}$.

Frequentist TS with the bootstrap is semi-parametric as it only requires specification of the mean structure and regularity conditions needed for bootstrap consistency (Chatterjee and Bose, 2005). In addition, it avoids specification of a prior and potentially expensive computation (e.g., MCMC). If there is historical data or scientific evidence that can be used to construct an informative prior, this information can be incorporated into frequentist TS via data augmentation (DA). We illustrate using a simple version of DA; other more sophisticated approaches are possible. Suppose we wish to use an informative prior ρ on $\boldsymbol{\Gamma}$. We posit a working prior model for the error $\epsilon_1, \epsilon_2, \ldots \sim_{\text{i.i.d.}} F_\epsilon$. Let $M \in \mathbb{Z}_+$ be a positive integer which reflects the number of 'prior samples' we wish to generate. Let $\mathcal{D}_0 = \emptyset$, at time $t = 1$, upon observing $\mathbf{X}_1$ we then draw $\widetilde{\gamma}_1^1 \sim \rho(\gamma)$ and set $A_1 = \arg\max_a \psi(\mathbf{X}_1, a)^{\mathrm{T}}\widetilde{\gamma}_1^1$ and subsequently observe Y_1. In addition, draw a second sample as follows. Set $\widetilde{\mathbf{X}}_1 =$

$\mathbf{X}_1$, draw $\widetilde{\gamma}_1^2 \sim \rho(\gamma)$, $\widetilde{\epsilon}_1 \sim F_\epsilon$, and $\widetilde{A}_1 \sim \text{Uniform}(\mathcal{A})$, and set $\widetilde{Y}_1 = \psi(\widetilde{\mathbf{X}}_1, \widetilde{A}_1)^\intercal \widetilde{\gamma}_1^2 + \widetilde{\epsilon}_1$. We continue to generate data in this way so that after m steps we have data $\mathcal{D}_m = \left\{(\mathbf{X}_i, A_i, Y_i), (\widetilde{\mathbf{X}}_i, \widetilde{A}_i, \widetilde{Y}_i)\right\}_{i=1}^m$. Once m is sufficiently large so that $\widehat{\gamma}_m$ is well-defined from $\mathcal{D}_m$, at iterations $t = m+1, m+2, \ldots$ we proceed as follows. We observe $\mathbf{X}_t$, compute the bootstrap estimator $\widehat{\gamma}_{t-1}^{(b)}$, set $A_t = \arg\max_a \psi(\mathbf{X}_t, a)^\intercal \widehat{\gamma}_{t-1}^{(b)}$ and observe Y_t. If $t \leq M$, we construct a second sample in which we set $\widetilde{\mathbf{X}}_t = \mathbf{X}_t$, draw $\widetilde{\epsilon}_t \sim F_\epsilon$, $\widetilde{\gamma}_t \sim \rho(\gamma)$, and $A_t \sim \text{Uniform}(\mathcal{A})$, and set $\widetilde{Y}_t = \psi(\widetilde{\mathbf{X}}_t, A_t)^\intercal \widetilde{\gamma}_t + \widetilde{\epsilon}_t$.

The preceding algorithm generates a set of M artificial samples from the 'prior.' Each sample was generated at an observed context value and, in this way, avoided having to posit a model for the contexts. However, if one were willing to posit a context model, it would have been possible to simply generate these M samples before collecting any data. This idea of simulating artificial data from a prior is general and applies to more general decision problems, e.g., Markov decision processes.

6.4 Thompson Sampling in more general settings

We have thus far discussed TS for a simple two-arm clinical trial and for a linear contextual bandit. We now illustrate how TS can be applied in multi-stage (possibly non-Markov) decision problems (Tsiatis et al., 2019) and infinite horizon Markov decision processes (MDPs; Puterman, 2014).

6.4.1 TS for multi-stage decision problems

We consider an adaptive sequential multiple assignment randomized trial (SMART, Lavori and Dawson, 2004; Murphy, 2005a) with T treatment stages and a planned enrollment size of n subjects. We assume that subjects arrive in cohorts of size k and that $n = km$ so that there are a total of m cohorts. To simplify notation, we assume that one cohort finishes the trial before the next one begins (for a treatment of the more general setting with overlapping and random cohort sizes, see Manschot et al., 2023).

The observed data after the ℓth cohort completes the trial is

$$\mathcal{D}_\ell = \{(\mathbf{X}_{1,i}, A_{1,i}, Y_{1,i}, \mathbf{X}_{2,i}, A_{2,i}, Y_{2,i}, \ldots, \mathbf{X}_{T,i}, A_{T,i}, Y_{T,i})\}_{i=1}^{\ell k},$$

which comprises ℓk trajectories, one per subject, where $\mathbf{X}_{1,i} \in \mathbb{R}^p$ is baseline information for subject i, $A_{t,i} \in \mathcal{A} = \{1, \ldots, K\}$ is the intervention assigned to subject i at time t, $\mathbf{X}_{t,i} \in \mathbb{R}^p$ contains interim information collected on subject i during the course of treatment $A_{t-1,i}$ for $t = 2, \ldots, T$, and $Y_{t,i} \in \mathcal{Y} \subseteq \mathbb{R}$ is an immediate (momentary) outcome measured on subject i after treatment $A_{t,i}$. The trajectories need not be independent across subjects as accumulated data on past subjects is used in treatment selection. We omit a subscript i when discussing a generic subject, i.e., $(\mathbf{X}_1, A_1, Y_1, \mathbf{X}_2, A_2, Y_2, \ldots, \mathbf{X}_T, A_T, Y_T)$.

Let $\mathbf{H}_1 = \mathbf{X}_1$ and $\mathbf{H}_t = (\mathbf{H}_{t-1}, A_{t-1}, Y_{t-1}, \mathbf{X}_t)$ for $t \geq 2$. Thus, $\mathbf{H}_t$ represents the available information to inform treatment selection for a subject in the trial at time t. In many contexts, the set of allowable treatments depends on a subject's health status (van der Laan and Petersen, 2007), e.g., in the context of schizophrenia, one cannot prescribe a type I anti-psychotic to a subject with tardive dyskinesia (Lieberman et al., 2005). We operationalize such constraints as a sequence of functions $\boldsymbol{\zeta} = \{\zeta_t\}_{t=1}^T$ with $\zeta_t : \operatorname{dom} \mathbf{H}_t \to 2^{\mathcal{A}}$ so that $\zeta_t(\mathbf{h}_t) \subseteq \mathcal{A}$ is the set of allowable treatments for a subject with history $\mathbf{H}_t = \mathbf{h}_t$.

A treatment regime, in this context is a sequence of decision rules $\boldsymbol{\pi} = (\pi_1, \pi_2, \ldots, \pi_T)$ such that $\pi_t : \mathcal{H}_t \to \mathcal{A}$ and $\pi_t(\mathbf{h}_t) \in \zeta_t(\mathbf{h}_t)$ for all $\mathbf{h}_t \in \operatorname{dom} \mathbf{H}_t$, $t = 1, 2, \ldots, T$. An optimal treatment regime maximizes the expectation of the cumulative outcome, $\sum_{t=1}^T Y_t$, if applied to select treatments in the target population. The optimal regime is formalized using potential outcomes. As in previous sections, write $\overline{\boldsymbol{a}}_t = (a_1, \ldots, a_t)$. Let $\mathbf{H}_t^{\overline{\boldsymbol{a}}_{t-1}}$ be the potential history at time t under treatment sequence $\overline{\boldsymbol{a}}_{t-1}$ and $Y_t^{\overline{\boldsymbol{a}}_t}$ the potential outcome at time t under treatment sequence $\overline{\boldsymbol{a}}_t$; for convenience, we define $\mathbf{H}_1^{\overline{\boldsymbol{a}}_0} \equiv \mathbf{H}_1$. The potential outcome at time t under a sequence of decision rules $\overline{\boldsymbol{\pi}}_t = (\pi_1, \ldots, \pi_t)$ is

$$Y_t^{\overline{\boldsymbol{\pi}}_t} = \sum_{\overline{a}_t} Y_t^{\overline{\boldsymbol{a}}_t} \prod_{v=1}^{t} 1\left\{\pi_v\left(\mathbf{H}_v^{\overline{\boldsymbol{a}}_{v-1}}\right) = a_v\right\}.$$

The value of a regime $\boldsymbol{\pi}$ is $V(\boldsymbol{\pi}) = \mathbb{E}\left(\sum_{v=1}^{T} Y_v^{\overline{\boldsymbol{\pi}}_v}\right)$, and the optimal regime, $\boldsymbol{\pi}^{\text{opt}}$, satisfies $V(\boldsymbol{\pi}^{\text{opt}}) \geq V(\boldsymbol{\pi})$ for all feasible regimes $\boldsymbol{\pi}$.

To identify $\boldsymbol{\pi}^{\text{opt}}$ from the data-generating model, we make the following standard assumptions. Define

$$\mathcal{W} = \left\{\left(\mathbf{H}_t^{\overline{\boldsymbol{a}}_{t-1}}, Y_t^{\overline{\boldsymbol{a}}_t}\right) : \overline{\boldsymbol{a}}_t \in \mathcal{A}^t, a_v \in \zeta_v(\mathbf{H}_v^{\overline{\boldsymbol{a}}_{v-1}}) \,\forall\, 1 \leq v \leq t\right\}_{t=1}^{T}$$

to be the set of realizable (feasible) potential outcomes. We assume the following conditions hold: (C1) strong ignorability, $\mathcal{W} \perp A_t | \mathbf{H}_t$ for all $t = 1, \ldots, T$; (C2) positivity, there exists $\epsilon > 0$ such that $P(A_t = a | \mathbf{H}^t = \mathbf{h}_t) \geq \epsilon$ for all $\mathbf{h}_t \in \operatorname{dom} \mathbf{H}_t$, $a \in \zeta_t(\mathbf{h}_t)$, and $t = 1, \ldots, T$; and (C3) consistency, $\mathbf{H}_t = \mathbf{H}_t^{\overline{\mathbf{A}}_{t-1}}$ and $Y_t = Y_t^{\overline{\mathbf{A}}_t}$ for all $t = 1, \ldots, T$, i.e., the observed history and outcomes are the potential history and outcomes under treatment actually assigned. We also assume that there are not multiple versions of treatment or interference among subjects (Tsiatis et al., 2019). In the context of a SMART, (C1) and (C2) can be guaranteed by design. In practice, the (approximate) validity of the other conditions must be argued on the basis of the underlying science and implementation of the trial (see Tsiatis et al., 2019; Hernán and Robins, 2020, and references therein). Hereafter, we implicitly assume these conditions hold.

We characterize the optimal regime, $\boldsymbol{\pi}^{\text{opt}}$, using dynamic programming (Bellman, 1952). Define the Q-function at stage-T as

$$Q_T(\mathbf{h}_T, a_T) = \mathbb{E}\left(Y_T \middle| \mathbf{H}_T = \mathbf{h}_T, A_T = a_T\right),$$

and recursively for $t = T-1, T-2, \ldots, 1$ define

$$Q_t(\mathbf{h}_t, a_t) = \mathbb{E}\left\{Y_t + \max_{a_{t+1} \in \zeta_{t+1}(\mathbf{H}_{t+1})} Q_{t+1}(\mathbf{H}_{t+1}, a_{t+1}) \middle| \mathbf{H}_t = \mathbf{h}_t, A_t = a_t\right\}.$$

It follows that an optimal regime is given by $\pi_t^{\text{opt}}(\mathbf{h}_t) = \arg\max_{a_t \in \zeta_t(\mathbf{h}_t)} Q_t(\mathbf{h}_t, a_t)$ (see Murphy, 2005b; Schulte et al., 2014). Thus, given data after ℓ cohorts, one can construct an estimator of $\boldsymbol{\pi}^{\text{opt}}$ by constructing estimators $\widehat{Q}_{t,\ell}$ of Q_t for $t = 1, \ldots, T$, and subsequently $\widehat{\pi}_{t,\ell}(\mathbf{h}_t) = \arg\max_{a_t \in \zeta_t(\mathbf{h}_t)} \widehat{Q}_{t,\ell}(\mathbf{h}_t, a_t)$. We illustrate this approach using parametric models for the Q-functions, though more flexible non-parametric models are possible (Ernst et al., 2005).

For each t we posit a working model $Q_t(\mathbf{h}_t, a_t; \boldsymbol{\theta}_t)$ indexed by $\boldsymbol{\theta}_t \in \boldsymbol{\Theta}_t \subseteq \mathbb{R}^{q_t}$. We assume that $Q_t(\mathbf{h}_t, a_t; \boldsymbol{\theta}_t)$ is defined and continuously differentiable for all $\boldsymbol{\theta}_t$ in an open set that contains $\boldsymbol{\Theta}_t$. Define $\widehat{\boldsymbol{\theta}}_{T,\ell}$ as the solution to the so-called conditional least-squares score equation

$$\sum_{i=1}^{\ell k} \{Y_{T,i} - Q_T(\mathbf{H}_{T,i}, A_{T,i}; \boldsymbol{\theta}_T)\} \nabla_{\boldsymbol{\theta}_T} Q_T(\mathbf{H}_{T,i}, A_{T,i}; \boldsymbol{\theta}_T) = 0, \tag{6.3}$$

and similarly, for $t = T-1, T-2, \ldots, 1$ define $\widehat{\boldsymbol{\theta}}_{t,\ell}$ as the solution to

$$\sum_{i=1}^{\ell k} \left\{ Y_{t,i} + \max_{a_{t+1}} Q_{t+1}(\mathbf{H}_{t+1,i}, a_{t+1}; \widehat{\boldsymbol{\theta}}_{t+1,\ell}) - Q_t(\mathbf{H}_{t,i}, A_{t,i}; \boldsymbol{\theta}_t) \right\} \times \quad \nabla_{\boldsymbol{\theta}_t} Q_t(\mathbf{H}_{t,i}, A_{t,i}; \boldsymbol{\theta}_t) = 0. \tag{6.4}$$

The estimated optimal regime using data from the first ℓ cohorts is thus $\widehat{\pi}_{t,\ell}(\mathbf{h}_t) = \arg\max_{a_t \in \zeta_t(\mathbf{h}_t)} Q_t(\mathbf{h}_t, a_t; \widehat{\boldsymbol{\theta}}_{t,\ell})$.

We use the preceding estimating equations with the multiplier bootstrap to implement a frequentist version of TS. However, in early cohorts, the estimating equations will not have unique solutions so one needs a base strategy to begin. One natural approach is to use uniform randomization at each stage for a fixed number of cohorts, say L, so that for any subject i in cohort $\ell \leq L$ with history $\mathbf{H}_{t,i}$ will be assigned treatment $A_{t,i} \sim \text{Uniform}\{\zeta_t(\mathbf{H}_{t,i})\}$. For a subject i in cohort $\ell = L+1, \ldots, m$ draw $\lambda_{i,1}, \ldots, \lambda_{i,(\ell-1)k} \sim_{i.i.d.} \text{Exp}(1)$, compute $\widehat{\boldsymbol{\theta}}^{(b)}_{T,\ell-1,i}$ as the solution to

$$\sum_{j=1}^{(\ell-1)k} \lambda_{i,j} \left\{ Y_{T,j} - Q_T(\mathbf{H}_{T,j}, A_{T,j}; \boldsymbol{\theta}_T) \right\} \nabla_{\boldsymbol{\theta}_T} Q_T(\mathbf{H}_{T,j}, A_{T,j}; \boldsymbol{\theta}_T) = 0,$$

and, recursively, compute $\widehat{\boldsymbol{\theta}}^{(b)}_{t,\ell-1,i}$ for $t = T-1, \ldots, 1$ as the solution to

$$\sum_{j=1}^{(\ell-1)k} \lambda_{i,j} \left\{ Y_{t,j} + \max_{a_{t+1}} Q_{t+1}(\mathbf{H}_{t+1,j}, a_{t+1}; \widehat{\boldsymbol{\theta}}^{(b)}_{t+1,\ell-1,i}) - Q_t(\mathbf{H}_{t,j}, A_{t,j}; \boldsymbol{\theta}_t) \right\} \times \nabla_{\boldsymbol{\theta}_t} Q_t(\mathbf{H}_{t,j}, A_{t,j}; \boldsymbol{\theta}_t) = 0.$$

Thus, a subject i in cohort $\ell = L+1, \ldots, m$ with history $\mathbf{H}_{t,i}$ at time t, is assigned treatment $A_{t,i} = \arg\max_{a_t \in \zeta_t(\mathbf{H}_{t,i})} Q_t(\mathbf{H}_{t,i}, a_t; \widehat{\boldsymbol{\theta}}^{(b)}_{t,\ell-1,i})$.

The version of TS for multi-stage decision problems we describe uses the estimated sampling distribution of parameters indexing the Q-functions in place of a proper posterior distribution. To see this, let $\widehat{P}_{t,\ell}$ denote the estimated sampling distribution of $\widehat{\boldsymbol{\theta}}_{t,\ell-1}$ based on the multiplier bootstrap applied to data from the first $\ell - 1$ cohorts. For a subject with history $\mathbf{H}_t = \mathbf{h}_t$ in cohort ℓ and any $a \in \zeta_t(\mathbf{h}_t)$ the event $A_t = a$ is equivalent to the event $a = \arg\max_{a_t \in \zeta_t(\mathbf{h}_t)} Q_t(\mathbf{h}_t, a_t; \widehat{\boldsymbol{\theta}}^{(b)}_{t,\ell-1})$ which occurs with probability

$$\int 1\left\{ a = \arg\max_{a_t \in \zeta_t(\mathbf{h}_t)} Q_t(\mathbf{h}_t, a_t; \boldsymbol{\theta}) \right\} d\widehat{P}_{t,\ell-1}(\boldsymbol{\theta}).$$

In a fully-Bayesian approach, $\widehat{P}_{t,\ell-1}$ would be replaced by the posterior distribution over $\boldsymbol{\theta}_t$ given data on the first $\ell - 1$ cohorts.

In some settings, one may wish to incorporate prior information into frequentist TS for multi-stage decision problems. One way to do this is to posit a prior for the joint trajectory distribution, $(\mathbf{X}_1, A_1, Y_1, \mathbf{X}_2, A_2, Y_2, \ldots, \mathbf{X}_T, A_T, Y_T)$ and then to simulate data from this prior to augment the observed data; i.e., one can simulate J i.i.d. trajectories under the prior as a kind of zeroth cohort. This can be an effective strategy for folding in domain knowledge or historical data when it is available at the trajectory level.

Remark 1. We did not use partial information of subjects within a cohort; e.g., if the enrollment and/or completion times of the stages vary across subjects within a cohort, it is possible to use data from subjects who have advanced further in the trial to inform the treatment decisions for subjects at earlier stages. This can increase efficiency though at the expense of more complex bookkeeping. See Norwood et al. (2022) for details.

6.4.2 TS for MDPs

In decision problems with a long or indefinite time horizon one needs to impose more structure on the data-generating model than in the preceding section to facilitate extrapolation in time. Most commonly, one assumes that the data are from a stationary and homogeneous MDP (Sutton, 1997). We present a frequentist version of TS in this setting. However, we first discuss the construction of a homogeneous and stationary MDP from raw (possibly non-Markov) data. This is a critically important issue in application but has received little attention in the precision medicine literature (see Wang et al., 2017; Ma et al., 2023, for references).

6.4.2.1 Pre-processing and the Markov assumption

As in the preceding section, we consider longitudinal data on n subjects in a sequential randomized trial.[1] However, we now assume that subjects enroll in a single cohort and that the treatment decisions are aligned in time for all subjects in the cohort. At any time t, the raw observed data are of the form

$$\{(\mathbf{X}_{1,i}, A_{1,i}, Y_{1,i}, \mathbf{X}_{2,i}, A_{2,i}, Y_{2,i}, \ldots, \mathbf{X}_{t,i}, A_{t,i}, Y_{t,i})\}_{i=1}^{n}, \tag{6.5}$$

which comprises n trajectories of the form $(\mathbf{X}_1, A_1, Y_1, \mathbf{X}_2, A_2, Y_2, \ldots, \mathbf{X}_t, A_t, Y_t)$, where $\mathbf{X}_1 \in \mathbb{R}^p$ are baseline measurements, $\mathbf{A}_t \in \mathcal{A} = \{1, 2, \ldots, K\}$ is the assigned intervention at time t, $\mathbf{X}_t \in \mathcal{X}$ are interim measurements taken during the course of A_t, and $Y_t \in \mathcal{Y} \subseteq [0, 1]$ are outcomes coded so that higher values are better. Let the history $\mathbf{H}_t$ be defined as in the preceding section and let $\mathbf{\Pi}$ denote the class of feasible regimes. We write $Y_t^{\boldsymbol{\pi}}$ to denote the potential outcome at time t under $\boldsymbol{\pi} \in \mathbf{\Pi}$.

For any $\boldsymbol{\pi} \in \mathbf{\Pi}$ an $t \geq 1$ write $\underline{\boldsymbol{\pi}}_t = (\pi_t, \pi_{t+1}, \ldots)$. Given history $\mathbf{H}_t = \mathbf{h}_t$ and $\boldsymbol{\pi} \in \mathbf{\Pi}$, define the state-value function at time t as

$$V_t(\boldsymbol{\pi}, \mathbf{h}_t) = V_t(\underline{\boldsymbol{\pi}}_t, \mathbf{h}_t) = \mathbb{E}\left(\sum_{v \geq 0} \gamma^v Y_{t+v}^{\boldsymbol{\pi}} \middle| \mathbf{H}_t = \mathbf{h}_t\right),$$

where $\gamma \in (0, 1)$ is a discount factor. The optimal feasible regime, $\boldsymbol{\pi}^{\text{opt}} \in \mathbf{\Pi}$, satisfies $V_t(\boldsymbol{\pi}^{\text{opt}}, \mathbf{h}_t) \geq V_t(\boldsymbol{\pi}, \mathbf{h}_t)$ for all $\boldsymbol{\pi} \in \mathbf{\Pi}$ and $\mathbf{h}_t \in \operatorname{dom} \mathbf{H}_t$. It is clear that without additional structure, one cannot recover $\boldsymbol{\pi}^{\text{opt}}$ from n trajectories of length t as in (6.5) even as $n \to \infty$ (as one will have no information about $\underline{\boldsymbol{\pi}}_{t+1}^{\text{opt}}$). The most common approach to estimating $\boldsymbol{\pi}^{\text{opt}}$ in practice is to assume that, after some suitable transformation, the observed data can be represented as a homogeneous MDP; we now describe how such a transformation might be constructed.

Assume that there exists a sequence of summary functions $\{\psi_t\}_{t \geq 1}$ with $\psi_t : \operatorname{dom} \mathbf{H}_t \to \mathcal{S} \subseteq \mathbb{R}^q$ and we call $\mathbf{S}_t = \psi_t(\mathbf{H}_t)$ the state of the system at time t. For example, the state might be constructed by concatenating interim measurements, treatments, and outcomes over a fixed look-back period (Ma et al., 2023), taking a weighted average over past measurements (Laber and Staicu, 2018), or using data-driven feature selection, e.g., using recurrent neural networks (Wang et al., 2018). We assume that the summary function induces a homogeneous MDP so that

$$\mathbf{S}^{t+1} \perp (\mathbf{H}^{t-1}, A_{t-1}, Y_{t-1}) \big| (\mathbf{S}^t, A^t),$$

and the conditional distribution of $\mathbf{S}_{t+1}$ given $(\mathbf{S}_t, A_t)$ does not depend on time t. We also assume that the summary is such that $Y_t = u(\mathbf{S}_t, A_t, \mathbf{S}_{t+1})$ for some fixed and known

[1] We omit a discussion of the necessary causal assumptions in this section delaying a formal statement of these assumptions to the the next section.

function $u : \mathcal{S}\times\mathcal{A}\times\mathcal{S} \rightarrow \mathcal{Y}$, and that there exists function $\upsilon : \mathcal{S} \rightarrow 2^{\mathcal{A}}$ such that $\upsilon\{\psi_t(\mathbf{h}_t)\} = \zeta_t(\mathbf{h}_t)$ for all $\mathbf{h}_t \in \operatorname{dom}\mathbf{H}_t$ and all t. Let $\mathbf{\Pi}_{\mathcal{M}}$ denote the set of maps, $\varpi : \mathcal{S} \rightarrow \mathcal{A}$, such that $\varpi(\mathbf{s}) \in \upsilon(\mathbf{s})$ for all $\mathbf{s} \in \mathcal{S}$. Let Y_t^{ϖ} denote the potential outcome under $\varpi \in \mathbf{\Pi}_{\mathcal{M}}$. For each t, $\mathbf{h}_t \in \operatorname{dom}\mathbf{H}_t$, and $a_t \in \zeta_t(\mathbf{h}_t)$ define

$$Q_t^{\text{opt}}(\mathbf{h}_t, a_t) = \sup_{\boldsymbol{\pi}\in\mathbf{\Pi}} \mathbb{E}\left\{\sum_{v=0}^{\infty} \gamma^v Y_{t+v}^{\boldsymbol{\pi}} \big| \mathbf{H}_t = \mathbf{h}_t, A_t = a_t\right\},$$

then it follows (e.g., see Puterman, 2014; Bertsekas, 2012) that

$$Q_t^{\text{opt}}(\mathbf{h}_t, a_t) = \\ \sup_{\boldsymbol{\pi}\in\mathbf{\Pi}} \mathbb{E}\left\{Y_t^{\boldsymbol{\pi}} + \gamma \max_{a_{t+1}\in\zeta_t(\mathbf{H}_{t+1})} Q_{t+1}^{\text{opt}}(\mathbf{H}_{t+1}, a_{t+1}) \big| \mathbf{H}_t = \mathbf{h}_t, A_t = a_t\right\},$$

and an optimal decision strategy based on the raw data, say $\boldsymbol{\pi}^{\text{opt}}$, is given by $\pi_t^{\text{opt}}(\mathbf{h}_t) = \arg\max_{\boldsymbol{a}_t\in\zeta_t(\mathbf{h}_t)} Q_t^{\text{opt}}(\mathbf{h}_t, a_t)$. If $\{(Y_{t+1}, \max_{a_{t+1}\in\zeta_{t+1}(\mathbf{H}_{t+1})} Q_{t+1}^{\text{opt}}(\mathbf{H}_{t+1}, a_{t+1})\} \perp \mathbf{H}_t | (\mathbf{S}_t, A_t)$, then it follows that $Q_t^{\text{opt}}(\mathbf{h}_t, a_t)$ depends on $\mathbf{h}_t$ only through $\mathbf{s}_t = \psi_t(\mathbf{h}_t)$ and therefore $\pi_t^{\text{opt}}(\mathbf{h}_t)$ depends on $\mathbf{h}_t$ only through $\psi_t(\mathbf{h}_t)$ (Wang et al., 2017). Furthermore, the optimal value starting from $\mathbf{H}_t = \mathbf{h}_t$ satisfies

$$\begin{aligned} V_t^{\text{opt}}(\mathbf{h}_t) &= Q_t^{\text{opt}}\{\mathbf{h}_t, \pi_t^{\text{opt}}(\mathbf{h}_t)\} \\ &= \mathbb{E}\left\{\sum_{v=0}^{\infty} \gamma^v Y_{t+v}^{\boldsymbol{\pi}^{\text{opt}}} \big| \mathbf{H}_t = \mathbf{h}_t\right\} \\ &= \mathbb{E}\left\{\sum_{v=0}^{\infty} \gamma^v Y_{t+v}^{\boldsymbol{\pi}^{\text{opt}}} \big| \mathbf{S}^t = \psi_t(\mathbf{h}_t)\right\} \\ &= \sup_{\boldsymbol{\varpi}\in\mathbf{\Pi}_{\mathcal{M}}^{\infty}} \mathbb{E}\left\{\sum_{v=0}^{\infty} \gamma^v Y_{t+v}^{\boldsymbol{\varpi}} \big| \mathbf{S}^t = \psi_t(\mathbf{h}_t)\right\} \\ &= \sup_{\varpi\in\mathbf{\Pi}_{\mathcal{M}}} \mathbb{E}\left\{\sum_{v=0}^{\infty} \gamma^v Y_{t+v}^{\varpi} \big| \mathbf{S}^t = \psi_t(\mathbf{h}_t)\right\} \end{aligned} \tag{6.6}$$

where $\mathbf{\Pi}_{\mathcal{M}}^{\infty}$ is the space of sequences in $\mathbf{\Pi}_{\mathcal{M}}$ and the last equality follows from the fact that the best treatment in a state $\mathbf{S}^t = \mathbf{s}$ does not depend on t (see Puterman, 2014, for additional details). Let ϖ^{opt} attain the sup in (6.6). It follows that the reduced process

$$\{(\mathbf{S}_{1,i}, A_{1,i}, Y_{1,i}, \mathbf{S}_{2,i}, A_{2,i}, Y_{2,i}, \ldots, \mathbf{S}_{t,i}, A_{t,i}, Y_{t,i})\}_{i=1}^{n} \tag{6.7}$$

comprises trajectories from a homogeneous MDP and that $\pi_t^{\text{opt}}(\mathbf{h}_t) = \varpi^{\text{opt}}\{\psi_t(\mathbf{h}_t)\}$ is optimal; i.e., $V_t(\boldsymbol{\pi}^{\text{opt}}, \mathbf{h}_t) \geq V_t(\boldsymbol{\pi}, \mathbf{h}_t)$ for all $\boldsymbol{\pi} \in \mathbf{\Pi}$ and $\mathbf{h}_t \in \operatorname{dom}\mathbf{H}_t$. Furthermore, $\boldsymbol{\pi}^{\text{opt}}$ can be estimated using only the data from the reduced process (6.7) as we describe in the next section. Constructing a suitable reduced process that is parsimonious, homogeneous, Markov, and has the same optimal regime as the original process is not trivial. While data-driven methods for constructing the maps ψ_t exist (Wang et al., 2017; Ma et al., 2023), this is more often done using *ad hoc* transformations and justified using clinical theory.

6.4.2.2 Q-learning in MDPs

We assume that the observed data (possibly after transformation) are of the form

$$\{(\mathbf{S}_{1,i}, A_{1,i}, \mathbf{S}_{2,i,}, A_{2,i}, \ldots, \mathbf{S}_{t,i}, A_{t,i}, \mathbf{S}_{t+1,i})\}_{i=1}^{n},$$

which comprise n trajectories, one for each subject, of the form $(\mathbf{S}_1, A_1, \mathbf{S}_2, A_2, \ldots, \mathbf{S}_t, A_t, \mathbf{S}_{t+1})$, where: $\mathbf{S}_t \in \mathcal{S} \subseteq \mathbb{R}^q$ is a summary of the subject's health status at time t and $A_t \in \mathcal{A} = \{1, 2, \ldots, K\}$ is the treatment assigned at time t. In the context of MDPs, the term action is often used in place of treatment; we shall use the terms interchangeably. We assume that there exists a fixed function $u : \mathcal{S} \times \mathcal{A} \times \mathcal{S} \to \mathbb{R}$, so that the outcome $Y_t = u(\mathbf{S}_t, A_t, \mathbf{S}_{t+1})$ captures the utility associated with the state-treatment-next state triple $(\mathbf{S}_t, A_t, \mathbf{S}_{t+1})$.

We assume that the data-generating model is a homogeneous MDP so that for any measurable set $\mathcal{B} \subseteq \mathcal{S}$ and time t

$$P\left(\mathbf{S}_{t+1} \in \mathcal{B} \middle| \mathbf{S}_1, \ldots, \mathbf{S}_t, A_1, \ldots, A_t\right) = P\left(\mathbf{S}_{t+1} \middle| \mathbf{S}_t, A_t\right)$$

with probability one, and the probability does not depend on t.

We assume that there exists a set-valued function $\nu : \mathcal{S} \to 2^{\mathcal{A}}$ so that $\nu(\mathbf{s}) \subseteq \mathcal{A}$ is the set of allowable treatments for a subject in state $\mathbf{s}$; we assume $\nu(\mathbf{s})$ is non-empty for all $\mathbf{s} \in \mathcal{S}$. A treatment regime in this context is a map $\pi : \mathcal{S} \to \mathcal{A}$ that satisfies $\pi(\mathbf{s}) \in \nu(\mathbf{s})$ for all $\mathbf{s} \in \mathcal{A}$. Let $\mathbf{\Pi}$ denote the set of all treatment regimes. Under a regime $\pi \in \mathbf{\Pi}$, a subject with $\mathbf{S}_t = \mathbf{s}$ at time t will be recommended treatment $\pi(\mathbf{s})$. An optimal treatment regime maximizes expected discounted cumulative utility if used to select treatments for patients in the target population. As in previous sections, we formalize this definition using potential outcomes. Let $\mathbf{S}_t^{\overline{\boldsymbol{a}}_{t-1}}$ denote the potential state under treatment sequence $\overline{\boldsymbol{a}}_{t-1} = (a_1, \ldots, a_{t-1})$; for convenience, we follow the notational convention that $\mathbf{S}_1^{\overline{\boldsymbol{a}}_0} \equiv \mathbf{S}_1$. The potential outcome under treatment sequence $\overline{\boldsymbol{a}}_t$ is thus

$$Y_t^{\boldsymbol{a}_t} = u\left(\mathbf{S}_t^{\overline{\boldsymbol{a}}_{t-1}}, a_t, \mathbf{S}_{t+1}^{\overline{\boldsymbol{a}}_t}\right),$$

and the potential outcome at time t under a regime π is

$$Y_t^{\pi} = \sum_{\overline{\boldsymbol{a}}_t} Y_t^{\overline{\boldsymbol{a}}_t} \prod_{v=1}^{t-1} 1\left\{\pi(\mathbf{S}_v^{\overline{\boldsymbol{a}}_{v-1}}) = a_v\right\}.$$

For any $\mathbf{s} \in \mathcal{S}$ and regime π define the state-value function

$$V(\pi, \mathbf{s}) = \mathbb{E}\left(\sum_{v \geq 0} \gamma^v Y_{t+v}^{\pi} \middle| \mathbf{S}_t = \mathbf{s}\right),$$

where $\gamma \in (0, 1)$ is a discount factor. The optimal regime, π^{opt}, satisfies $V(\pi^{\text{opt}}, \mathbf{s}) \geq V(\pi, \mathbf{s})$ for all $\mathbf{s} \in \mathcal{S}$ and $\pi \in \mathbf{\Pi}$. To identify π^{opt} in terms of the data-generating model we make use of the following causal assumptions which mirror those made in previous sections. Let

$$\mathcal{W} = \left\{\left(\mathbf{S}_t^{\overline{\boldsymbol{a}}_{t-1}}, Y_t^{\overline{\boldsymbol{a}}_t}\right) : \overline{\boldsymbol{a}}_t \in \mathcal{A}^t,\, a_v \in \nu(\mathbf{S}_v^{\overline{\boldsymbol{a}}_{v-1}})\, \forall\, 1 \leq v \leq t\right\}_{t \geq 1};$$

we assume: (C1) strong ignorability, $\mathcal{W} \perp A_t | (\overline{\mathbf{S}}_t, \overline{\mathbf{A}}_{t-1})$, for all $t \geq 1$; (C2) positivity, there exists $\epsilon > 0$ such that $P(A_t = a | \overline{\mathbf{S}}_t, \overline{\mathbf{A}}_{t-1}) \geq \epsilon$ for all $a \in \nu(\mathbf{S}_t)$ with probability one; and (C3) consistency, $\mathbf{S}_t = \mathbf{S}_t^{\overline{\mathbf{A}}_{t-1}}$ for all t. In addition, we assume that there is no interference nor are there multiple versions of treatment. We note that because $Y_t = u(\mathbf{S}_t, A_t, \mathbf{S}_{t+1})$ it follows from (C3) that $Y_t = Y_t^{\overline{\boldsymbol{a}}_t}$. For any $\mathbf{s} \in \mathcal{S}$ and $a \in \nu(\mathbf{s})$, define the optimal Q-function as

$$Q(\mathbf{s}, a) = \sup_{\pi \in \mathbf{\Pi}} \mathbb{E}\left(\sum_{v \geq 0} \gamma^v Y_{t+v}^{\pi} \middle| \mathbf{S}_t = \mathbf{s}, A_t = a\right),$$

then it follows (see Ertefaie and Strawderman, 2018) under (C1)–(C3) that

$$Q(\mathbf{s}, a) = \mathbb{E}\left\{Y_t + \gamma \max_{a_{t+1}\in\nu(\mathbf{S}_{t+1})} Q(\mathbf{S}_{t+1}, a_{t+1})\big|\mathbf{S}_t = \mathbf{s}, A_t = a\right\}, \tag{6.8}$$

where, critically, the expectation is taken with respect to the data-generating model rather than a counterfactual distribution. Let $\psi : \mathcal{S} \times \mathcal{A} \to \mathbb{R}^d$ be an arbitrary function of state. It follows that

$$\begin{aligned} Q(\mathbf{S}_t, A_t) &= \mathbb{E}\left\{Y_t + \gamma \max_{a_{t+1}\in\nu(\mathbf{S}_{t+1})} Q(\mathbf{S}_{t+1}, a_{t+1})\Big|\mathbf{S}_t, A_t\right\} \\ \Longrightarrow 0 &= \mathbb{E}\left\{Y_t + \gamma \max_{a_{t+1}\in\nu(\mathbf{S}_{t+1})} Q(\mathbf{S}_{t+1}, a_{t+1}) - Q(\mathbf{S}_t, A_t)\Big|\mathbf{S}_t, A_t\right\} \\ \Longrightarrow 0 &= \mathbb{E}\left[\left\{Y_t + \gamma \max_{a_{t+1}\in\nu(\mathbf{S}_{t+1})} Q(\mathbf{S}_{t+1}, a_{t+1}) - Q(\mathbf{S}_t, A_t)\right\}\psi(\mathbf{S}_t, A_t)\right], \end{aligned}$$

where the last equality follows from multiplying the second equality by $\psi(\mathbf{S}_t, A_t)$ and taking an expectation. Q-learning uses this last equality to construct an estimating function for the Q-function. We illustrate this idea using a linear model for the Q-function of the form $Q(\mathbf{s}, a) = \phi(\mathbf{s}, a)^{\mathrm{T}}\boldsymbol{\theta}$ where $\phi : \mathcal{S} \times \mathcal{A} \to \mathbb{R}^d$ is a feature vector and $\boldsymbol{\theta} \in \boldsymbol{\Theta} \subseteq \mathbb{R}^d$ is a vector of unknown coefficients. We take $\psi(\mathbf{s}, a) = \nabla_{\boldsymbol{\theta}} Q(\mathbf{s}, a; \boldsymbol{\theta}) = \phi(\mathbf{s}, a)$, and construct $\widehat{\boldsymbol{\theta}}_{t,n}$ as the solution to

$$\begin{aligned} 0 = \sum_{i=1}^{n}\sum_{v=1}^{t} &\left\{Y_{t,i} + \gamma \max_{a_{t+1}\in\nu(\mathbf{S}_{t+1,i})} \phi(\mathbf{S}_{t+1,i}, a_{t+1})^{\mathrm{T}}\boldsymbol{\theta} - \phi(\mathbf{S}_{t,i}, A_{t,i})^{\mathrm{T}}\boldsymbol{\theta}\right\} \\ &\times \phi(\mathbf{S}_{t,i}, A_{t,i}), \end{aligned} \tag{6.9}$$

so that the estimated optimal regime is $\widehat{\pi}_{t,n}(\mathbf{s}) = \arg\max_{a\in\nu(\mathbf{s})} Q(\mathbf{s}, a; \widehat{\boldsymbol{\theta}}_{t,n})$.

To implement TS in this context we again use the estimated sampling distribution of $\widehat{\boldsymbol{\theta}}_{t,n}$, (based on an asymptotic approximation in which n grows large). To select a treatment at time $t+1$, we draw $\lambda_{1,n}, \ldots, \lambda_{n,n} \sim_{i.i.d.} \mathrm{Exp}(1)$, compute $\widetilde{\boldsymbol{\theta}}_{t,n}$ as the solution to

$$\begin{aligned} 0 = \sum_{i=1}^{n}\lambda_{i,n}\sum_{v=1}^{t} &\left\{Y_{t,i} + \gamma \max_{a_{t+1}\in\nu(\mathbf{S}_{t+1,i})} \phi(\mathbf{S}_{t+1,i}, a_{t+1})^{\mathrm{T}}\boldsymbol{\theta} - \phi(\mathbf{S}_{t,i}, A_{t,i})^{\mathrm{T}}\boldsymbol{\theta}\right\} \\ &\times \phi(\mathbf{S}_{t,i}, A_{t,i}), \end{aligned}$$

and assign treatments at time point $t+1$ according to the regime $\widetilde{\pi}_t(\mathbf{s}) = \arg\max_{a\in\nu(\mathbf{s})} Q(\mathbf{s}, a; \widetilde{\boldsymbol{\theta}}_{t,n})$; i.e., $A_{t+1,i} = \arg\max_{a\in\nu(\mathbf{S}_{t+1,i})} \psi(\mathbf{S}_{t+1,i}, A_{t+1,i})^{\mathrm{T}}\widetilde{\boldsymbol{\theta}}_{t,n}$, for $i = 1, \ldots, n$.

The preceding version of TS uses a single bootstrap resample at each time point. An alternative is to compute a separate resample for each subject, i.e., for subject j, we draw $\lambda_{1,n,j}, \ldots, \lambda_{n,n,j} \sim_{i.i.d.} \mathrm{Exp}(1)$, compute $\widetilde{\boldsymbol{\theta}}_{t,n,j}$ as the solution to

$$\begin{aligned} 0 = \sum_{i=1}^{n}\lambda_{i,n,j}\sum_{v=1}^{t} &\left\{Y_{t,i} + \gamma \max_{a_{t+1}\in\nu(\mathbf{S}_{t+1,i})} \phi(\mathbf{S}_{t+1,i}, a_{t+1})^{\mathrm{T}}\boldsymbol{\theta} - \phi(\mathbf{S}_{t,i}, A_{t,i})^{\mathrm{T}}\boldsymbol{\theta}\right\} \\ &\times \phi(\mathbf{S}_{t,i}, A_{t,i}), \end{aligned}$$

and set $A_{t+1,j} = \arg\max_{a\in\nu(\mathbf{S}_{t+1,i})} \phi(\mathbf{S}_{t+1,j}, a)^{\mathrm{T}}\widetilde{\boldsymbol{\theta}}_{t,n,j}$. This approach, while computationally more expensive, often provides better balance in terms of treatment allocation across subject states.

6.4.3 Inference for TS in MDPs

Statistical inference under adaptive sampling, i.e., when accumulated are used to select interventions, is markedly more complex than non-adaptive sampling (Lai and Wei, 1982; Zhan et al., 2021; Zhang et al., 2020, 2022). Intuitively, a key challenge is ensuring sufficient information generation across the entire state-action (state-treatment) space $\mathcal{S} \times \mathcal{A}$. An adaptive algorithm attempting to maximize cumulative reward may quickly become concentrated around an optimal regime so that little data is available for estimation and inference about the performance of other regimes of interest (say business-as-usual, or a less intensive regime, etc.). In this section, we introduce some basic technical tools that are often useful for analyzing TS in MDPs (as well as in other settings such as bandits or partially observable MDPs).

We treat the number of subjects, n, as fixed and consider asymptotic approximations as the number of time points, t, grows large. As in the preceding section, to simplify notation, we assume that subjects are aligned in time. Let $\mathcal{F}_t$ denote the σ-algebra generated by $\{(\mathbf{S}_{1,i}, A_{1,i}, \mathbf{S}_{2,i,}, A_{2,i}, \ldots, \mathbf{S}_{t-1,i}, A_{t-1,i}, \mathbf{S}_{t,i})\}_{i=1}^{n}$, and for any $\boldsymbol{\theta}$ define

$$u_t(\theta) = \sum_{i=1}^{n} \left\{ Y_{t,i} + \gamma \max_{a_{t+1}} \phi(\mathbf{S}_{t+1,i}, a_{t+1})^{\mathsf{T}}\boldsymbol{\theta} - \phi(\mathbf{S}_{t,i}, A_{t,i})^{\mathsf{T}}\boldsymbol{\theta} \right\} \phi(\mathbf{S}_{t,i}, A_{t,i}).$$

The Q-learning estimating equations (6.9) can thus be written as $\mathcal{U}_t(\boldsymbol{\theta}) = 0$, where

$$\mathcal{U}_t(\boldsymbol{\theta}) = \sum_{v=1}^{t} u_v(\boldsymbol{\theta}).$$

Suppose that the model is correctly specified so that $Q(\mathbf{s}, a) = \phi(\mathbf{s}, a)^{\mathsf{T}}\boldsymbol{\theta}^*$ for some $\boldsymbol{\theta}^* \in \boldsymbol{\Theta}$ and all $(\mathbf{s}, a) \in \mathcal{S} \times \mathcal{A}$. Then it follows that $\mathcal{U}_t(\boldsymbol{\theta}^*)$ is a Martingale with respect to the filtration $\{\mathcal{F}_t\}_{t\geq 1}$ as

$$\begin{aligned}
\mathbb{E}\left\{\mathcal{U}_t(\boldsymbol{\theta}^*)\middle|\mathcal{F}_t\right\} &= \mathbb{E}\left\{u_t(\boldsymbol{\theta}^*)\middle|\mathcal{F}_t\right\} + \mathcal{U}_{t-1}(\boldsymbol{\theta}^*) \\
&= \mathbb{E}\left[\sum_{i=1}^{n} \left\{ Y_{t,i} + \gamma \max_{a_{t+1}} \phi(\mathbf{S}_{t+1,i}, a_{t+1})^{\mathsf{T}}\boldsymbol{\theta}^* - \phi(\mathbf{S}_{t,i}, A_{t,i})^{\mathsf{T}}\boldsymbol{\theta}^* \right\} \phi(\mathbf{S}_{t,i}, A_{t,i})\middle|\mathcal{F}_t\right] \\
&\quad + \mathcal{U}_{t-1}(\boldsymbol{\theta}^*) \\
&= \mathbb{E}\left[\sum_{i=1}^{n} \left\{ Y_{t,i} + \gamma \max_{a_{t+1}} Q(\mathbf{S}_{t+1,i}, a_{t+1}) - Q(\mathbf{S}_{t,i}, A_{t,i}) \right\} \phi(\mathbf{S}_{t,i}, A_{t,i})\middle|\mathcal{F}_t\right] \\
&\quad + \mathcal{U}_{t-1}(\boldsymbol{\theta}^*) \\
&= \mathbb{E}\left[\sum_{i=1}^{n} \left\{ Y_{t,i} + \gamma \max_{a_{t+1}} Q(\mathbf{S}_{t+1,i}, a_{t+1}) - Q(\mathbf{S}_{t,i}, A_{t,i}) \right\} \phi(\mathbf{S}_{t,i}, A_{t,i})\middle|\mathbf{S}_t, A_t\right] \\
&\quad + \mathcal{U}_{t-1}(\boldsymbol{\theta}^*) \\
&= \mathcal{U}_{t-1}(\boldsymbol{\theta}^*).
\end{aligned}$$

Thus, $\mathcal{U}_t(\boldsymbol{\theta})$ is a Martingale estimating function (MEF; Godambe, 1991; Heyde, 1997; Hwang and Basawa, 2014), and the operating characteristics of $\widehat{\boldsymbol{\theta}}_{t,n}$ can be derived through properties of the functions $\boldsymbol{\theta} \mapsto \mathcal{U}_t(\boldsymbol{\theta})$. Our focus will be on conditions under which $\Sigma_{t,n}^{-1/2}(\boldsymbol{\theta}^*)\left\{\widehat{\boldsymbol{\theta}}_{t,n} - \boldsymbol{\theta}^*\right\} \rightsquigarrow \mathrm{N}(0, I_d)$ as $t \to \infty$, where $\Sigma_{t,n}(\boldsymbol{\theta}^*)$ is a (possibly random) scaling matrix. The conditions we provide are standard in MEF-theory. While these conditions are seemingly mild, they can be difficult to verify in practice.

Let $||J||_F = \sqrt{\text{trace}(J^\top J)}$ denote the Frobenius norm. Define $\xi_t(\boldsymbol{\theta}^*) \triangleq \text{Var}\{u_t(\boldsymbol{\theta}^*)|\mathcal{F}_t\} = \mathbb{E}\{u_t(\boldsymbol{\theta})u_t(\boldsymbol{\theta})^\top|\mathcal{F}_t\}$. We assume (C1) that $||\xi_t(\boldsymbol{\theta}^*)|| \to \infty$ almost surely, as $t \to \infty$. Condition (C1) is a regularity condition which ensures sufficient information is generated across the state-action space. To see this, write

$$\text{Var}\{u_t(\boldsymbol{\theta}^*)|\mathcal{F}_t\} = \sum_{i=1}^{n} \mathbb{E}\{\delta_{t,i}^2(\boldsymbol{\theta}^*)|\mathbf{S}_{t,i}, A_{t,i}\}\, \phi(\mathbf{S}_{t,i}, A_{t,i})\phi(\mathbf{S}_{t,i}, A_{t,i})^\top,$$

where $\delta_{t,i}(\boldsymbol{\theta}) = Y_{t,i} + \gamma \max_{a_{t+1}} Q(\mathbf{S}_{t+1,i}, a_{t+1}) - Q(\mathbf{S}_{t,i}, A_{t,i})$ is the temporal difference error. If we assume that $\mathbb{E}\{\delta_{t,i}^2(\boldsymbol{\theta}^*)|\mathbf{S}_{t,i}, A_{t,i}\}$ is bounded below by some constant $c > 0$ with probability one, then a sufficient condition for (C1) is that the mininum eigenvalue of $\sum_{v=1}^{t}\sum_{i=1}^{n} \phi(\mathbf{S}_{v,i}, A_{v,i})\phi(\mathbf{S}_{v,i}, A_{v,i})^\top$ diverges to ∞, a condition that appears commonly in asymnptotics for time-series and other stochastic regression settings (Lai and Wei, 1982).

The second condition we require is (C2) that the MEF is regular, i.e., $\boldsymbol{\theta}^*$ is an interior point of $\boldsymbol{\Theta}$, $\mathcal{U}_t(\boldsymbol{\theta})$ is continuously differentiable almost everywhere in a neighborhood $\boldsymbol{\theta}^*$, and for any sequence $\overline{\boldsymbol{\theta}}_t$ converging in probability to $\boldsymbol{\theta}^*$ as $t \to \infty$, we have

$$\left|\left|\xi_t^{-1/2}(\boldsymbol{\theta}^*)\left\{\nabla_{\boldsymbol{\theta}}\mathcal{U}_t(\overline{\boldsymbol{\theta}}_t) - \nabla_{\boldsymbol{\theta}}\mathcal{U}_t(\boldsymbol{\theta}^*)\right\}\xi_t^{-1/2}(\boldsymbol{\theta}^*)\right|\right| \to_p 0,$$

as $t \to \infty$. Condition (C2) is a smoothness condition that rules out the possibility of multiple optimal treatments in any state (at such points, the max operator is not differentiable). It is possible to weaken this condition but at the expense of more complex asymptotic arguments (see Laber et al., 2014).

The third condition we require is (C3) that there exists a constant (non-stochastic) matrix $\boldsymbol{\Omega} \in \mathbb{R}^{d\times d}$ such that

$$\xi_t^{-1/2}(\boldsymbol{\theta}^*)\nabla_{\boldsymbol{\theta}}\mathcal{U}_t(\boldsymbol{\theta}^*)\xi_t^{-1/2}(\boldsymbol{\theta}^*) \to_p \boldsymbol{\Omega},$$

as $t \to \infty$. Condition (C3) is a regularity condition that can typically be verified using strong laws for dependent data (Prakasa Rao, 1987).

Finally, we require (C4) that $-\{\xi_t(\boldsymbol{\theta}^*)\}^{-1/2}\mathcal{U}_t(\boldsymbol{\theta}^*) \rightsquigarrow \text{N}(0, I_d)$. This condition can be established using a Martingale central limit theorem (Hall and Heyde, 2014).

Under (C1)–(C4) and mild moment conditions, it can be shown (Hwang, 2015) that $\boldsymbol{\Omega}\xi_t^{1/2}(\boldsymbol{\theta}^*)\left(\widehat{\boldsymbol{\theta}}_t - \boldsymbol{\theta}^*\right) \rightsquigarrow N(0, I_d)$, which is the desired result with $\Sigma_{t,n}^{-1/2}(\boldsymbol{\theta}^*) = \boldsymbol{\Omega}\xi_t^{1/2}(\boldsymbol{\theta}^*)$. This shows that $\widehat{\boldsymbol{\theta}}_{t,n} = O_p(||\xi_t^{-1/2}(\boldsymbol{\theta}^*)||)$, which in turn can be used to derive the (asymptotic) rate of the cumulative regret. To use this result to construct a confidence set for $\boldsymbol{\theta}^*$, we can use a projection interval as follows. Suppose that if $\boldsymbol{\theta}^*$ were known, one could construct a consistent estimator $\widehat{\boldsymbol{\Sigma}}_{t,n}^{-1/2}(\boldsymbol{\theta}^*)$ of $\boldsymbol{\Sigma}_{t,n}^{-1/2}(\boldsymbol{\theta}^*)$. Let $\chi_{d,1-\alpha}^2$ be the upper $(1-\alpha)\times 100\%$ percentile of a chi-squared distribution with d-degrees of freedom and define

$$\boldsymbol{\Gamma}_{t,n,1-\alpha} = \left\{\boldsymbol{\Theta} \in \boldsymbol{\Theta} : \widehat{\Sigma}_{t,n}^{-1/2}(\boldsymbol{\theta})\left(\widehat{\boldsymbol{\theta}}_{t,n} - \boldsymbol{\theta}\right) \le \chi_{d,1-\alpha}^2\right\}.$$

It follows that $P\{\boldsymbol{\theta}^* \in \Gamma_{t,n,1-\alpha}\} \ge 1-\alpha+o_P(1)$. The set $\Gamma_{t,n,1-\alpha}$ is thus a valid (asymptotic) confidence region for $\boldsymbol{\theta}^*$ which in turn can be used to construct projection sets for other functions of $\boldsymbol{\theta}^*$, e.g., the value of the optimal regime (see also Zhang et al., 2022).

6.5 Open problems and ongoing work

Our goal in this chapter was to introduce TS as a flexible and extensible methodology for adaptive clinical trials especially in the context of mobile- and tele-health. However, despite a long history of empirical and theoretical study, there are a number of pressing open problems associated with TS. One such problem is statistical efficiency. The estimating equations we described are used widely in practice but they need not lead to the smallest asymptotic variance among the class of regular MEFs. Furthermore, if the posited class of models for the Q-function is misspecified, the solution to the MEF need not recover the projection of the true Q-function on the model class (see Baird, 1995; Leete and Laber, 2022). An important open question is how to construct the estimating equations to obtain efficiency and the projection property. In principle, the efficient weights for the estimating equations can be obtained using the theory of optimal MEFs (Hwang and Basawa, 2011). However, the efficient weights depend on the unknown system dynamics and the cost of estimating the optimal weights risks further misspecification and/or inflated variance (Leete and Laber, 2022).

Another important open problem is interim analysis and optimal stopping for adaptive experiments under TS. In theory, one could obtain (approximate) joint asymptotic normality for the estimated parameters at multiple pre-specified analysis points and subsequently derive stopping boundaries (Jennison and Turnbull, 1999). However, the derivations of these boundaries are likely to be intricate.

Lastly, we note that TS may fail to perform well if the underlying system is non-stationary. One *ad hoc* approach is to limit the look-back period and only use estimating equations constructed from recent data. An important problem is how to adaptively choose the look-back period to optimally balance bias and variance.

Part II

Estimation of Optimal Treatment Strategies

Chapter 7

Constructing and Evaluating Optimal Treatment Sequences: An Introductory Guide for Bayesians

David A. Stephens

In this chapter, we discuss Bayesian approaches to forming optimal treatment sequences derived from observational data. We show how plausible standard approaches do not give the correct quantification of treatment sequence effectiveness, and how frequentist solutions can be adapted to yield valid Bayesian solutions. For simplicity, we restrict attention to the case when the number of treatment intervals m is fixed and finite. We explain how the classical methods of G-computation, Q-learning, and marginal structural modelling via inverse probability weighting for inferring optimal static and dynamic treatment sequences can be adapted to become full Bayesian procedures. The advantage of adopting a fully Bayesian approach is that it gives a complete representation of uncertainty in inference, and properly quantifies the performance of estimated optimal (and sub-optimal) regimes.

The Bayesian approach to learning optimal treatment regimes is a developing literature that is mainly founded in the parametric, and flexible but still model-based paradigm; a recent review of Bayesian methodology applied to the causal setting can be found in Oganisian and Roy (2021). An introduction to classical Bayesian approaches is given by Saarela et al. (2015), who used a posterior predictive approach that requires the specification of parametric distributions for outcomes and intermediate covariates, as described in section 7.4. More recently, Murray et al. (2018) proposed a Bayesian adaptation to Q-learning (see section 7.3.6). Hua et al. (2022) proposed a Bayesian joint model for the sequence of interventions and clinical measurements, including intermediary covariates and the final outcome, largely adopting the parametric paradigm. More akin to frequentist semi-parametric approaches, Arjas and Saarela (2010) used Bayesian nonparametric regression and backward induction. Guan et al. (2020) deploy another nonparametric policy search approach in a clinical setting. Recently, a Bayesian weighting method (see section 7.6) for inferring optimal DTRs via dynamic marginal structural models (MSMs, see Orellana et al. (2010)) was developed by Rodriguez Duque et al. (2023). We summarize the key elements of these approaches in later sections but begin with an introduction and an illustrative example.

7.1 Introduction

To discover the optimal treatment regime from observational data in the Bayesian framework, we need first to construct the appropriate inference and decision-theoretic formulation. In the usual setting, longitudinal data $(X_k, A_k), k = 1, \ldots, m$, and a terminal outcome Y at stage m, are observed on a random sample of size n from some homogeneous population, and serve to inform the choice of an optimal treatment regime for future patients.

The principal challenge in determining the optimal strategy from observational data is the mis-match between the target of inference and the data-generating model. Typically the inference target is some quantity defined in a hypothetical experimental world where

DOI: 10.1201/9781003216223-7

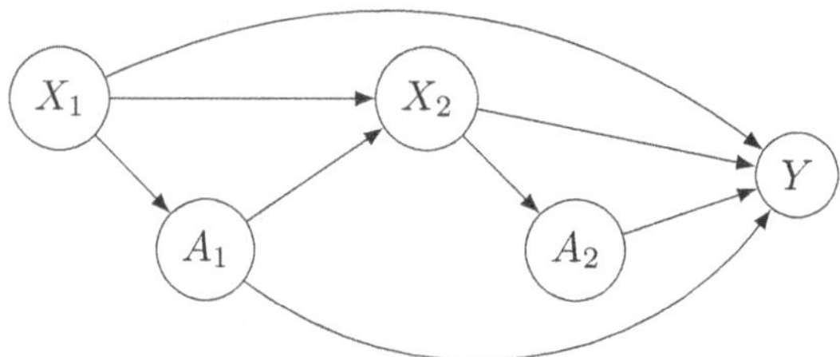

Figure 7.1 *Two stage example with mediation of the effect of* A_1 *via* X_2 *which is blocked in an outcome regression of* Y *on* (X_1, A_1, X_2, A_2).

treatment is assigned by intervention, independently of patient characteristics. The observed data, however, arise in the observational world where treatment is received via a mechanism which does depend on patient characteristics, so that any observed treatment impact is confounded. This difference between experimental target and observational reality can be overcome by modelling, by means of assumed connections between the two worlds or appropriate extrapolation from one to the other.

The second challenge is in constructing the inference model. The Bayesian statistical framework is usually based on parametric constructions so that a likelihood can be constructed and the Bayesian posterior distribution computed. The challenge for parametric analyses is that any parametric model is prone to mis-specification, which can lead to incorrect inference.

7.2 An Illustrative Example

In the following example, we illustrate how apparently plausible standard forms of analysis fail to give the correct quantification of the effect of a sequence of treatments.

Consider two binary treatments (A_1, A_2) and a single outcome generated by the data-generating model with $X_1 \sim \text{Normal}(1, 1)$, $A_1 \sim \text{Bernoulli}\{\text{expit}(-2 + X_1)\}$ at the first stage, and $X_2 \sim \text{Normal}(-3 + X_1 + A_1, 1)$ and $A_2 \sim \text{Bernoulli}\{\text{expit}(2 - X_2)\}$ at the second stage, with outcome model $Y \sim \text{Normal}(X_1 + A_1 + X_2 + A_2, 1)$. The data-generating model can be represented by the directed acyclic graph (DAG) in Figure 7.1.

This data-generating mechanism is notable in three respects: first, there is the possibility of confounding of the effect of treatment as X_1 and X_2 are causes of both the observed treatments A_1 and A_2 and the outcome Y; secondly, the effect of A_1 on Y is both direct (due to the arrow $A_1 \longrightarrow Y$) and indirect (due to the paths $A_1 \longrightarrow X_2 \longrightarrow Y$ and $A_1 \longrightarrow X_2 \longrightarrow A_2 \longrightarrow Y$); thirdly, the path $A_1 \longrightarrow X_2 \longrightarrow A_2$ indicates that the assignment of A_1 influences the later assignment of A_2. Thus, the effect of A_1 is mediated through later variables. The full likelihood derived from this DAG is useful as a probabilistic representation of the data structure, and often necessary for correct adjustment; it would typically be the basis of Bayesian inference. However, the number of terms in the specification can be large, which renders the likelihood quite complex to specify, and inference and decision-making often lack robustness to mis-specification.

Suppose we aim to discover the optimal treatment sequence, that is, which pattern (a_1, a_2) optimizes (for simplicity, maximizes) the expected outcome. We can conceive of this problem in two ways.

(i) *Static problem:* for any specified sequence (a_1, a_2), evaluate the outcome that would be expected under that sequence. Report the sequence that maximizes the expected outcome. More generally, report the expected outcome for all sequences under consideration, and report (say) and order of preference for the sequences, and the degree of suboptimality that each treatment sequence represents.

(ii) *Dynamic problem:* design a sequence of decision rules (d_1, d_2), that, for each subject, take as input the available information (h_1, h_2) up to time points 1 and 2 respectively, such that the optimal treatment sequence is determined on an individual-level basis using the personalized information available. That is, for each individual

$$a_1^{\text{opt}} = d_1(x_1) \qquad a_2^{\text{opt}} = d_2(x_1, a_1, x_2),$$

where d_1 and d_2 are *decision rules*, that is, functions that take the arguments as input, and return an optimally selected treatment allocation for each time point. In this dynamic formulation, treatments are individualized by applying d_1 and d_2 to individual-level histories. Note that we may also study dynamic strategies at the population level by replacing the individual-level calculation with a sample average.

It is important to note that the observed data are assumed not to arise from any optimal allocation process, but merely from the data-generating process encapsulated in Figure 7.1. We will give a general formulation in section 7.3.

7.2.1 *The Optimal Static Treatment Sequence*

We consider the static case first. Using counterfactual notation, we seek the sequence $(a_1^{\text{opt}}, a_2^{\text{opt}})$ given by

$$(a_1^{\text{opt}}, a_2^{\text{opt}}) = \arg\max_{(a_1,a_2)} \mathbb{E}[Y(a_1, a_2)].$$

Here the expectation is taken over the study population, which is characterized by subject characteristics summarized in (X_1, X_2). Thus the optimal static treatment sequence is optimal at the *population* level.

The first aspect that distinguishes the analysis here from a standard Bayesian analysis is that, in contrast to the data-generating mechanism from Figure 7.1, the target of inference is based on a DAG where the treatments arise by *intervention*, that is, where the treatments are fixed at the required levels directly, and not as a result of the observation process captured by Figure 7.1. The pertinent DAG for the desired calculation is one where the arrows $X_1 \longrightarrow A_1$ and $X_2 \longrightarrow A_2$ are absent; see Figure 7.2. In this DAG, if X_1 and X_2 are conditioned upon (as would be the case in the typical regression model), the effect of treatment (a_1, a_2) is only manifested via direct paths.

In the corresponding 'experimental' (interventional) model, intervening to set $(A_1, A_2) = (a_1, a_2)$ yields the expected (counterfactual) outcome, denoted $\mathbb{E}[Y(a_1, a_2)]$, we have by standard calculations that

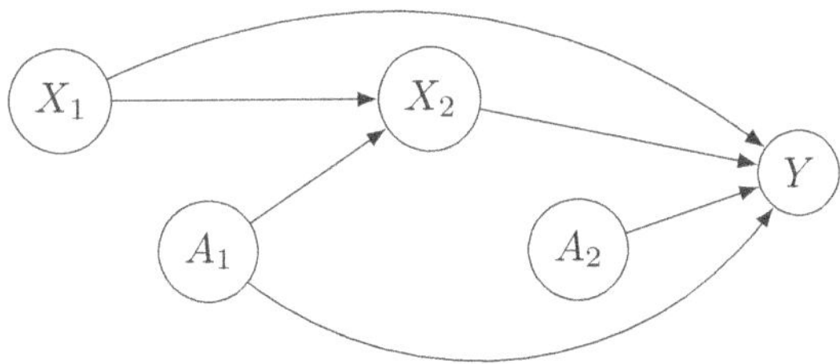

Figure 7.2 *Two stage example with intervention to set the value of A_1 and A_2.*

$$\begin{aligned}
\mathbb{E}[Y(a_1,a_2)] &= \mathbb{E}_{X_1,X_2}[X_1 + a_1 + X_2 + a_2] \\
&= 1 + a_1 + a_2 + \mathbb{E}_{X_1}[\mathbb{E}_{X_2|X_1}[X_2|X_1]] \\
&= 1 + a_1 + a_2 + \mathbb{E}_{X_1}[-3 + X_1 + a_1] \\
&= -1 + 2a_1 + a_2.
\end{aligned}$$

That is, $\mathbb{E}[Y(0,0)] = -1, \mathbb{E}[Y(1,0)] = 1, \mathbb{E}[Y(0,1)] = 0, \mathbb{E}[Y(1,1)] = 2$, and we have that

$$\mathbb{E}[Y(0,0)] < \mathbb{E}[Y(0,1)] < \mathbb{E}[Y(1,0)] < \mathbb{E}[Y(1,1)]$$

which establishes the preference ordering on the fixed (pre-specified) treatment patterns.

7.2.2 A Standard Bayesian Analysis for the Static Case

A Bayesian formulation would target the posterior distribution for the expected counterfactual $\mathbb{E}[Y(a_1,a_2)]$, or the corresponding posterior predictive distribution, or Bayesian estimators of these quantities derived from these distributions. We proceed assuming the form of the outcome model is known. An obvious method of analysis for the observational data involves the regression of Y on the treatment and confounder data (X_1, A_1, X_2, A_2) simultaneously. This can readily be achieved via standard Bayesian analysis using the linear model. A correctly specified outcome model alone, however, consistently estimates the coefficients of (X_1, A_1, X_2, A_2) as $(1,1,1,1)$, and produces posterior distributions that centre at these values. This posterior distribution can be used to construct posterior predictive distributions for the hypothetical outcomes at any combination of treatments, and an estimate of the expected counterfactual can be constructed from this posterior predictive.

Using the regression model to recover counterfactual outcomes relies upon a plug-in estimate of the posterior mean, which in large samples is equivalent to the frequentist (OLS) estimator given by

$$\frac{1}{n}\sum_{i=1}^{n}(\widehat{\beta}_0 + X_{i1}\widehat{\beta}_1 + a_1\widehat{\beta}_2 + X_{i2}\widehat{\beta}_3 + a_2\widehat{\beta}_4).$$

As $n \longrightarrow \infty$, this quantity converges in probability to

$$1 + \mathbb{E}[X_1] + a_1 + \mathbb{E}[X_2] + a_2.$$

In the data-generating model, $\mathbb{E}[X_1] = 1$ and

$$\begin{aligned}
\mathbb{E}[X_2] &= \mathbb{E}_{X_1,A_1}[\mathbb{E}_{X_2|X_1,A_1}[X_2|X_1,A_1]] \\
&= \mathbb{E}_{X_1,A_1}[-3 + X_1 + A_1] \\
&= \mathbb{E}_{X_1}[-3 + X_1 + \text{expit}(-2 + X_1)] \\
&= -2 + \mathbb{E}_{X_1}[\text{expit}(-2 + X_1)] \simeq -1.69.
\end{aligned}$$

Therefore the counterfactual outcomes are inconsistently estimated using this Bayesian strategy. The issue arises due to the confounding that is present in the data-generating process, but also due to mediation of the effect of A_1 through X_2. The probability limit of the Bayesian estimator is (approximately) $-0.69 + a_1 + a_2$, and none of the counterfactual outcomes or contrasts are correctly estimated, and although the optimal (outcome maximizing) treatment sequence $(a_1, a_2) = (1, 1)$ is correctly recovered, the ordering of the treatment patterns is not correctly recovered; to optimize the expected potential outcome, the treatment pattern (1,0) is preferred to pattern (0,1), as $\mathbb{E}[Y(1,0)] > \mathbb{E}[Y(0,1)]$, whereas the using the outcome regression method the estimated versions are equal. Thus, a standard likelihood-based approach cannot recover the targets of inference in cases where there is mediation of the effect of past treatments.

A Bayesian solution can be constructed using an auxiliary variable approach. The key issue that compromises the above calculation is that in the observed data X_2 is influenced by A_1, which itself is caused by X_1, whereas the target of inference requires X_2 to be determined by an experimentally determined A_1 which is set at level a_1 when the static sequence (a_1, a_2) is being considered. However, having fitted a model to predict X_2 as a function of (X_1, A_1) that matches the data generating distribution, this model may then be used to generate auxiliary versions, $\widetilde{X}_2 \equiv \widetilde{X}_2(a_1)$, for each target treatment level a_1, by examining the posterior predictive distribution. Equipped with the auxiliary data, analysis can then be carried out regressing Y on $(X_1, A_1, \widetilde{X}_2(a_1), A_2)$. The procedure is summarized in Algorithm 7.1. This analysis produces a posterior distribution for the regression parameters, which can in turn be used to produce a predictive distribution for outcomes for every combination of (a_1, a_2), which can then be appropriately summarized.

7.2.3 *The Optimal Dynamic Treatment Sequence*

Optimal dynamic treatment sequences are typically constructed at the *individual* level. That is, for each point in the treatment sequence, it is desired to determine the optimal treatment to be allocated at that time point by taking into account information on the individual subject that is available at that instant. Such a process is termed *tailoring*. As described in section 7.2, at time point 1, the information available for tailoring is simply the value of $h_1 = x_1$; at time point 2, we may tailor on $h_2 = (x_1, a_1, x_2)$: tailoring rules will be denoted (d_1, d_2). However, it is evident from the earlier discussion that treatment decisions taken at stage 1 may affect treatment decisions at stage 2, and this influences how we formulate the construction of the dynamic strategy.

At the individual level, we still seek the optimal sequence $(a_1^{\text{opt}}, a_2^{\text{opt}})$, but note that as $a_2^{\text{opt}} = d_2(x_1, a_1, x_2)$, we may decide upon the optimal second stage treatment directly using the observed data. For example, using the linear model

$$\beta_{200} + \beta_{201}x_1 + \beta_{202}a_1 + \beta_{203}x_2 + a_2(\beta_{210} + \beta_{211}x_1 + \beta_{212}a_1 + \beta_{213}x_2)$$

or more compactly

$$h_{20}\beta_{20} + a_2 h_{21}\beta_{21},$$

where

$$\begin{aligned} \beta_{20} &= (\beta_{200}, \beta_{201}, \beta_{202}, \beta_{203})^\top & \qquad h_{20} &= (1, x_1, a_1, x_2) \\ \beta_{21} &= (\beta_{210}, \beta_{211}, \beta_{212}, \beta_{213})^\top & \qquad h_{21} &= (1, x_1, a_1, x_2) \end{aligned}$$

it is evident that

$$a_2^{\text{opt}} = \mathbf{1}\{\beta_{210} + \beta_{211}x_1 + \beta_{212}a_1 + \beta_{213}x_2 > 0\},$$

that is, the optimal second stage treatment sets $a_2 = 1$ if, for the individual concerned, the expected outcome increases under that setting, and sets $a_2 = 0$ otherwise. Therefore the tailoring rule is

$$d_2(h_{21}; \beta_{21}) = \mathbf{1}\{\beta_{210} + \beta_{211}x_1 + \beta_{212}a_1 + \beta_{213}x_2 > 0\}.$$

For the moment we assume that parameters β_{20} and β_{21} are known, but in practice an inferential step is necessary.

Having decided upon the optimal treatment at stage 2, we now attempt to construct the optimal treatment at stage 1. This step is more complicated; for each individual, we have computed their optimal stage 2 treatment as a_2^{opt}, but in general, this is not guaranteed to be identical to their *actual* stage 2 treatment A_2. Therefore, direct usage of the observed outcome Y in the assessment of a_1^{opt} is not possible, as Y is a consequence of the treatment sequence (A_1, A_2) and not (A_1, a_2^{opt}). A formulation is required that allows for the use of observed data to infer the optimal treatment at the first stage under hypothetical optimal treatment assignment at the second stage.

If, for binary treatments, the blip function is formed with a single, continuous tailoring variable x, then the form of the decision rule is

$$a^{\text{opt}} = \mathbf{1}\{\beta_0 + \beta_1 x > 0\} \equiv \mathbf{1}\{x > \theta\},$$

where $\theta = -\beta_0/\beta_1$ provided $\beta_1 > 0$. This indicates a more direct form of tailoring rule that relies on thresholding the tailoring variables, for example

$$\begin{aligned} d_2(h_2) &= \mathbf{1}\{(x_1 > \theta_{21}) \cap (x_2 > \theta_{22})\} \\ d_2(h_1) &= \mathbf{1}\{(x_1 > \theta_{11})\} \end{aligned}$$

where $(\theta_{11}, \theta_{21}, \theta_{22})$ are fixed thresholds. Rules defined using thresholds may be learned from the observed data by constructing the blip function directly in terms of the indicators of compatibility with the rule. For the two-stage case, we might fit the model with blip

$$\mathbf{1}\{(x_1 > \theta_{21}) \cap (x_2 > \theta_{22})\}\beta_{21}$$

and then make the decision to treat or not treat at stage 2 based on the sign of β_{21}. This leads to a non-linear dependence on θ_{21} and θ_{22} in the outcome mean model.

7.2.4 A Standard Bayesian Analysis for the Dynamic Case

A Bayesian solution using auxiliary variables can be constructed. Consider a collection of auxiliary response variables, $\widetilde{Y}$, one for each individual in the study, that represent the outcomes that would be observed if the individual was treated as per the observed data at stage 1, but then optimally treated at stage 2. First, note that for each individual, we have the decomposition

$$\mathbb{E}[Y(a_1, a_2^{\text{opt}})] = \mathbb{E}[Y(a_1, a_2)] + \{\mathbb{E}[Y(a_1, a_2^{\text{opt}})] - \mathbb{E}[Y(a_1, a_2)]\}$$

and, given the proposed model for the outcome used to deduce the optimal stage 2 treatment, we have that

$$\mathbb{E}[Y(a_1, a_2^{\text{opt}})] - \mathbb{E}[Y(a_1, a_2)] = (a_2^{\text{opt}} - a_2)h_{21}\beta_{21}.$$

This suggests that for each individual we should take

$$\widetilde{Y} = Y + (a_2^{\text{opt}} - a_2)h_{21}\beta_{21}.$$

Note that $\widetilde{Y} \geq Y$ almost surely; $\widetilde{Y} \equiv Y$ if, in fact, the individual did receive their optimal treatment at stage 2, and $\widetilde{Y} > Y$ if they were sub-optimally treated. Once the $\widetilde{Y}$ has been obtained, a further model can be developed to represent them. Using the decomposition

$$\mathbb{E}[Y(a_1, a_2^{\text{opt}})] = \mathbb{E}[Y(0, a_2^{\text{opt}})] + \{\mathbb{E}[Y(a_1, a_2^{\text{opt}})] - \mathbb{E}[Y(0, a_2^{\text{opt}})]\}$$

we may propose the conditional outcome model for $\widetilde{Y}$ with mean

$$\beta_{100} + \beta_{101}x_1 + a_2(\beta_{110} + \beta_{111}x_1) \equiv h_{10}\beta_{10} + a_1 h_{11}\beta_{11}$$

say, where

$$\beta_{10} = (\beta_{100}, \beta_{101})^\top \qquad h_{10} = (1, x_1)$$
$$\beta_{11} = (\beta_{110}, \beta_{111})^\top \qquad h_{11} = (1, x_1).$$

A key assumption in such a model is that under optimal treatment at stage 2, the variation in $\widetilde{Y}$ is due only to (x_1, a_1) but not the second-stage variables. Once a fit to the auxiliary outcomes $\widetilde{Y}$ has been obtained, the optimal first-stage decision is obtained using the tailoring rule d_1 where

$$d_1(h_{11}; \beta_{11}) = \mathbf{1}\{h_{11}\beta_{11} > 0\}.$$

A full Bayesian analysis based on this strategy is straightforward if the model parameters are now assumed to be unknown. The analysis is easiest to implement using a sampling-based approach, implemented as follows:

- sample the stage 2 posterior for (β_{20}, β_{21});
- for each individual, produce a sample from the optimal stage 2 treatment as a function of the sample from the stage 2 posterior

$$a_2^{\text{opt}} = \mathbf{1}\{h_{21}\beta_{21} > 0\};$$

- for each individual, produce a sample from the auxiliary outcome

$$\widetilde{Y} = Y + (a_2^{\text{opt}} - a_2)h_{21}\beta_{21};$$

- using the auxiliary outcomes, sample the stage 1 posterior for (β_{10}, β_{11});
- for each individual, produce a sample from the optimal stage 1 treatment as a function of the sample from the stage 1 posterior

$$a_1^{\text{opt}} = \mathbf{1}\{h_{11}\beta_{11} > 0\}.$$

This process results in a posterior sample for $(a_1^{\text{opt}}, a_2^{\text{opt}})$ for each individual, from which posterior probabilities of optimality on the possible combinations of treatments for all individuals can be estimated. Algorithm 7.2 describes the steps in the implementation. The posterior distributions can be used to deduce the optimal rule based on a tailored loss function. For the binary treatment case, the estimated probabilities form a 2×2 table for each individual, and the desired optimal dynamic rule will typically be the one that carries the highest posterior probability.

Note that for each individual the values

$$Y^{\text{opt}} = Y + (a_1^{\text{opt}} - a_1)h_{11}\beta_{11} + (a_2^{\text{opt}} - a_2)h_{21}\beta_{21}$$

may be constructed as further auxiliaries to represent outcomes that would have been observed under optimal treatment at each stage. From Algorithm 7.2, sampled values of $a_1^{\text{opt}}, a_2^{\text{opt}}, \beta_{11}$ and β_{21} can be converted into sampled values of Y^{opt} for each individual.

The suggested method for obtaining the auxiliary outcome $\widetilde{Y}$ could be replaced by a simple prediction from the fitted stage 2 model evaluated at (a_1, a_2^{opt}), that is, using both terms in the stage 2 outcome model rather than the treatment effect component only.

7.2.5 *Weaknesses in the Standard Bayesian Analysis*

The Bayesian approaches described in sections 7.2.2 and 7.2.4 use sampling-based approaches in a conventional fashion using auxiliary variable formulations. However, the analyses rely on assumptions that are typically regarded as overly strong compared with comparable frequentist analyses. The assumptions relate to the requirement for correct parametric specification.

1. *Mean model specification*: both static and dynamic approaches rely on regression models that must be correctly specified in order to achieve consistent estimation of the effect of treatment strategies.
2. *Sufficient adjustment for confounding and mediation*: part of the correct specification assumption relates to the need to ensure that all paths between the treatments and the outcome are accounted for correctly.
3. *Error distribution specification*: in order to construct a likelihood-based analysis, distributional assumptions need to be made for the various conditional models. In the case of binary (treatment) variables, this essentially amounts to the choice of link function in a binary regression. For continuous variables, the choices of link function and of the residual error model must be made.

7.3 Recap of the Causal Formulation

We now extend the illustrative example to multiple stages and give the analogous frequentist formulation. We assume that there are m treatment stages, observations of possible confounders X_k, observed treatments A_k, and possibly intermediate outcomes Y_k, for $k = 1, \ldots, m$.

7.3.1 Potential Outcomes and their Expectation

The expected potential outcome $\mathbb{E}[Y(\overline{a}_m)] = \mathbb{E}[Y(a_1, \ldots, a_m)]$ represents the expected response to treatment pattern $\overline{a}_m$. More generally, the treatment decision at each interval may be the result of a treatment decision $a_k = d_k(h_k)$. The potential outcome of interest may depend functionally on the terminal value Y_m alone, so that $Y(\overline{a}_m) \equiv Y_m(\overline{a}_m)$, or be some summary of intermediate outcomes vector across all stages, for example

$$Y(\overline{a}_m) \equiv \sum_{k=1}^{m} Y_k(\overline{a}_m).$$

We restrict attention to the case where the outcome of interest is a scalar, although this also can be readily generalized. The *value* function, $V(\cdot)$, is a function of the treatment pattern $\overline{a}_m$ or treatment decision rule pattern $\overline{d}_m$ to be optimized, i.e., $V(\overline{a}_m) = \mathbb{E}[Y(\overline{a}_m)]$ and

$$V(\overline{a}_m^{\text{opt}}) = \max_{\overline{d}_m} \mathbb{E}[Y(\overline{d}_m)].$$

7.3.2 Types of Treatment Strategies

As mentioned in section 7.2, there are two types of assessment that could be considered.

(i) *Fixed* strategies: these are strategies that are pre-determined, prior to any data observation apart from perhaps measurement of baseline covariates. The statistical challenge for assessing the relative advantages of fixed strategies is the quantification of the effect of intervention $\overline{a}_m$ in the presence of confounding.

(ii) *Dynamic* or *adaptive* strategies: these are strategies that determine treatment in a sequential fashion with the treatment at stage k allowed to depend on a patient's prior history, h_k. As well as accounting for confounding, the statistical challenge is to deduce the optimal strategy when it may not have been observed in the data for any individual.

In most cases, the optimal dynamic strategies are constructed from a *hyperopic* standpoint, with optimal decisions being those that maximize the terminal outcome, as opposed to *myopic* strategies that prioritize short-term or stagewise optimality.

7.3.3 Bellman Optimization for Dynamic Strategies

Most methods for discovering optimal dynamic treatment strategies use the *Bellman optimization* approach which utilizes the fact that the optimal treatment only arises if stagewise (hyperopic) optimality is ensured. For example, the optimal treatment sequence can only arise if, first, the stage m optimal treatment is selected; once a_m^{opt} or d_m^{opt} is deduced, the stage $m-1$ optimal treatment can be deduced, assuming optimal treatment is followed at interval m; this reverse-order recursion eventually returns the optimal sequence $\overline{a}_m^{\text{opt}}$ with, for $k = m, m-1, \ldots, 1$,

$$a_k^{\text{opt}} = \arg\max_a V_k(h_k, a)$$

which, when completed, yield the optimal sequence or rule.

7.3.4 Decomposing the Effect of Treatment

Many of the classical methods of analysis are based on sequential decompositions of the form

$$\mathbb{E}[Y(\overline{a}_m)] = \mathbb{E}[Y(\mathbf{0})] + \sum_{k=0}^{m-1} \mathbb{E}[Y(\overline{a}_{k+1}, \mathbf{0}) - Y(\overline{a}_k, \mathbf{0})] \tag{7.1}$$

that exploit the telescoping sum involving stagewise contrasts comparing treatment a to treatment 0 at that stage. For example if $m = 2$,

$$\begin{aligned}\mathbb{E}[Y(a_1, a_2)] = \mathbb{E}[Y(0,0)] &+ \mathbb{E}[Y(a_1, 0) - Y(0,0)] \\ &+ \mathbb{E}[Y(a_1, a_2) - Y(a_1, 0)].\end{aligned}$$

This decomposition can be adopted to yield a recursive assessment of the expected counterfactual of interest. The total effect of a given treatment pattern up to stage k, with zero treatment for stages $k+1, \ldots, m$, may always be decomposed as

$$\begin{aligned}\mathbb{E}[Y(\overline{a}_k, \mathbf{0})] &= \mathbb{E}[Y(\overline{a}_{k-1}, \mathbf{0})] + \mathbb{E}[Y(\overline{a}_k, \mathbf{0}) - Y(\overline{a}_{k-1}, \mathbf{0})] \\ &= \mu_{k0}(h_k; \beta_{k0}) + \mu_{k1}(h_k, a_k; \beta_{k1})\end{aligned} \tag{7.2}$$

say, with separate models proposed for the two components; however, in the observed data, we only have access to the terminal outcome Y, and not data adhering to treatment at level zero past stage k. The functional forms of $\mu_{k0}(\cdot)$ and $\mu_{k1}(\cdot, a)$ are quite general, but typically we might choose linear regression-like terms. The dependence of $\mu_{k1}(\cdot, a)$ on a may include polynomial terms in a, although in the binary treatment case the mean model decomposition can be rewritten

$$\mu_{k0}(h_k; \beta_{k0}) + a_k \mu_{k1}(h_k; \beta_{k1}).$$

The term $\mu_{k1}(h_k, a_k; \beta_{k1})$ that reflects the expected additional treatment contribution is sometimes termed the *blip* function, whereas the term $\mu_{k0}(h_k; \beta_{k0})$ is referred to as the expected (counterfactual) *treatment-free* model.

The usual solution involves the recursive computation of pseudo-outcomes at each stage. As in section 7.3.3 we proceed via backwards recursion: for stage $k = m, m-1, \ldots, 1$, with $\widetilde{Y}_m \equiv Y$, we

(i) fit the model in (7.2) to auxiliary $\widetilde{Y}_k$ to obtain parameter estimates $(\widehat{\beta}_{k0}, \widehat{\beta}_{k1})$;

(ii) compute the fitted value $\widehat{Y}_k = \mu_{k0}(h_k; \widehat{\beta}_{k0}) + \mu_{k1}(h_k, a_k; \widehat{\beta}_{k1})$;

(iii) compute the stage $k-1$ auxiliary outcome as the difference $\widetilde{Y}_{k-1} = \widetilde{Y}_k - \widehat{Y}_k$.

This recursion leads to a decomposition of the outcome along the lines of (7.1), and an estimate of the counterfactual outcome based on the quantity

$$\psi(\overline{a}_m) = \mu_{10}(h_1; \widehat{\beta}_{10}) + \sum_{k=1}^{m} \mu_{k1}(h_k, a_k; \widehat{\beta}_{k1})$$

that is

$$\widehat{\mathbb{E}}[Y(\overline{a}_m)] = \frac{\sum_{i=1}^{n} \mathbf{1}_{\overline{a}_m}(\overline{a}_{im})\psi_i(\overline{a}_{im})}{\sum_{i=1}^{n} \mathbf{1}_{\overline{a}_m}(\overline{a}_{im})}.$$

Provided the conditional treatment-free and treatment effect models $\mu_{k0}(h_k; \beta_{k0})$ and $\mu_{k1}(h_k, a_k; \beta_{k1})$ at each stage are correctly specified, this approach produces consistent estimates of $\mathbb{E}[Y(\overline{a}_m)]$.

7.3.5 *Structural Nested Mean Models*

In the assessment of dynamic strategies, stagewise consideration of the optimal sequence is necessary as indicated in section 7.2.4. The generalization of the procedure implemented there is encompassed in the *Structural Nested Mean Model* (SNMM, Robins (1994)), which decomposes the expected counterfactual outcome into stagewise assessments of the discrepancy between optimal and sub-optimal treatment patterns.

The decomposition of the expected counterfactual outcome utilizes a representation based on the stagewise optimal treatment, specifically

$$\mathbb{E}[Y(\overline{a}_m)] = \mathbb{E}[Y(\overline{a}_m^{\text{opt}})] - \sum_{k=1}^{m} \mathbb{E}[Y(\overline{a}_{k-1}, \underline{a}_{k-1}^{\text{opt}}) - Y(\overline{a}_k, \underline{a}_k^{\text{opt}})], \tag{7.3}$$

with the convention $\overline{a}_0 = \underline{a}_m^{\text{opt}} = \emptyset$. The term $\mathbb{E}[Y(\overline{a}_m^{\text{opt}})]$ represents the expected outcome under optimal treatment at every treatment stage; in the summation, the kth term represents the contrast, or expected difference, in outcome between optimal treatment a_k^{opt} and potential treatment a_k at stage k, assuming treatment $\overline{a}_{k-1}$ prior to interval k, and optimal treatment $\underline{a}_k^{\text{opt}}$ for intervals subsequent to interval k.

Note that, by construction, each of the terms in the summation is non-negative, as if a_k matches a_k^{opt}, then the term is identically zero. Thus, the form of (7.3) reflects the fact that the expected counterfactual outcome $\mathbb{E}[Y(\overline{a}_m)]$ is lower than $\mathbb{E}[Y(\overline{a}_m^{\text{opt}})]$ by an amount equal to the sum of discrepancies arising from sub-optimal treatment at each stage.

Next, a model is specified for the contrasts; typically, for the contrast models, a contrast against some baseline category is posited, and if treatment is on an ordinal scale, the value '0' is a natural one. For example, for $1 \leq k \leq m$, with the decomposition

$$\begin{aligned}
\mathbb{E}[Y(\overline{a}_{k-1}, \underline{a}_{k-1}^{\text{opt}}) - Y(\overline{a}_{k-1}, a_k, \underline{a}_{k+1}^{\text{opt}})] \\
&= \mathbb{E}[Y(\overline{a}_{k-1}, a_k^{\text{opt}}, \underline{a}_k^{\text{opt}}) - Y(\overline{a}_{k-1}, 0, \underline{a}_k^{\text{opt}})] \\
&\quad - \mathbb{E}[Y(\overline{a}_{k-1}, a_k, \underline{a}_k^{\text{opt}}) - Y(\overline{a}_{k-1}, 0, \underline{a}_k^{\text{opt}})]
\end{aligned}$$

reducing the modelling problem to one of specifying the form of

$$\mathbb{E}[Y(\overline{a}_{k-1}, a, \underline{a}_k^{\text{opt}}) - Y(\overline{a}_{k-1}, 0, \underline{a}_k^{\text{opt}})] \tag{7.4}$$

for arbitrary a, which measures the (unconfounded) effect of (potential) treatment a at the kth stage. The *blip* function form in (7.4) should depend on its arguments $(\overline{a}_{k-1}, a)$ but not $\underline{a}_k^{\text{opt}}$, and typically a conditional model based on history $h_k = (x_1, a_1, \ldots, x_{k-1}, a_{k-1}, x_k)$ as well as a is built. To complete the modelling, a model for the treatment-free counterfactual outcome

$$\mathbb{E}[Y(\overline{a}_{k-1}, 0, \underline{a}_k^{\text{opt}})]$$

is required; this can also depend on h_k. In general, the model for the expected counterfactual outcome at stage k takes the form

$$\mathbb{E}[Y(\overline{a}_{k-1}, 0, \underline{a}_k^{\text{opt}})] + \mathbb{E}[Y(\overline{a}_{k-1}, a, \underline{a}_k^{\text{opt}}) - Y(\overline{a}_{k-1}, 0, \underline{a}_k^{\text{opt}})]$$

or, in the conditional form $\mu_{k0}(h_k) + \mu_{k1}(h_k, a)$, say.

In the two-stage, binary treatment case example from section 7.2, we have

$$\begin{aligned}\mathbb{E}[Y(a_1, a_2)] = \mathbb{E}[Y(a_1^{\text{opt}}, a_2^{\text{opt}})] - \left\{\mathbb{E}[Y(a_1^{\text{opt}}, a_2^{\text{opt}}) - Y(a_1, a_2^{\text{opt}})]\right\} \\ - \left\{\mathbb{E}[Y(a_1, a_2^{\text{opt}}) - Y(a_1, a_2)]\right\}.\end{aligned}$$

For the contrast models, we might specify linear models

$$\begin{aligned}\mathbb{E}[Y(a_1, a_2) - Y(a_1, 0)] &= a_2(\mathbf{x}_2\beta_{21}) && \text{Stage 2} \\ \mathbb{E}[Y(a_1, a_2^{\text{opt}}) - Y(0, a_2^{\text{opt}})] &= a_1(\mathbf{x}_1\beta_{11}) && \text{Stage 1}\end{aligned}$$

where $\mathbf{x}_2$ depends on elements of $h_2 = (x_1, a_1, x_2)$, and $\mathbf{x}_1$ depends on elements of $h_1 = x_1$ with treatment-free models of a similar nature. In general, we have for (7.4) at stage k

$$\mathbb{E}[Y(\overline{a}_{k-1}, a_k, \underline{a}_k^{\text{opt}}) - Y(\overline{a}_{k-1}, 0, \underline{a}_k^{\text{opt}})] = a_k(\mathbf{x}_k\beta_{k1})$$

where $\mathbf{x}_k$ depends on h_k.

The discovery of the optimal dynamic strategy proceeds using the Bellman backwards stagewise approach. The stage k optimal treatment is determined as before by the tailoring rule

$$a_k^{\text{opt}} = \mathbf{1}\{\mathbf{x}_k\beta_{k1} > 0\},$$

where the stage k model needs to be fitted to the auxiliary outcome $\widetilde{Y}_k$ which is formed as in section 7.2.4 as

$$\widetilde{Y}_k = Y + \sum_{j=k+1}^{m} (a_j^{\text{opt}} - a_j)\mathbf{x}_{j1}\beta_{j1}. \tag{7.5}$$

In the frequentist analysis, estimation is carried out using OLS, with the β parameters replaced by their estimated values. A Bayesian analogue that extends the approach from section 7.2.4 is straightforward, and is detailed in section 7.5

7.3.6 *Dynamic Strategies using Q-learning*

Q-learning is a recursive procedure similar to that described in section 7.3.5 that repeatedly estimates stagewise optimal outcomes based using the Bellman optimization strategy. At the final interval m, the model

$$\begin{aligned}\mathbb{E}[Y(\overline{a}_m)] &= \mathbb{E}[Y(\overline{a}_{m-1}, 0)] + \{\mathbb{E}[Y(\overline{a}_{m-1}, a_m)] - \mathbb{E}[Y(\overline{a}_{m-1}, 0)]\} \\ &= \mu_{m0}(h_m; \beta_{m0}) + \mu_{m1}(h_m, a_m; \beta_{m1})\end{aligned} \tag{7.6}$$

is fitted to observed outcome data Y, parameters β_{m0} and β_{m1} estimated, the optimal estimated treatment rule

$$a_m^{\text{opt}} = \arg\max_a \mu_{m1}(h_m, a; \widehat{\beta}_{m1})$$

inferred, and the optimized outcome estimated as

$$\widetilde{Y}_m^{\text{opt}} = \mu_{m0}(h_m; \widehat{\beta}_{m0}) + \mu_{m1}(h_m, a_m^{\text{opt}}; \widehat{\beta}_{m1})$$

for each individual. Taking the $\widetilde{Y}_m^{\text{opt}}$ as auxiliary data, representing the outcome that would have been observed had the individual been optimally treated at the stage m, the model

$$\begin{aligned}\mathbb{E}[Y(\overline{a}_{m-1}, a_m^{\text{opt}})] \\ &= \mathbb{E}[Y(\overline{a}_{m-2}, 0, a_m^{\text{opt}})] \\ &\qquad + \{\mathbb{E}[Y(\overline{a}_{m-2}, a_{m-1}, a_m^{\text{opt}})] - \mathbb{E}[Y(\overline{a}_{m-2}, 0, a_m^{\text{opt}})]\} \\ &= \mu_{m-1,0}(h_{m-1}; \beta_{m-1,0}) + \mu_{m-1,1}(h_{m-1}, a_{m-1}; \beta_{m-1,1})\end{aligned} \tag{7.7}$$

is fitted to the $\widetilde{Y}_m^{\text{opt}}$ collection, parameters $\beta_{m-1,0}$ and $\beta_{m-1,1}$ estimated, the optimal treatment

$$a_{m-1}^{\text{opt}} = \arg\max_a \mu_{m-1,1}(h_{m-1}, a; \widehat{\beta}_{m-1,1})$$

determined, and the optimized outcome estimated as

$$\widetilde{Y}_{m-1}^{\text{opt}} = \mu_{m-1,0}(h_{m-1}; \widehat{\beta}_{m-1,0}) + \mu_{m-1,1}(h_{m-1}, a_{m-1}^{\text{opt}}; \widehat{\beta}_{m-1,1})$$

for each individual. This recursion continues until the entire optimal rule sequence is inferred according to the stagewise procedure

$$a_k^{\text{opt}} = \arg\max_a \mu_{k1}(h_k, a; \widehat{\beta}_{k1})$$

$k = 1, 2, \ldots, m$. In the binary treatment case, the rule for stage k simplifies as before to

$$a_k^{\text{opt}} = \mathbf{1}\{\mu_{k1}(h_k; \widehat{\beta}_{k1}) > 0\},$$

that is set $a_k^{\text{opt}} = 1$ if $\mu_{k1}(h_k; \widehat{\beta}_{k1}) > 0$, and set $a_k^{\text{opt}} = 0$ otherwise.

The Q-learning approach is very straightforward to implement, but its success relies upon the correct specification of the stagewise mean models at each of the m stages. A Bayesian version of the Q-learning procedure is straightforward to implement, with posterior sampling replacing point estimation at each stage, and the sampling of the auxiliary quantities from the relevant posterior predictive distributions.

7.4 Parametric Methods

Causal statements respect the temporal ordering, and hence the treatment decision at stage k is informed by the history h_k which includes all preceding covariates $x_1, \ldots, x_k$ and intermediate outcomes $y_1, \ldots, y_{k-1}$, as well as treatments assigned prior to stage k, $a_1, \ldots, a_{k-1}$. In the pure likelihood specification, it is sometimes useful for modelling purposes to retain the distinction between covariates and outcomes, even if subsequent treatment decisions treat the information equivalently.

7.4.1 Parametric Likelihood

Assuming a parametric specification, the likelihood for the observed data is readily factorized via the temporal ordering as

$$p(x_1)p(a_1|x_1)p(y_1|a_1, x_1)\left\{\prod_{k=2}^{m} p(x_k|h_{k-1}, a_{k-1})p(a_k|h_k)p(y_k|h_k, a_k)\right\}.$$

Building a model that permits inference requires the stagewise specification of the component models. There are three conditional models to specify: for $k = 1, 2, \ldots, m$ the models are

(i) $p(x_k|h_{k-1}, a_{k-1})$
(ii) $p(a_k|h_k)$
(iii) $p(y_k|h_k, a_k)$

each of which would be typically represented by a regression formulation. There are two things to note. First, the possible complexity of the stage k specified model increases with k, as the number of possible predictors grows linearly, with quadratic growth in interaction terms, etc. This results in a very complex structure overall. Secondly, the model in (i) that represents the stage k covariate distribution would usually be able to be omitted in any analysis, with the empirical distribution used in an estimation of the expected outcomes. However, if the conditional distribution of X_k depends functionally on any of $A_1, \ldots, A_{k-1}$, then there is the possibility of mediation of the effect of these past treatments via X_k, and any observed covariate value is subject to variation in past observed treatments. Therefore the assessment of the potential outcomes resulting from a given (hypothetical intervention) potential treatment sequence cannot be accurately assessed unless the mediation effect, and confounding, is adjusted for.

7.4.2 G-computation

Although a correct specification of the data-generating mechanism cannot yield consistent recovery of the counterfactual outcomes based on the original data alone, it can be used to create a synthetic (auxiliary) data set that allows correct inference to be recovered. The method described in section 7.2.2 illustrates this approach in two stages. In the synthetic data, we adhere to the DAG structure in Figure 7.2, but exploit the fact that the conditional model for X_2 given X_1 and A_1 is the same in Figure 7.2 as it is in Figure 7.1, so that this relationship is learnable from the observed data. In order to complete the estimation of the counterfactual outcomes, two auxiliary versions of X_2 are generated using the fitted predictive model at levels $A_1 = 0$ and $A_1 = 1$ respectively. Finally, the correct outcome regression of Y on the observed X_1, A_1 and A_2, and the two synthetic X_2 samples, is fitted and used to estimate the counterfactual outcomes. In the Bayesian setting, all steps are implemented using full posterior calculations.

This use of the auxiliary data that adheres to the target experimental or intervention-based design can be applied to account for mediation in more general settings provided the true data-generating DAG is known, and also provided the probabilistic specification in the parametric likelihood is correct. This approach is sometimes termed *G-computation*. It is reliant on knowledge of the models for the X and Y variables $p(x_k|h_{k-1}, a_{k-1})$ and $p(y_k|h_k, a_k)$ for $k = 1, 2$, but not modeling of treatment assignment mechanism at either stage.

The extension of the approach to m stages is conceptually straightforward, but is still reliant on correct specification of the stagewise models $p(x_k|h_{k-1}, a_{k-1})$. In addition, the number of auxiliary variables to be generated grows exponentially in m, and so the storage requirements become prohibitive if m is moderately large and all possible treatment patterns are to be assessed. A Bayesian sampling-based algorithm is presented in Algorithm 7.3.

7.5 Robust Linear Regression via G-estimation

The requirement for correct specification of all stagewise conditional mean models is a strong one. A mitigation strategy that may be used in the linear regression case is to employ *G-estimation*, which we describe first in its frequentist form.

7.5.1 G-estimation

Classical G-estimation modifies the regression/OLS estimating equation to yield an estimation procedure that allows for mis-specification of the treatment-free outcome component $\mu_{k0}(h_k;\beta_{k0})$, provided the treatment assignment model $p_k(a_k|h_k)$ is correctly specified.

The methodology can be used in any linear regression setting, and can be used for the assessment of static regimes, but is more typically used for the dynamic case, so we focus on that here. Suppose that the stage k mean model for auxiliary outcome $\widetilde{Y}_k$ (computed recursively using equation (7.5)) takes the form

$$\mu_k(h_k, a_k;\beta_k) = \mathbf{x}_{k0}\beta_{k0} + a_k\mathbf{x}_{k1}\beta_{k1},$$

where $\mathbf{x}_{k0}$ and $\mathbf{x}_{k1}$ are row vectors that depend on h_k. In this model, the effect of treatment at level a_k is captured via the blip model component $\mathbf{x}_{k1}\beta_{k1}$ that is separable in additive form from the treatment-free component $\mathbf{x}_{k0}\beta_{k0}$. In G-estimation, it is **always** necessary to assume that the blip model correctly captures the effect of treatment, so that the expected difference $\mathbb{E}[\widetilde{Y}_k - A_k\mathbf{x}_{k1}\beta_{k1}|H_k = h_k]$ does not depend on A_k even if it is not zero, as would be the case under complete correct specification. The OLS estimating equation at stage k for the method described in section 7.3.5 is

$$\sum_{i=1}^{n}\begin{pmatrix}\mathbf{x}_{ik0}^\top \\ a_{ik}\mathbf{x}_{ik1}^\top\end{pmatrix}\{\widetilde{y}_{ik} - \mu_k(h_{ik}, a_{ik};\beta_k)\} = \mathbf{0}.$$

In G-estimation, this equation is modified to

$$\sum_{i=1}^{n}\begin{pmatrix}\mathbf{x}_{ik0}^\top \\ (a_{ik} - \pi_k(h_{ik};\widehat{\alpha}_k))\mathbf{x}_{k1}^\top\end{pmatrix}\{\widetilde{y}_{ik} - \mu_k(h_{ik}, a_{ik};\beta_k)\} = \mathbf{0}, \tag{7.8}$$

where $\pi_k(h_k;\alpha_k) = \mathbb{E}[A_k|h_k]$ is the modelled expected value for the stage k treatment, with parameter α_k, resulting from the conditional treatment model $p_k(a_k|h_k)$.

Consistent estimation of treatment effect parameter β_{k1} may now be achieved if either the treatment-free model, $\mu_{k0}(h_k;\beta_{k0})$, or the treatment assignment model $p_k(a_k|h_k)$ is correctly specified; this follows as the second component of (7.8) has expectation zero if either of these assumptions holds. This is a form of *double robustness*. Estimation of $\mathbb{E}[Y(\mathbf{0})]$ requires correct specification of the baseline treatment-free model, however, for the assessment of the optimal treatment pattern, estimation of this quantity is typically not required.

Doubly robust estimation can also be achieved in an equivalent *augmented* regression, based on the augmented mean model

$$\mathbf{x}_{k0}\beta_{k0} + a_k\mathbf{x}_{k1}\beta_{k1} + \pi_k(h_k;\widehat{\alpha}_k)\mathbf{x}_{k1}\phi_k, \tag{7.9}$$

where ϕ_k is parameter vector of the same dimension as β_{k1}. The third term in (7.9) is used to match the estimating equation in (7.8).

The G-estimation approach has been widely applied in settings where the component stagewise models are linear. Similar methods can be derived in the log-linear outcome case by modification of the estimating equation, but the method is complicated to implement in more general cases.

7.5.2 Bayesian G-estimation

The construction in (7.9) is important as it facilitates a Bayesian version of G-estimation in a straightforward fashion, without only slight deviation from fully Bayesian principles. The Bayesian linear model analysis based on the augmented mean model can proceed in standard fashion, with posterior distributions for $(\beta_{k0}, \beta_{k1}, \phi_k)$ at each stage computed using the usual prior-to-posterior calculations. These posteriors define the posterior distributions on the optimal dynamic rules d_k which can deployed for new individuals. The stagewise auxiliary outcomes can be computed using (7.5), and the stagewise optimal treatments sampled as functions of the stagewise posteriors. Algorithm 7.4 presents the overall strategy.

As in the earlier Bayesian analyses, computation of the posterior distribution at each stage relies on correct parametric specification of the blip model as $\mathbf{x}_{k1}\beta_{k1}$, and at least one of the treatment-free counterfactual model as $\mathbf{x}_{k0}\beta_{k0}$ and the treatment assignment model $p(a_k|h_k)$, as well as distributional assumptions that permit the construction of the stage k likelihood function.

7.5.3 Justification for Two-step Bayesian Estimation

The Bayesian implementation in Algorithm 7.4 adheres to standard Bayesian principles in every aspect apart from the use of the plug-in estimates of parameters $\alpha_k, k = 1, \ldots, m$ for the treatment assignment models. As indicated in the algorithm, it is certainly possible to compute posterior distributions for these parameters. However, it is now widely accepted that it is not necessary or desirable to reflect the posterior uncertainty in these nuisance parameters in the computation of the outcome model posteriors, at least in the fully parametric setting. Formal arguments based on decision-theoretic principles can be made, as can arguments based on modularized inference that allow for deviation from the use of the full likelihood. Heuristically, we argue as follows: G-estimation based on adjustment under correct specification is only valid at the single (true) value of conditional expectation $\mathbb{E}[A_k|h_k; \alpha_k]$ where α_k takes its (true) data-generating value. Therefore we are in fact forced to use a plug-in method based on a Bayesian (or indeed any consistent) estimate rather than to propagate the uncertainty via a full posterior distribution. For any given data set, there is a single 'best guess' at the true value of α_k that provides correct adjustment, and therefore this value should be used in a plug-in calculation. See Zigler and Dominici (2014), and Stephens et al. (2023) for an extensive discussion.

7.6 Breaking Confounding using Reweighting

Reweighting may also be used to resolve the problem of mediation and confounding effects. Different forms of weighting can be used, the most common form being based on inverse probability weights, but more general forms can be implemented within a regression setting. We discuss first frequentist formulations of reweighting.

7.6.1 Inverse Probability Weighting

The inverse probability weighting (IPW) method breaks the confounding by reweighting the observational data to yield an effectively unconfounded sample in which the effect of treatment can be assessed. When applied in the static case, the weight attached to observation Y_i is proportional to the reciprocal of

$$p(\overline{a}_{im}|h_m) = p(a_{i1}|h_{i1}) \prod_{k=2}^{m} p(a_{ik}|h_{ik})$$

with each component model represented parametrically. This form of inverse weighting can be implemented for continuous exposures, but we restrict attention to the binary treatment case. In the two-stage case from the example from section 7.2, the probability weight attached to an individual with observation pattern (a_{i1}, a_{i2}) is proportional to

$$w(a_{i1}, a_{i2}) = \frac{1}{p(a_{i1}, a_{i2}|x_{i1}, x_{i2})} = \frac{1}{p_1(a_{i1}|x_{i1})p_2(a_{i2}|x_{i1}, a_{i1}, x_{i2})}$$

with the two conditional models typically parameterized, with parameters α_1 and α_2, say, estimated by likelihood methods. In a frequentist moment-based calculation, the IPW estimator of counterfactual outcome for target treatment sequence (a_1, a_2) is

$$\widehat{\mathbb{E}}[Y(a_1, a_2)] = \frac{1}{n} \sum_{i=1}^{n} \frac{\mathbf{1}_{a_1}(A_{i1}) \mathbf{1}_{a_2}(A_{i2}) Y_i}{p_1(a_1|X_{i1}; \widehat{\alpha}_1) p_2(a_2|X_{i1}, a_1, X_{i2}; \widehat{\alpha}_2)} \tag{7.10}$$

which utilizes the observed data by including all individuals whose observed treatment pattern matches the target sequence, and taking a weighted average of them, with weights determined by the observed treatment sequence.

A similar moment-based estimator can be obtained using a weighted linear regression using a mean model that does not reflect the data generating model, but rather is misspecified, say, as

$$\mathbb{E}[Y|A_1, A_2] = \beta_0 + \beta_1 A_1 + \beta_2 A_2 + \beta_3 A_1 A_2$$

say, and uses case weights $w(a_{i1}, a_{i2}), i = 1, \ldots, n$. The weighted least-squares solution is given by

$$\widehat{\beta} = \arg\min_{\beta} \sum_{i=1}^{n} w(a_{i1}, a_{i2}; \widehat{\alpha})(y_i - \beta_0 - \beta_1 a_{i1} - \beta_2 a_{i2} - \beta_3 a_{i1} a_{i2})^2 \tag{7.11}$$

which can be solved analytically, after initial estimation of $\alpha = (\alpha_1, \alpha_2)$ using likelihood-based approaches. As usual, the weighted least-squares can be justified as maximum likelihood estimation with the form in (7.11) regarded as a negative log-likelihood for β based on a conditional model for the outcome assuming heteroscedastic Gaussian errors. To match the estimator in (7.10), the model

$$\mathbb{E}[Y|A_1, A_2] = \beta_0 + \beta_1 \mathbf{1}_{a_1}(A_1) \mathbf{1}_{a_2}(A_2)$$

can be used.

A doubly robust estimator that relies on weighting was detailed by Bang and Robins (2005) (with erratum Bang and Robins (2008)). For a single stage setting and a binary treatment, and similar to the augmentation in equation 7.9, a regression model of the form

$$\mathbf{x}_0 \beta_0 + a \mathbf{x}_1 \beta_1 + \frac{1-a}{1 - \pi(x; \widehat{\alpha})} \phi_0 + \frac{a}{\pi(x; \widehat{\alpha})} \phi_1 \tag{7.12}$$

that is fitted using ordinary least squares returns a consistent estimator of the expected counterfactual outcome $\mathbb{E}[Y(a)]$ if either the regression component $\mathbf{x}_0 \beta_0 + a \mathbf{x}_1 \beta_1$ or the treatment model $\pi(x; \widehat{\alpha})$ is correctly specified. The last two terms of equation (7.12) augment the regression in such a way that the resulting estimating equation for $\mathbb{E}[Y(a)]$ matches the IPW estimating equation. For the estimator in (7.10), the augmentation term for estimating the static regime $\mathbb{E}[Y(a_1, a_2)]$ takes the form

$$\frac{\mathbf{1}_{a_1}(A_1) \mathbf{1}_{a_2}(A_2)}{p_1(a_1|X_{i1}) p_2(a_2|X_{i1}, a_1, X_{i2}; \widehat{\alpha}_2)}.$$

For the assessment of dynamic strategies, reweighting can be used in a stagewise fashion to deduce the optimal stagewise strategy. Analysis proceeds in the usual Bellman fashion, for stages $m, m-1, \ldots, 2, 1$ with the impact of treatment at stage k assessed using a weighted regression for auxiliary outcome $\widetilde{Y}_k$ with stage k weight

$$p(\overline{a}_{ik}|h_k) = p(a_{i1}|h_{i1}) \prod_{j=2}^{k} p(a_{ij}|h_{ij})$$

and component models fitted in the same way as for the static strategies.

Inverse probability weighting requires correct specification of the treatment assignment mechanism at each treatment stage, and it can be argued that modelling the treatment assignment process as a function of history is more straightforward than modelling auxiliary outcome values as is necessary for G-computation, G-estimation, or Q-learning. There is no need to specify a model for the intermediate or terminal outcomes, although the weighted regression approach demonstrates that the manner in which a nuisance model may be introduced to reduce the variance of the estimated counterfactual values in the terminal outcome model.

7.6.2 *Dynamic Weighted Ordinary Least Squares (dWOLS)*

For discrete-valued treatments, more general forms of weight can be proposed based on the *balancing principle.* The overall objective of reweighting is to adjust the observed joint distribution of A and X such that in the reweighted distribution A and X are independent. For the single time point setting, the joint distribution can be written $p(a,x) = p(x)p(a|x)$; the objective of reweighting is to construct a new joint distribution, $p^W(a,x)$, by using a multiplicative factor $w(a,x) > 0$ that operates pointwise on the support of A and X such that

$$p^w(a,x) \equiv \frac{p(x)p(a|x)w(a,x)}{\sum_t \int p(s)p(t|s)w(s,t)\,ds} = p^w(a)p^w(x)$$

that is, such that in the resulting joint distribution A and X are independent, with the constraint that the marginal distribution of X does not change, that is, $p^w(x) = p(x)$. This implies the requirement that the product $p(a|x)w(a,x)$ does not depend on x. For the IPW case with binary treatments, we have

$$p(a|x)w(a,x) = \pi(x)^a(1-\pi(x))^{1-a}\left(\frac{1}{\pi(x)}\right)^a\left(\frac{1}{1-\pi(x)}\right)^{1-a} = 1$$

for $a = 0, 1$, so the relation holds, but the relation also holds if the weight function is chosen to be $w(a,x) = |a - p(a|x)|$ and other forms of weights. This formulation forms the basis of dynamic weighted ordinary least squares (dWOLS, Wallace and Moodie (2015)) that allows weighted regression methods to be used to estimate static and dynamic regimes via reweighting.

7.6.3 *Inverse Weighting for Strategies Based on Thresholds*

The approach of reweighting can be applied to the dynamic problem based on thresholds as described in section 7.2.3. Suppose for simplicity that a single tailoring variable, X, is available at each time point, and that the decision rule at stage k, d_k, is an indicator of whether the tailoring variable meets a thresholding criterion, say $X_k \in \mathcal{R}_k$ where $\mathcal{R}_k$ depends on some fixed thresholding parameters θ_k (for example, we might consider $X_k > 2.1, X_k < -1.6$ or $1 < X_k < 1.5$). To assess the value, $V(\bar{d}_m)$, of the dynamic rule $\bar{d}_m$, we may use an IPW approach applied to compatibility with the decision rules rather than with the target treatments. That is, we may estimate the expected value of the dynamic rule by assessing, at each interval, whether a subject is compatible with the decision rule and recording new indicators $Z_k, k = 1, \ldots, m$, with observed values z_k, where $Z_k = \mathbf{1}\{X_k \in \mathcal{R}_k\}$, and using the estimate of the counterfactual outcome for adhering to the thresholding rule

$$\widehat{\mathbb{E}}[Y(\bar{d}_m)] = \frac{1}{n}\sum_{i=1}^{n}\left\{\prod_{k=1}^{m}\frac{\mathbf{1}_1(z_{ik})}{\varphi_k(h_{ik};\widehat{\eta}_k)}\right\}y_i,$$

where $\varphi_k(h_k; \eta)$ is the estimated stage k conditional probability that $Z_k = 1$ given history h_k.

7.6.4 Bayesian Implementation of Weighting Methods

It is instructive to recap precisely how reweighting methods break confounding. Comparing the data-generating DAG in Figure 7.1 with the targeted interventional (experimental) DAG in Figure 7.2, we see that the associated distributions can be written as

$$p^{\mathcal{O}}(x_1, a_1, x_2, a_2, y) = p(x_1)p(a_1|x_1)p(x_2|x_1, a_1)p(a_2|x_2)p(y|x_1, a_1, x_2, a_2)$$

in the first case, and

$$p^{\mathcal{E}}(x_1, a_1, x_2, a_2, y) = p(x_1)p(a_1)p(x_2|x_1, a_1)p(a_2)p(y|x_1, a_1, x_2, a_2)$$

in the second case. Therefore we can write

$$\begin{aligned} p^{\mathcal{E}}(x_1, a_1, x_2, a_2, y) &= \frac{p^{\mathcal{E}}(x_1, a_1, x_2, a_2, y)}{p^{\mathcal{O}}(x_1, a_1, x_2, a_2, y)} p^{\mathcal{O}}(x_1, a_1, x_2, a_2, y) \\ &= \frac{p(a_1)p(a_2)}{p(a_1|x_1)p(a_2|x_2)} p^{\mathcal{O}}(x_1, a_1, x_2, a_2, y) \qquad (7.13) \end{aligned}$$

in which the term

$$w(x_1, a_1, x_2, a_2) = \frac{p(a_1)p(a_2)}{p(a_1|x_1)p(a_2|x_2)}$$

acts to reweight points in the support of the observational joint distribution to match the experimental distribution. This justifies the form of the weight that appears in equation (7.10), as there the counterfactual expectation is taken with respect to the experimental joint distribution, based on data from the observational joint distribution.

The Bayesian approach to weighting can be justified from two perspectives. First, the approach can be regarded as a standard Bayesian approach based on a weighted likelihood that for independent and identically distributed outcome data would take the form

$$\mathcal{L}(\beta) = \prod_{i=1}^{n} f(y_i|x_i, a_i; \beta)^{nw_i}$$

where the case weights $w_1, \ldots, w_n$ are scaled to sum to one. The use of weighted likelihood is not universally accepted as a legitimate (parametric) Bayesian calculation, as the likelihood does not arise from a de Finetti-type representation. Nevertheless, in large samples, the behaviour of the posterior distribution computed from the weighted likelihood is satisfactory. Note also that the augmented regression approach given in equation (7.12) can be used to formulate Bayesian inference with a standard (non-weighted) likelihood, albeit one that exploits the plug-in strategy from section 7.5.3. See Graham et al. (2016).

A second justification can be obtained by considering a collection of auxiliary variables, Y^w say, that represent outcomes that would have been observed under the hypothetical experimental/interventional data generating setting where allocation of treatment is independent of confounding, as in Figure 7.2. The auxiliary variables can be sampled using *importance resampling*, based on equation (7.13): we consider a set of weights $\{w_1, \ldots, w_n\}$ computed as

$$w_i \propto \frac{1}{p(a_{i1}|x_{i1})p(a_{i2}|x_{i2})}$$

where the conditional treatment models are assumed correctly specified. Then $(Y_i^w, X_i^w, A_i^w), i = 1, \ldots, n$ are obtained by sampling with replacement from the observed data according to the discrete distribution $\{w_1, \ldots, w_n\}$. By design, in the auxiliary data, confounding is removed by the reweighting, and analysis can proceed according to an unweighted likelihood model for the Y^w.

7.7 Relaxation of Parametric Assumptions

All of the methods described in earlier sections rely upon parametric distributional assumptions relating to the residual errors in the outcome or auxiliary outcome models. That is, the residual errors are typically assumed to be Gaussian, so that the Bayesian analysis can proceed using the Gaussian likelihood. This is one of the weaknesses identified in section 7.2.5, and is a much stronger assumption than is typically made in the frequentist literature, although it is typically not too harmful. The distributional assumptions may be relaxed using Bayesian nonparametric approaches. One relatively straightforward non-parametric formulation is based on a computational strategy often referred to as the Bayesian bootstrap, which we describe in the next section.

7.7.1 The Bayesian Bootstrap

The classical formulation of the Bayesian bootstrap (Rubin, 1981) assumes that the data points are realizations from a multinomial model on the finite set of real values $\{z_1, \ldots, z_n\}$ – the observed data – with unknown probability $\varpi = (\varpi_1, \ldots, \varpi_n)$, and assuming a priori that $\varpi \sim \textit{Dirichlet}\,(\alpha, \ldots, \alpha)$, then, a posteriori $\varpi \sim \textit{Dirichlet}\,(\alpha + 1, \ldots, \alpha + 1)$, that is, the posterior distribution on the unknown data generating distribution is a Dirichlet distribution on $\{z_1, \ldots, z_n\}$. Conditional on a draw ϖ from the posterior distribution, samples from the posterior predictive can be made by drawing independently from $\{z_1, \ldots, z_n\}$ with associated probabilities $\{\varpi_1, \ldots, \varpi_n\}$. The Bayesian bootstrap is obtained under the improper specification $\alpha = 0$.

The Bayesian bootstrap is a consequence of a non-parametric prior being placed on the unknown distribution function of the data, F, with inference for F following using a standard Bayesian calculation. Specifically, the non-parametric prior is the *Dirichlet process*, where under the prior $F \sim DP\,(\alpha, G_0)$ where $\alpha > 0$ is the *concentration parameter* and G_0 is the *base measure* that acts as a prior expectation for the unknown F. In light of data $(z_1, \ldots, z_n)$, the resulting posterior distribution of F is also a Dirichlet process, $DP\,(\alpha_n, G_n)$, where $\alpha_n = \alpha + n$ and

$$G_n(.) = \frac{\alpha}{\alpha + n} G_0(.) + \frac{1}{\alpha + n} \sum_{i=1}^{n} \delta_{z_i}(\cdot).$$

A random draw from the posterior distribution on F provides a (conditional) distribution from which the observables may be drawn independently. If $\alpha \longrightarrow 0$, a sample from the posterior distribution is simply a single draw ϖ from the Dirichlet$(1, \ldots, 1)$ distribution, that essentially places a random probability symmetrically on the n observed data.

To utilize the Bayesian bootstrap for semi-parametric inference, suppose that in the frequentist calculation we have the estimate for generic parameter β determined either by a loss-minimization using loss function $\ell(\cdot, \cdot)$, or as a solution to an estimating equation based on estimating function $u(\cdot, \cdot)$. These two formulations cover almost all cases that are used in the causal literature. In the former case, a posterior sample for the parameter β can then be derived by solving

$$\beta(\varpi) = \arg\min_b \sum_{i=1}^{n} \varpi_i \ell\,(z_i, b) \tag{7.14}$$

whereas in the latter, we must solve the weighted estimating equation

$$\beta(\varpi) : \sum_{i=1}^{n} \varpi_i u\left(z_i, \beta\right) = 0. \tag{7.15}$$

In both cases, $\beta(\varpi)$ is obtained via a *deterministic* transformation of ϖ. A sample from the posterior distribution for β can be obtained by repeatedly drawing $\varpi \sim \text{Dirichlet}\,(1, \ldots, 1)$ and obtaining the solutions to (7.14) or (7.15).

7.7.2 The Bayesian Bootstrap for Evaluating Treatment Sequences

The Bayesian bootstrap has now been extensively deployed in settings related to semi-parametric causal inference and in the construction and evaluation of optimal treatment sequences: see, for example, Chamberlain and Imbens (2003), Saarela et al. (2015), Saarela et al. (2016), Graham et al. (2016). A justification of this as a fully Bayesian posterior sampling procedure for performing inference under mis-specification is given in Stephens et al. (2023). The Bayesian bootstrap can be extended to consider non-limiting cases, where $\alpha > 0$, in a reasonably straightforward fashion. The formulation above assumes a univariate data problem, but this can be easily extended to consider conditional distributions in a regression setting, for example, for the modelling of an outcome conditional on treatment and confounders, or a treatment conditional on confounders, as required in each of the algorithms used to construct Bayesian optimal treatment strategies. For example, in Algorithm 7.2, the posterior sampling of β parameters at each stage can be performed using the Bayesian bootstrap rather than using a Gaussian posterior, and then the optimal treatments are determined by transforming the posterior samples in the same way as in the parametric case.

One issue to be noted in the stagewise analysis on which the algorithms depend is that some care needs to be taken when deploying the Bayesian bootstrap for two-step analysis as discussed in section 7.5.3. Specifically, when plugging in treatment parameter estimates, $\widehat{\alpha}_k$, to provide adjustment based on equation (7.9), the Bayesian bootstrap solution requires that the estimate be derived from a weighted estimation procedure based on the *same* draw of weights used to estimate the model parameters. That is, a draw $\varpi \sim \text{Dirichlet}\,(1, \ldots, 1)$ is used to estimate the parameter α_k using a loss-minimization step, or equivalently maximum likelihood for the correctly specified treatment model,

$$\alpha_k(\varpi) = \arg\max_{s} \sum_{i=1}^{n} \varpi_i \log p(a_{ik}|h_{ik}; s) \tag{7.16}$$

and then parameter β_k estimated using weighted least squares

$$\beta_k(\varpi) = \arg\min_{b_0, b_1, t} \sum_{i=1}^{n} \varpi_i(\widetilde{y}_{ik} - \mathbf{x}_{ik0} b_0 - a_{k_i} \mathbf{x}_{ik1} b_1 - \pi_k(h_{ik}; \alpha_k(\varpi))\mathbf{x}_{ik1} t)^2 \tag{7.17}$$

based on the **same** draw of ϖ. In this way, the posterior uncertainty in the unknown joint data generating distribution is correctly converted into posterior uncertainty concerning the quantity of interest. An algorithm to implement the Bayesian bootstrap-based construction of an optimized individual strategy is given in Algorithm 7.5. The Bayesian bootstrap can also be applied to the reweighting adjustment methods from section 7.6, with the adjustment weights forming part of the objective function ℓ or the estimating function u associated with the outcome model, with the Dirichlet weights multiplying each contribution as in (7.16) and (7.17).

7.8 Discussion

The Bayesian approach to optimal treatment sequence assessment and construction is advantageous as it can provide a more complete assessment of the treatment strategies being considered by fully reporting their associated uncertainties. Principles that are applied in frequentist analysis can be easily developed in a Bayesian analogue. In the Bayesian calculation, there is no reliance on asymptotic quantification of uncertainty, although this can come at the cost of making parametric assumptions. For most Bayesians, given the complexity of the system under study, this is an acceptable compromise. However, even the parametric assumptions can be relaxed if computational strategies based on Bayesian non-parametric assumptions are utilized. The Bayesian bootstrap and similar algorithms can be deployed to carry out fully Bayesian inference under less stringent assumptions that concern the conditional mean model specification for the outcome, and assumptions about the treatment assignment mechanism.

Algorithm 7.1: Bayesian algorithm for assessing a two-stage static treatment sequence

Data: (X_1, A_1, X_2, A_2, Y) random sample of size n

Fit Bayesian regression model with parameters γ to X_2 given (X_1, A_1) data.
Obtain posterior sample $\gamma^{(l)}, l = 1, \ldots, L$ of size L from posterior $\pi_n(\gamma)$.
for $l = 1, \ldots, L$ **do**
  foreach Target level a_1 **do**
    Sample $\widetilde{X}_2(a_1)$ from the posterior predictive distribution derived from $\pi_n(\gamma)$ at (X_1, a_1).
    Fit Bayesian regression model with parameters β to Y given $(X_1, A_1, \widetilde{X}_2^{(l)}, A_2)$ data, with conditional mean $m(\cdot; \beta)$, to obtain posterior $\pi_n^{(l)}(\beta)$.
    Obtain single posterior sample $\beta^{(l)}$ from posterior $\pi_n^{(l)}(\beta)$.
    foreach Target level a_2 **do**
      For each individual, sample an outcome $Y^{(l)}(a_1, a_2)$ from the posterior predictive distribution based on the mean $m(\cdot; \beta^{(l)})$.
    end
  end
end
For all (a_1, a_2), $\{Y^{(l)}(a_1, a_2), l = 1, \ldots, L\}$ form posterior sample of counterfactual outcomes for each individual.

Algorithm 7.2: Bayesian algorithm for determining a two-stage optimal dynamic treatment sequence

Data: (X_1, A_1, X_2, A_2, Y) random sample of size n

/* Start at stage 2 */

for Stage 2 analysis **do**

Fit Bayesian linear model

$$h_{20}\beta_{20} + a_2 h_{21}\beta_{21}$$

to outcome data.

Obtain posterior sample $(\beta_{20}^{(l)}, \beta_{21}^{(l)}), l = 1, \ldots, L$ of size L from posterior $\pi_n(\beta_{20}, \beta_{21})$.

for l in 1:L **do**

Compute optimal Stage 2 treatment for each individual, for each posterior sample

$$a_2^{\text{opt}(l)} = \mathbf{1}\{h_{21}\beta_{21}^{(l)} > 0\} \qquad l = 1, \ldots, L$$

Compute auxiliary outcomes for each individual, for each posterior sample

$$\widetilde{Y}^{(l)} = Y + (a_2^{\text{opt}(l)} - a_2)h_{21}\beta_{21}^{(l)}; \qquad l = 1, \ldots, L$$

end

end

/* End at stage 1 */

for Stage 1 analysis **do**

for l in 1:L **do**

Fit Bayesian linear model

$$h_{10}\beta_{10} + a_1 h_{11}\beta_{11}$$

to auxiliary data set $\widetilde{Y}^{(l)}$.

Obtain single posterior sampled value $(\beta_{10}^{(l)}, \beta_{11}^{(l)})$ from posterior distribution.

Compute optimal Stage 1 treatment for each individual

$$a_1^{\text{opt}(l)} = \mathbf{1}\{h_{11}\beta_{11}^{(l)} > 0\}.$$

end

end

Algorithm 7.3: Bayesian algorithm for assessing an m-stage static treatment sequence

Data: $((X_k, A_k), k = 1, \ldots, m, Y)$ random sample of size n
for $k = 2, \ldots, m$ **do**
  Fit Bayesian regression model with parameters γ_k to X_k given (H_{k-1}, A_{k-1}) data.
  Obtain posterior sample $\gamma_k^{(l)}, l = 1, \ldots, L$ of size L from posterior $\pi_n(\gamma_k)$.
end
Identify set $\mathcal{A}$ of treatment configurations to be evaluated.
for $l = 1, \ldots, L$ **do**
  foreach Target configuration $\overline{a}_m \in \mathcal{A}$ **do**
    for $k = 2, \ldots, m$ **do**
      For each individual, sample an auxiliary $\widetilde{X}_k^{(l)}(\overline{a}_{k-1})$ from the posterior predictive distribution for stage k using posterior sample $\gamma_k^{(l)}$.
    end
  end
  Fit Bayesian regression model with parameters β to Y given X_1, auxiliary data $\widetilde{X}^{(l)}$, and observed treatments $A_1, \ldots, A_m$, with conditional mean $m(\cdot;\beta)$, to obtain posterior $\pi_n^{(l)}(\beta)$.
  Obtain single posterior sample $\beta^{(l)}$ from posterior $\pi_n^{(l)}(\beta)$.
  For each individual, sample an outcome $Y^{(l)}(\overline{a}_m)$ from the posterior predictive distribution based on the mean $m(\cdot;\beta^{(l)})$.
end
For all $\overline{a}_m \in \mathcal{A}$, $\{Y^{(l)}(\overline{a}_m), l = 1, \ldots, L\}$ form posterior sample of counterfactual outcomes for each individual.

Algorithm 7.4: Bayesian algorithm for assessing an m-stage dynamic treatment sequence using G-estimation.

Data: $((X_k, A_k), k = 1, \ldots, m, Y)$ random sample of size n

Set $\widetilde{Y}_m^{(l)} = Y$ for $l = 1, \ldots, L$.

for $k = m, m-1, \ldots, 1$ **do**

  Fit Bayesian regression model with parameters α_k to A_k given H_k data.

  Obtain posterior sample $\alpha_k^{(l)}, l = 1, \ldots, L$ of size L from posterior $\pi_n(\alpha_k)$.

  Compute Bayesian estimate $\widehat{\alpha}_k$.

  Compute stage k Bayesian posterior based on the augmented mean model

$$\mathbf{x}_{k0}\beta_{k0} + a_k\mathbf{x}_{k1}\beta_{k1} + \pi_k(h_k; \widehat{\alpha}_k)\mathbf{x}_{k1}\phi_k$$

  and auxiliary outcomes $\widetilde{Y}_k$. Generate single sample from the posterior $\pi_n^{(l)}(\beta_k)$, computed using lth auxiliary data set $\widetilde{Y}_k^{(l)}$

  for $l = 1, \ldots, L$ **do**

    Compute sample of stage k optimal treatments

$$a_k^{\text{opt}(l)} = \mathbf{1}\{\mathbf{x}_{k1}\beta_{k1}^{(l)} > 0\}.$$

    for each individual.

    Sample/compute stage $k-1$ auxiliary outcome

$$\widetilde{Y}_{k-1}^{(l)} = Y + \sum_{j=k}^{m}(a_j^{\text{opt}(l)} - a_j)\mathbf{x}_{j1}\beta_{j1}^{(l)}.$$

    from the posterior predictive distribution.

  end

end

For each individual, the posterior samples $\{\overline{a}_m^{\text{opt}(l)}, l = 1, \ldots, L\}$ describe the uncertainty in optimal strategies.

For each individual, $\{\widetilde{Y}_0^{(l)}, l = 1, \ldots, L\}$ summarize the hypothetical optimized outcomes.

Algorithm 7.5: Bayesian algorithm for assessing an m-stage dynamic treatment sequence using G-estimation based on the Bayesian bootstrap.

Data: $((X_k, A_k), k = 1, \dots, m, Y)$ random sample of size n

Set $\widetilde{Y}_m^{(l)} = Y$ for $l = 1, \dots, L$.

for $k = m, m-1, \dots, 1$ **do**

  for $l = 1, \dots, L$ **do**

    Sample $\varpi^{(l)} \sim Dirichlet(1, \dots, 1)$.

    Compute posterior sampled version $\alpha_k^{(l)}$ by solving the weighted likelihood problem

$$\alpha_k^{(l)} = \arg\max_s \sum_{i=1}^n \varpi_i^{(l)} \log p(a_{ik} | h_{ik}; s)$$

    Compute posterior sampled version $\beta_k^{(l)}$ by solving the weighted least squares problem

$$\beta_k^{(l)} = \arg\min_{b_0, b_1, t} \sum_{i=1}^n \varpi_i (\widetilde{y}_{ik} - \mathbf{x}_{ik0} b_0 - a_{ik} \mathbf{x}_{ik1} b_1 - \pi_k(h_{ik}; \alpha_k^{(l)}) \mathbf{x}_{ik1} t)^2$$

    Compute stage auxiliary outcomes $\widetilde{Y}_k^{(l)}$.

    Compute sample of stage k optimal treatments

$$a_k^{\text{opt}(l)} = \mathbf{1}\{\mathbf{x}_{k1} \beta_{k1}^{(l)} > 0\}.$$

    for each individual.

    Sample/compute stage $k-1$ auxiliary outcome

$$\widetilde{Y}_{k-1}^{(l)} = Y + \sum_{j=k}^m (a_j^{\text{opt}(l)} - a_j) \mathbf{x}_{j1} \beta_{j1}^{(l)}.$$

    from the posterior predictive distribution.

  end

end

For each individual, the posterior samples $\{\overline{a}_m^{\text{opt}(l)}, l = 1, \dots, L\}$ describe the uncertainty in optimal strategies.

For each individual, $\{\widetilde{Y}_0^{(l)}, l = 1, \dots, L\}$ summarize the hypothetical optimized outcomes.

Chapter 8

Measurement Error in Adaptive Treatment Strategies

Michael Wallace

8.1 Introduction

Measurement error describes when an observed value of a variable differs from the value we wish to observe. Suppose, for example, that we believe systolic blood pressure (SBP) is an important variable in determining the efficacy of a treatment. A hypothetical patient visits their clinician, who measures their SBP. The number that results is our observed value of the patient's blood pressure, and in a typical analysis would enter into our models and equations on the (implicit) assumption that it is the 'true' value we wished to observe. Unfortunately, this assumption is likely violated, as it is in a large variety of settings (Murray et al., 1993; Thiébaut et al., 2007; Ferrari et al., 2007; Zeger et al., 2000).

To understand this we must first ask a rather fundamental question: what is the 'truth'? When we measure a patient's blood pressure what, precisely, do we want to observe? Is it the patient's blood pressure at that precise moment in time? Is it their average blood pressure over the previous day, week, or even month? Depending on the answer we may encounter smaller, or larger, differences between our single observation and the 'truth' we are searching for.

The consequences of measurement error are complex and often difficult to anticipate, and a wide literature has developed around it (Carroll et al., 2006; Buonaccorsi, 2010; Gustafson, 2004; Yi, 2017). Despite this, however, it is often overlooked (Shaw et al., 2018), and common misconceptions concerning its effects abound. It is tempting, for example, to imagine that if our measurement error is 'random', then its effects will 'average out' in large enough samples. Those with some more thorough exposure to the topic, meanwhile, may be familiar with the appealing but rarely valid result that measurement error at worst causes attenuation in effect estimates. The reality is much more complex.

There are few general rules when it comes to the consequences of measurement error, even in the relatively familiar waters of parameter estimation in regression modeling. It can lead to over- or under-estimation of effect sizes, deviation from desired Type I and II error rates, and even reverse the sign of estimated effects (Keogh et al., 2020).

Much of the established literature on measurement error may translate to the context of precision medicine, especially when analysis techniques grounded in more established statistical theory are used. However, the precision medicine framework also introduces a number of complexities that require explicit handling. Errors may arise in tailoring covariates, treatments, or the outcome, each with different implications. Moreover, the typical goal of a precision medicine problem - estimation of a treatment rule for future patients - must be approached with care. Despite the ubiquity of measurement error - especially in healthcare settings - the literature exploring it in the context of precision medicine is extremely limited.

In this chapter, we will provide an introduction to measurement error and the various roles it can play in a precision medicine analysis. Through a variety of simulation studies, we

DOI: 10.1201/9781003216223-8

will demonstrate the impact measurement error can have in this framework, and how that impact varies depending on which model components are measured imprecisely. While our primary focus will be on the consequences of measurement error, we will also briefly discuss - and demonstrate - correction methods when error-prone tailoring variables are observed. Overall, this chapter should serve as motivation for discussions surrounding measurement error in the precision medicine framework.

8.2 Methodological Background

We begin with introductory material concerning measurement error, dynamic treatment regimes, and the interaction between the two.

8.2.1 Measurement Error: General Framework

Before we can discuss the implications of measurement error in the specific context of precision medicine, we first establish some important ideas from the more general measurement error literature. This section, while by no means a comprehensive introduction to the topic, will establish some concepts and results upon which the subsequent discussion in the precision medicine framework will rely. The interested reader is strongly encouraged to review the broader measurement error literature, in particular the papers by Keogh et al. (2020) and Shaw et al. (2020), which provide an accessible introduction to measurement error, its effects, and methods for its correction.

We assume that for every measurement there is some 'true' value we wish to observe. These true values will be represented by their standard notation (such as X, A, and Y for tailoring, treatment, and outcome variables). In many cases, the definition of 'truth' may be subjective and/or implied through context. In our motivating example of systolic blood pressure, we might let X denote the average SBP of a patient over the preceding day, week, month, or longer. In practice, defining the true value should be carefully done in consultation with experts in the problem under study.

Next, we must establish the relationship between the truth and what is actually observed. The simplest, and most intuitive of these so-called measurement error models is known as *classical additive* measurement error (Cochran, 1968), and may be considered when variables are continuous. Here, we suppose that $X^\dagger = X + U$ is observed (suppressing patient-specific notation), where the superscript $\dagger$ notation is used to denote the error-prone surrogate of the corresponding true value.[1] Here, U denotes a random measurement error component, independent of X, with mean zero and constant variance. It is also assumed that the outcome Y is indepenent of $X^\dagger$ conditional on X. This last assumption is that of *non-differential* error, which is most likely to be violated in settings where data are gathered after the outcome is known. For example, if we asked someone their smoking habits subsequent to a diagnosis of lung cancer we may expect that diagnosis (the outcome) to affect the accuracy of the reported data. We shall only consider non-differential error, which is usually reasonable when data are gathered longitudinally as is common in our setting.

Measurement error may of course take many other forms. The simplest modification to classical additive error is when the mean of U is not non-zero, giving rise to *systematic* or *biased* error. Errors may also be multiplicative instead of additive (such as when larger true values are associated with larger errors). We may even consider *Berkson* error (Berkson, 1950) where, instead of assuming $X^\dagger = X + U$ with U independent of X, we suppose $X = X^\dagger + U$ with U independent of $X^\dagger$. The precise form of one's measurement error will inform both the problems it can cause and the solutions needed for its handling. When

[1]The measurement error literature more commonly uses a superscript $*$ to denote the observed measurement, but this notation is reserved for potential outcomes in this book.

considering continuous variables, we shall limit our attention to classical additive error, including some cases of systematic error.

When variables are categorical (such as the binary treatments we shall consider) our error model structures must change. In this context, measurement error is often instead termed *misclassification*, to reflect fundamental differences in how errors may arise. For a binary variable, for example, we may define the familiar concepts of sensitivity $P(A^\dagger = 1|A = 1)$ and specificity $P(A^\dagger = 0|A = 0)$, or the related positive predictive value $PPV = P(A = 1|A^\dagger = 1)$ and the negative predictive value $NPV = P(A = 0|A^\dagger = 0)$. We may also consider situations where agreement between A and $A^\dagger$ depends on other variables, such as if patients with more severe symptoms are more (or less) likely to adhere to their prescribed treatment.

Having established some of the possible error structures we might consider, we can now explore how measurement error (or misclassification) may undermine an analysis. Returning to the case of classical additive measurement error in a continuous variable, we present a simple illustration of its possible effects. Consider a simple linear regression model of the form $E[Y|X = x] = \beta_0 + \beta_X x$ where, instead of x, an error prone $x^\dagger = x + u$ is observed where U is independent of X with mean zero and constant variance. If we conducted a so-called *naive* analysis, proceeding as if $x^\dagger = x$ and fitting the model $E[Y|X^\dagger = x^\dagger] = \beta_0^\dagger + \beta_X^\dagger x^\dagger$, then we would find $\beta_X^\dagger = \frac{Var(X)}{Var(X)+Var(U)}\beta_X$. A naive analysis therefore results in an *attenuated* estimate of β_X (see Section 3.1 of Keogh et al. (2020)).

A similar result may be observed in the case of a continuous outcome regressed on a single binary covariate measured with error. If we consider the model $E[Y|A = a] = \beta_0 + \beta_A a$ and instead fit $E[Y|A^\dagger = a^\dagger] = \beta_0^\dagger + \beta_A^\dagger a^\dagger$ we again find (assuming the misclassification is independent of Y) attenuation in our parameter, with $\beta_A^\dagger = (PPV + NPV - 1)\beta_A$ (see Section 3.1 of Gustafson (2004)).

In these very simple settings, therefore, the effects of measurement error may be anticipated through knowledge of either the variance of the error term in the continuous case or the positive and negative predictive values in the binary case. Some argue that such attenuated effects may be tolerated, for example because underestimation of an effect may be seen as less of a concern than an overestimation of an effect. Whether or not one subscribes to this viewpoint, it is nevertheless a dangerous over-simplification of the problems measurement error can cause. As soon as we deviate from the very simple (and strong) assumptions of the preceding examples, such as by considering confounders, or non-linear outcome models, the impact of measurement error becomes much harder to predict. The precision medicine framework can also complicate how we react to the effects of measurement error, which we shall discuss in Section 8.2.3.

These simple examples do, however, indicate how we may begin to correct for the effects of measurement error. If we know, for example, that our naive analysis leads to an attenuated effect estimate through $\beta_X^\dagger = \frac{Var(X)}{Var(X)+Var(U)}\beta_X$, then this would suggest that if we could find estimates of the variances of X and U (denoted $\hat{\sigma}_X^2, \hat{\sigma}_U^2$) we could use these and our naive estimate $\hat{\beta}_X^\dagger$ to form a 'corrected' estimate $\hat{\beta}_X = \frac{\hat{\sigma}_X^2+\hat{\sigma}_U^2}{\hat{\sigma}_U^2}\hat{\beta}_X^\dagger$. A similar approach could be employed to adjust an attenuated parameter estimate in the case of a binary variable subject to misclassification through estimation of the positive and negative predicted values.

We may think of σ_U^2, or NPV and PPV, as describing the size or severity of the error, and key to understanding the impacts of - and correction for - measurement error is estimation of these statistics. For this, we will usually require some auxiliary data. Auxiliary data come in various forms, and may afford us the opportunity to estimate both the size and structure of the measurement error. The ideal auxiliary data are *validation* data, where we observe the true X on a subset of our sample. Validation data may be very expensive, or often impossible, to obtain, and so a more common alternative are *replicate* data. As the name implies, replicate data (or simply *replicates*) arise when we are able to take measurements more than once on at least some individuals. Replicate measurements are typically assumed to be independent and identically distributed error-prone observations of the true value. More generally, *instrumental* data - correlated with X but whose errors are independent of the errors in $X^\dagger$ - may be used. In this chapter, we will focus on situations where replicate data are observed, as these are typically the most likely to be available in practice.

The type of auxiliary data available is one of several factors that affects what methods may be used to correct for the effects of measurement error or misclassification in an analysis. We have already seen that in the case of single covariates measured with error (or subject to misclassification) that it may be possible to simply adjust the naive estimate of a model parameter if we have knowledge of the variance of the error or the positive and negative predictive values for our data. (We would also need to take steps to adjust inferential statistics, such as standard errors, to account for the uncertainty in the measurement error estimation process.) More complex analyses, such as those featuring multiple covariates, non-continuous outcome variables, non-linear models, and so on, each require unique handling.

One of the more popular methods for measurement error correction is known as *regression calibration* (Carroll and Stefanski, 1990; Gleser, 1990). Widely applicable, it offers unbiased estimates in the case of linear regression of a continuous outcome on covariates measured with error, if either the measurement error model is known or its parameters consistently estimated. Regression calibration uses auxiliary data to form an estimate of the true value we wish to observe, and this estimate may then be used in place of the true value in a standard analysis. A common method for determining the estimated true value is the so-called *best linear unbiased predictor* (BLUP). For X subject to measurement error, potentially in the presence of variables Z measured without error, then the BLUP is given by

$$X^{RC} = \mu_X + \begin{bmatrix} \Sigma_{XX^\dagger} & \Sigma_{XZ} \end{bmatrix} \begin{bmatrix} \Sigma_{X^\dagger X^\dagger} & \Sigma_{X^\dagger Z} \\ \Sigma_{ZX^\dagger} & \Sigma_{ZZ} \end{bmatrix}^{-1} \begin{bmatrix} X^\dagger - \mu_X \\ Z \quad \mu_Z \end{bmatrix}$$

where μ_A and Σ_{AB} denote the mean of A and the covariance between A and B, respectively. The terms in this expression may be estimated from the data, making use of auxiliary data (such as replicates). Our analysis would then proceed as normal, with our estimate of X^{RC} used in place of X.

Numerous other correction techniques are available, with varying degrees of complexity and theoretical properties. With our focus primarily on the consequences of failing to correct for error, we shall not consider correction methods beyond a simple illustration of regression calibration in Section 8.4.1. An excellent introduction to many of the most commonly-used correction methods is provided in Shaw et al. (2020).

Finally, we have hitherto not discussed the possibility of measurement error in the outcome itself. Errors in the outcome are typically viewed with less concern, as their impact may often be comparatively limited. For example, suppose our outcome Y is subject to classical additive error where $y^\dagger = y + u_Y$ is observed with u_Y independent of Y with zero mean and constant variance. In this scenario, $E[Y^\dagger|X = x] = E[Y|X = x]$ and so if we wish to estimate parameters in a model of the form $E[Y|X = x] = \beta_0 + \beta_X x$ (for example) then a naive analysis using $y^\dagger$ in place of y will be unbiased.

While this would seem to suggest that error in the outcome can be more safely ignored, the reality is again far more complex. First, even in the idealized setting above, our analysis will lack power as $Var(Y^\dagger|X) = Var(Y|X) + Var(U_Y)$. Moreover, systematic measurement error will likely lead to biased parameter estimates, while the effects of more complex error structures are even harder to predict.

8.2.2 Dynamic Treatment Regime Estimation

We shall pursue precision medicine through the framework of dynamic treatment regimes (DTRs): sequences of treatment decision rules taking tailoring variables as input and outputting individualized treatment recommendations (Murphy, 2003; Lavori and Dawson, 2004). Our goal is to identify the optimal DTR: the sequence of decision rules that maximize the expected outcome (assuming that larger values of Y are preferred). Numerous approaches have been developed for this task (see Chakraborty and Moodie (2013), and Kosorok and Moodie (2015) for comprehensive discussions) but we will focus on the method of dynamic weighted ordinary least squares (dWOLS, Wallace and Moodie (2015)). As the name suggests, this approach is grounded in weighted ordinary least squares regression, offering relatively straightforward implementation within an analytical framework already familiar to most practitioners. While many users will likely prefer to code this method themselves, it is also implemented in the R package DTRreg (Wallace et al., 2017; Simoneau et al., 2020), which includes extensions of the original dWOLS method to survival outcomes (Simoneau et al., 2019) and continuous treatments (Schulz and Moodie, 2020), as well as the related method of G-estimation (Robins, 2004). With its foundation in well-explored theory, dWOLS may be readily adapted or modified to handle issues arising from measurement error, which have already been extensively studied in the context of regression modeling.

We first illustrate dWOLS in the case of a single binary treatment decision $A \in \{0, 1\}$ and continuous tailoring variable X. A may represent any binary treatment decision, such as two treatment options or an intervention versus standard care. For simplicity, we shall refer to $A = 1$ and $A = 0$ as representing 'treatment' and 'no treatment', respectively. Consider an outcome, Y, modeled as:

$$E[Y|x, a] = \beta_0 + \beta_1 x + a(\beta_2 + \beta_3 x) - a^{opt}(\beta_2 + \beta_3 x)$$

where a^{opt} is the optimal treatment for an individual with an observed tailoring variable value of x. In the above model it may be easily verified that $a^{opt} = 1_{\{\beta_2+\beta_3>0\}}$. We note that, because a^{opt} is a function of model parameters and x (but not a), this outcome model can be re-framed as

$$E[Y|x, a] = f(x; \phi) + a(\psi_0 + \psi_1 x) \tag{8.1}$$

where we have decomposed it into two components described as follows:

- $f(x; \phi)$ is the *treatment-free* component as it denotes the expected outcome if $a = 0$.
- $a(\psi_0 + \psi_1 x)$ is the *blip* component corresponding to the expected change in outcome for the observed treatment compared to if $a = 0$.

By compartmentalizing the outcome in this way, we can see that identifying a^{opt} requires the identification of the *blip parameters* ψ_0, ψ_1, whereas ϕ are nuisance parameters and are not required for treatment identification.

To estimate the model parameters in (8.1), we may carry out a standard regression analysis, regressing Y on the terms in models proposed for the treatment-free and blip components as in any other regression problem. If a and x are independent, then correct specification of the blip model is sufficient to ensure consistent estimation of the blip parameters. However, if we are unwilling to make this assumption then the full outcome model - that is, both the blip and treatment-free models - must be correctly specified.

Model flexibility may be gained by generating a weighted dataset which restores covariate balance between X and A. dWOLS approaches this by estimating a *treatment* model which describes the relationship between A and X. The resulting propensity scores $\pi(a|x) = P(A = 1|X = x)$ are then used to construct weights of the form $w(a, x) = |a - \pi(a|x)|$, which gives more weight to individuals who received a low probability treatment is given their observed x. A weighted regression of the outcome on the terms in the blip and treatment-free models, using these weights, will then yield consistent estimators of ψ_0 and ψ_1 if at least one of the treatment or treatment-free models are correctly specified. This *double robustness* property is shared by several related methods, including G-estimation (Robins, 2004) and augmented inverse probability of treatment weighting (Zhang et al., 2012). Having obtained estimates $\hat{\psi}_0$ and $\hat{\psi}_1$ of the blip model parameters, the optimal treatment rule is then estimated as $\hat{a}^{opt} = 1_{\{\hat{\psi}_0+\hat{\psi}_1 x>0\}}$.

This approach readily extends to the multi-stage treatment case, where we suppose a sequence of treatment decisions is to be made. As illustration, we consider a two-stage example with a single tailoring variable at each stage, denoted x_1 and x_2, and binary treatments denoted a_1 and a_2. We use a_k^{opt} to denote the optimal stage k treatment. We consider an outcome model of the form

$$\begin{aligned} E[Y|x_1, a_1, x_2, a_2] = \phi_0 + \phi_1 x_1 - \left[a_1^{opt}(\psi_{10} + \psi_{11}x_1) - a_1(\psi_{10} + \psi_{11}x_1)\right] \\ - \left[a_2^{opt}(\psi_{20} + \psi_{21}x_2) - a_2(\psi_{20} + \psi_{21}x_2)\right] \end{aligned} \tag{8.2}$$

where $a_k^{opt} = 1_{\{\psi_{k0}+\psi_{k1}x_k\}}$. Here, $\phi_0 + \phi_1 x_1$ is the expected outcome if treatment at both stages is optimal, and the remaining terms (in square brackets) correspond to what is 'lost' at each stage if $a_k \neq a_k^{opt}$ (that is, if treatment is non-optimal). These quantities are often referred to as *regrets*, and we refer to (8.2) as a regret-based formulation of the outcome. The regret-based formulation may be thought of as equal to an optimal outcome minus the effects of non-optimal treatment, which is equivalent to an *advantage*-based formulation where the advantage (equal to the negative of the regret) reflects what is gained from the use of an optimal treatment compared to a non-optimal one. We shall proceed with the regret-based presentation for consistency with the extant dWOLS literature.

In the multi-stage case, dWOLS proceeds recursively, beginning at the final stage and working backwards towards the first. This process is necessary as in many situations the treatment decisions at earlier stages may have consequences for treatment decisions made later. For example, a treatment available at stage one may appear effective in the short term, but it may also undermine the efficacy of treatments that might come later. By starting with the final treatment decision and working backward, we are able to optimize each treatment decision while accounting for its potential effects on future stages.

In our example, we start with the estimation of the stage two blip parameters ψ_{20}, ψ_{21}. We can see how this is, effectively, a single-stage problem by re-framing the outcome model as

$$E[Y|x_1, a_1, x_2, a_2] = f_2(x_1, a_1, x_2; \phi) + a_2(\psi_{20} + \psi_{21}x_2) \tag{8.3}$$

recalling, again, that a_2^{opt} is a function of x_2 and not a_2. This is analogous to (8.1), where we see that we again have a treatment-free component $f_2(h_2; \phi)$ and a blip component. It is therefore sufficient to find ψ_{20}, ψ_{21} to determine a_2^{opt}. We start by specifying models for the treatment-free and blip components of (8.3), as well as estimating propensity scores for the second stage treatment $\pi_2(a_2|h_2)$ via (for example) logistic regression. dWOLS then proceeds as before with a weighted regression of Y on the terms specified in the treatment-free and blip models, with weights $w(a_2, h_2) = |a_2 - \pi_2(a_2|h_2)|$. This returns estimates of the second stage blip parameters, which may be used to estimate $\hat{a}_2^{opt} = 1_{\{\hat{\psi}_{20}+\hat{\psi}_{21}x_2>0\}}$. Again, the blip parameter estimators are doubly robust: consistent if at least one of the treatment-free or treatment models is correctly specified (although in practice it is unlikely we would be able to fully identify the treatment-free model; see Section 8.3.2 for a more detailed illustration).

To estimate the stage one model parameters we must first construct a *pseudo-outcome* that, in effect, removes the influence of any stage two variables. In this case, we define the stage one pseudo-outcome

$$\tilde{y}_1 = y + (\hat{a}_2^{opt} - a_2)(\hat{\psi}_{20} + \hat{\psi}_{21}x_2)$$

which equals the expected outcome if the stage two treatment were - potentially contrary to fact - optimal. This construction allows us to the identify the optimal stage one treatments conditional on the stage two treatment being optimal, helping ensure that our stage one treatment decision does not undermine what can be achieved at stage two.

By comparison with (8.2) we may see that $\tilde{y}_1$ can then be modeled as

$$E[\tilde{Y}_1|x_1, a_1] = \phi_0 + \phi_1 x_1 - \left[a_1^{opt}(\psi_{10} + \psi_{11}x_1) - a_1(\psi_{10} + \psi_{11}x_1)\right]$$

and, by a similar argument as used to derive (8.3), may be re-framed into the familiar treatment-free and blip components as

$$E[\tilde{Y}_1|x_1, a_1] = f_1(x_1; \phi) + a_1(\psi_{10} + \psi_{11}x_1).$$

This represents another single-stage problem and may be tackled similarly: specifying models for $f_1(x_1; \phi)$, the blip, and the treatment model for A_1 and conducting a weighted ordinary least squares regression with $\tilde{y}_1$ to estimate ψ_{10}, ψ_{11}.

8.2.3 Measurement Error and DTR Estimation

In Section 8.2.1 we discussed some simple illustrations of the impact of measurement error in regression analyses. It is therefore clear that dWOLS, being itself grounded in weighted least squares regression, may also be undermined if variables are measured with error. Of course, any statistical method is susceptible to measurement error, but we are able to leverage the familiar (and relatively simple) methodology underpinning dWOLS to both anticipate – and correct for – its effects.

While dWOLS largely simplifies the problem of DTR estimation to that of a sequence of weighted linear regressions, there are various subtleties when it comes to understanding measurement error in the specific context of precision medicine. Here, we focus on errors in continuous tailoring variables, binary treatments, and continuous outcomes. We shall consider each of these separately, assuming measurement error (or misclassification) is present in precisely one of these variables, with all others measured correctly. While in reality, one may reasonably expect errors in multiple variables simultaneously, we hope that focusing on each model component individually will help articulate some of the more nuanced implications of measurement error in the precision medicine framework.

8.2.3.1 Errors in Tailoring Variables

A defining feature of precision medicine is that treatment rules are formed based on tailoring variables. In the single-stage example of the preceding section, our optimal rule was "$a^{opt} = 1$ if $\psi_0 + \psi_1 x > 0$, $a^{opt} = 0$ otherwise", and our problem was one of estimating ψ_0 and ψ_1. Clearly, if our tailoring variable is subject to measurement error, and by extension our estimates of ψ_0, ψ_1 are biased, we have no guarantee that the estimated treatment rule will be the correct one. Moreover, unlike the simple linear regression example discussed in Section 8.2.1, it is not only the ψ_1, the parameter associated with x that is of interest; we require both ψ_0 and ψ_1 to form our treatment rule.

In the single-stage case we may first view this as a standard linear regression problem, and thus any measurement error correction method appropriate for that context may be applied if our outcome model is correctly specified. For example, if replicate measurements are available, then regression calibration may be applied as it would for any other linear regression scenario.

If our treatment-free model is misspecified, however, the implications for the double robustness property of dWOLS are less obvious. Recall that the goal of weighting in dWOLS is to establish covariate balance between A and X, which is achieved through the estimation of the relationship between these two variables. If X is not observed, however, then while our outcome Y may be assumed to depend on the true X, the treatment will likely depend on $X^{\dagger}$. For example, if we were interested in the relationship between blood pressure and resting heart rate, then while heart rate should depend on the true underlying SBP, any treatment decisions made by a physician will be based on observable (i.e., error-prone) data.

Spicker and Wallace (2020) explored this problem and found that regression calibration may still be applied, with the BLUP of X used throughout the entire analysis in place of X. Notably, this includes using X^{RC}, and not $X^{\dagger}$ in the treatment model. While this does not return the fully consistent estimators of the error-free setting, it has been shown that this approach should lead to "approximately consistent" results as long as at least one of the treatment or treatment-free models is correctly specified.

While estimation in the single-stage setting may therefore be handled with relative ease, the recursive nature of the multistage case introduces an additional complication. As discussed in Section 8.2.2, dWOLS proceeds by constructing pseudo-outcomes which aim to remove the influence of any stage two variables that may interfere with the stage one analysis. If we consider the two-stage example characterized in (8.2), then in the error-free setting we may consider the 'remainder'

$$\hat{r}_2 - r_2 = (\hat{a}_2^{opt} - a_2)(\hat{\psi}_{20} + \hat{\psi}_{21}x_2) - (a_2^{opt} - a_2)(\psi_{20} + \psi_{21}x_2), \tag{8.4}$$

where r_2 denotes the stage two regret. If our blip parameters and treatment rule are correctly estimated then (8.4) reduces to zero and permits use of $\tilde{y}_1$ for valid stage one parameter estimation.

In contrast, if we observe $x_2^{\dagger}$ instead of x_2, only the former can be used in the construction of $\hat{r}_2$, and so even if the blip parameters and treatment rule are correctly estimated (such as through the use of regression calibration as described above), the expression (8.4) reduces to

$$\hat{r}_2 - r_2 = (a_2^{opt} - a_2)\psi_{21}(x_2^{\dagger} - x_2)$$

and thus even with perfect stage two estimation, the error in $x_2^{\dagger}$ results in a stage one pseudo-outcome that is not independent of the stage two variables. We will investigate the impact of this in Section 8.4.3.

The preceding discussion has focused solely on the estimation of model parameters and, by extension, the optimal treatment rule. An equally (if not more) important question concerns the implementation of our results for future patients. We cannot limit ourselves to considering measurement error in our analysis; we must also consider its presence in the variables we will use to make treatment decisions in practice.

Notably, this concern persists even in the case where we know the true optimal treatment rule. For example, suppose it is known that we should prescribe an intervention if the three-month average SBP exceeds 130, and otherwise continue with standard care. A patient with a long-term average blood pressure below 130 may nevertheless have a high measurement on the day they visit their physician and be prescribed a non-optimal therapy.

One quantity of interest may therefore be the probability that, given an observed $x^{\dagger}$, a patient receives the incorrect treatment. For example, in the case of a single tailoring variable if the true optimal treatment rule is of the form "$a^{opt} = 1$ if $x > \tau$" for some treatment threshold τ, then $P(X < \tau | x^{\dagger} > \tau)$ (or $P(X > \tau | x^{\dagger} < \tau)$) gives the probability that a patient would receive the incorrect treatment if their treatment decision was based on the observed $x^{\dagger}$.

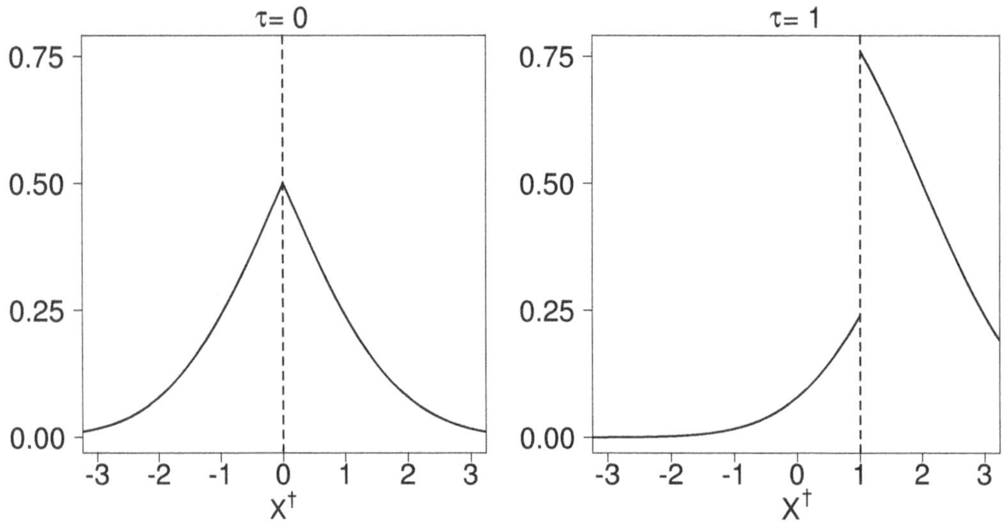

Figure 8.1 *Probability a patient receives the incorrect treatment if $X^\dagger$ is used for the treatment decision instead of X where $X^\dagger = X + U$ with $X, U \sim N(0,1)$ when the treatment threshold (dashed line) is either 0 (left) or 1 (right).*

In very simple cases such probabilities may be computed directly. For example, if $X \sim N(\mu_X, \sigma_X^2)$ and $X^\dagger = X + U$ with $U \sim N(0, \sigma_U^2)$, then if we observe $X^\dagger = x^\dagger$ it may be shown that

$$X | X^\dagger = x^\dagger \sim N\left(\frac{\sigma_X^2 x^\dagger + \sigma_U^2 \mu_X}{\sigma_X^2 + \sigma_U^2}, \frac{\sigma_X^2 \sigma_U^2}{\sigma_X^2 + \sigma_U^2}\right).$$

This can lead to results that can seem initially counter-intuitive. In Figure 8.1 we present the probability of mistreatment for various values of $x^\dagger$ for an example where X and U are both $N(0,1)$. We consider two possible treatment thresholds of $\tau = 0$ and $\tau = 1$. In the former case, the mistreatment probability is symmetric about the treatment threshold, as we might expect. In the latter case, however, we see that the probability of mistreatment is much higher for observed values of $x^\dagger$ that are slightly above the treatment threshold than for values that are slightly below it. This is because for this particular setup, it is relatively unlikely for such a large true x to occur: it is more likely that an observation slightly greater than one is due to measurement error than because x was also greater than one.

Real-world scenarios will of course be far more complex, but the preceding results demonstrate the care that must be taken when tailoring treatment decisions based on error-prone observations in even the simplest settings. When tailoring variables are measured with error, there is in effect a 'ceiling' on how well any treatment rule can perform in practice, and as such obtaining auxiliary data - such as replicate measurements - is just as important when implementing our decision rules as for when estimating them.

8.2.3.2 Treatment Misclassification

While it is not uncommon to use prior treatments as tailoring variables for future treatment decisions, we shall not consider this possibility. Nevertheless, while misclassification in the treatment may seem a simpler problem than an error in tailoring variables, it also requires careful attention.

Indeed, the mere structure of the misclassification itself may not always be obvious. In practice, we may have up to three treatment measures. We would normally know what was prescribed, and in some cases, the patient may report their treatment adherence. Both, one, or neither of these two measures may align with a third: what treatment regime was truly followed? We must think carefully about how these observations may relate.

In the case where a patient reports their behaviour, we may denote this as $A^\dagger$ and assume it is dependent on the true A (with both, in turn, depending on what was prescribed). In contrast, if we consider the simpler case where our only measurement is of what was prescribed, then it may be more reasonable to assume that the true A depends on the error-prone $A^\dagger$.

We shall limit ourselves to the latter case and, working within the binary treatment setting, we may view a patient as adherent or non-adherent to therapy. The mechanisms of adherence will vary on a case by case basis. For example, in some circumstances, patients may have access to the treatment they were not prescribed, whereas in others they might not. Additionally, (non-) adherence may depend on other covariates, most notably the tailoring variable. This may be particularly plausible in settings where the tailoring variable is a marker of symptom severity or some other predictor of the health outcome of the patient. Clearly, in such circumstances, the potential impact on our analysis and estimated treatment rules could be severe.

As mentioned in Section 8.2.1, when considering a simple linear regression model of the form $E[Y|A=a] = \beta_0 + \beta_A a$, misclassification in a binary covariate A results in attenuation of the associated parameter estimate. In our framework, meanwhile, our focus is on the blip component of our outcome, such as $a(\psi_0 + \psi_1 x)$ in our simple single stage setting. Here, the parameters associated with A are precisely those in the blip, and as our focus is on the treatment rule $a^{opt} = 1_{\{\psi_0+\psi_1 x>0\}}$, we observe that if *all* blip parameters are attenuated by the same factor then the resulting treatment rule will still be valid. We will demonstrate this principle in Section 8.5.

Similar to the case of measurement error in the tailoring variable, misclassification of A has implications in the multi-stage setting in the construction of pseudo-outcomes. We again consider (8.4), the difference between the stage two regret and its estimate. Even with full knowledge of ψ_0, ψ_1, and a^{opt}, in the case where $a^\dagger$ is observed instead of a, this expression reduces to

$$\hat{r}_2 - r_2 = (a_2 - a_2^\dagger)(\hat{\psi}_{20} + \hat{\psi}_{21} x_2).$$

and, as in the case of error in the tailoring variable, our stage one pseudo-outcome may be 'contaminated' by stage two variables.

Finally, we should again consider the implementation of our estimate treatment rules on future patients. Our work in this chapter assumes that our goal is to estimate the true treatment rule, assuming future patients will be fully adherent to their prescribed treatments. While in more traditional analyses we may wish to ignore non-adherence altogether (taking an intention-to-treat approach), the limitations we have highlighted in this section, along with the results presented in Section 8.5, demonstrate that this is not necessarily a valid strategy in the dynamic treatment regime framework.

8.2.3.3 Errors in the Outcome

Measurement error in the outcome may typically be overlooked in a more standard regression analysis, although as always there are exceptions. Within our framework, the result noted in Section 8.2.1 may extend to analyses of a single-stage treatment problem, with classical additive error in Y leading to more uncertain, but unbiased, parameter estimates. Interestingly, our model setup can afford some additional flexibility. Suppose $Y^\dagger = Y + U_Y$ with $U_Y \sim N(\upsilon_Y, \sigma^2_{UY})$, independent of Y. If υ_Y is non-zero, reflecting systematic error, a naive analysis that uses $Y^\dagger$ in place of Y should only be affected in the estimation of the intercept term. As this does not interact with treatment (and so does not enter our blip model), the resulting blip parameter and optimal treatment estimator will remain unbiased.

While the preceding scenario would be of similarly little concern in a standard regression analysis where the relationship between X and Y was of primary interest, the same cannot be said if we allow the error in $Y^\dagger$ to depend on X itself. If we suppose $U_Y \sim N(\upsilon_Y X, \sigma^2_{UY})$, for example, then a dWOLS analysis of an outcome model of the form $E[Y|A = a, X = x] = \phi_0 + \phi_1 x + a(\psi_0 + \psi_1 x)$ should still produce consistent blip parameter estimators as the error in $Y^\dagger$ will be 'absorbed' by the ϕ_1 nuisance parameter. Should the error in Y depend on the treatment, however, then our estimation of the blip parameters will be unreliable.

As in the preceding settings, the construction of pseudo-outcomes in the multistage case is also problematic. If we construct

$$\tilde{y}_1 = y^\dagger + (\hat{a}_2^{opt} - a_2)(\hat{\psi}_{20} + \hat{\psi}_{21} x_2)$$

then any dependence of $y^\dagger$ on x_2 or a_2 that is not captured by the regret component will be carried over to stage one. As such, our stage one analysis may once again be compromised.

8.3 Simulation Studies: General Setup

We will now explore the impact of measurement errors in the tailoring and outcome variables, and misclassification in a binary treatment, through various simulation studies. For ease of exposition, we will first summarize the general structure of these simulations in a fully error-free setting. We will consider both one-stage and two-stage example. While analysis of the second stage of the two-stage case is equivalent to that of a single stage problem, we believe that exploring a simpler one stage example separately will help add clarity. This will also allow us, when considering the two stage case, to focus our attention on the impact of the various errors on the estimation of stage one parameters through the construction of pseudo-outcomes. All of our simulation setups are deliberately simplistic; we will not consider error-free confounders or multiple tailoring variables. We will also use a relatively large sample size of $n = 1,000$ in our estimation procedures. Our focus in this work is to highlight some of the principles underlying measurement error within the precision medicine and dynamic treatment regime framework, so that these principles may be better anticipated and understood in more complex, realistic settings. We make no guarantees about the applicability of our results to more general problems, and stress that measurement error in any real-world analysis will require careful and bespoke handling.

8.3.1 One Stage

Our one-stage case will consider a continuous outcome Y dependent on a single tailoring covariate X and binary treatment A. We generate $X \sim N(0, 1)$ while treatment will depend on X through $P(A = 1|X = x) = \left[1 + \exp(1 - x + 0.5x^2)\right]^{-1}$ and as such is amenable to estimation via logistic regression. The outcome is generated as

$$Y \sim -1 + X + X^2 + A(\psi_0 + \psi_1 X) + N(0, 1)$$

so that the optimal treatment rule is $a^{opt} = 1$ if $\psi_0 + \psi_1 x > 0$ and $a^{opt} = 0$ otherwise. We set $\psi_0 = -0.5$ and $\psi_1 = 1$ so the treatment rule may be viewed more simply as $a^{opt} = 1$ if $X > -\psi_0/\psi_1 = 0.5$ and $a^{opt} = 0$ otherwise. We refer to $\tau = -\psi_0/\psi_1$ as the treatment threshold.

Recall the double robustness property of dWOLS: assuming the blip model is correctly specified, then as long as at least one of the treatment or treatment-free models is correctly specified a weighted regression of Y on the terms in the outcome model with weights $w = |a - \hat{\pi}(a|x)|$ will result in the consistent estimation of the blip parameters. We will explore this double robustness property by conducting four analyses, where either (1) both treatment and treatment-free models are misspecified; (2) only the treatment-free model misspecify;

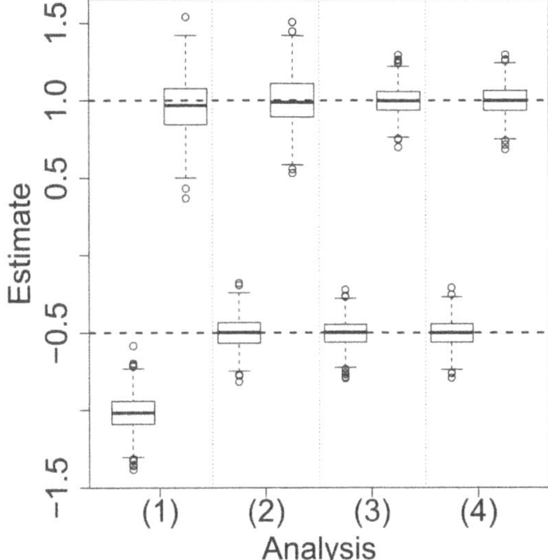

Figure 8.2 *Estimates of blip parameters $\psi_0 = -0.5$ (lower boxes and dashed line) and $\psi_1 = 1$ (upper boxes and dashed line) in the error-free setting. 'Analysis' corresponds to which of the treatment and treatment-free models is correctly specified: (1) neither correct; (2) treatment correct; (3) treatment-free correct; (4) both correct. Results from 1,000 simulated datasets of size $n = 1,000$.*

(3) only the treatment model is misspecified; or (4) both treatment and treatment-free models are correctly specified. Misspecification of the treatment or treatment free model is accomplished through the omission of the quadratic term in x.

As an illustration of analysis in the error-free setting, we generate 1,000 datasets each of size $n = 1,000$ and use dWOLS to estimate the blip model parameters for each of the four analyses. The resulting blip parameter estimates are summarized in Figure 8.2, where the double robustness of the method is apparent.

While dWOLS is fundamentally a tool for parameter estimation, we should also consider the performance of an analysis in terms of making future treatment decisions. For every simulated dataset used for parameter estimation (which we shall term *training* datasets) we will also generate testing, or *tailoring* datasets of size $m = 10,000$. The tailoring datasets will allow us to simulate what may be observed were our estimated treatment rules to be applied to a future cohort of similar patients.

One important metric will be the mistreatment probability: the probability that a randomly selected future patient will receive the incorrect treatment if the estimated optimal treatment rule $\hat{a}^{opt} = 1_{\{\hat{\psi}_0+\hat{\psi}_1 x\}}$ is used instead of the true optimal rule. While this can be calculated theoretically in some circumstances through knowledge of the distribution of X and the true and estimated treatment rules, we shall limit ourselves to empirical estimation in our tailoring datasets for easier and more direct comparison across cases. In our error-free analyses, the median mistreatment probabilities across our 1,000 tailoring datasets were 16.2% 1.9%, 1.8%, and 1.8% for analyses (1)-(4) respectively. It is important to note that even in the idealized, error-free setting, our estimates will still deviate slightly from the true treatment rule and, by extension, we will see some patients treated non-optimally. In cases where the estimators are unbiased, then greater uncertainty in those estimators will inflate the mistreatment probability. This will be particularly relevant in situations where measurement error does not bias our estimators but does add uncertainty to the estimation process.

While the probability of mistreatment is an intuitive metric, it is also a rather simplistic one. We will therefore also consider the expected 'cost' of mistreated patients in terms of the expected outcome we are hoping to maximize across the population. This is an important consideration as the difference in outcome between a correctly and incorrectly treated patient is $\psi_0 + \psi_1 x$, which may be very small - especially for those close to the true treatment threshold.

To capture the cost of mistreatment, in each tailoring dataset we will calculate what we term the *regret percentage*

$$r_{\%} = 100 \times \frac{\sum_i (a_i^{opt} - \hat{a}_i^{opt})(\psi_0 + \psi_1 x_i)}{\sum_i |\psi_0 + \psi_1 x_i|},$$

where we are summing over individuals indexed by i. The numerator reflects the regret of our estimated treatment: what is 'lost' from the outcome if the estimated treatment is non-optimal. The denominator, meanwhile, represents the difference in outcome if a patient is optimally treated versus non-optimally treated. Note that the numerator is non-negative as either $\psi_0 + \psi_1 x_i > 0$ and $a_i^{opt} = 1$, or $\psi_0 + \psi_1 x_i < 0$ and $a_i^{opt} = 0$.

This metric therefore expresses the total loss in the expected outcome resulting from non-optimal treatment assignment as a percentage of the maximum possible loss when comparing fully optimal treatment with fully non-optimal treatment. An $r_{\%}$ of 0% occurs if the estimated and observed optimal treatments coincide for all patients in the dataset, while an $r_{\%}$ of 100% indicates our estimated treatment was universally non-optimal. In our error-free simulations, we observed $r_{\%}$ values of 4.65% when both models were misspecified, while it was just 0.05% when at least one of the treatment or treatment-free models was correct. These results demonstrate how a mistreatment probability of around 2% may nevertheless have a very small impact on our outcome: slight bias in our estimated treatment rules may result in patients receiving the 'wrong' treatment, but only for patients close to the true treatment threshold and thus with small values of $\psi_0 + \psi_1 x$.

It is important to recognize that interpretation of mistreatment probabilities and $r_{\%}$ should be done with care, especially when comparing across different data generation procedures. A mistreatment probability of 2% or a regret percentage of 0.05% are small in absolute terms but are a by-product of our large sample sizes and good parameter estimation. These metrics should be compared within the context of our various simulation examples, and not considered in isolation as evidence of the performance one might expect more generally.

8.3.2 Two Stages

In the two-stage case, we consider a single tailoring variable at each stage. We generate $X_1 \sim N(0, 1)$ and $X_2 \sim N(A_1, 1)$, allowing the second stage tailoring variable to depend on the first stage treatment. Treatment is assumed to depend on the corresponding stage's tailoring variable, with $P(A_k = 1|X_k = x_k) = \left[1 + \exp(1 - x_k + 0.5x_k^2)\right]^{-1}$, $k = 1, 2$. The outcome Y is generated following the regret-based structure introduced in Section 8.2.2 as

$$\begin{aligned} Y \sim -1 + X_1 + X_1^2 &+ \left[A_1(\psi_{10} + \psi_{11}X_1) - A_1^{opt}(\psi_{10} + \psi_{11}X_1)\right] \\ &+ \left[A_2(\psi_{20} + \psi_{21}X_2) - A_2^{opt}(\psi_{20} + \psi_{21}X_2)\right] \\ &+ N(0, 1). \end{aligned}$$

In the two-stage case we set $\psi_{k0} = -0.5$ and $\psi_{k1} = -1$ so that $a_k^{opt} = 1$ if $x_k < -0.5$ (reversing the threshold direction from our one-stage case). Note that, within this regret-based outcome modeling framework the treatment-free model at both stages depends on the a_k^{opt} terms we are trying to estimate. While it is unrealistic to correctly specify these in a real-world analysis, as our focus is on the effects of measurement error we will continue to pursue four analysis strategies with none, one, or both treatment and treatment-free models are correctly specified. Mis-specification of the treatment models, as before, will be accomplished through omission of the x_k^2. Mis-specification of the treatment-free models, meanwhile, will be achieved through the use of models that are simply linear in x_1 at stage one and linear in x_1 and x_2 at stage two, omitting the x_1^2 and a_k^{opt} terms.

Analysis using dWOLS will begin at stage two, as described in Section 8.2.2. Logistic regression is used to estimate the relationship between A_2 and X_2 to form the weights $w(a_2|x_2) = |a_2 - \hat{\pi}(a_2|x_2)|$. Then, a weighted least squares regression of the outcome on the terms in the treatment-free and blip models will be used to estimate the stage two blip parameters and associated treatment rule $\hat{a}_2^{opt} = 1_{\{\hat{\psi}_{20}+\hat{\psi}_{21}x_2\}}$. These will be used to form the stage one pseudo-outcome

$$\tilde{y}_1 = y + (\hat{a}_2^{opt} - a_2)(\hat{\psi}_{20} + \hat{\psi}_{21}x_2)$$

which will be analyzed similarly. Model mis-specification will be consistent across stages: the treatment or treatment-free models will be mis-specified at stage one if and only if they are mis-specified at stage two.

Because the second stage case is analogous to a single-stage problem, our two-stage simulations will focus primarily on the results of the stage one analysis. We will review the stage one blip parameter and threshold estimates, as well as the probability of a patient receiving the wrong stage one treatment and the stage one regret percentages. Stage two results will be mentioned if they appear informative.

As an illustration, we again simulate 1,000 datasets of size $n = 1,000$, each accompanied by a tailoring dataset of size $m = 10,000$. The results concerning stage one blip parameter estimates are similar to the one-stage case - albeit with greater variability arising from the additional complexities and uncertainties in this example. This is reflected in the mistreatment probabilities in our tailoring dataset, averaging around 3.2% when predicting stage one treatment and 2.7% when predicting stage two treatment. The regret percentages are still small in absolute terms, averaging around 0.1% and 0.15% at stages one and two, respectively.

When interpreting these results we must keep in mind that, in practice, stage one treatment may have consequences for stage two that are not captured by stage-specific performance metrics. For example, an incorrect decision at stage one may not result in a substantial loss in terms of stage one regret, but it may result in a patient's stage two treatment being less beneficial than it might have been had they received an optimal treatment at stage one. While our focus will lie primarily on the impact of errors on the accuracy of our stage one analyses, these 'knock on' effects should not be overlooked.

8.4 Measurement Error in Tailoring Variables

Having established our general simulation framework in the error-free setting, we now begin our exploration of the impact of measurement error in precision medicine by exploring errors in the tailoring variables. As discussed in Section 8.2.3.1, such error is not merely a concern in estimation, but also when implementing treatment rules for future patients. In addition to the simulations in Section 8.3 where both the training and tailoring datasets assumed error-free observations were available, we will therefore consider three further analyses: training on an error-prone dataset but tailoring on an error-free one, training on an error-free dataset but tailoring on an error-prone one, and training and tailoring both using error-prone tailoring variables. We will explore the consequences of measurement error in tailoring variables on naive analyses and future treatment, as well as explore the use of regression calibration as a relatively straightforward measurement error correction technique in this setting.

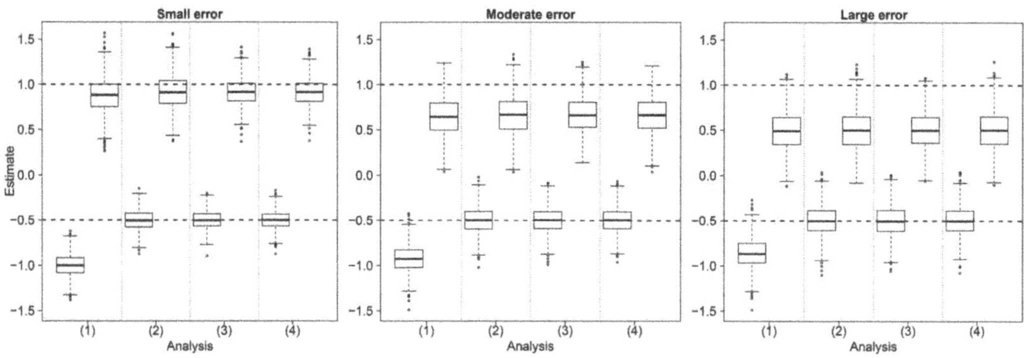

Figure 8.3 *Estimates of blip parameters $\psi_0 = -0.5$ (lower boxes and dashed line) and $\psi_1 = 1$ (upper boxes and dashed line) when the tailoring variable is subject to low (left), medium (centre) or hight (right) measurement error. 'Analysis' corresponds to which of the treatment and treatment-free models is correctly specified: (1) neither correct; (2) treatment correct; (3) treatment-free correct; (4) both correct. Results from 1,000 simulated datasets of size $n = 1,000$.*

8.4.1 One Stage: Naive Analysis

Having generated the true tailoring variable X, we will also generate an error-prone surrogate $X^\dagger = X + U_X$ subject to classical, additive, unbiased measurement error with $U \sim N(0, \sigma^2_{UX})$. We will simulate datasets with measurement error of various sizes, setting $\sigma^2_{UX} = 0.1, 0.5, 1$ which we will describe as small, moderate, and large measurement error respectively. Treatment A will depend either on X or $X^\dagger$ depending on which of our training and tailoring datasets are assumed error-free or error-prone. In the error-prone case, the dependency between A and $X^\dagger$ will be fully analogous to the error-free case, with $P(A = 1|X^\dagger = x^\dagger) = \left[1 + \exp(1 - x^\dagger + 0.5(x^\dagger)^2)\right]^{-1}$. The outcome is assumed to depend on X regardless of the context, and is therefore unchanged from the error-free setting outlined in Section 8.3.1.

Estimation is conducted using either x or $x^\dagger$ depending on the analysis setup. Estimation in the error-prone settings will be conducted using $x^\dagger$ in place of x throughout, replicating a naive analysis where measurement error is present but ignored. As in the error-free case, results are derived from 1,000 pairs of training and tailoring datasets of size $n = 1,000$ and $m = 10,000$, respectively.

Before considering the impact of measurement error on future treatment, we first summarize the blip parameters resulting from naive analyses when measurement error is present. These are summarized in Figure 8.3, where the impact of measurement error is apparent even in the case where σ^2_{UX} has its lowest value of 0.1. While the estimates of ψ_0 are largely unaffected, the estimates of ψ_1 are attenuated across our simulations. The attenuation factor is consistent with what is observed in the case of measurement error in simple linear regression: our ψ_1 estimates are approximately equal to the true ψ_1 values scaled by a factor of $\frac{Var(X)}{Var(X)+\sigma^2_{UX}}$. As $Var(X) = 1$ throughout our simulations, this results in naive estimates of ψ_1 of around 0.91, 0.67, and 0.5 in the low, moderate, and large error settings.

As discussed in Section 8.2.3.1, such attenuation in our DTR setting may have more severe consequences than a more traditional analysis where merely the relationship between outcome and covariate is of interest. Because our estimators of ψ_0 remain consistent, the bias in our estimator of ψ_1 leads to inaccurately estimated treatment thresholds. Compared to a true threshold of $\tau = 0.5$, our naive analyses result in estimated thresholds of around 0.55, 0.75, and 1 in the low, moderate, and large error scenarios. These biases will have

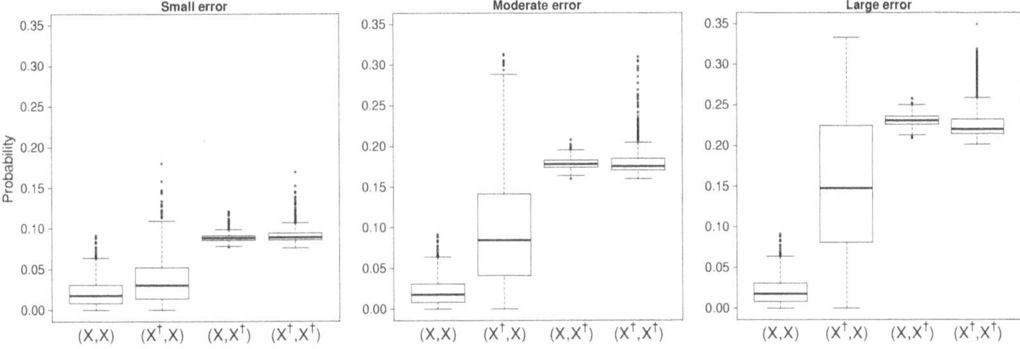

Figure 8.4 *Probability of mistreatment when a treatment rule estimated from a training dataset is used to make treatment decisions for a tailoring dataset. Variables in parentheses indicate (Training, Tailoring) where X denotes the true value and $X^\dagger$ denotes an error-prone observation. Results from 1,000 simulated training/tailoring pairs of size $n = 1,000$ (training) and $m = 10,000$ (tailoring).*

clear implications for the accuracy of future treatment decisions, whether they are based on X or $X^\dagger$.

We explore this using our tailoring datasets, first examining the mistreatment probabilities resulting from the implementation of the estimated optimal treatment rules. We consider four scenarios based on whether X or $X^\dagger$ is used at the training and/or tailoring stage. Results are summarized in Figure 8.4, where we limit attention to analysis (4) where both the treatment and treatment-free models are correctly specified. This therefore represents a best-case scenario, although results where only one of these models was correctly specified were largely similar.

Several patterns are evident in these results. First, as we would expect, performance worsens as the size of the measurement error increases. We also observe the consequences of the bias in our naive analyses when the results are applied to error-free tailoring variables, with mistreatment probabilities averaging as high as 0.15 in the large error case.

When using $X^\dagger$ for making treatment decisions, meanwhile, the mistreatment probabilities are substantially higher, but not greatly affected by whether the estimation was based on X or $X^\dagger$. This reflects how making treatment decisions based on error-prone tailoring variables can be hugely problematic. Indeed, even if the true optimal treatment rule were known, naive application of it to error-prone observations would result in similar mistreatment rates to those observed in our simulation results.

Also of interest in these results is the variability. Unsurprisingly, we see greater volatility when training on $X^\dagger$ compared to training on X. Somewhat more interesting, however, is the far greater volatility observed when tailoring on X compared to $X^\dagger$ (especially when we train on $X^\dagger$).

These patterns speak to another - perhaps less obvious - consequence of measurement error in this setting. The variance of X is smaller than that of $X^\dagger$, which creates a more 'sensitive' decision-making process. When we tailor based on $X^\dagger$ we observe a reliably large mistreatment probability: we cannot expect to do better than what the error in our tailoring variable will allow. The greater variability in $X^\dagger$ also makes it difficult for our analyses to perform *much* worse on this metric as there is effectively too much 'noise' in the data generation process. In contrast, when tailoring on X we may see a very strong performance if the estimated threshold is close to the truth, but a very poor one if it is not.

The regret percentages from these simulations exhibit similar patterns. When training on $X^\dagger$ and tailoring on the true X, the average loss due to mistreatment was around 0.3%, 2.2% and 6% for small, moderate, and large errors respectively. However, these were subject to substantial uncertainty, with 25% of simulated datasets resulting in a regret percentage of at least 12% in the large error case. When tailoring on $X^\dagger$, meanwhile, it made little difference whether estimation was based on a true or error-prone variable, with both averaging regret percentages of around 2%, 8% and 12% across our three error settings. There was comparatively very little variation in these results.

8.4.2 One Stage: Regression Calibration

As expected, naive analysis when tailoring variables are measured with error results in biased blip parameter estimates, misestimated optimal treatment rules, and incorrect treatment decisions. The preceding results, owing to the simplicity of the setup, demonstrated somewhat predictable effects of measurement error in the form of attenuation in the estimates of ψ_1. In theory, such attenuation may be accounted for by applying a post-hoc correction to the naive estimates based on knowledge of the size of the measurement error. Here, however, we present an illustration of the slightly more complex - but far more versatile - measurement error correction technique of regression calibration.

As outlined in Section 8.2.1, regression calibration proceeds by constructing regression calibration estimates X^{RC} of X using auxiliary data, such as replicates. These may be computed directly, or using tools available in many standard statistical software packages. Once estimated, a dWOLS analysis proceeds as normal, simply using the regression calibration estimates in place of X throughout.

We apply this procedure on 1,000 simulated datasets where independent, identically distributed replicate measures are assumed available on all individuals. The resulting blip parameter and treatment threshold estimates appear approximately consistent when at least one of the treatment or treatment-free models is correctly specified. This replicates existing work on this topic (Spicker and Wallace, 2020) and we do not present those results here.

Instead, we consider the impact of these improved estimates on future treatment decisions, particularly when it may be possible to gather replicate (or other auxiliary) data. In such cases, we could then construct regression calibration estimates of X not for the purposes of analysis, but simply for the purposes of assigning treatment. Analogous to the results summarized in Figure 8.4 we compare mistreatment probabilities based on whether the training or tailoring datasets used X or regression calibration estimates. Results are summarized in Figure 8.5. Overall, while we observe similar patterns to the naive analyses,

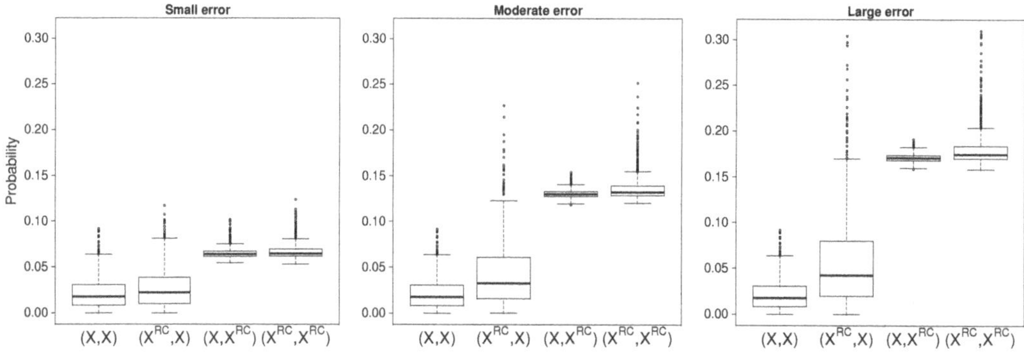

Figure 8.5 *Probability of mistreatment when a treatment rule estimated from a training dataset is used to make treatment decisions for a tailoring dataset. Variables in parentheses indicate (Training, Tailoring) where X denotes the true value and X^{RC} denotes the corresponding regression calibration estimate. Results from 1,000 simulated training/tailoring pairs of size $n = 1,000$ (tailoring) and $m = 10,000$ (tailoring).*

the performance when using regression calibration estimates are markedly improved. This improvement is reflected in the regret percentages: even in the large error setting non-optimal treatments resulted in an average loss of just 0.5% when treatment rules were estimated using regression calibration estimates and implemented using the true X. When only error-prone variables are available in the tailoring dataset, meanwhile, we again face limitations that would not be overcome even with knowledge of the true optimal rule. However, the regret percentages are still substantially improved, averaging around 8% in the worst-case scenario of large error. These results would of course only improve if more replicates – and thus more accurate estimates of the true X – were available.

8.4.3 Two Stages

The preceding results demonstrate that when the tailoring variable is measured with error a naive analysis will result in inaccurate blip parameter estimates and misidentified optimal treatment rules. These biases can however, be largely accounted for through the use of regression calibration.

In the two-stage case we can therefore expect analogous issues in the estimation of the stage two blip parameters, with the analysis at stage one undermined not only by an error in $X_1^\dagger$ but also in the construction of the stage one pseudo-outcome as discussed in Section 8.2.3.1.

A fully naive analysis of a two-stage problem with measurement errors in both X_1 and X_2 simply result in poor performance at stage two and even worse performance at stage one, and we do not present such results here. We instead focus on the impact of errors in X_2 that manifest solely through the construction of the stage one pseudo-outcome.

We therefore construct a two stage simulation study as per the setup described in Section 8.3.2 as follows. First, only the stage two tailoring variable X_2 is measured with error, with $X_2^\dagger = X_2 + U_{X_2}$ and U_{X_2} having mean zero and constant variance set to 0.1, 0.5, and 1. We will ignore estimation of the stage two model parameters, and instead construct our stage one pseudo-outcome using the true ψ_{20}, ψ_{21} and a_2^{opt} values. As described in Section 8.2.3.1, our stage one pseudo-outcome will therefore depend on a remainder term of the form $(a_2^{opt} - a_2)\psi_{21}(x_2^\dagger - x_2)$, which would equal zero if no measurement errors were present. We then conduct a stage one dWOLS analysis as normal, where the stage one tailoring variable is generated without error.

Generating 1,000 simulated training and tailoring datasets, as usual, the stage one blip parameter estimates are summarized in Figure 8.6. The estimates still exhibit bias despite knowledge of the true stage two model parameters and the stage one variables being measured without error. The impact of this bias is fairly limited, however, with the corresponding treatment threshold estimates biased by around 10% in even the most extreme measurement error scenario. This produces a mistreatment probability of only 3.4% in the tailoring dataset (just 0.6% higher than when X_2 is measured without error) and a negligible loss in terms of regret percentage.

While this is somewhat encouraging news, it nevertheless demonstrates how errors may propagate through a multi-stage process and interfere with analysis at stages even where no error is present. In more complex scenarios, or analyses with a greater number of stages, this may lead to far more pronounced effects.

8.4.4 Summary

The results presented in this section demonstrate that measurement errors in tailoring variables can have a substantial impact. A fully naive analysis, even in an extremely simple - and largely idealized - single-stage problem, can produce biased blip parameter estimates which in turn lead to inaccurate identification of the optimal treatment rule. These problems

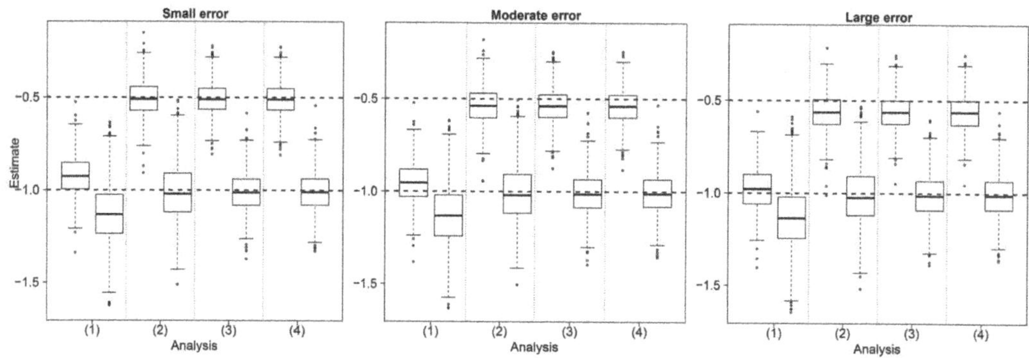

Figure 8.6 *Estimates of stage one blip parameters* $\psi_{10} = -0.5$ *(upper boxes and dashed line) and* $\psi_{11} = -1$ *(lower boxes and dashed line) when the second stage tailoring variable is subject to low (left), medium (centre) or hight (right) measurement error. True stage two blip parameters used in the construction of stage one pseudo-outcome, stage one tailoring variable measured without error. 'Analysis' corresponds to which of the treatment and treatment-free models is correctly specified: (1) neither correct; (2) treatment correct; (3) treatment free correct; (4) both correct. Results from 1,000 simulated datasets of size* $n = 1,000$.

may only be compounded in multi-stage problems, where errors in variables in later stages can undermine analysis at earlier stages through contamination of the pseudo-outcome. The implications of measurement error in tailoring variables are also not limited to the analysis stage, with the application of decision rules using error-prone data similarly problematic. The well-established measurement error correction method of regression calibration, however, offers considerable potential in such settings.

8.5 Misclassification in the Treatment

We now consider measurement error in the treatment which, occurring in a binary variable, we will refer to as misclassification. In this section, we will consider situations where patients were assigned one of the two possible treatments, but some patients were non-adherent. As such, the error-prone $A^{\dagger}$ (or $A_k^{\dagger}$) will denote the treatment that a patient was prescribed, while A (or A_k) will denote what treatment was actually followed. We do not consider the scenario where a patient may report a treatment behavior that is different from what was prescribed. Within this framework it is assumed that A (or A_k) may depend on $A^{\dagger}$ (or $A_k^{\dagger}$), but not vice-versa.

8.5.1 One Stage

Starting with the single-stage case, we assume that X (and Y) are measured without error. We construct the error-prone treatment variable $A^{\dagger}$ with $P(A^{\dagger} = 1|X = x) = \left[1 + \exp(1 - x + 0.5x^2)\right]^{-1}$. In our first simulations we generate the true A through specification of the positive predictive value $PPV = P(A = 1|A^{\dagger} = 1)$ and negative predictive value $NPV = P(A = 0|A^{\dagger} = 0)$. We set PPV and NPV to be 0.95, 0.9, and 0.75 to reflect small, moderate, and large degrees of misclassification respectively. We also considered scenarios where $PPV \neq NPV$, to reflect situations, where adherence rates varied based on prescribed treatment, which generated similar results. Our outcome is generated as in the error-free case: in particular, noting that it is assumed that Y depends on the true A and not the error-prone $A^{\dagger}$.

We continue to consider four analyses where none, one, or both the treatment and treatment-free models are correctly specified, with mis-specification accomplished through

Table 8.1 *Median (median squared error) of blip parameters* $(\psi_0, \psi_1) = (-0.5, 1)$ *and treatment thresholds* $\tau = 0.5$ *when treatment subject to misclassification.* $PV = P(A = a|A^\dagger = a)$: *positive and negative predictive values,* $\lambda = PPV + NPV - 1$ *attenuation factor. Rows correspond to which of the treatment and treatment-free models is correctly specified: (1) neither correct; (2) treatment correct; (3) treatment-free correct; (4) both correct. Results from 1,000 simulated datasets of size* $n = 1,000$.

	$PV = 0.95, \lambda = 0.9$			$PV = 0.9, \lambda = 0.8$			$PV = 0.75, \lambda = 0.5$		
	$\hat{\psi}_0$	$\hat{\psi}_1$	$\hat{\tau}$	$\hat{\psi}_0$	$\hat{\psi}_1$	$\hat{\tau}$	$\hat{\psi}_0$	$\hat{\psi}_1$	$\hat{\tau}$
(1)	-0.966	0.849	1.130	-0.913	0.747	1.216	-0.763	0.453	1.685
	(0.217)	(0.027)	(0.397)	(0.171)	(0.064)	(0.512)	(0.069)	(0.299)	(1.405)
(2)	-0.450	0.895	0.500	-0.399	0.796	0.500	-0.248	0.496	0.499
	(0.005)	(0.018)	(0.004)	(0.011)	(0.044)	(0.005)	(0.064)	(0.254)	(0.014)
(3)	-0.450	0.897	0.501	-0.400	0.800	0.499	-0.252	0.498	0.496
	(0.005)	(0.012)	(0.004)	(0.010)	(0.040)	(0.005)	(0.062)	(0.252)	(0.014)
(4)	-0.450	0.899	0.501	-0.401	0.800	0.502	-0.251	0.501	0.493
	(0.005)	(0.012)	(0.004)	(0.011)	(0.040)	(0.004)	(0.062)	(0.249)	(0.013)

the omission of the x^2 term. All of these will be carried out as naive analyses, using $a^\dagger$ wherever we might wish to use a. Note that this is therefore correct for the treatment model, as it is assumed $A^\dagger$ is dependent on X, but not in the construction of the blip, which depends on A.

The blip parameter and treatment threshold estimates for 1,000 simulated datasets are summarized in Table 8.1. As discussed in Section 8.2.1, in a standard linear regression problem misclassification in a binary covariate results in effect estimates attenuated by a factor of $\lambda = PPV + NPV - 1$. This result is reflected in our simulations when at least one of the treatment or treatment-free models is correctly specified. Most pertinently, in these cases estimates of both ψ_0 and ψ_1 are attenuated by this same factor, resulting in accurate threshold estimates. While we still see an increase in mistreatment probabilities and outcome loss due to the greater uncertainty when misclassification rates are highest, these are not particularly severe. Even with $PPV = NPV = 0.75$ we observe an average mistreatment rate of around 4% and an average regret percentage of just 0.3% in our tailoring datasets.

The preceding results, while encouraging, rely on the assumption that A depends only on $A^\dagger$. We now explore the scenario where adherence depends on the tailoring covariate X. We allow the positive and negative predictive values to vary by individual, so that they both increase with X. These probabilities are modeled so that, on average, the PPV and NPV values across each sample will be approximately 0.95, 0.9, and 0.75.

The resulting blip parameter and treatment threshold estimates (Table 8.2) demonstrate that covariate-dependent adherence results in dramatically biased blip parameter and treatment threshold estimates. We also experienced multiple sign errors in the high misclassification case, with 10-20% of our estimated ψ_1 values being less than zero and resulting in a treatment rule that assigns $a^{opt} = 1$ if $x < \hat{\tau}$ instead of if $x > \hat{\tau}$. In our tailoring datasets, the application of our estimated treatment rules results in mistreatment probabilities of around 11%, 25% and 31% in the small, moderate, and large misclassification settings respectively. The associated loss in expected outcomes is also substantial, averaging around 2%, 12% and 22%.

8.5.2 *Two Stages*

It is clear from the preceding results that if misclassification directly depends on X then our analyses become extremely unreliable, and so we do not consider this scenario in the two-stage case. We will, however, briefly present results of a two-stage simulation where at both stages we again generate misclassified treatments through the specification of the

Table 8.2 *Median (median squared error) of blip parameters* $(\psi_0, \psi_1) = (-0.5, 1)$ *and treatment thresholds* $\tau = 0.5$ *when treatment subject to misclassification dependent on the tailoring variable.* $\overline{PV}$ = *positive and negative predictive values across the sample. Rows correspond to which of the treatment and treatment-free models is correctly specified: (1) neither correct; (2) treatment correct; (3) treatment-free correct; (4) both correct. Results from 1,000 simulated datasets of size* $n = 1,000$.

	$\overline{PV} = 0.95$			$\overline{PV} = 0.9$			$\overline{PV} = 0.75$		
	$\hat{\psi}_0$	$\hat{\psi}_1$	$\hat{\tau}$	$\hat{\psi}_0$	$\hat{\psi}_1$	$\hat{\tau}$	$\hat{\psi}_0$	$\hat{\psi}_1$	$\hat{\tau}$
(1)	-1.074	0.502	2.134	-1.136	0.316	3.438	-1.237	0.129	6.755
	(0.330)	(0.248)	(2.671)	(0.404)	(0.468)	(8.631)	(0.543)	(0.758)	(39.123)
(2)	-0.500	0.583	0.847	-0.534	0.357	1.513	-0.628	0.118	4.004
	(0.005)	(0.173)	(0.121)	(0.006)	(0.414)	(1.026)	(0.017)	(0.778)	(12.280)
(3)	-0.492	0.555	0.888	-0.553	0.360	1.534	-0.669	0.170	3.749
	(0.004)	(0.198)	(0.151)	(0.005)	(0.410)	(1.069)	(0.029)	(0.689)	(10.557)
(4)	-0.497	0.594	0.839	-0.531	0.352	1.509	-0.629	0.128	4.356
	(0.003)	(0.165)	(0.115)	(0.004)	(0.420)	(1.019)	(0.017)	(0.761)	(14.872)

Table 8.3 *Median (median squared error) of stage one blip parameters* $(\psi_{10}, \psi_{11}) = (-0.5, -1)$ *and treatment thresholds* $\tau_1 = 0.5$ *when treatment subject to misclassification.* $PV = P(A_k = a_k | A_k^\dagger = a_k), k = 1, 2$*: positive and negative predictive values. 'Analysis' corresponds to which of the treatment and treatment-free models is correctly specified: (1) neither correct; (2) treatment correct; (3) treatment-free correct; (4) both correct. Results from 1,000 simulated datasets of size* $n = 1,000$.

	$PV = 0.95$			$PV = 0.9$			$PV = 0.75$		
	$\hat{\psi}_{10}$	$\hat{\psi}_{11}$	$\hat{\tau}_1$	$\hat{\psi}_{10}$	$\hat{\psi}_{11}$	$\hat{\tau}_1$	$\hat{\psi}_{10}$	$\hat{\psi}_{11}$	$\hat{\tau}_1$
(1)	-0.942	-1.028	-0.918	-0.909	-0.928	-0.986	-0.778	-0.634	-1.246
	(0.195)	(0.012)	(0.175)	(0.167)	(0.015)	(0.237)	(0.077)	(0.134)	(0.556)
(2)	-0.480	-0.920	-0.526	-0.457	-0.817	-0.561	-0.334	-0.518	-0.652
	(0.005)	(0.015)	(0.014)	(0.006)	(0.035)	(0.019)	(0.028)	(0.232)	(0.055)
(3)	-0.479	-0.914	-0.528	-0.455	-0.814	-0.563	-0.33	-0.513	-0.640
	(0.005)	(0.01)	(0.009)	(0.005)	(0.034)	(0.014)	(0.029)	(0.237)	(0.042)
(4)	-0.478	-0.910	-0.53	-0.455	-0.814	-0.566	-0.328	-0.514	-0.639
	(0.005)	(0.010)	(0.009)	(0.005)	(0.035)	(0.014)	(0.030)	(0.236)	(0.041)

positive and negative predictive values independently of the tailoring variable. We set these to 0.95, 0.9, and 0.75 as before, with the same misclassification rates for both stages.

We have already seen that the effect of misclassification on a single stage analysis was to bias the blip parameter estimates by a similar factor, resulting in reliable treatment threshold estimates. In the two stage-setting, therefore, even if treatment at stage two is subject to misclassification, we may still expect $\hat{a}_2^{opt}$ to reasonably approximate a_2^{opt}. Our key concern, as outlined in Section 8.2.3.2, is the differences between a_2 and $a_2^\dagger$ undermining the presumed independence between our stage one pseudo-outcome and stage two variables. This concern is borne out by our results (Table 8.3). Despite the stage two estimation resulting in valid estimates, differences between a_2 and $a_2^\dagger$ nevertheless interfere with our stage one analysis and bias our results. While the effects are relatively limited in absolute terms, it speaks (as was the case in Section 8.4.3) to the additional considerations that must be addressed when conducting multi-stage analyses.

8.5.3 Summary

These results demonstrate that while misclassification of the treatment results in biased blip parameter estimates, if that bias is similar across all parameters the resulting treatment rules should remain valid. Essential to this is that the probability the observed and true treatments differ does not depend on the tailoring variable; otherwise a naive analysis is compromised. In the multi-stage setting, meanwhile, the preceding property means that analysis at the final stage may often remain valid in the presence of misclassified treatment. However, if misclassified treatments are used in the formation of pseudo-outcomes for earlier stages of analysis, those analyses will be undermined.

8.6 Measurement Error in the Outcome

In our final set of simulations we consider the case where the treatment and tailoring variables are measured correctly, but there is an error in the outcome. We simulate an error-prone outcome $Y^\dagger = Y + U_Y$ where U_Y is normally distributed independently of Y with constant variance. We will investigate the impact of varying structures for the mean of U_Y, including systematic errors that depend on other variables in our analysis.

8.6.1 One Stage

In our single-stage simulations, we will generate an outcome subject to four measurement error structures: (i) $E[U_Y] = 0$; (ii) $E[U_Y] = \upsilon_Y$; (iii) $E[U_Y|X = x] = \upsilon_Y x$; and (iv) $E[U_Y|A = a] = \upsilon_Y a$ where υ_Y is a constant that controls the size of the error. Structure (i) therefore corresponds to (unbiased) classical additive measurement error, while structures (ii)-(iv) correspond to various forms of systematic error. We will generate data according to three levels of measurement error severity, with small, moderate, and large errors corresponding to where $\upsilon_Y/SD(Y) = 0.1, 0.5, 1$ and $Var(U_Y)/Var(Y) = 0.1, 0.5, 1$. Note that our 'large' error case therefore has both the largest systematic error as well as the largest error variance, so is relatively extreme.

As usual, we generate 1,000 training and tailoring dataset pairs, using $y^\dagger$ in place of y in our analyses. For brevity, we only consider analysis where both the treatment and treatment-free models are correctly specified (analysis (4) of preceding sections). The results from error structures (i)-(iii) were as expected, with the only impact of the error being to add imprecision, but not inaccuracy, to our blip parameter estimates. This is particularly encouraging when the error depends on X where, as anticipated, this impacts the nuisance parameters in the treatment-free model, leaving the all-important blip parameters largely unaffected.

Also expected was the poor performance seen in our simulations when the measurement error depended on the treatment A, summarized in Figure 8.7. While in our low error scenario, the effects were fairly limited (unsurprising given the weak relationship between U_Y and A in that setting), our moderate and large error setups returned substantially biased estimates of ψ_0 and, by extension unreliable optimal treatment threshold estimates. In applying these estimated rules to our tailoring datasets, average mistreatment rates of 20% and 40% were observed in the two larger error scenarios.

8.6.2 Two Stages

In the two-stage case our attention shifts to the impact of error in the outcome on the construction of the stage one pseudo-outcome. Except for the error-prone $Y^\dagger = Y + U_Y$, we generate data identically to the two stage error-free setting (recalling in particular that $X_2 \sim N(A_1, 1)$). Here, error structures (i) and (ii) are unchanged, corresponding to unbiased error and systematic error independent of other variables. Error structures (iii) and (iv), meanwhile, are generated to depend on the stage two variables X_2 and A_2, respectively.

As in the single stage case, unbiased and constant systematic error (error structures (i) and (ii)) do not present any new concerns: blip parameter estimates remain unbiased, albeit with greater uncertainty. If the error depends on A, meanwhile, then we have already seen

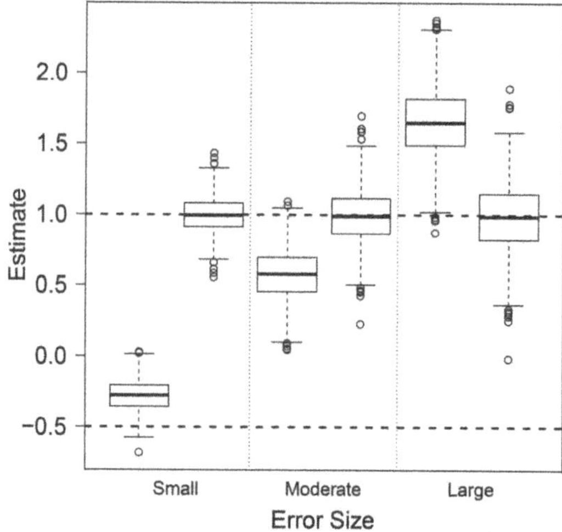

Figure 8.7 *Estimates of blip parameters* $\psi_0 = -0.5$ *(lower boxes and dashed line) and* $\psi_1 = 1$ *(upper boxes and dashed line) when the outcome is subject to error dependent on A. 'Analysis' corresponds to both correct. Results from 1,000 simulated datasets of size* $n = 1,000$.

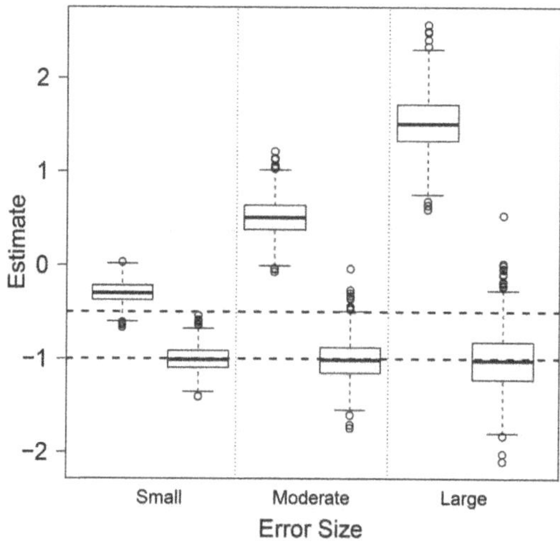

Figure 8.8 *Estimates of stage one blip parameters* $\psi_{10} = -0.5$ *(upper boxes and dashed line) and* $\psi_{11} = -1$ *(lower boxes and dashed line) when the outcome is subject to error dependent on* X_2. *'Analysis' corresponds to both correct. Results from 1,000 simulated datasets of size* $n = 1,000$.

that our stage two estimation is compromised and, as such, there would be little utility in pursuing a multi-stage analysis.

We therefore highlight the case where the error in Y depends on the stage two tailoring variable. The resulting stage one blip parameters are summarized in Figure 8.8. As expected, while measurement error in the outcome may safely depend on the tailoring variable in a single-stage analysis, the multi-stage case is not so accommodating. As we saw when constructing pseudo-outcomes using error-prone x_2 variables, bias is observed in the ψ_{10} estimates, reflecting the dependence of X_2 on A_1 entering the stage one pseudo-outcome through $Y^{\dagger}$.

8.6.3 Summary

At least some of the common perceptions concerning measurement error in the outcome may therefore be translated into the precision medicine framework. In particular, the classical additive (unbiased) error does not interfere with our blip parameter estimates beyond the usual increase in uncertainty. Meanwhile, the ability to accommodate some forms of systematic error by virtue of their impact being restricted to the parameters of the treatment-free model, may afford some additional resilience. As always, care must be taken in analyzing and understanding one's measurement error structures, paying particular attention to whether the error may truly be assumed to only interfere with the nuisance parameters in our model. This is especially true in any multi-stage problem, where the impact of errors on the construction of pseudo-outcomes must again be anticipated.

8.7 Discussion

Measurement error presents a complex and often inescapable challenge in biostatistical research. While many features of established measurement error theory is applicable in the precision medicine framework, there are numerous additional considerations that require careful handling. In this chapter we have provided an introductory overview of the problem of measurement error in the specific application of dynamic treatment regime estimation, while also discussing broader considerations within precision medicine more generally.

By breaking down our problem into errors in tailoring variables, misclassification in the treatment, and errors in the outcome, we have demonstrated how each of these cases can cause different problems requiring potentially distinct solutions. When the tailoring variable is measured with error we have shown that the oft-cited maxim relating measurement error to attenuation of effects does not easily translate to this framework. Even in our most simplistic of settings, where the effect of error is indeed to attenuate the parameter estimates associated with that variable, this is nevertheless a substantial limitation to optimal treatment rule estimation. With our estimated rule depending on multiple parameters, attenuation in one (but not another) will result in inaccurate treatment decisions. A contrasting result is found in the presence of misclassified treatments. Here, under certain conditions, the effect of misclassification is to attenuate all parameters by the same factor and, as such, reasonable treatment rules may still be estimated.

One condition of this result, however, is that misclassification does not depend on the tailoring variable. In general, we have shown that dependency between the errors and other model components must be very carefully assessed. This is particularly evident when considering errors in the outcome, where even errors that are dependent on the tailoring variable may be accommodated in a single stage problem if their only effect is to bias nuisance parameters in our model. Conversely, if our error structure results in interference with the blip then our analysis will be compromised.

The multistage case is, predictably, far more complex. We have seen how even in a two-stage example errors may propagate backwards through our analysis, and these issues will only compound further in situations with more stages. Of particular concern are errors that may not cause bias in a one-stage setting, but could interfere with multi-stage analysis. These may easily be overlooked, or provide a false sense of security, especially if a naive appeal to established measurement error theory is made.

Beyond the problem of parameter estimation and treatment rule identification, measurement errors must also be considered in the application of precision medicine. Basing a treatment decision on an error-prone variable, for example, may result in a patient receiving a non-optimal treatment even if the treatment rule was correctly identified. While beyond the scope of this work, a related question concerns treatment (non-) adherence. If it is known that certain variables may be predictors of lower (or higher) adherence with prescribed treatments, this is information that could potentially be used to better tailor our treatment decisions.

While our focus has been on the consequences of leaving measurement error unaccounted for, we have demonstrated that regression calibration may be successfully employed in some dynamic treatment regime estimation settings when using dynamic weighted ordinary least squares. This method has been shown to be much more widely applicable. Correction techniques for other dynamic treatment regime methods, meanwhile, require further exploration.

The simplicity of our simulation setups must not, however, be underestimated. We considered only linear models with a single tailoring variable and no confounders. Our sample sizes were generous. We only generated errors in one model component at a time, whereas simultaneous errors are more realistic (and more problematic). Our error structures themselves have also been simplistic. While several of the results in this chapter may hold more broadly, they should not be carelessly generalized to any real-world problem. Rather, we hope this work highlights that while there are some contexts where there is cause for optimism, measurement error must never be ignored. In practice, we would strongly advise conducting similar simulation studies based on hypothesized error structures to investigate their potential effects.

Ultimately, the best remedy for the problems caused by measurement error is to avoid – or at least minimize – it in the first place. We repeat the familiar advice that investing in good measurements at the data collection phase should be a top priority in any study. Being aware of measurement errors at the design stage may help inform more efficient resource management (such as taking fewer, but more accurate, measurements), or highlight the need for auxiliary data such as replicated observations. These steps not only help minimize the effects of measurement error but also help ensure correction techniques may be put to good use. This is as true in precision medicine as in any other context.

Chapter 9

Nonparametric Heterogeneous Treatment Effect Estimation in Repeated Cross Sectional Designs

Xinkun Nie, Chen Lu, Stefan Wager

9.1 Introduction

Difference-in-differences is an increasingly popular observational study design for estimating causal effects from repeated cross-sections (e.g., Angrist and Pischke, 2008; Bertrand et al., 2004; Card and Krueger, 1994; Lechner, 2011; Obenauer and von der Nienburg, 1915). For an overview of applying difference-in-differences methods in public health, see Dimick and Ryan (2014), Gertler et al. (2011) and Wing et al. (2018) for a review. Recently, several authors have employed it to study public health policy and implications due to COVID-19 (Brodeur et al., 2021; Goodman-Bacon and Marcus, 2020).

A standard design with cross-sectional data is as follows: we conduct a survey or draw a sample for some outcome (e.g., medical expenditure) from two comparable states (or cities, regions, etc.). The first state later enacts some health policy of interest (e.g., encouragement of Medicare enrollment) and the second state doesn't. We then draw another sample from both states at a time after the health policy has been implemented in the first state. The simplest difference-in-differences estimator assumes global parallel trends: if neither state had enacted the policy, then their trends would have evolved in the same way. It would then attribute any difference in trends between the two states to the effect of the policy change.

In this paper, we focus on flexibly estimating treatment effect heterogeneity in the above design. There are two main challenges. The first challenge involves representing and targeting heterogeneity effectively without assuming specific functional forms. The second challenge involves relaxing the classic assumption of "global parallel trends", which is unlikely to hold when there is heterogeneity explained by covariates. In particular, states may have changing subgroups of people that exhibit markedly different trends on their own. For example, when studying the effect of enrollment in Medicare on medical expenditure, we may find that there are subgroups within states (e.g., based on age, income or gender) that have different baseline trends; then, if the two states under comparison have different proportions of these subgroups, the global parallel trends assumption immediately becomes questionable. Instead, we may want to control for these covariates, and only assume parallel trends once we have conditioned on them (e.g., Abadie, 2005; Acemoglu and Angrist, 2001; Blundell et al., 2004; Heckman et al., 1998).

Throughout the paper, we work in the following formal setup. We observe n independent samples (S_i, T_i, X_i, Y_i), where the state indicator $S_i \in \{0, 1\}$ denotes whether the i-th individual is in the control or exposed state, $T_i \in \{0, 1\}$ denotes the time of the observation (pre- vs. post-intervention), $X_i \in \mathbb{R}^d$ is a set of potential confounders and $Y_i \in \mathbb{R}^d$ is the outcome of interest. Only samples in the "exposed" state and "post" time period to get treated, i.e., we can write the treatment or exposure indicator as $W_i = S_i T_i$. Following the potential outcomes framework (Imbens and Rubin, 2015), let $Y_i(0)$ and $Y_i(1)$ denote

DOI: 10.1201/9781003216223-9

the control and treated potential outcomes and suppose we observe $Y_i = Y_i(W_i)$. We are interested in estimating the heterogeneous treatment effect is $\tau(x)$, defined as the expected treatment effect is conditional on covariates $X_i = x$ and on X_i treated:

$$\tau(x) = \mathbb{E}[Y(1) \mid X_i = x, S_i = 1, T_i = 1] - \mathbb{E}[Y(0) \mid X_i = x, S_i = 1, T_i = 1]. \tag{9.1}$$

Because $\mathbb{E}[Y(0) \mid X_i = x, S_i = 1, T_i = 1]$ is not observed, we impose a parallel trends assumption conditional on covariates, so that

$$\begin{aligned} \mathbb{E}[Y(0) \mid X_i = x, S_i = 1, T_i = 1] &= \mathbb{E}[Y(0) \mid X_i = x, S_i = 1, T_i = 0] \\ &+ \mathbb{E}[Y(0) \mid X_i = x, S_i = 0, T_i = 1] - \mathbb{E}[Y(0) \mid X_i = x, S_i = 0, T_i = 0], \end{aligned} \tag{9.2}$$

which then allows us to identify the conditional average treatment effect on the treated as follows,

$$\begin{aligned} \tau(x) = \mathbb{E}[Y_i \mid X_i = x,\ S_i = 1,\ T_i = 1] - \mathbb{E}[Y_i \mid X_i = x,\ S_i = 1,\ T_i = 0] \\ - \mathbb{E}[Y_i \mid X_i = x,\ S_i = 0,\ T_i = 1] + \mathbb{E}[Y_i \mid X_i = x,\ S_i = 0,\ T_i = 0]. \end{aligned} \tag{9.3}$$

As discussed in Abadie (2005), (9.2) may be more credible than the standard parallel trends assumption that holds without conditioning on X_i as it enables us to control for known sources of confounding.

A classical approach to estimating $\tau(x)$ would be to employ flexible nonparametric modeling of the treatment effect function. A common practice is to employ a two-way fixed effect linear model with interactions for Y_i in terms of X_i, S_i, T_i of the form

$$Y \sim \beta_x^\top X + \beta_s^\top XS + \beta_t^\top XT + \beta_{s,t}^\top XST, \tag{9.4}$$

then interpreting $\hat{\tau}(x) = \hat{\beta}_{s,t}^\top x$ as the treatment effect (e.g., Anzia and Berry, 2011). However, the estimator (9.4) is not justified by a nonparametric version of the assumption (9.2) due to the assumed linear functional forms on $\tau(x)$ and on any confounding effects of X_i that affect the outcome Y_i (Angrist and Pischke, 2008; Ding and Li, 2019; Keele and Minozzi, 2013; Lechner, 2011). These constraining assumptions can be difficult to satisfy in practice.

In this paper, we aim to flexibly estimate the treatment effect function $\tau(X)$ given only the assumption (9.2) along with a relevant form of overlap. As a direct consequence of (9.2), the data generating process can be written as the following generic specification:

$$Y_i = b(X_i) + S_i \cdot \xi(X_i) + T_i \cdot \rho(X_i) + T_i \cdot S_i \cdot \tau(X_i) + \varepsilon_i, \tag{9.5}$$

where the joint distribution of $\{T_i,\ X_i,\ S_i\}$ may be arbitrary and

$$\begin{aligned} \xi(x) = \mathbb{E}[Y_i \mid X_i = x,\ S_i = 1, T_i = 0] - \mathbb{E}[Y_i \mid X_i = x,\ S_i = 0, T_i = 0], \\ \rho(x) = \mathbb{E}[Y_i \mid X_i = x,\ S_i = 0, T_i = 1] - \mathbb{E}[Y_i \mid X_i = x,\ S_i = 0, T_i = 0], \end{aligned} \tag{9.6}$$

are the conditional effect of S alone and T alone, and $\mathbb{E}[\varepsilon_i \mid X_i, S_i, T_i] = 0$. We note that all the conditional effect function $b(\cdot), \xi(\cdot), \rho(\cdot), \tau(\cdot)$ can be nonparametric funcitons. One naive way to estimate $\tau(\cdot)$ in this model is as follows. Recall our expression for $\tau(x)$ in (9.2). From that expression, one might attempt to estimate

$$g(z) = g(x, s, t) = \mathbb{E}[Y_i \mid X_i = x,\ S_i = s,\ T_i = t] \tag{9.7}$$

for the four pairs of s and t on the corresponding subsets of the data, and then estimate $\hat{\tau}(x) = \hat{g}(x, 1, 1) - \hat{g}(x, 1, 0) - \hat{g}(x, 0, 1) + \hat{g}(x, 0, 0)$. However, this approach is often not robust. As an example where this method might fail, consider a high dimensional linear model, $Y_i(s,t) = X_i^\top \beta_{s,t} + \epsilon_i(s,t)$, with $X_i, \beta_{s,t} \in \mathbb{R}^d$, and $\mathbb{E}[\epsilon_i(s,t) \,|\, X_i] = 0$. We might consider fitting the Lasso (Tibshirani, 1996) for each $\hat{\beta}(s,t)$ separately, and estimate $\hat{\tau}(x) = x^\top(\hat{\beta}(1,1) - \hat{\beta}(1,0) - \hat{\beta}(0,1) + \hat{\beta}(0,0))$. However, the lasso regularizes each $\hat{\beta}(s,t)$ towards 0 separately, which might result in $\hat{\beta}(1,1) - \hat{\beta}(1,0) - \hat{\beta}(0,1) + \hat{\beta}(0,0)$ being regularized away from 0, even when $\tau(x) = 0$ everywhere. See Künzel et al. (2019) and Nie and Wager (2021) for a similar discussion on the T-Learner for the CATE.

We seek to build a robust estimator for $\tau(\cdot)$. To this end, we start by considering the case where the underlying treatment effect $\tau(x)$ is constant and the only challenge is to eliminate confounding. We start by developing an orthogonal transformation of (9.5) that generalizes the transformation of Robinson (1988) for the conditionally linear model. This representation allows us to build a transformed regression estimator (TR) to estimate the constant treatment effect. Our TR estimator achieves the parametric $1/\sqrt{n}$ rate of convergence while allowing for slower estimation rates on all nuisance components. The $1/\sqrt{n}$ rate of convergence in the TR estimator allows valid asymptotic confidence interval construction, while we still enable flexible nonparametric estimation on the nuisance components (e.g., without linearity assumptions). We further discuss the properties of the transformed regression estimator when the underlying linearity assumption is misspecified. We then build upon the transformed regression construction and propose a heterogeneous treatment effect estimator for $\tau(\cdot)$ and show empirically the proposal is advantageous comparing to existing baselines.

Compared to the standard difference-in-differences design, we do not assume the panel setting where every individual is observed both before and after the treatment. In that particular case, one could apply any of the existing heterogeneous treatment effect estimators (e.g., Athey et al., 2019; Hill, 2011; Künzel et al., 2019; Nie and Wager, 2021) by taking the difference between the outcomes from the two time periods as the new outcome variable. In our setting, we make the less stringent assumption of conditional parallel trends, and allow covariate shifts for the two-time periods which makes the setting significantly more challenging. Adapting advances in semiparametric efficiency theory and leveraging flexible nonparametric machine learning methods for this task are our main methodological contribution.

9.2 Related Work

The difference-in-differences approach to treatment effect estimation was popularized by Card and Krueger (1994), and has since become ubiquitous in the social sciences. Angrist and Pischke (2008) and Lechner (2011) provides a textbook treatment and a broad literature review. Building on Abadie (2005), we are here most interested in extensions of classical difference-in-differences methods that leverage covariate information to make the parallel trends assumption more plausible. Several authors have also recently extended difference-in-differences analyses in other complementary directions. Arkhangelsky (2018) and Athey and Imbens (2006) consider difference-in-differences type designs where there may be non-additive treatment effects. Abadie et al. (2010), Arkhangelsky et al. (2019), Athey et al. (2018), Ben-Michael et al. (2021), Xu (2017) and Li and Li (2019) develop methods that can be applied in the panel setting in which the same individuals are observed in both the pre- and post-periods, whereas in our setting we observe separately cross-sectional data in each period.

Most of the existing literature with repeated cross sections, including Abadie (2005), Li and Li (2019), Sant'Anna and Zhao (2020), Chang (2020), assume that there is no covariate shift across cross-sections from the same state: they require that the joint distribution of (X_i, S_i) does not vary with T_i, i.e., that $(X_i,\, S_i) \perp\!\!\!\perp T_i$. Our approach does not require this assumption (see Proposition 1 and the following comment), as this assumption may be hard to justify with cross-sectional data where we are not able to survey exactly the same people in the pre- and post periods. For example, in a ride-sharing application, Lu et al. (2018) estimates the effects of a dynamic pricing feature on drivers' behaviors by leveraging a natural experiment where a software bug temporarily disables a dynamic pricing feature for certain drivers. In this case, we may expect the distribution of the covariates X_i for active drivers varies both with exposure S_i and time T_i.

Methodologically, we build on a large body of work in nonparametric estimation of heterogeneous treatment effects. One approach is to reduce the "regularization bias" that might occur. Examples of this line of work include Athey and Imbens (2016), Hahn et al. (2020), and Shalit et al. (2017). Another approach, the one we choose to adopt, is to develop meta-learning procedures that do not depend on a specific machine learning method. Key examples of such works are Künzel et al. (2019) and Nie and Wager (2021). Our decomposition of $\tau(x)$ is conceptually similar to the orthogonal moments constructions from Robinson (1988), and more broadly, from Belloni et al. (2011), Bickel et al. (1993), Newey (1994), Scharfstein et al. (1999), van der Laan and Rubin (2006) and others.

In the difference-in-differences design, flexible modeling and estimation that goes beyond the standard two-way fixed effects and linearity assumptions have also drawn considerable interest. Abadie (2005) considers inverse propensity stratification-based methods. Another approach considers more flexible outcome models, see (e.g., Heckman et al., 1998; Meyer, 1995). Recently, Chang (2020), Sant'Anna and Zhao (2020) and Zimmert (2018) proposed doubly robust variants of the approach of Abadie (2005) also allows for heterogeneity in $\tau(x)$.

9.3 An Orthogonal Transformation for the Repeated Cross Sections

The key orthogonality property of our proposed heterogeneous treatment effect estimator relies on a new decomposition for the outcome model (9.2) motivated by Robinson (1988). The conditional probabilities of an observation being in state S_i or time period T_i conditionally on $X_i = x$ play a central role in our analysis (Rosenbaum and Rubin, 1983). We write these quantities as

$$s(x) = \mathbb{P}[S_i = 1 \,|\, X_i = x], \quad t(x) = \mathbb{P}[T_i = 1 \,|\, X_i = x]. \tag{9.8}$$

We write $e_{s,t}(X_i) = \mathbb{E}[S_i = s, T_i = t \,|\, X_i]$. We also write $m(x) = \mathbb{E}[Y_i \,|\, X_i = x]$ for the conditional response function marginalizing over T_i and S_i, and

$$\begin{aligned} \varsigma(x) &= \mathbb{E}[Y_i \,|\, X_i = x,\, S_i = 1] - \mathbb{E}[Y_i \,|\, X_i = x,\, S_i = 0], \\ \nu(x) &= \mathbb{E}[Y_i \,|\, X_i = x,\, T_i = 1] - \mathbb{E}[Y_i \,|\, X_i = x,\, T_i = 0], \end{aligned} \tag{9.9}$$

for the conditional effect of S marginalizing over T and S respectively. We write the conditional covariance of S_i and T_i as

$$\Delta(x) = e_{1,1}(x) - s(x)t(x). \tag{9.10}$$

Finally, for convenience, we let $Z_i = (X_i, S_i, T_i)$. Given this notation, we can verify the following (the derivation is given in the Supplementary Materials).

Proposition 1. *Suppose we have access to an independent and identically distributed sequence of tuples Y_i and $Z_i = (X_i,\, S_i,\, T_i)$. Under the model (9.2), our data-generating distribution admits a representation*

$$Y_i = m(X_i) + A(Z_i)\nu(X_i) + B(Z_i)\varsigma(X_i) + C(Z_i)\tau(X_i) + \epsilon_i, \tag{9.11}$$

where $\mathbb{E}[\epsilon_i \mid Z_i] = 0$, *and*

$$
\begin{aligned}
A(Z_i) &= \left(1 - \frac{\Delta^2(X_i)}{s(X_i)(1-s(X_i))t(X_i)(1-t(X_i))}\right)^{-1} \cdot \\
&\quad \left(T_i - t(X_i) - \frac{\Delta(X_i)(S_i - s(X_i))}{s(X_i)(1-s(X_i))}\right), \\
B(Z_i) &= \left(1 - \frac{\Delta^2(X_i)}{s(X_i)(1-s(X_i))t(X_i)(1-t(X_i))}\right)^{-1} \cdot \\
&\quad \left(S_i - s(X_i) - \frac{\Delta(X_i)(T_i - t(X_i))}{t(X_i)(1-t(X_i))}\right), \\
C(Z_i) &= S_i T_i - e_{1,1}(X_i) - \left(s(X_i) + \frac{\Delta(X_i)}{t(X_i)}\right) A(Z_i) - \\
&\quad \left(t(X_i) + \frac{\Delta(X_i)}{s(X_i)}\right) B(Z_i).
\end{aligned}
\tag{9.12}
$$

Furthermore, all terms in the above decomposition are orthogonal in the following sense:

$$
\begin{aligned}
&\mathbb{E}[A(Z) \mid X] = \mathbb{E}[B(Z) \mid X] = \mathbb{E}[C(Z) \mid X] = 0, \\
&\mathbb{E}[A(Z) \mid X,\, S] = \mathbb{E}[C(Z) \mid X,\, S] = 0, \\
&\mathbb{E}[B(Z) \mid X,\, T] = \mathbb{E}[C(Z) \mid X,\, T] = 0, \\
&\mathbb{E}[B(Z)C(Z) \mid X] = \mathbb{E}[A(Z)C(Z) \mid X] = 0.
\end{aligned}
\tag{9.13}
$$

The key property of this representation is the orthogonality property (9.13), which will enable flexible estimation of treatment effects at parametric rates as discussed in the following section. In the setting of Abadie (2005) and Sant'Anna and Zhao (2020), assumption gives $T_i \perp\!\!\!\perp S_i \mid X_i$, which implies $\Delta(X_i) = 0$. As an immediate corollary to Proposition 1, this decomposition then simplifies to a functional form closely reminiscent of Robinson's transformation (Robinson, 1988):

$$
\begin{aligned}
Y_i = m(X_i) &+ (S_i - s(X_i))\varsigma(X_i) + (T_i - t(X_i))\nu(X_i) \\
&(S_i T_i - t(X_i)S_i - s(X_i)T_i + s(X_i)t(X_i))\tau(X_i) + \epsilon_i.
\end{aligned}
\tag{9.14}
$$

More generally, we see that when $\Delta(X_i)$ is close to 0, all expressions underlying (10.10) and (9.12) are well-conditioned, and we expect estimation using (10.10) to be stable. Conversely, if T_i and S_i are highly correlated conditionally on X_i, then $\Delta^2(X_i) \approx s(X_i)(1 - s(X_i))t(X_i)(1 - t(X_i))$ and (9.12) could become unstable; this is as expected, because if S_i and T_i are highly correlated, then we do not expect their interaction effect to be well identified.

Finally, we note that all nuisance components in the decomposition above are marginal quantities, and thus can be estimated using all of the data. This property is desirable for empirical performance as it is more data efficient when we need to estimate them in a small-sample regime.

9.4 The Transformed Regression Estimator

As a building block of our proposed heterogeneity treatment effect estimator, we first consider estimation in a setting where the treatment effect itself is constant $\tau(x) = \tau$ in the representation (10.10), but all other nuisance components defined above, i.e., $m(x)$, $\nu(x)$, $\varsigma(x)$, $s(x)$, $t(x)$ and $\Delta(x)$, may vary with x. The standard approach to estimating τ in this setting is to write a two-way fixed effect model of the form

$$
Y \sim \beta_x^\top X + \beta_s S + \beta_t T + \beta_{s,t} ST \tag{9.15}
$$

and to interpret the coefficient on ST as an estimate of the treatment effect. However, as shown in our experiments, this simple linear regression-based approach to treatment effect estimation may be severely biased in the setting where the linear model (9.15) is misspecified.

Here, we propose the **transformed regression (TR)** estimator with cross-fitting (shown in Algorithm 9.1). The method is based on the decomposition (10.10), which is motivated by a decomposition used by Robinson (1988) to estimate parametric components in partial linear models. Robinson's decomposition has also been used in many other recent works, such as in Athey et al. (2019) for causal forests, Robins (2004) for G-estimation, as well as in Chernozhukov et al. (2018) and Zhao et al. (2017). The transformed regression estimator, motivated by Robinson, also has good theoretical properties. In Theorem 2, we show that the transformed regression estimator is $\sqrt{n}$-consistent and asymptotically normal under considerably more generality than simply running an OLS regression with the model (9.15). We note that cross-fitting helps avoid overfitting of the estimates and also serves as a proof technique to show $\sqrt{n}$-consistency on τ. Having $\sqrt{n}$–consistency on τ enables us to build valid asymptotic confidence intervals for τ, while we still allow nonparametric estimation on the nuisance components without imposing linearity assumptions such as in (9.15). The proof of the theorem is in the Supplementary Materials.

Theorem 2. *Under the conditions of Proposition 1, suppose furthermore that $\tau(x) = \tau$ is constant and that the following conditions hold:*

1. *Overlap: the conditional probabilities $e_{s,t}(x)$ are bounded away from 0 by some small $\eta > 0$ for all values of t, s and x.*
2. *Consistency: for any estimated nuisance parameter $\hat{\mu}(x)$, such as $\hat{m}(x)$, $\hat{\nu}(x)$ and $\hat{\varsigma}(x)$, we have that:*
$$\sup_x |\hat{\mu}(x) - \mu(x)| \to_p 0$$
3. *Risk decay: for any estimated nuisance parameter $\hat{\mu}(x)$, we have:*
$$\mathbb{E}\left[(\hat{\mu}(x) - \mu(x))^2\right] = o\left(\frac{1}{\sqrt{n}}\right)$$
4. *Boundedness: all the nuisance parameters are uniformly bounded:*
$$\sup_x |\mu(x)|\ , \quad \sup_x |\hat{\mu}(x)| < M$$
for some constant $M < \infty$.

Then, writing $\hat{\tau}_{TR}$ as the transformed regression estimator obtained using Algorithm 9.1, and $\hat{\tau}^*$ as the transformed regression estimator with oracle nuisance parameters, we have

$$\sqrt{n}(\hat{\tau}_{TR} - \hat{\tau}^*) \xrightarrow{p} 0, \quad \sqrt{n}(\hat{\tau}^* - \tau) \xrightarrow{d} \mathcal{N}(0, V_{TR}),$$

where

$$V_{TR} = \frac{\mathbb{E}[\sigma^2(z)C^2(z)]}{\mathbb{E}[C^2(z)]^2}, \tag{9.16}$$

and $\sigma(z)^2 = \operatorname{Var}[\epsilon_i \mid Z_i = z]$. In the case when $T_i \perp\!\!\!\perp S_i \mid X_i$, and $\sigma^2(z) = \sigma^2$ is constant, the expression for V_{TR} simplifies to $V_{TR} = \sigma^2/\mathbb{E}[t(x)(1-s(x))t(x)(1-s(x))]$.

In step 3 of Algorithm 9.1, $\varsigma(x)$ and $\nu(x)$ can be estimated with methods for heterogeneous treatment effect estimation. In our simulations, we use causal forests (Athey et al., 2019), but we note that other estimators in the literature can also be used here (e.g., Athey et al., 2019; Hill, 2011; Künzel et al., 2019; Nie and Wager, 2021).

Algorithm 9.1: Transformed Regression Estimator (TR)

1 Split the data into Q roughly equal folds, $\mathcal{I}_1$, $\mathcal{I}_2$, ..., $\mathcal{I}_K$, with K fixed, to be used for cross-fitting.

2 For each fold $\mathcal{I}_k$, fit $\hat{m}^{-\mathcal{I}_k}(x), \hat{s}^{-\mathcal{I}_k}(x), \hat{t}^{-\mathcal{I}_k}(x)$ and $\hat{e}_{1,1}^{-\mathcal{I}_k}(x)$, with data not in $\mathcal{I}_k$, using any supervised learning method for prediction accuracy (the superscript of $-\mathcal{I}_k$ denotes using data not in the k-th fold).

3 Estimate $\hat{\nu}^{-\mathcal{I}_k}(x)$ as a heterogeneous "treatment effect" of S_i while ignoring T_i; and estimate $\hat{\varsigma}^{-\mathcal{I}_k}(x)$ as a "treatment effect" of T_i ignoring S_i. Both can leverage methods designed for heterogeneous treatment estimation in the single cross-section case.

4 Construct $\hat{A}^{-\mathcal{I}_k}(z)$, $\hat{B}^{-\mathcal{I}_k}(z)$, $\hat{C}^{-\mathcal{I}_k}(z)$ and $\hat{\Delta}^{-\mathcal{I}_k}(x)$, where $z = (x, s, t)$, using the estimated nuisance parameters following (9.12). Then, for $j \in \mathcal{I}_k$, obtain point estimates $\hat{C}^{-\mathcal{I}_k}(Z_j)$ and

$$\hat{H}^{-\mathcal{I}_k}(Z_j) = Y_j - \Big(\hat{m}^{-\mathcal{I}_k}(X_j) + \hat{A}^{-\mathcal{I}_k}(Z_j)\hat{\nu}^{-\mathcal{I}_k}(X_j) + \tag{9.17}$$

$$\hat{B}^{-\mathcal{I}_k}(Z_j)\hat{\varsigma}^{-\mathcal{I}_k}(X_j)\Big). \tag{9.18}$$

5 Run OLS on $\hat{H}^{-\mathcal{I}_k}(Z_j)$ against $\hat{C}^{-\mathcal{I}_k}(Z_j)$ to produce

$$\hat{\tau}^{-\mathcal{I}_k} = \frac{\sum_{j \in \mathcal{I}_k} \hat{H}^{-\mathcal{I}_k}(Z_j)\hat{C}^{-\mathcal{I}_k}(Z_j)}{\sum_{j \in \mathcal{I}_k} \hat{C}^{-\mathcal{I}_k}(Z_j)^2} \tag{9.19}$$

6 Combine predictions from different folds $\mathcal{I}_k$:

$$\hat{\tau}_{TR} = \sum_{i=k}^{K} \frac{|\mathcal{I}_k|}{n} \hat{\tau}^{-\mathcal{I}_k} \tag{9.20}$$

If we ever want to use the transformed regression estimator which assumes a constant treatment effect, it is important to understand how it behaves under misspecification. Interestingly, as shown in Proposition 3, even when $\tau(x)$ is not constant, the transformed regression estimator converges to a weighted average of $\tau(x)$ with positive weights, mirroring the findings in Crump et al. (2009) and Li et al. (2018). The proof for Proposition 3 is found in the Supplementary Materials.

Proposition 3. *If we use the transformed regression estimator from Algorithm 9.1, and the conditions from Theorem 2 are satisfied, then*

$$\sqrt{n}(\hat{\tau}_{TR} - \bar{\tau}) \xrightarrow{d} \mathcal{N}(0, V_{TR}), \quad \bar{\tau} = \frac{\mathbb{E}[C^2(z)\tau(x)]}{\mathbb{E}[C^2(z)]}, \tag{9.21}$$

where V_{TR} is the same variance term from Theorem 2.

We also note that when in the setting of Abadie (2005), where $T_i \perp\!\!\!\perp S_i \,\big|\, X_i$ and so $\Delta(X_i) = 0$, the above simplifies to:

$$\bar{\tau} = \frac{\mathbb{E}[[s(x)(1 - s(x))t(x)(1 - t(x))] \cdot \tau(x)]}{\mathbb{E}[s(x)(1 - s(x))t(x)(1 - t(x))]}.$$

When $\tau(x)$ is not constant, the transformed regression estimator can thus be thought of as a weighted mean of the treatment effect, where more weight is given to the data points that are likely to appear with all four (S_i, T_i) pairs.

9.5 Estimating Treatment Heterogeneity with Repeated Cross Sectional Data

In this section, we relax the assumption from the previous section that the underlying treatment effect is constant, and aim to estimate the heterogeneous treatment effect. We propose a flexible nonparametric estimator in the difference-in-differences setup that draws inspiration from recent advances in heterogeneous treatment effect estimation in the single cross-section case.

We adapt our estimator of a constant causal parameter τ into an estimator for a heterogeneous treatment function $\tau(x)$, by turning the estimation equation underlying the former estimator into a loss function. The R-learner (Nie and Wager, 2021) follows this strategy to derive a heterogeneous treatment effect estimator from Robinson's decomposition (Robinson, 1988) in the setting of a single cross-section. We follow the same strategy here with repeated cross-sectional data. Using the decomposition from (10.10), we can estimate treatment effect heterogeneity with the following algorithm **R-DiD**:

Algorithm 9.2: Heterogeneous Treatment Effect Estimation with Cross Sectional Data (R-DiD)

1 Split the data into K roughly-equal folds $\mathcal{I}_1$, ..., $\mathcal{I}_K$ for cross-fitting.

2 Following steps 2 to 4 of Algorithm 9.1, estimate the nuisance parameters $\hat{m}^{-\mathcal{I}_k}(x)$, $\hat{\varsigma}^{-\mathcal{I}_k}(x)$, $\hat{\nu}^{-\mathcal{I}_k}(x))$, $\hat{A}^{-\mathcal{I}_k}(z)$, $\hat{B}^{-\mathcal{I}_k}(z)$, $\hat{C}^{-\mathcal{I}_k}(z)$ using data not in the k-th fold. Also following step 4 of Algorithm 9.1, produce point estimates $\hat{C}^{-\mathcal{I}_k}(Z_j)$ and $\hat{H}^{-\mathcal{I}_k}(Z_j)$ according to (9.17) for $j \in \mathcal{I}_k$.

3 Estimate the cross-fitted heterogeneous treatment effect $\hat{\tau}^{(-\mathcal{I}_k)}(\cdot)$ for data in $\mathcal{I}_k$ as

$$\hat{\tau}^{(-\mathcal{I}_k)}(\cdot) = \arg\min_{\tau} \left\{ \frac{1}{|\mathcal{I}_k|} \sum_{j \in \mathcal{I}_k} \left(\hat{H}^{-\mathcal{I}_k}(Z_j) - \hat{C}^{-\mathcal{I}_k}(Z_j)\tau(X_j) \right)^2 + \Lambda_n(\tau(\cdot)) \right\},$$

where $\Lambda_n(\cdot)$ is some regularization term. For $j \in \mathcal{I}_k$, use $\hat{\tau}^{(-\mathcal{I}_k)}(X_j)$ as the estimate for $\tau(X_j)$.

Recall from the last section that when the treatment effect $\tau(x)$ is constant, the transformed regression estimator achieves $\sqrt{n}$ rate for estimating the treatment effect parameter τ. When $\tau(x)$ is a nonparametric function, we can no longer achieve $\sqrt{n}$ parametric rates. Instead, we aim to show a quasi-oracle result, i.e., even if estimating the nuisance components $m(x)$, $\nu(x)$, $\varsigma(x)$, $\Delta(x)$, $s(x)$ and $t(x)$ have a slow convergence rate, we can still achieve fast nonparametric rates on the treatment effect function $\tau(x)$ as if we had known these nuisance components perfectly. See Chernozhukov et al. (2018); Luedtke and van der Laan (2016b); van der Laan and Dudoit (2003) for similar developments. In this work, we leverage the recent result from Foster and Syrgkanis (2019) that generalizes the quasi-oracle bounds in Nie and Wager (2021).

In particular, for any treatment effect function $\tilde{\tau}$ and nuisance function $\tilde{\mu}$ where the nuisance function $\mu(x)$ includes $m(x)$, $\nu(x)$, $\varsigma(x)$, $\Delta(x)$, $s(x)$ and $t(x)$, define the loss function

$$L(\tilde{\tau}, \tilde{\mu}) = \mathbb{E}[(Y - \tilde{m}(X) - \tilde{A}(Z)\tilde{\nu}(X) - \tilde{B}(Z)\tilde{\varsigma}X - \tilde{C}(Z)\tilde{\tau})^2]. \tag{9.22}$$

Suppose in Algorithm 2, instead of leveraging cross-fitting to learn nuisance components, we use sample splitting, i.e. we split the data in half, and use the first half to learn all the nuisance components $\hat{\mu}$, and use the second half to estimate $\hat{\tau}$. The following then holds as a direct consequence of Theorem 1 in Foster and Syrgkanis (2019).

Theorem 4. *Suppose the conditional probabilities $e_{s,t}(x)$ are bounded away from 0 by some constant $\eta > 0$ for all values of t, s and x, and the outcome $|Y|$ is bounded by M. Suppose further that $K = 2$ in Algorithm 9.2, and let $\hat{\tau} = \hat{\tau}^{(-2)}$ be the treatment effect estimate on the first fold. Suppose there exist rate functions r_n such that*

$$\|\hat{\mu} - \mu\|_{L_2}^4 = O_p(r(n)) \tag{9.23}$$

and

$$L(\hat{\tau}, \hat{\mu}) - L(\tau, \hat{\mu}) = O_p(r(n)), \tag{9.24}$$

then

$$\|\hat{\tau} - \tau\|_{L_2(P)}^2 = O_p(\eta^{-16} M^4 r(n)) \tag{9.25}$$

for all nuisance parameter $\mu(x)$ including $m(x)$, $\nu(x)$, $\varsigma(x)$, $\Delta(x)$, $s(x)$ and $t(x)$.

The theorem above shows that the required learning rate on the nuisance components is only at a 4th-order growth rate compared to the learning rate on the target parameter τ. Note that if the nuisance components μ were known, (9.24) would be in terms of $L(\hat{\tau}, \mu) - L(\tau, \mu)$. We refer readers to Section 4 in Foster and Syrgkanis (2019) to see that in the case of empirical risk minimization, the cost to relate these quantities gets absorbed, and the same conclusion holds. The proof of the theorem relies on the orthogonality results from Proposition 1 and is included in the Supplementary Materials.

9.6 Simulation Study

In this section, we test the validity of our methods in a variety of simulation setups where the true underlying treatment effect can be both constant and non-constant. In the simulations, we generate n i.i.d. samples X_i of dimension p from some underlying distribution P; the pre/post-treatment time indicator T_i and the state indicator S_i are generated with a multinomial distribution over the four pairs $(T_i, S_i) \in \{(1,1), (1,0), (0,1), (0,0)\}$. The outcomes Y_i are generated from (9.5) with $\epsilon_i \mid X_i \sim \mathcal{N}(0, 1)$. Next, we present results in the case where the underlying treatment effect is constant as well in the case where it is heterogeneous.

We compare five methods in estimating heterogeneous treatment effects, four of which serve as baselines. **OLS** is as shown in (9.4). The **T**-Learner runs a separate regression for each of the four conditional quantities in (9.2) with a regression forest and follows (9.2) to build the estimate $\hat{\tau}$ from the four separate regressions. The **CF-time** learner runs a causal forest to learn the time-wise treatment effect in the treated location, i.e.

$$\mathbb{E}[Y_i \mid X_i = x, S_i = 1, T_i = 1] - \mathbb{E}[Y_i \mid X_i = x, S_i = 1, T_i = 0],$$

and then runs another causal forest to learn the time-wise treatment effect in the control location, i.e.

$$\mathbb{E}[Y_i \mid X_i = x, S_i = 0, T_i = 1] - \mathbb{E}[Y_i \mid X_i = x, S_i = 0, T_i = 0],$$

and subtracts the two estimates. On the other hand, The **CF-state** learner runs a causal forest to learn the state-wise treatment effect in the treated time period, i.e.

$$\mathbb{E}[Y_i \mid X_i = x, S_i = 1, T_i = 1] - \mathbb{E}[Y_i \mid X_i = x, S_i = 0, T_i = 1],$$

and then runs another causal forest to learn the time-wise treatment effect in the control period, i.e.

$$\mathbb{E}[Y_i \mid X_i = x, S_i = 1, T_i = 0] - \mathbb{E}[Y_i \mid X_i = x, S_i = 0, T_i = 0],$$

and subtracts the two estimates.

We compare the above four baselines with the **R-DiD** estimator outlined in Algorithm 9.2. In particular, we note that causal forests (Athey et al., 2019) can be understood as an instantiation of the R-learner with random forests, and can be used in Step 3 of Algorithm 9.2.[1] All regressions in all of the methods under comparison are implemented with regression forests from the package `grf` (Athey et al., 2019). In Algorithm 9.2, we take $\hat{H}$ as the "outcome" and $\hat{C}$ as the "treatment" in a causal forest. Along with **CF-time** and **CF-state**, they are all implemented with the package `grf`. We consider the following four setups:

Setup A $X_i \sim \mathcal{N}(0, \mathrm{I}_{d\times d})$; easy treatment effect $\tau(x) = x_4 + 0.5x_5$; easy conditional effects $\rho(x) = 1/(1+\exp(x_3)) + 4x_5^2$, $\xi(X) = 1/(1+\exp(x_4)) + 3x_6^2$; easy baseline $b(x) = \max(x_1 + x_2, 0) + 4x_6^2$; constant propensity for S_i: $s(x) = 0.6$, but constant propensity for T_i, $t(x) = 0.4$, and S_i is independent from T_i.

Setup B $X_i \sim \mathcal{N}(0, \mathrm{I}_{d\times d})$; easy treatment effect $\tau(x) = 0.5(x_1 + x_2 + x_3)$; challenging conditional effects $\rho(x) = 5(sin(x_1 x_2 \pi) + 2(x_3 - 0.5)^2)$ and $\xi(x) = 5(sin(x_1 x_2 \pi) + 2x_5^2)$. There is no baseline effect, i.e. $b(x) = 0$; propensities are constant $s(x) = t(x) = 0.5$, with S_i and T_i independent.

Setup C $X_i \sim \mathcal{N}(0, \mathrm{I}_{d\times d})$; there exists no time or state effect: $\rho(x) = \xi(x) = 0$, but highly correlated baseline effect $b(x) = 2\sin(1.5x_1)$ and propensities, where $e_{1,1}(x) = 0.5 + 0.5(1 - 6\eta)\sin(1.5x_1)$, and $e_{s,t}(x) = (1 - e_{1,1}(x))/3$, for $(s,t) \neq (1,1)$; $\tau = 1$.

Setup D $X_i \sim \mathcal{N}(0, \mathrm{I}_{d\times d})$; easy non-constant treatment effect $\tau(x) = 3x_1 + 2x_4$; easy conditional effects $\rho(X) = 2x_5$, $\xi(X) = 0$; easy baseline $b(x) = \max(x_1 + x_2 + x_4 + x_6, 0)$; non-constant propensity for S_i: $s(x) = \min(\max(\eta, (1/(1+\exp(-0.5x_3)))), 1-\eta)$, and non-constant propensity for T_i, $t(x) = \min(\max(\eta, (1/(1+\exp(-0.5x_2)))), 1-\eta)$, and S_i is independent from T_i. This is a well-specified setup for OLS.

The results of the simulations are shown in Table 9.1. For each of the n values, we draw n training data points and another separate n testing data points. We report results on this independent testing set. We run the experiments 200 times, and the mean squared error of each algorithm is shown below. Our proposal **R-DiD** performs well, while in simulation setup D, we see that OLS performs particularly well given it's a well-specified setup. However, in practice, it is less conceivable to have a well-specified setup, and our algorithm shines due to its flexibility to model nonparametrically and robustness towards estimation errors in nuisance components.

9.7 Application

To test our methods in practice, we revisit a study from Angrist and Kugler (2008) on the effect of import restrictions on self-employment incomes. The context is as follows: Columbia was one of the major suppliers of cocaine to North America and Europe before the 2000s. Before 1994, Columbia relied on coca leaf supplies from Bolivia and Peru, which it then refined to produce cocaine. Starting from 1994, a series of interdictions made by the United States and local militaries disrupted the air bridge that brought the coca leaves

[1] For more discussions on the connection between the causal forests and the R-learner, see Section 1.3 in (Athey and Wager, 2019).

Table 9.1 *Simulation results on mean squared error on an independent test set comparing our proposal* ***R-DiD*** *against four other baselines in different simulation setups, with varying training sample size n and dimensions p. Results are averaged across 200 independent runs.*

Setup	n	p	R-DiD	CF-time	CF-state	T	OLS
A	1000	6	**1.01**	3.83	3.29	7.8	15.05
A	1000	12	**1.11**	4.7	3.56	8.64	23.85
A	2000	6	**0.61**	2.53	1.93	5.09	7.75
A	2000	12	**0.67**	2.7	2.02	5.63	11.61
B	1000	6	**2.69**	14.1	15.18	40.8	38.66
B	1000	12	**2.78**	15.25	19.55	49.38	64.63
B	2000	6	**2.07**	8.8	8.71	32.56	18.19
B	2000	12	**1.66**	10.22	9.73	37.25	28.92
C	1000	6	**0.03**	0.04	0.04	0.27	0.55
C	1000	12	**0.02**	0.03	0.04	0.29	0.78
C	2000	6	**0.02**	**0.02**	**0.02**	0.22	0.36
C	2000	12	**0.02**	**0.02**	**0.02**	0.21	0.46
D	1000	6	1.92	1.64	2.73	2.34	**0.18**
D	1000	12	2.37	1.97	3.11	2.78	**0.32**
D	2000	6	1.17	1.01	1.94	1.65	**0.09**
D	2000	12	**1.34**	1.45	1.35	**1.34**	1.4

to Columbian refiners. As a result, coca cultivation shifted to Columbia's rural areas. The study from Angrist and Kugler (2008) then examines, among other things, the effect of the restriction of coca import on self-employment incomes in Columbia. The authors define self-employment income as income from individual short-term contract from the sale of domestically produced goods, and from agricultural productions. The authors conclude that the decrease in imports has a positive effect on self-employment incomes.

The dataset includes repeated cross-section survey data and contains the following information about individuals: gender, age, number of families members, immigrant status, marital status, and whether they lived in rural or urban areas, which we use as covariates X_i. The individuals come from one of three coca-growing regions (Bolivar, Cauca and Narino), or one of thirteen non-growing regions (Atlantico, Sucre, Cordoba, Santander, Boyaca, Caldas, Risaralda, Quindio, Tolima, Huilda, Antioquia, Choco, Valle de Cauca); see map in Angrist and Kugler (2008) for details. The dataset also includes a number of demilitarized zones, which we omit in our analysis.[2] Individuals from growing regions are classified as exposed, with $S_i = 1$, and those in non-growing regions classified as non-exposed, with $S_i = 0$, because of the increase in coca production could only benefit those in growing regions. As for time periods, we take 1993 as the pre-treatment period, with $T_i = 0$; because air interdictions occurred throughout 1994, we take 1995 as the post-treatment period, with $T_i = 1$. The outcomes are the log self-employment incomes, Y_i.

We first fit the treatment effect function $\tau(x)$ using the heterogeneous effect estimator **R-DiD** as in Algorithm 9.2. Figure 9.1 provides a histogram of the estimated treatment effects. We see that there appears to be heterogeneity in the treatment, as the histogram exhibits two distinct masses.

Beyond heterogeneity estimates, we compare a few different methods for the estimation of average treatment effects in this setup. In Appendix 9.8, we describe the augmented

[2]It was suggested that being a demilitarized zone may have an effect on the incomes of people from that region. Moreover, the demilitarized zones were exclusively growing regions. If we were to include the indicator of whether an individual is from a demilitarized region as one of our covariates, all such individuals would be in the treated group, hence violating overlap.

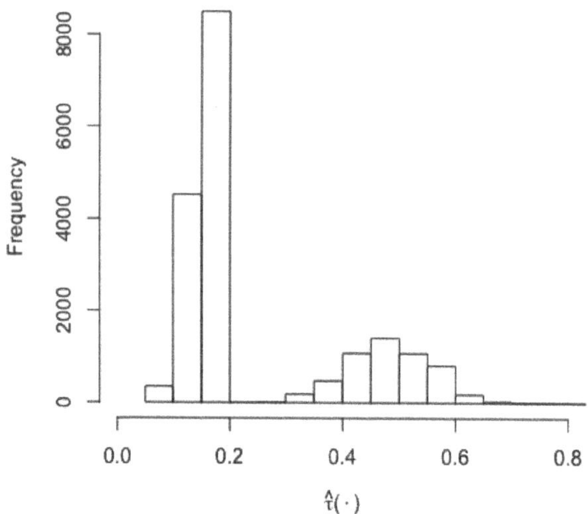

Figure 9.1 *Histogram of $\hat{\tau}(\cdot)$ fitted using Algorithm 9.2 on the dataset from Angrist and Kugler (2008). We see that there appears to be heterogeneity in the treatment: the treatment effects lie in two groups, one around* 0.1 *and the other around* 0.5. *Our results in Table 9.3 suggest that these two groups are treatment effects for people living in urban and rural areas respectively.*

Table 9.2 *Average treatment effect estimates in the difference-in-differences setup with data from Angrist and Kugler (2008), where* 1993 *is the pre-treatment year and* 1995 *is the post-treatment year. The first three methods assume a constant treatment effect $\tau(x) = \tau$, and the latter two allow for treatment heterogeneity. The OLS method is most similar to the method used by Angrist and Kugler (2008). We see that AIPW and AMLE, which allow for heterogeneity in the treatment effects, both obtain a lower point estimate than the other methods, which all assume the underlying effect is constant. This may suggest that there exists heterogeneity in the treatment effects.*

Estimator	Estimate	Std. err
Sample Means	0.279	0.059
OLS	0.274	0.031
TR	0.275	0.031
AMLE	0.234	0.031
AIPW	0.258	0.031

inverse propensity estimator (**AIPW**) that builds upon the heterogeneous treatment effect estimates from Algorithm 9.2. An alternative approach is **AMLE**, which builds upon the Augmented Minimax Linear Estimation (AMLE) approach of Hirshberg and Wager (2021) by constructing balancing weights. See an earlier working paper (Lu et al., 2019) for details on this estimator and comparison with **AIPW**. We also compare our **TR** estimator that assumes constant treatment effects, as well as **Sample Means** by taking the empirical means of (9.3), and the standard **OLS** as in (9.15).[3] See Table 9.2 for result comparisons.

Table 9.2 shows the results for estimating average treatment effects. There exists a non-trivial difference between the estimated effect from methods that allow for heterogeneity in

[3]Note that OLS is the method used in Angrist and Kugler (2008), except we use the data in 1995 as the post-treatment period, but Angrist and Kugler (2008) use the data from 1995 up until 2000 as the post-treatment period and assumed a fixed effect for each of the year-treatment interaction.

Table 9.3 *This table gives evidence that suggests the existence of heterogeneity in the treatment effect from the dataset of Angrist and Kugler (2008). The first row is obtained by running the AMLE method on only individuals who live in the urban area; the second row comes from running AMLE on individuals who live in the rural area. As shown, there seems to be a much larger treatment effect on individuals living in rural areas than on individuals in urban areas.*

Estimand	Estimate	Std. err
ATE Urban	0.102	0.035
ATE Rural	0.582	0.057

Table 9.4 *Treatment effect estimates with data from Angrist and Kugler (2008), where* 1998 *is the pretreatment year and* 2000 *is the post-treatment year. All the methods suggest that there is negligible treatment effect.*

Estimator	Estimate	Std. err
Sample Means	-0.009	0.047
OLS	0.004	0.023
TR	0.012	0.023
AMLE	0.008	0.023
AIPW	0.007	0.023

$\tau(x)$ and those that do not, which suggests that there is a weighting effect going on when the likelihood of state and treatment time indicators vary with covariates. All the methods suggest that there is a positive effect of air interdictions on the log self-employment income, as found in Angrist and Kugler (2008). Recall that, when the treatment effect is non-constant, **TR** obtains estimates of weighted average treatment effects, given by Proposition 3. Because **TR** is giving significantly different results from the non-constant effect methods, we suspect that in this dataset the treatment effect varies with covariates. We also note that, in this case, the **OLS** estimator is fairly closely aligned with the **TR** estimator, suggesting that assuming linear nuisance components did not have too big an effect on our estimation of τ. However, it may have been difficult to argue a-priori that the linear specification used by **OLS** would be innocuous here.

As further evidence of treatment heterogeneity, Table 9.3 shows average effects obtained by **AMLE**, separately for urban and rural regions. Thus, estimates provided by the transformed regression estimator should not necessarily be interpreted as average treatment effects, and may instead better be interpreted as targeting a weighted estimand following the discussion in Section 9.4.

As a final sanity check, we also run a placebo analysis with the years 1998 and 2000 as the pre- and post-treatment period, and we use our methods to check if there was an effect in these years. It is encouraging that all the methods suggest there is a negligible effect on the treatment effect, as shown in Table 9.4.

9.8 Appendix: Augmented IPW for Cross Sectional data

Given our proposed heterogeneous treatment effect estimator, one direct way to construct an average treatment effect estimator is by building on results for doubly robust estimation as developed in Chernozhukov et al. (2016). In order to do so, we first note that the average treatment parameter can be written as a weighted average of outcomes using inverse-probability-style weights as follows: $\tau = \mathbb{E}[\gamma(Z_i)Y_i]$ with

$$\gamma(Z_i) = \gamma(X_i,\, S_i,\, T_i) = \frac{T_i S_i}{e_{1,1}(X_i)} - \frac{(1-T_i)S_i}{e_{0,1}(X_i)} - \frac{T_i(1-S_i)}{e_{1,0}(X_i)} + \frac{(1-T_i)(1-S_i)}{e_{0,0}(X_i)}. \tag{9.26}$$

Recall $g(z) = \mathbb{E}[Y_i \,|\, X_i = x,\, S_i = s,\, T_i = t]$. The result of Chernozhukov et al. (2016) imply that if we obtain good estimates both of $\hat{g}$ and the inverse-probability-style weights outlined above, then we can obtain semi parametrically efficient estimates of τ using the doubly robust form such as in Augmented Inverse Propensity Weighitng (AIPW) (Robins and Rotnitzky, 1995). We will refer to this algorithm as **AIPW**, which takes on the following steps:

1. Following the cross-fitting steps 2 to 4 of Algorithm 9.1, estimate the nuisance parameters $\hat{m}^{-\mathcal{I}_k}(x)$, $\hat{\varsigma}^{-\mathcal{I}_k}(x)$, $\hat{\nu}^{-\mathcal{I}_k}(x))$, $\hat{A}^{-\mathcal{I}_k}(z)$, $\hat{B}^{-\mathcal{I}_k}(z)$, $\hat{C}^{-\mathcal{I}_k}(z)$ using data not in the $\mathcal{I}_k$, where $\mathcal{I}_1$, ..., $\mathcal{I}_K$ are the K folds of the data. In the same way, fit nonparametric regressions for the propensities $\hat{e}_{1,1}^{-\mathcal{I}_k}(x)$, $\hat{e}_{1,0}^{-\mathcal{I}_k}(x)$, $\hat{e}_{0,1}^{-\mathcal{I}_k}(x)$ and $\hat{e}_{0,0}^{-\mathcal{I}_k}(x)$.
2. Run step 3 of Algorithm 9.2 to obtain cross-fitted point estimates $\hat{\tau}(X_j) = \hat{\tau}^{-\mathcal{I}_k}(X_j)$, for each $j \in \mathcal{I}_k$.
3. For each $j \in \mathcal{I}_k$, produce the cross-fitted point estimates:

$$\begin{aligned} \hat{g}(Z_j) &= \hat{m}^{-\mathcal{I}_k}(X_j) + \hat{A}^{-\mathcal{I}_k}(Z_j)\hat{\nu}^{-\mathcal{I}_k}(X_j) \\ &\quad + \hat{B}^{-\mathcal{I}_k}(Z_j)\hat{\varsigma}^{-\mathcal{I}_k}(X_j) + \hat{C}^{-\mathcal{I}_k}(Z_j)\hat{\tau}^{-\mathcal{I}_k}(X_j) \end{aligned} \tag{9.27}$$

   and

$$\hat{\gamma}(Z_j) = \frac{T_j S_j}{\hat{e}_{1,1}^{-\mathcal{I}_j}(X_j)} - \frac{(1-T_j)S_j}{\hat{e}_{0,1}^{-\mathcal{I}_j}(X_j)} - \frac{T_j(1-S_j)}{\hat{e}_{1,0}^{-\mathcal{I}_j}(X_j)} + \frac{(1-T_j)(1-S_j)}{\hat{e}_{0,0}^{-\mathcal{I}_j}(X_j)}. \tag{9.28}$$

4. Estimate the average treatment effect $\mathbb{E}[\tau(x)]$ as:

$$\hat{\tau}_{DR} = \frac{1}{n}\sum_{i=1}^{n}\Big(\hat{\tau}(X_i) + \hat{\gamma}(Z_i)(Y_i - \hat{g}(Z_i))\Big). \tag{9.29}$$

Abadie (2005) and Sant'Anna and Zhao (2020) explored a special case of this approach in cases where (X_i, S_i) are independent from T_i. As a result, only the estimate of the single propensity $s(x)$ is needed to perform a similar estimation, as opposed to the quantity $\gamma(x, s, t)$.

While plug-in estimation with the doubly robust score admits for algorithmically simple estimation of the average treatment effect, probabilities $e_{1,1}(x)$ etc. may get quite small, and so inverting even slightly inaccurate propensity estimates may result in instability.

9.9 Appendix: Supplemental Materials

9.9.1 Proof of Proposition 1

Assuming parallel trends conditioning on covariates X_i as in (9.2), Y_i can be written from (9.5) as follows:

$$\begin{aligned} Y_i &= (1 - T_i - S_i + T_i S_i)g(X_i, 0, 0) + (T_i - T_i S_i)g(X_i, 0, 1) \\ &\quad + (S_i - T_i S_i)g(X_i, 1, 0) + T_i S_i g(X_i, 1, 1) + \epsilon_i \end{aligned} \tag{9.30}$$

where $g(x,\ s,\ t) = \mathbb{E}[Y_i \mid X_i = x, S_i = s, T_i = t]$. We could then write the above as:

$$Y_i = g(X_i, 0, 0) + T_i\rho(X_i) + S_i\xi(X_i) + T_iS_i\tau(X_i) + \epsilon_i \tag{9.31}$$

where ρ and ξ are defined as in (9.6). Note that ultimately, we want a decomposition of the following form:

$$Y_i = D(Z_i) \cdot m(X_i) + A(Z_i) \cdot \nu(X_i) + B(Z_i) \cdot \varsigma(X_i) + C(Z_i) \cdot \tau(X_i) + \epsilon_i \tag{9.32}$$

we thus seek coefficients A, B, C and D. Note that we have the following expressions:

$$\begin{aligned}
m(X_i) =& e_{0,0}(X_i)g(X_i, 0, 0) + e_{0,1}(X_i)g(X_i, 0, 1) + e_{1,0}(X_i)g(X_i, 1, 0) + \\
& e_{1,1}(X_i)g(X_i, 1, 1) \\
\nu(X_i) =& \frac{e_{1,1}(X_i)}{t(X_i)} g(X_i, 1, 1) + \frac{e_{0,1}(X_i)}{t(X_i)} g(X_i, 0, 1) \\
& - \frac{e_{1,0}(X_i)}{(1 - t(X_i))} g(X_i, 1, 0) - \frac{e_{0,0}(X_i)}{(1 - t(X_i))} g(X_i, 0, 0) \\
\varsigma(X_i) =& \frac{e_{1,1}(X_i)}{s(X_i)} g(X_i, 1, 1) + \frac{e_{1,0}(X_i)}{s(X_i)} g(X_i, 1, 0) \\
& - \frac{e_{0,1}(X_i)}{(1 - s(X_i))} g(X_i, 1, 0) - \frac{e_{0,0}(X_i)}{(1 - s(X_i))} g(X_i, 0, 0) \\
\tau(X_i) =& g(X_i, 0, 0) - g(X_i, 0, 1) - g(X_i, 1, 0) + g(X_i, 1, 1).
\end{aligned}$$

Equating the coefficients from (9.32) and (9.30), we have that:

$$\begin{aligned}
& D(Z_i)e_{0,0}(X_i) - A(Z_i)\frac{e_{0,0}(X_i)}{(1 - t(X_i))} - B(Z_i)\frac{e_{0,0}(X_i)}{(1 - s(X_i))} + C(Z_i) \\
& = 1 - T_i - S_i + T_iS_i \\
& D(Z_i)e_{0,1}(X_i) + A(Z_i)\frac{e_{0,1}(X_i)}{t(X_i)} - B(Z_i)\frac{e_{0,1}(X_i)}{(1 - s(X_i))} - C(Z_i) \\
& = T_i - T_iS_i \\
& D(Z_i)e_{1,0}(X_i) - A(Z_i)\frac{e_{1,0}(X_i)}{(1 - t(X_i))} + B(Z_i)\frac{e_{1,0}(X_i)}{s(X_i)} - C(Z_i) \\
& = S_i - T_iS_i \\
& D(Z_i)e_{1,1}(X_i) + A(Z_i)\frac{e_{1,1}(X_i)}{t(X_i)} + B(Z_i)\frac{e_{1,1}(X_i)}{s(X_i)} + C(Z_i) \\
& = T_iS_i.
\end{aligned}$$

Summing the equations, we get that $D \equiv 1$. We can then reformulate our objective as:

$$Y_i = m(X_i) + A(Z_i) \cdot \nu(X_i) + B(Z_i) \cdot \varsigma(X_i) + C(Z_i) \cdot \tau(X_i) + \epsilon_i \tag{9.33}$$

which is the final form expressed in the proposition. We re-express the components as:

$$\begin{aligned}
\nu(x) &= \rho(x) + \frac{e_{1,1}(x)}{t(x)}\tau(x) + \left(\frac{e_{1,1}(x)}{t(x)} - \frac{e_{1,0}(x)}{(1 - t(x))}\right)\xi(x) \\
\varsigma(x) &= \xi(x) + \frac{e_{1,1}(x)}{t(x)}\tau(x) + \left(\frac{e_{1,1}(x)}{s(x)} - \frac{e_{0,1}(x)}{(1 - s(x))}\right)\rho(x) \\
m(x) &= g(x, 0, 0) + (e_{1,1}(x) + e_{1,0}(x))\xi(x) + (e_{1,1}(x) + e_{0,1}(x)\rho(x) + \\
& \quad e_{1,1}(x)\tau(x)
\end{aligned}$$

equating coefficients of (9.33) and (9.31), we have:

$$\frac{e_{1,1}(X_i)}{t(X_i)}A(Z_i)+\frac{e_{1,1}(X_i)}{s(X_i)}B(Z_i)+C(Z_i)=T_iS_i-e_{1,1}(X_i)$$
$$\left(\frac{e_{1,1}(X_i)}{t(X_i)}-\frac{e_{1,0}(X_i)}{(1-t(X_i))}\right)A(Z_i)+B(Z_i)=S_i-s(X_i)$$
$$A(Z_i)+\left(\frac{e_{1,1}(X_i)}{s(X_i)}-\frac{e_{0,1}(X_i)}{(1-s(X_i))}\right)B(Z_i)=T_i-t(X_i).$$

Let us define $\Delta_s(x)=e_{1,1}(x)/s(x)-e_{0,1}(x)/(1-s(x))$ and $\Delta_t(x)=e_{1,1}(x)/t(x)-e_{1,0}(x)/(1-t(x))$. The second and third equations become:

$$\Delta_t(X_i)A(Z_i)+B(Z_i)=S_i-s(X_i)$$
$$A(Z_i)+\Delta_s(X_i)B(Z_i)=T_i-t(X_i)$$

which gives us:

$$A(Z_i)=\frac{1}{1-\Delta_t(X_i)\cdot\Delta_s(X_i)}(T_i-t(X_i)-\Delta_s(X_i)\cdot(S_i-s(X_i)))$$
$$B(Z_i)=\frac{1}{1-\Delta_t(X_i)\cdot\Delta_s(X_i)}(S_i-s(X_i)-\Delta_t(X_i)\cdot(T_i-t(X_i)))$$
$$C(Z_i)=T_iS_i-e_{1,1}(X_i)-\frac{e_{1,1}(X_i)}{t(X_i)}A(Z_i)-\frac{e_{1,1}(X_i)}{s(X_i)}B(Z_i).$$

To obtain the expressions in (9.12), we just have to get rid of the conditional expectations form above, and it is easy to check that we will obtain the desired forms. Now we check (9.13). First, note that:

$$\mathbb{E}[A(Z_i)\mid X_i]$$
$$=f(X_i)^{-1}\left(\mathbb{E}[T_i\mid X_i]-t(X_i)-\frac{\Delta(X_i)(\mathbb{E}[S_i\mid X_i]-s(X_i))}{s(X_i)(1-s(X_i))}\right)$$

where $f(X_i)=1-\frac{\Delta^2(X_i)}{s(X_i)(1-s(X_i))t(X_i)(1-t(X_i))}$. Because $\mathbb{E}T_i\mid X_i=t(X_i)$ and $\mathbb{E}[S_i\mid X_i]=s(X_i)$, the above expression evaluates to zero. Similarly, we can show $\mathbb{E}[B(Z_i)\mid X_i]=\mathbb{E}[C(Z_i)\mid X_i]=0$. For terms such as $\mathbb{E}[A(Z)\mid X,S]$, note that

$$\mathbb{E}[A(Z_i)\mid X_i,S_i=1]$$
$$=f(X_i)^{-1}\left(\mathbb{E}[T_i\mid X_i,S_i=1]-t(X_i)-\frac{\Delta(X_i)}{s(X_i)}\right).$$

Because $\mathbb{E}[T_i\mid X_i,S_i=1]=e_{1,1}(X_i)/s(X_i)$, the above also evaluates to zero. Similarly, we can show that $\mathbb{E}[A(Z_i)\mid X_i,S_i=0]$ and $\mathbb{E}[B(Z_i)\mid X_i,T_i]=0$. For $\mathbb{E}[C(Z)\mid X,S]$, note that:

$$\mathbb{E}[B(Z_i)\mid X_i,S_i=1]=f(X_i)^{-1}\left(1-s(X_i)-\frac{\Delta(X_i)(\frac{e_{1,1}(X_i)}{s(X_i)}-t(X_i))}{t(X_i)(1-t(X_i))}\right)$$
$$=1-s(X_i).$$

Thus we have

$$\mathbb{E}[C(Z_i)\mid X_i,S_i=1]=\frac{e_{1,1}(X_i)}{s(X_i)}-\frac{e_{1,1}}{s(X_i)}(1-s(X_i))-e_{1,1}(X_i)=0,$$

and $\mathbb{E}[C(Z_i) \mid X_i, S_i = 0] = 0$ and $\mathbb{E}[C(Z_i) \mid X_i, T_i] = 0$ can be checked similarly. To check $C(Z_i)$ is uncorrelated with $A(Z_i)$ given X_i:

$$
\begin{aligned}
&\mathbb{E}[C(Z_i)A(Z_i) \mid X_i] \\
&= \mathbb{E}_{S_i,T_i}\left[A(Z_i)\big(S_iT_i - e_{1,1}(X_i) - \frac{e_{1,1}(X_i)}{t(X_i)}A(Z_i) - \frac{e_{1,1}(X_i)}{s(X_i)}B(Z_i)\big)\right] \\
&= \mathbb{E}_{S_i,T_i}\left[\frac{1}{f(X_i)}\big(T_i - t(X_i)\big)\big(T_iS_i - e_{1,1}(X_i)\big)\right] \\
&\quad - \mathbb{E}_{S_i,T_i}\left[\frac{\Delta(X_i)}{f(X_i)s(X_i)(1-s(X_i))}(S_i - s(X_i))(T_iS_i - e_{1,1}(X_i))\right] \\
&\quad - \mathbb{E}_{S_i,T_i}\left[\frac{e_{1,1}(X_i)}{t(X_i)f(X_i)^2}\cdot\left\{(T_i - t(X_i))^2\right.\right. \\
&\qquad\qquad - 2\frac{\Delta(X_i)}{s(X_i)(1-s(X_i))}(T_i - t(X_i))(S_i - s(X_i)) \\
&\qquad\qquad \left.\left. + \frac{\Delta(X_i)^2}{s(X_i)^2(1-s(X_i))^2}(S_i - s(X_i))^2\right\}\right] \\
&\quad + \mathbb{E}_{S_i,T_i}\left[\frac{e_{1,1}(X_i)}{s(X_i)f(X_i)^2}\cdot\left\{\frac{\Delta(X_i)}{t(X_i)(1-t(X_i))}(T_i - t(X_i))^2\right.\right. \\
&\qquad - \frac{\Delta(X_i)^2}{s(X_i)(1-s(X_i))t(X_i)(1-t(X_i))}(T_i - t(X_i))(S_i - s(X_i)) \\
&\qquad \left.\left. - (T_i - t(X_i))(S_i - s(X_i)) + \frac{\Delta(X_i)}{s(X_i)(1-s(X_i))}(S_i - s(X_i))^2\right\}\right] \\
&= \frac{e_{1,1}(X_i)}{f(X_i)}\left((1 - t(X_i)) - \frac{\Delta(X_i)}{s(X_i)} - (1 - t(X_i)) + \frac{\Delta(X_i)}{s(X_i)}\right) \\
&= 0
\end{aligned}
$$

where the third equality follows by noting that

$$
\begin{aligned}
\mathbb{E}[(T_i - t(X_i))^2 \mid X_i] &= t(X_i)(1 - t(X_i), \\
\mathbb{E}[(S_i - s(X_i))^2 \mid X_i] &= s(X_i)(1 - s(X_i)), \\
\mathbb{E}[(T_i - t(X_i))(S_i - s(X_i)) \mid X_i] &= \Delta(X_i).
\end{aligned}
$$

We can similarly check that $\mathbb{E}[C(Z_i)B(Z_i) \mid X_i] = 0$.

9.9.2 Proof of Theorem 2

First we prove the statement $\sqrt{n}(\hat{\tau}_{TR} - \hat{\tau}^*) \xrightarrow{p} 0$, where $\hat{\tau}_{TR}$ is the transformed regression estimator and $\hat{\tau}^*$ is the transformed regression estimator with oracle nuisance parameters. From (9.20), we see that

$$
\sqrt{n}(\hat{\tau}_{TR} - \hat{\tau}^*) = \sqrt{n}\left(\sum_{k=1}^{K}\frac{|\mathcal{I}_k|}{n}\hat{\tau}^{-\mathcal{I}_k} - \hat{\tau}^*\right) = \sum_{k=1}^{K}\frac{|\mathcal{I}_k|}{n}\cdot\sqrt{n}(\hat{\tau}^{-\mathcal{I}_k} - \hat{\tau}^*). \tag{9.34}
$$

Because each $|\mathcal{I}_k|/n$ is approximately $1/K$, which is fixed as n grows, and the number of folds K is also fixed, $\sqrt{n}(\hat{\tau}_{TR} - \hat{\tau}^*) \xrightarrow{p} 0$ will follow if we show that $\sqrt{n}(\hat{\tau}^{-\mathcal{I}_k} - \hat{\tau}^*) \rightarrow_p 0$.

The proof consists of two steps. Firstly, we show that, if two nuisance parameters $\mu(x)$ and $\nu(x)$, estimated by $\hat{\mu}^{-\mathcal{I}_k}(x)$ and $\hat{\nu}^{-\mathcal{I}_k}(x)$ respectively, satisfy conditions 2, 3 and 4 from above, then the estimation of their product $\mu(x)\cdot\nu(x)$ by $\hat{\mu}^{-\mathcal{I}_k}(x)\cdot\hat{\nu}^{-\mathcal{I}_k}(x)$, and their sum $\mu(x)+\nu(x)$ by $\hat{\mu}^{-\mathcal{I}_k}(x)+\hat{\nu}^{-\mathcal{I}_k}(x)$, also satisfy conditions 2, 3, and 4. As a result, the estimate of $\hat{H}^{-\mathcal{I}_k}(x)$ and $\hat{C}^{-\mathcal{I}_k}(x)$, by sums and products of other nuisance parameters, such as $\hat{m}^{-\mathcal{I}_k}(x)$ and $\hat{e}_{1,1}^{-\mathcal{I}_k}(x)$, also satisfies the conditions listed above. Secondly, we show the desired result, assuming that $\hat{H}^{-\mathcal{I}_k}(x)$ and $\hat{C}^{-\mathcal{I}_k}(x)$ satisfy the conditions above.

We start with the first step. Assume that $\hat{\mu}^{-\mathcal{I}_k}(x)$ and $\hat{\mu}^{-\mathcal{I}_k}(x)$ satisfy conditions 2 to 4. We want to estimate $\mu(x)\cdot\nu(x)$ by $\hat{\mu}^{-\mathcal{I}_k}(x)\cdot\hat{\nu}^{-\mathcal{I}_k}(x)$, and $\mu(x)+\nu(x)$ by $\hat{\mu}^{-\mathcal{I}_k}(x)+\hat{\nu}^{-\mathcal{I}_k}(x)$. Consistency and boundedness comes easily from the consistency and boundedness of $\hat{\mu}^{-\mathcal{I}_k}(x)$ and $\hat{\mu}^{-\mathcal{I}_k}(x)$. Risk decay comes as follows:

$$
\begin{aligned}
&\mathbb{E}[(\hat{\mu}^{-\mathcal{I}_k}(x)\cdot\hat{\nu}^{-\mathcal{I}_k}(x)-\mu(x)\cdot\nu(x))^2]\\
&=\mathbb{E}\left[\left(\frac{1}{2}(\hat{\mu}+\mu)(\hat{\nu}-\nu)+\frac{1}{2}(\hat{\nu}+\nu)(\hat{\mu}-\mu)\right)^2\right]\\
&=\mathbb{E}\left[\left(\frac{1}{2}(\hat{\mu}+\mu)(\hat{\nu}-\nu)\right)^2\right]+\mathbb{E}\left[\left(\frac{1}{2}(\hat{\nu}+\nu)(\hat{\mu}-\mu)\right)^2\right]\\
&\quad+\mathbb{E}\left[\left(\frac{1}{2}(\hat{\mu}+\mu)(\hat{\nu}-\nu)\right)\left(\frac{1}{2}(\hat{\nu}+\nu)(\hat{\mu}-\mu)\right)\right]\\
&\le 2\left(\mathbb{E}\left[\left(\frac{1}{2}(\hat{\mu}+\mu)(\hat{\nu}-\nu)\right)^2\right]+\mathbb{E}\left[\left(\frac{1}{2}(\hat{\nu}+\nu)(\hat{\mu}-\mu)\right)^2\right]\right)\\
&\le M^2\left(\mathbb{E}\left[(\hat{\mu}-\mu)^2\right]+\mathbb{E}\left[(\hat{\nu}-\nu)^2\right]\right)\\
&=o\left(\frac{1}{\sqrt{n}}\right)
\end{aligned}
$$

where we used the assumption that the nuisance parameters are all bounded by M. Risk decay for $\mu+\nu$ follows similarly. Recall we want to show the following:

$$
\begin{aligned}
\hat{\tau}^{-\mathcal{I}_k}-\hat{\tau}^* &= \frac{\frac{1}{n}\sum_{j\in\mathcal{I}_k}\hat{H}^{-\mathcal{I}_k}(Z_j)\hat{C}^{-\mathcal{I}_k}(Z_j)}{\frac{1}{n}\sum_{j\in\mathcal{I}_k}\hat{C}^{-\mathcal{I}_k}(Z_j)^2}-\frac{\frac{1}{n}\sum_{j\in\mathcal{I}_k}H(Z_j)C(Z_j)}{\frac{1}{n}\sum_{j\in\mathcal{I}_k}C(Z_j)^2}\\
&=o_p\left(\frac{1}{\sqrt{n}}\right),
\end{aligned}
\tag{9.35}
$$

which will follow if we can show that

$$
\frac{1}{n}\sum_{j\in\mathcal{I}_k}\hat{H}^{-\mathcal{I}_k}(Z_j)\hat{C}^{-\mathcal{I}_k}(Z_j)-\frac{1}{n}\sum_{j\in\mathcal{I}_k}H(Z_j)C(Z_j)=o_p(\frac{1}{\sqrt{n}})
\tag{9.36}
$$

and

$$
\frac{1}{n}\sum_{j\in\mathcal{I}_k}\hat{C}^{-\mathcal{I}_k}(Z_j)^2-\frac{1}{n}\sum_{j\in\mathcal{I}_k}C(Z_j)^2=o_p(\frac{1}{\sqrt{n}}).
\tag{9.37}
$$

Because with these bounds, and noting the Taylor expansion of $f(x,y)=\frac{x}{y}$ at some point x_0 and $y_0\neq 0$ is given by:

$$
f(x,y)=f(x_0,y_0)+\frac{1}{y_0}\cdot(x-x_0)-\frac{x_0}{y_0^2}\cdot(y-y_0)+O\left((x-x_0)^2+(y-y_0)^2\right)
$$

we have that:

$$\begin{aligned}
\hat{\tau}_{\mathcal{I}_k} - \hat{\tau}^* &= \frac{\frac{1}{n}\sum_{j\in\mathcal{I}_k}\hat{H}^{-\mathcal{I}_k}(Z_j)\hat{C}^{-\mathcal{I}_k}(Z_j)}{\frac{1}{n}\sum_{j\in\mathcal{I}_k}\hat{C}^{-\mathcal{I}_k}(Z_j)^2} - \frac{\frac{1}{n}\sum_{j\in\mathcal{I}_k}H(Z_j)C(Z_j)}{\frac{1}{n}\sum_{j\in\mathcal{I}_k}C(Z_j)^2} \\
&= f\left(\frac{1}{n}\sum_{j\in\mathcal{I}_k}\hat{H}^{-\mathcal{I}_k}(Z_j)\hat{C}^{-\mathcal{I}_k}(Z_j), \frac{1}{n}\sum_{j\in\mathcal{I}_k}\hat{C}^{\mathcal{I}_k}(X_j)^2\right) \\
&\quad - f\left(\frac{1}{n}\sum_{j\in\mathcal{I}_k}H(Z_j)C(Z_j), \frac{1}{n}\sum_{j\in\mathcal{I}_k}C(Z_j)^2\right) \\
&= \frac{1}{\frac{1}{n}\sum_{j\in\mathcal{I}_k}C(Z_j)^2}\cdot\left(\frac{1}{n}\sum_{j\in\mathcal{I}_k}\hat{H}^{-\mathcal{I}_k}(Z_j)\hat{C}^{-\mathcal{I}_k}(Z_j)\right. \qquad (9.38)\\
&\quad \left. - \frac{1}{n}\sum_{j\in\mathcal{I}_k}H(Z_j)C(Z_j)\right) - \frac{\frac{1}{n}\sum_{j\in\mathcal{I}_k}H(Z_j)C(Z_j)}{\left(\frac{1}{n}\sum_{j\in\mathcal{I}_k}C(Z_j)^2\right)^2} \\
&\quad \cdot\left(\frac{1}{n}\sum_{j\in\mathcal{I}_k}\hat{C}^{\mathcal{I}_k}(X_j)^2 - \frac{1}{n}\sum_{j\in\mathcal{I}_k}C(Z_j)^2\right) + o_p\left(\frac{1}{n}\right) \\
&= o_p\left(\frac{1}{\sqrt{n}}\right)
\end{aligned}$$

where Slutsky's theorem is used in the last equality. Let us first check (9.36). Note that:

$$\begin{aligned}
&\frac{1}{n}\sum_{j\in\mathcal{I}_k}\hat{H}^{-\mathcal{I}_k}(Z_j)\hat{C}^{-\mathcal{I}_k}(Z_j) - \frac{1}{n}\sum_{j\in\mathcal{I}_k}H(Z_j)C(Z_j) && (9.39)\\
&= \frac{1}{n}\sum_{j\in\mathcal{I}_k}H(Z_j)\big(\hat{C}^{-\mathcal{I}_k}(Z_j) - C(Z_j)\big) && (9.40)\\
&\quad + \frac{1}{n}\sum_{j\in\mathcal{I}_k}C(Z_j)\big(\hat{H}^{-\mathcal{I}_k}(Z_j) - H(Z_j)\big) && (9.41)\\
&\quad + \frac{1}{n}\sum_{j\in\mathcal{I}_k}\big(\hat{H}^{-\mathcal{I}_k}(Z_j) - H(Z_j)\big)\big(\hat{C}^{-\mathcal{I}_k}(Z_j) - C(Z_j)\big). && (9.42)
\end{aligned}$$

We check that the three terms above are small. For (9.40), we first check that $H(Z_j)\big(\hat{C}^{-\mathcal{I}_k}(Z_j) - C(Z_j)\big)$ has mean zero. Note that

$$\begin{aligned}
&\mathbb{E}[H(Z_j)\big(\hat{C}^{-\mathcal{I}_k}(Z_j) - C(Z_j)\big)] \\
&= \mathbb{E}\Big[\big(\tau(X_i)C(Z_i) + \epsilon_i\big)\big(e_{1,1}(X_i) + J(X_i)A(Z_i) + K(X_i)B(Z_i)\big) \\
&\quad - \Big(\tau(X_i)C(Z_i) + \epsilon_i\Big)\Big(\hat{e}_{1,1}^{-\mathcal{I}_k}(X_i) + \hat{J}^{-\mathcal{I}_k}(X_i)\hat{A}^{-\mathcal{I}_k}(Z_i) \\
&\quad + \hat{K}^{-\mathcal{I}_k}(X_i)\hat{B}^{-\mathcal{I}_k}(Z_i)\Big)\Big] \\
&= \mathbb{E}[\tau(X_i)\hat{J}^{-\mathcal{I}_k}(X_i)\hat{A}^{-\mathcal{I}_k}(Z_i)C(Z_i)] \\
&\quad + \mathbb{E}[\tau(X_i)\hat{K}^{-\mathcal{I}_k}(X_i)\hat{B}^{-\mathcal{I}_k}(Z_i)C(Z_i)],
\end{aligned}$$

where $J(X_i) = e_{1,1}(X_i)/t(X_i)$ and $K(X_i) = e_{1,1}(X_i)/s(X_i)$ and we similarly define the cross-fitted analogue $\hat{J}^{-)_k}(\cdot)$ and $\hat{K}^{-\sqcap_k}(\cdot)$. Many terms above vanished because of (9.13). We will just show that

$$\mathbb{E}[\tau(X_i)\hat{J}^{-\mathcal{I}_k}(X_i)\hat{A}^{-\mathcal{I}_k}(Z_i)C(Z_i)] = 0, \tag{9.43}$$

and the argument for $\mathbb{E}[\tau(X_i)\hat{K}^{-\mathcal{I}_k}(X_i)\hat{B}^{-\mathcal{I}_k}(Z_i)C(Z_i)]$ is identical. Note that

$$\tau(X_i)\hat{J}^{-\mathcal{I}_k}(X_i)\hat{A}^{-\mathcal{I}_k}(Z_i) = \hat{L}^{-\mathcal{I}_k}(X_i) + \hat{N}^{-\mathcal{I}_k}(X_i)T_i + \hat{P}^{-\mathcal{I}_k}(X_i)S_i, \tag{9.44}$$

where

$$\begin{aligned}
\hat{L}^{-\mathcal{I}_k}(X_i) &= \tau(X_i)\hat{J}^{-\mathcal{I}_k}(X_i)\cdot\frac{1}{\hat{f}^{-\mathcal{I}_k}(X_i)}\left(\frac{\hat{\Delta}^{-\mathcal{I}_k}(X_i)}{1-\hat{s}^{-\mathcal{I}_k}(X_i)} - \hat{t}^{-\mathcal{I}_k}(X_i)\right),\\
\hat{N}^{-\mathcal{I}_k}(X_i) &= \tau(X_i)\hat{J}^{-\mathcal{I}_k}(X_i)\cdot\frac{1}{\hat{f}^{-\mathcal{I}_k}(X_i)},\\
\hat{P}^{-\mathcal{I}_k}(X_i) &= -\tau(X_i)\hat{J}^{-\mathcal{I}_k}(X_i)\cdot\frac{1}{\hat{f}^{-\mathcal{I}_k}(X_i)}\frac{\hat{\Delta}^{-\mathcal{I}_k}(X_i)}{\hat{s}^{-\mathcal{I}_k}(X_i)\left(1-\hat{s}^{-\mathcal{I}_k}(X_i)\right)}.
\end{aligned}$$

Thus, again by (9.13), we have

$$\begin{aligned}
\mathbb{E}[\hat{L}^{-\mathcal{I}_k}(X_i)C(Z_i)] &= \mathbb{E}[\mathbb{E}[\hat{L}^{-\mathcal{I}_k}(X_i)C(Z_i) \mid -\mathcal{I}_k]]\\
&= \mathbb{E}[\mathbb{E}[\hat{L}^{-\mathcal{I}_k}(X_i)\mathbb{E}[C(Z_i) \mid X_i] \mid -\mathcal{I}_k]]\\
&= 0
\end{aligned}$$

where the first line conditions on the data not in fold $\mathcal{I}_k$. Similarly, we have that

$$\mathbb{E}[\hat{N}^{-\mathcal{I}_k}(X_i)T_iC(Z_i)] = \mathbb{E}[\hat{P}^{-\mathcal{I}_k}(X_i)S_iC(Z_i)] = 0.$$

Hence we know that $\mathbb{E}[\tau(X_i)\hat{J}^{-\mathcal{I}_k}(X_i)\hat{A}^{-\mathcal{I}_k}(Z_i)C(Z_i)]$, and subsequently $\mathbb{E}[H(Z_j)(\hat{C}^{-\mathcal{I}_k}(Z_j) - C(Z_j))]$, are all zero. Now we are ready to show that (9.40) is $o_p(\frac{1}{\sqrt{n}})$:

$$\begin{aligned}
&\mathbb{E}\left[\left(\frac{1}{n}\sum_{j\in\mathcal{I}_k} H(Z_j)\left(\hat{C}^{-\mathcal{I}_k}(Z_j) - C(Z_j)\right)\right)^2\right] && (9.45)\\
&= \frac{|\mathcal{I}_k|}{n}\frac{1}{n}\mathbb{E}[H(Z_j)^2(\hat{C}^{-\mathcal{I}_k}(Z_j) - C(Z_j))^2] && (9.46)\\
&\le \frac{|\mathcal{I}_k|}{n}\frac{M^2}{n}\mathbb{E}[(\hat{C}^{-\mathcal{I}_k}(Z_j) - C(Z_j))^2] && (9.47)\\
&= o\left(\frac{1}{n^{3/2}}\right) && (9.48)
\end{aligned}$$

where the first equality is precisely because all terms of the form $H(Z_j)(\hat{C}^{-\mathcal{I}_k}(Z_j) - C(Z_j))$ have mean zero, and the bound comes from the risk decay assumption. To show (9.41) is $o_p(\frac{1}{\sqrt{n}})$, the argument is exactly the same as the one we gave above: the only difference being we have to check that the term $C(Z_j)(\hat{H}^{-\mathcal{I}_k}(Z_j) - H(Z_j))$ has mean zero. Note that:

$$\begin{aligned}
&\mathbb{E}[C(Z_j)(\hat{H}^{-\mathcal{I}_k}(Z_j) - H(Z_j))]\\
&= \mathbb{E}\Bigg[C(Z_i)\big(m(X_i) + \nu(X_i)A(Z_i) + \varsigma(X_i)B(Z_i)\big)
\end{aligned}$$

$$- C(Z_i)(\hat{m}_{1,1}^{-\mathcal{I}_k}(X_i) + \hat{\nu}^{-\mathcal{I}_k}(X_i)\hat{A}^{-\mathcal{I}_k}(Z_i) + \hat{\varsigma}^{-\mathcal{I}_k}(X_i)\hat{B}^{-\mathcal{I}_k}(Z_i))\Big]$$
$$= \mathbb{E}-\hat{\nu}^{-\mathcal{I}_k}(X_i)\hat{A}^{-\mathcal{I}_k}(Z_i)C(Z_i) + \mathbb{E}[-\hat{\varsigma}^{-\mathcal{I}_k}(X_i)\hat{B}^{-\mathcal{I}_k}(Z_i)C(Z_i)],$$

where terms vanish in the last equality because of (9.13). Again we just have to show that $\hat{\nu}^{-\mathcal{I}_k}(X_i)\hat{A}^{-\mathcal{I}_k}(Z_i)C(Z_i)$ and $\hat{\varsigma}^{-\mathcal{I}_k}(X_i)\hat{B}^{-\mathcal{I}_k}(Z_i)C(Z_i)$ have mean zero, which follows exactly the same argument as we used for (9.43). Thus (9.41) is also $o_p(\frac{1}{\sqrt{n}})$. We only have to check that (9.42) is $o_p(\frac{1}{\sqrt{n}})$, which follows by Cauchy-Schwarz and the risk decay assumption:

$$\begin{aligned}
&\frac{1}{n}\sum_{j\in\mathcal{I}_k}(\hat{H}^{-\mathcal{I}_k}(Z_j) - H(Z_j))(\hat{C}^{-\mathcal{I}_k}(Z_j) - C(Z_j)) \\
&\le \left(\frac{1}{n}\sum_{j\in\mathcal{I}_k}\left(\hat{H}^{-\mathcal{I}_k}(Z_j) - H(Z_j)\right)^2\right)^{\frac{1}{2}}\left(\frac{1}{n}\sum_{j\in\mathcal{I}_k}\left(\hat{C}^{-\mathcal{I}_k}(Z_j) - C(Z_j)\right)^2\right)^{\frac{1}{2}} \\
&= o_p\left(\frac{1}{\sqrt{n}}\right).
\end{aligned}$$

Thus we have finished checking (9.36). We proceed to check (9.37). Note that:

$$\frac{1}{n}\sum_{j\in\mathcal{I}_k}\hat{C}^{-\mathcal{I}_k}(Z_j)^2 - \frac{1}{n}\sum_{j\in\mathcal{I}_k}C(Z_j)^2 \tag{9.49}$$
$$= 2\cdot\frac{1}{n}\sum_{j\in\mathcal{I}_k}C(Z_j)(\hat{C}^{-\mathcal{I}_k}(Z_j) - C(Z_j)) \tag{9.50}$$
$$+ \frac{1}{n}\sum_{j\in\mathcal{I}_k}(\hat{C}^{-\mathcal{I}_k}(Z_j) - C(Z_j))^2. \tag{9.51}$$

The second term above is immediately $o_p(\frac{1}{\sqrt{n}})$ because of the risk decay assumption. Thus we only have to check that (9.50) is $o_p(\frac{1}{\sqrt{n}})$, which will follow exactly the same argument for (9.40), once we show that $C(Z_j)(\hat{C}^{-\mathcal{I}_k}(Z_j) - C(Z_j))$ has mean zero. Note then

$$\begin{aligned}
&\mathbb{E}[C(Z_j)\mathbb{E}[\hat{C}^{-\mathcal{I}_k}(Z_j) - C(Z_j)]] \\
&= \mathbb{E}\Big[- C(Z_i)(e_{1,1}(X_i) + J(X_i)A(Z_i) + K(X_i)B(Z_i)) \\
&\quad + C(Z_i)(\hat{e}_{1,1}^{-\mathcal{I}_k}(X_i) + \hat{J}^{-\mathcal{I}_k}(X_i)\hat{A}^{-\mathcal{I}_k}(Z_i) + \hat{K}^{-\mathcal{I}_k}(X_i)\hat{B}^{-\mathcal{I}_k}(Z_i))\Big] \\
&= \mathbb{E}[\hat{J}^{-\mathcal{I}_k}(X_i)\hat{A}^{-\mathcal{I}_k}(Z_i)C(Z_i)] + \mathbb{E}[\hat{K}^{-\mathcal{I}_k}(X_i)\hat{B}^{-\mathcal{I}_k}(Z_i)C(Z_i)],
\end{aligned}$$

where terms vanish in the last equality because of (9.13). Following the same argument for showing (9.43), we can show that the two terms above are both zero. Thus $C(Z_j)(\hat{C}^{-\mathcal{I}_k}(Z_j) - C(Z_j))$ indeed has mean zero and so is $o_p(\frac{1}{\sqrt{n}})$, so we have finished showing $\sqrt{n}(\hat{\tau}_{TR} - \hat{\tau}^*) \xrightarrow{p} 0$.

Now we show that $\sqrt{n}(\hat{\tau}^* - \tau) \xrightarrow{d} \mathcal{N}(0, V_{TR})$, where $V_{TR} = \frac{\mathbb{E}[\sigma^2(z)C^2(z)]}{\mathbb{E}[C^2(z)]^2}$. Note that

$$\sqrt{n}(\hat{\tau}^* - \tau) = \frac{\sqrt{n}(\frac{1}{n}\sum_{i=1}^n H(Z_i)C(Z_i) - (\frac{1}{n}\sum_{i=1}^n C(Z_i)^2)\tau)}{\frac{1}{n}\sum_{i=1}^n C(Z_i)^2} \tag{9.52}$$

$$= \frac{\sqrt{n}(\frac{1}{n}\sum_{i=1}^{n}\epsilon_i C(Z_i))}{\frac{1}{n}\sum_{i=1}^{n}C(Z_i)^2} \tag{9.53}$$

$$\xrightarrow{d} \frac{1}{\mathbb{E}[C(z)^2]} \cdot \mathcal{N}(0, \mathbb{E}[\sigma(z)^2 C(z)^2]) \tag{9.54}$$

$$\stackrel{d}{=} \mathcal{N}(0, \frac{\mathbb{E}[\sigma^2(z)C^2(z)]}{\mathbb{E}[C^2(z)]^2}) \tag{9.55}$$

where (9.54) uses Slutsky's theorem and the central limit theorem. The desired result then follows.

9.9.3 *Proof of Proposition 3*

The proof of Proposition 3 is essentially the same as that of the Theorem 2: by exactly the same argument, we know that $\sqrt{n}(\hat{\tau}_{TR} - \hat{\tau}^*) \xrightarrow{p} 0$, where $\hat{\tau}^*$ is the transformed regression estimator with oracle nuisance parameters. Then we just have to show $\sqrt{n}(\hat{\tau}^* - \bar{t}) \xrightarrow{d} \mathcal{N}(0, V_{TR})$, where $V_{TR} = \frac{\mathbb{E}[\sigma^2(z)C^2(z)]}{\mathbb{E}[C^2(z)]^2}$, which follows from the following calculation:

$$\sqrt{n}(\hat{\tau}^* - \bar{\tau}) = \frac{\sqrt{n}(\frac{1}{n}\sum_{i=1}^{n}H(Z_i)C(Z_i) - (\frac{1}{n}\sum_{i=1}^{n}C(Z_i)^2)\bar{\tau})}{\frac{1}{n}\sum_{i=1}^{n}C(Z_i)^2} \tag{9.56}$$

$$= \frac{\sqrt{n}(\frac{1}{n}\sum_{i=1}^{n}\epsilon_i C(Z_i))}{\frac{1}{n}\sum_{i=1}^{n}C(Z_i)^2} \tag{9.57}$$

$$\xrightarrow{d} \frac{1}{\mathbb{E}[C(z)^2]} \cdot \mathcal{N}(0, \mathbb{E}[\sigma(z)^2 C(z)^2]) \tag{9.58}$$

$$\stackrel{d}{=} \mathcal{N}\left(0, \frac{\mathbb{E}[\sigma^2(z)C^2(z)]}{\mathbb{E}[C^2(z)]^2}\right) \tag{9.59}$$

where (9.58) uses Slutsky's theorem and the central limit theorem.

9.9.4 *Proof of Theorem 4*

Following the notation in Foster and Syrgkanis (2019), we first define directional derivatives: we define $D_f(F)(f)[h] = \frac{d}{dt}F(f + th)|_{t=0}$ for a pair fo functions f, h. We define $D_f^k(F)(f)[h_1, \ldots, h_k] = \frac{\partial^k}{\partial t_1 \ldots \partial t_k}F(f + t_1 h_1 + \ldots + t_k h_k)|_{t_1 = \ldots = t_k = 0}$. Next, we check Assumptions 1-4 stated in Foster and Syrgkanis (2019). First, we check Assumption 2 on the first-order optimality.

$$\begin{aligned}
&D_\tau L(\tau, \mu)[\tau' - \tau] \\
&= -2\mathbb{E}[(Y - m(X) - A(Z)\nu(X) - B(Z)\varsigma(X) - C(Z)\tau(Z))C(Z) \\
&\quad (\tau'(X) - \tau(X))] \\
&= -2\mathbb{E}[\mathbb{E}[(Y - m(X) - A(Z)\nu(X) - B(Z)\varsigma(X) - C(Z)\tau(Z))C(Z) \\
&\quad (\tau'(X) - \tau(X)) \mid Z]] \\
&= -2\mathbb{E}[\mathbb{E}[\epsilon C(Z)(\tau'(X) - \tau(X)) \mid Z]] = 0
\end{aligned}$$

due to the fact that $\mathbb{E}[\epsilon \mid Z] = 0$ from Proposition 1.

Next, we check Assumption 1. Note that we have to check it with directional derivative with respect to all nuisance components $m(x), \nu(x), \varsigma(x), s(x), t(x), \Delta(x)$. By symmetry, we only need to check it with $m(x), \nu(x), s(x), \Delta(x)$.

$$
\begin{aligned}
&D_m D_\tau L(\tau, \{m(x), \nu(x), \varsigma(x), s(x), t(x), \Delta(x)\})[\tau' - \tau, m' - m] \\
&= -2d\mathbb{E}[(Y - (m(X) + t_m(m'(X) - m(X)) - A(Z)\nu(X) - B(Z)\varsigma(X) \\
&\quad - C(Z)(\tau(X) + t_\tau(\tau'(X) - \tau(X))))C(Z) \\
&\quad (\tau'(X) - \tau(X))]/dt_m|_{t_m=0,t_\tau=0} \\
&= -2\mathbb{E}[(m'(X) - m(X))C(Z)(\tau'(X) - \tau(X))] \\
&= -2\mathbb{E}[\mathbb{E}[(m'(X) - m(X))C(Z)(\tau'(X) - \tau(X)) \mid X]] \\
&= -2\mathbb{E}[(m'(X) - m(X))(\tau'(X) - \tau(X))\mathbb{E}[C(Z) \mid X]] \\
&= 0
\end{aligned}
$$

where the last equality follows from $\mathbb{E}[C(Z) \mid X] = 0$ as in Proposition 1.

Next, we check

$$
\begin{aligned}
&D_\nu D_\tau L(\tau, \{m(x), \nu(x), \varsigma(x), s(x), t(x), \Delta(x)\})[\tau' - \tau, \nu' - \nu] \\
&= -2d\mathbb{E}[(Y - m(X) - A(Z)(\nu(X) + t_\nu(\nu'(X) - \nu(X))) - B(Z)\varsigma(X) \\
&\quad - C(Z)(\tau(X) + t_\tau(\tau'(X) - \tau(X))))C(Z) \\
&\quad (\tau'(X) - \tau(X))]/dt_\nu|_{t_\nu=0,t_\tau=0} \\
&= -2\mathbb{E}[A(Z)(\nu'(X) - \nu(X))C(Z)(\tau'(X) - \tau(X))] \\
&= -2\mathbb{E}[\mathbb{E}[A(Z)(\nu'(X) - \nu(X))C(Z)(\tau'(X) - \tau(X)) \mid X]] \\
&= -2\mathbb{E}[(\nu'(X) - \nu(X))(\tau'(X) - \tau(X))\mathbb{E}[A(Z)C(Z) \mid X]] \\
&= 0
\end{aligned}
$$

where the last equality follows from $\mathbb{E}[A(Z)C(Z) \mid X] = 0$ as in Proposition 1.

Before we continue, we define

$$
\begin{aligned}
A_{t_\Delta}(Z_i) = &\left(1 - \frac{(\Delta + t_\Delta(\Delta' - \Delta))^2(X_i)}{s(X_i)(1 - s(X_i))t(X_i)(1 - t(X_i))}\right)^{-1} \\
&\left(T_i - t(X_i) - \frac{(\Delta + t_\Delta(\Delta' - \Delta))(S_i - s(X_i))}{s(X_i)(1 - s(X_i))}\right)
\end{aligned}
$$

and similarly, we define $B_{t_\Delta}(Z_i), C_{t_\Delta}(Z_i)$. We further define

$$
\begin{aligned}
M_{t_\Delta,t_\tau}(Z) = &Y - m(X) - A_{t_\Delta}(Z)\nu(X) - B_{t_\Delta}(Z)\varsigma(X) - C_{t_\Delta}(Z)(\tau(X) \\
&+ t_\tau(\tau'(X) - \tau(X)))
\end{aligned}
$$

and

$$
M(Z) = Y - m(X) - A(Z)\nu(X) - B(Z)\varsigma(X) - C(Z)\tau(X).
$$

We check

$$
\begin{aligned}
&D_\Delta D_\tau L(\tau, \{m(x), \nu(x), \varsigma(x), s(x), t(x), \Delta(x)\})[\tau' - \tau, \Delta' - \Delta] \\
&= -2d\mathbb{E}[M_{t_\Delta,t_\tau}(Z)C_{t_\Delta}(Z)(\tau'(X) - \tau(X))]/dt_\Delta|_{t_\Delta=0,t_\tau=0} \\
&= -2\mathbb{E}\left[C(Z)(\tau'(X) - \tau(X))\frac{\partial M_{t_\Delta,0}(Z)}{\partial t_\Delta}\bigg|_{t_\Delta=0}\right] \\
&\quad - 2\mathbb{E}\left[M(Z)(\tau'(X) - \tau(X))\frac{\partial C_{t_\Delta}(Z)}{\partial t_\Delta}\bigg|_{t_\Delta=0}\right].
\end{aligned}
$$

For the second term, we notice that $\mathbb{E}[M(Z) \mid Z] = 0$ from Proposition 1, and so

$$\begin{aligned}
&-2\mathbb{E}\left[M(Z)(\tau'(X) - \tau(X))\frac{\partial C_{t_\Delta}(Z)}{\partial t_\Delta}\bigg|_{t_\Delta=0}\right] \\
&= -2\mathbb{E}\left[\mathbb{E}\left[M(Z)(\tau'(X) - \tau(X))\frac{\partial C_{t_\Delta}(Z)}{\partial t_\Delta}\bigg|_{t_\Delta=0} \,\Big|\, Z\right]\right] \\
&= -2\mathbb{E}\left[(\tau'(X) - \tau(X))\frac{\partial C_{t_\Delta}(Z)}{\partial t_\Delta}\bigg|_{t_\Delta=0} \mathbb{E}[M(Z) \mid Z]\right] \\
&= 0.
\end{aligned}$$

For the first term,

$$\begin{aligned}
&-2\mathbb{E}\left[C(Z)(\tau'(X) - \tau(X))\frac{\partial M_{t_\Delta,0}(Z)}{\partial t_\Delta}\bigg|_{t_\Delta=0}\right] \\
&= 2\mathbb{E}\left[C(Z)(\tau'(X) - \tau(X))\left(\frac{\partial A_{t_\Delta}(Z)\nu(X)}{\partial t_\Delta}\bigg|_{t_\Delta=0} + \frac{\partial B_{t_\Delta}(Z)\varsigma(X)}{\partial t_\Delta}\bigg|_{t_\Delta=0}\right.\right. \\
&\left.\left.+ \frac{\partial C_{t_\Delta}(Z)\tau(X)}{\partial t_\Delta}\bigg|_{t_\Delta=0}\right)\right].
\end{aligned}$$

First, we note that

$$\begin{aligned}
&\frac{\partial A_{t_\Delta}(Z)\nu(X)}{\partial t_\Delta}\bigg|_{t_\Delta=0} \\
&= \frac{\partial\left(1 - \frac{(\Delta + t_\Delta(\Delta' - \Delta))^2(X)}{s(X)(1-s(X))t(X)(1-t(X))}\right)^{-1}}{\partial t_\Delta}\Bigg|_{t_\Delta=0}\Bigg(T - t(X) \\
&\quad - \frac{\Delta(X)\big(S - s(X)\big)}{s(X)(1 - s(X))}\Bigg)\nu(X) \\
&\quad + \left(1 - \frac{\Delta^2(X)}{s(X)(1 - s(X))t(X)(1 - t(X))}\right)^{-1} \\
&\quad \cdot \frac{\partial\left(T - t(X) - \frac{(\Delta(X) + t_\Delta(\Delta'(X) - \Delta))\big(S - s(X)\big)}{s(X)(1-s(X))}\right)}{\partial t_\Delta}\Bigg|_{t_\Delta=0}\nu(X) \\
&= f_1(X)A(Z) + f_2(X)f_3(X, S)
\end{aligned}$$

for some function f_1, f_2, f_3. The upshot is that

$$\begin{aligned}
&2\mathbb{E}\left[C(Z)(\tau'(X) - \tau(X))\left(\frac{\partial A_{t_\Delta}(Z)\nu(X)}{\partial t_\Delta}\bigg|_{t_\Delta=0}\right)\right] \\
&= 2\mathbb{E}[C(Z)(\tau'(X) - \tau(X))f_1(X)A(Z)] + 2\mathbb{E}[C(Z)(\tau'(X) - \tau(X)) \\
&\qquad f_2(X)f_3(X, S)] \\
&= 2\mathbb{E}[\mathbb{E}[C(Z)(\tau'(X) - \tau(X))f_1(X)A(Z) \mid X]] \\
&\qquad + 2\mathbb{E}[\mathbb{E}[C(Z)(\tau'(X) - \tau(X))f_2(X)f_3(X, S) \mid X, S]] \\
&= 2\mathbb{E}[(\tau'(X) - \tau(X))f_1(X)\mathbb{E}[C(Z)A(Z) \mid X]] \\
&\qquad + 2\mathbb{E}[(\tau'(X) - \tau(X))f_2(X)f_3(X, S)\mathbb{E}[C(Z) \mid X, S]] \\
&= 0 + 0 = 0
\end{aligned}$$

where the second to the last equality follows from $\mathbb{E}[C(Z) \mid X, S] = 0$ and $\mathbb{E}[C(Z)A(Z) \mid X] = 0$ from Proposition 1.

Following a similar argument, we can show that

$$2\mathbb{E}\left[C(Z)(\tau'(X) - \tau(X))\left(\frac{\partial B_{t_\Delta}(Z)\varsigma(X)}{\partial t_\Delta}\bigg|_{t_\Delta=0}\right)\right] = 0.$$

Note that

$$\begin{aligned}
&\frac{\partial C_{t_\Delta}(Z)\tau(X)}{\partial t_\Delta}\bigg|_{t_\Delta=0} \\
&= -\frac{\partial A_{t_\Delta}(Z)}{\partial t_\Delta}\bigg|_{t_\Delta=0}\left(s(X) + \frac{\Delta(X)}{t(X)}\right) - A(Z)\left(\frac{\Delta'(X) - \Delta(X)}{t(X)}\right)\tau(X) \\
&\quad - \frac{\partial B_{t_\Delta}(Z)}{\partial t_\Delta}\bigg|_{t_\Delta=0}\left(t(X) + \frac{\Delta(X)}{s(X)}\right) - B(Z)\left(\frac{\Delta'(X) - \Delta(X)}{s(X)}\right)\tau(X).
\end{aligned}$$

It's immediate from the previous arguments that

$$2\mathbb{E}\left[C(Z)\left(\frac{\partial B_{t_\Delta}(Z)}{\partial t_\Delta}\bigg|_{t_\Delta=0}\right) \mid X\right] = 0$$

and

$$2\mathbb{E}[C(Z)(\frac{\partial A_{t_\Delta}(Z)}{\partial t_\Delta}\bigg|_{t_\Delta=0}) \mid X] = 0,$$

and from Proposition 1, again we use the fact that and $\mathbb{E}[C(Z)A(Z) \mid X] = 0$ and $\mathbb{E}[C(Z)B(Z) \mid X] = 0$, we then conclude that

$$2\mathbb{E}[C(Z)(\tau'(X) - \tau(X))(\frac{\partial C_{t_\Delta}(Z)\tau(X)}{\partial t_\Delta}\bigg|_{t_\Delta=0}) = 0.$$

We can then conclude

$$D_\Delta D_\tau L(\tau, \{m(x), \nu(x), \varsigma(x), s(x), t(x), \Delta(x)\})[\tau' - \tau, \Delta' - \Delta] = 0.$$

An almost identical derivation can be taken to show that

$$D_s D_\tau L(\tau, \{m(x), \nu(x), \varsigma(x), s(x), t(x), \Delta(x)\})[\tau' - \tau, s' - s] = 0.$$

We have now concluded showing Assumption 2 from Foster and Syrgkanis (2019) holds.

To show Assumption 3 holds, we have

$$\begin{aligned}
&\frac{d^2}{dt_1 t_2}\mathbb{E}[(Y - m(X) - A(Z)\nu(X) - B(Z)\varsigma(X) - C(Z)(\bar{\tau}(X) \\
&\quad + t_1(\tau' - \tau) + t_2(\tau' - \tau)))^2] \\
&= 2C(Z)^2(\tau' - \tau)^2.
\end{aligned}$$

Given $s(X) + \frac{\Delta(X)}{t(X)} = \Omega(\eta)$ and $|A(Z)| = \Omega(\eta)$, etc., we have $C(Z) = \Omega(\eta^2)$. Thus, $\lambda = \Omega(\eta^4)$ and $\kappa = 0$ in Assumption 3.

To show Assumption 4 holds, we can check that

$$\begin{aligned}
&D_m^2 D_\tau L(\tau, \{\bar{m}(x), \nu(x), \varsigma(x), s(x), t(x), \Delta(x)\})[\tau' - \tau, m' - m, m' - m] \\
&= 0.
\end{aligned}$$

$$D_{\nu}^{2} D_{\tau} L(\tau, \{m(x), \bar{\nu}(x), \varsigma(x), s(x), t(x), \Delta(x)\})[\tau' - \tau, \nu' - \nu, \nu' - \nu]$$
$$= 0.$$
$$D_{\varsigma}^{2} D_{\tau} L(\tau, \{m(x), \nu(x), \bar{\varsigma}(x), s(x), t(x), \Delta(x)\})[\tau' - \tau, \varsigma' - \varsigma, \varsigma' - \varsigma] = 0.$$

Finally, we can check that

$$D_{\Delta}^{2} D_{\tau} L(\tau, \{m(x), \nu(x), \varsigma(x), s(x), t(x), \bar{\Delta}(x)\})[\tau' - \tau, \Delta' - \Delta, \Delta' - \Delta]$$
$$= O(M^2/\eta^4) \left\|\tau' - \tau\right\|_{L_2(P)} \left\|\Delta' - \Delta\right\|_{L_2(P)}$$

and this similarly holds when we take derivative with respect to $s(X)$ or $t(X)$. We conclude that $\beta_2 = O(M^2/\eta^4)$ in Assumption 4.

The result then directly follows from Theorem 1 in Foster and Syrgkanis (2019).

Chapter 10

Semiparametric Doubly Robust Targeted Double Machine Learning: A Review

Edward H. Kennedy

10.1 Introduction

In this review, we cover the basics of efficient nonparametric parameter estimation (also called functional estimation), with a focus on parameters that arise in causal inference problems. We review both efficiency bounds (i.e., what is the best possible performance for estimating a given parameter?) and the analysis of particular estimators (i.e., what is this estimator's error, and does it attain the efficiency bound?) under weak assumptions.

We consider the standard setup for functional estimation problems. Namely, we suppose we observe a sample of independent observations $(Z_1, ..., Z_n)$ all identically distributed according to some unknown probability distribution $\mathbb{P}$, which is assumed to lie in some model (i.e., set of distributions) $\mathcal{P}$. Importantly, the goal is *not* to estimate all of $\mathbb{P}$, or even an individual component of $\mathbb{P}$ such as a regression or density function. Instead, the goal is to estimate some structured combination of components, called a *target parameter* or *functional* $\psi : \mathcal{P} \mapsto \mathbb{R}^q$. A functional can be viewed as a map from the model to some space, which we take as the reals for simplicity (we will often focus on $q = 1$, since extensions to the multivariate $q \geq 2$ setup are typically straightforward).

We will see throughout this review that the special structure of functionals, being combinations of components of $\mathbb{P}$, endows this estimation problem with many interesting nuances. For example, fast $\sqrt{n}$ rates of convergence can be achieved in nonparametric models, in stark contrast to the problems of nonparametric regression or density estimation.

By now, there are many reviews and resources available on the topic of parameter estimation in modern flexible nonparametric models, e.g., Bickel et al. (1993), van der Vaart (2000), van der Vaart (2002), van der Laan and Robins (2003), Tsiatis (2006), Kosorok (2008), van der Laan and Rose (2011), Petersen and van der Laan (2014), Kennedy (2016), Chernozhukov et al. (2018), Kennedy (2018), Díaz (2020), and Hines et al. (2022), among others. In this review, we put special emphasis on minimax-style efficiency bounds, worked examples, and practical shortcuts for easing derivations. We gloss over most technical details, in the interest of highlighting important concepts and providing intuition for main ideas.

10.1.1 Notation

We write counterfactual outcomes as Y^a, i.e., the value of Y that would have been observed had we set $A = a$. At times we subscript expectations and other quantities with the distribution under which they are taken, i.e., $\mathbb{E}_P(Y \mid X = x)$ for an expectation under distribution P. When the distribution is clear from context, we sometimes omit subscripts; in general, quantities without subscripts are meant to be taken under some generic P in the model, or else under the true distribution $\mathbb{P}$. We denote convergence in distribution by $\rightsquigarrow$ and convergence in probability by $\xrightarrow{p}$. We use standard big-oh and little-oh notation, i.e., $X_n = O_{\mathbb{P}}(r_n)$ means X_n/r_n is bounded in probability and $X_n = o_{\mathbb{P}}(r_n)$ means $X_n/r_n \xrightarrow{p} 0$. To ease

DOI: 10.1201/9781003216223-10

notation we sometimes omit arguments for functions of multiple arguments, e.g., $\varphi = \varphi(z; P)$ when the arguments are clear or secondary to the discussion. We use $\mathbb{P}_n$ to denote the empirical measure so that sample averages are written as $\mathbb{P}_n(f) = \mathbb{P}_n\{f(Z)\} = \frac{1}{n}\sum_i f(Z_i)$. For a possibly random function $\widehat{f}$, we similarly write $\mathbb{P}(\widehat{f}) = \mathbb{P}\{\widehat{f}(Z)\} = \int \widehat{f}(z)\, d\mathbb{P}(z)$, and we let $\|\widehat{f}\|^2 = \int \widehat{f}(z)^2\, d\mathbb{P}(z)$ denote the squared $L_2(\mathbb{P})$ norm.

10.2 Setup: Target Parameters & Model Assumptions

10.2.1 Examples of Functionals

Here we give a list of examples of functionals, some of which arise from causal inference problems, and some of which do not. Many (but certainly not all) functionals in causal inference and missing data take the form of regression functions averaged over covariate distributions.

Example 1. (Regression function) Suppose $Z = (X, Y)$. The regression of Y on X is given by $\psi = \psi(x) = \mathbb{E}(Y \mid X = x)$.

Example 2. (Average treatment effect) Suppose $Z = (X, A, Y)$ for confounders X, treatment A, and outcome Y. Then under causal positivity, consistency, and no unmeasured confounding assumptions, the mean outcome if all in the population were treated at level $A = a$ is identified as the expected regression function

$$\psi = \mathbb{E}(Y^a) = \mathbb{E}\{\mathbb{E}(Y \mid X, A = a)\},$$

where we use the convention $\mathbb{E}(Y \mid X, A = a) \equiv \mu_a(X)$ for $\mu_a(x) = \mathbb{E}(Y \mid X = x, A = a)$, so the outer expectation in the above is over the marginal distribution of X. Corresponding contrasts are identified as $\mathbb{E}(Y^1 - Y^0) = \mathbb{E}\{\mathbb{E}(Y \mid X, A = 1) - \mathbb{E}(Y \mid X, A = 0)\}$, for example.

Remark 2 (Identifying Assumptions). Since the focus of this work is on statistical estimation and inference, rather than identification, we only briefly mention causal identifying assumptions, as in the previous example. The discussion in subsequent sections holds for the parameters of interest defined purely in statistical terms, regardless of whether the causal assumptions hold (excepting statistical assumptions like positivity, which we also mostly gloss over).

Example 3. (Mean missing outcome) Suppose $Z = (X, A, AY)$ for covariates X, missing indicator A, and outcome Y (which is only observed when $A = 1$). Then under positivity and missing at random assumptions, the mean outcome in the population is identified as the expected regression function

$$\psi = \mathbb{E}(Y) = \mathbb{E}\{\mathbb{E}(Y \mid X, A = 1)\}.$$

This is mathematically equivalent to the mean outcome if all were treated at level $A = 1$ from the previous example, and so statistical methods are identical.

Example 4. (Variance-weighted treatment effect) Suppose $Z = (X, A, Y)$ for confounders X, treatment A, and outcome Y. Then under causal positivity, consistency, and no unmeasured confounding assumptions, a variance-weighted average treatment effect is identified as

$$\psi = \mathbb{E}\{w(X)\mathbb{E}(Y^1 - Y^0 \mid X)\} = \frac{\mathbb{E}\{\text{cov}(A, Y \mid X)\}}{\mathbb{E}\{\text{var}(A \mid X)\}}$$

for weights $w(X) = \text{var}(A \mid X)/\mathbb{E}\{\text{var}(A \mid X)\}$ (Robins et al., 2008; Li et al., 2011).

Example 5. (Stochastic intervention effect) Suppose $Z = (X, A, Y)$ for confounders X, treatment A, and outcome Y. Then under positivity, consistency, and no unmeasured confounding assumptions, the mean outcome if treatments were sampled as $A \sim dG(a \mid x)$ for everyone in the population is identified as

$$\psi = \mathbb{E}\{\mathbb{E}(Y \mid X, A^*)\} = \int\int \mathbb{E}(Y \mid X = x, A = a)\; dG(a \mid x)\; d\mathbb{P}(x).$$

We refer to Díaz and van der Laan (2012); Haneuse and Rotnitzky (2013); Young et al. (2014), and Kennedy (2019) for further discussion.

Example 6. (Instrumental variable effects) Suppose $Z = (X, R, A, Y)$ for confounders X, instrumental variable (IV) R, treatment A, and outcome Y. Then under positivity, consistency, IV-unconfoundedness, exclusion, instrumentation, and monotonicity assumptions, the average treatment effect among compliers with $A^{r=1} > A^{r=0}$ is given by

$$\begin{aligned}\psi &= \mathbb{E}(Y^{a=1} - Y^{a=0} \mid A^{r=1} > A^{r=0}) \\ &= \frac{\mathbb{E}\{\mathbb{E}(Y \mid X, R = 1) - \mathbb{E}(Y \mid X, R = 0)\}}{\mathbb{E}\{\mathbb{E}(A \mid X, R = 1) - \mathbb{E}(A \mid X, R = 0)\}}.\end{aligned}$$

Replacing monotonicity with an effect homogeneity assumption, the same statistical functional instead represents an effect on the treated (Ogburn et al., 2015). Under a different effect homogeneity assumption, the related but different ratio estimand

$$\psi = \mathbb{E}\left\{\frac{\mathbb{E}(Y \mid X, R = 1) - \mathbb{E}(Y \mid X, R = 0)}{\mathbb{E}(A \mid X, R = 1) - \mathbb{E}(A \mid X, R = 0)}\right\}$$

identifies the average treatment effect (Wang and Tchetgen Tchetgen, 2018).

Example 7. (Time-varying treatment effects) Suppose $Z = (X_1, A_1, ..., X_t, A_t, ..., X_T, A_T, Y)$ for time-varying confounders X_t, treatments A_t, and final outcome Y. Then under consistency, with sequential versions of positivity and no unmeasured confounding assumptions, the mean outcome if all in the population followed the treatment sequence $\overline{a}_T = (a_1, ..., a_T)$ is identified as

$$\psi = \mathbb{E}(Y^{\overline{a}_T}) = \int \cdots \int \mathbb{E}(Y \mid \overline{X}_T = \overline{x}_T, \overline{A}_T = \overline{a}_T) \prod_{t=1}^{T} d\mathbb{P}(x_t \mid \overline{x}_{t-1}, \overline{a}_{t-1}).$$

This is known as Robins' g-formula (Robins, 1986; Robins and Hernán, 2009; van der Laan and Robins, 2003). The projection of this quantity (as a function of $\overline{a}_T$) onto an approximating *marginal structural model* $g(\overline{a}_T; \beta)$ is given by

$$\psi = \arg\min_{\beta \in \mathbb{R}^p} \int w(\overline{a}_T)\Big\{\mathbb{E}(Y^{\overline{a}_T}) - g(\overline{a}_T; \beta)\Big\}^2\, d\nu(\overline{a}_T)$$

where $\mathbb{E}(Y^{\overline{a}_T})$ is identified via the expression above, w is a specified weight function and ν is a dominating measure for the distribution of $\overline{A}_T$.

Example 8. (Mediation effects) Suppose $Z = (X, A, M, Y)$ for confounders X, treatment A, mediator M, and outcome Y. Then under positivity, consistency, and no unmeasured confounding assumptions for (A, M), the controlled direct effect of treatment A, keeping the mediator fixed at $M = m$, is identified by

$$\begin{aligned}\mathbb{E}(Y^{a,m} - Y^{a',m}) = \mathbb{E}\{&\mathbb{E}(Y \mid X, A = a, M = m) \\ &- \mathbb{E}(Y \mid X, A = a', M = m)\}.\end{aligned}$$

Indirect effects can be identified analogously (Pearl, 2009; Imai et al., 2010; Tchetgen Tchetgen and Shpitser, 2012). The natural direct effect of treatment, when the mediator is set to what it would have been under $A = a$, is identified by

$$\begin{aligned}\mathbb{E}(Y^{a,M^a} - Y^{a',M^a}) &= \mathbb{E}\{\mathbb{E}(Y \mid X, A = a, M = m) \\ &\quad - \mathbb{E}\int \mathbb{E}(Y \mid X, A = a', M = m)\, d\mathbb{P}(m \mid X, A = a).\end{aligned}$$

with indirect effects again identified similarly. Natural mediation effects require weaker positivity assumptions than controlled effects.

Example 9. (Treatment effect bounds) Suppose $Z = (X, A, Y)$ for confounders X, treatment A, and outcome Y. Then under consistency and positivity assumptions, the average treatment effect is bounded within

$$\psi = [\psi_\ell, \psi_u] = \mathbb{E}\{\mathbb{E}(Y \mid X, A = a)\} \pm \delta\mathbb{P}(A \neq a)$$

as long as $|\mathbb{E}(Y^a \mid X, A = a) - \mathbb{E}(Y^a \mid X, A \neq a)| \leq \delta$ (note this is weaker than no unmeasured confounding, which implies $\delta = 0$) (Richardson et al., 2014; Luedtke et al., 2015).

Example 10. (Expected density) Let Z have density p. Then the expected density is

$$\psi = \mathbb{E}\{p(Z)\} = \int p(z)^2\, dz.$$

This functional is a staple of the classical functional estimation literature and arises in tuning parameter selection in density estimation (Bickel and Ritov, 1988; Birgé and Massart, 1995).

Example 11. (Entropy) Let Z have density p. Then the entropy is

$$\psi = -\int p(z) \log p(z)\, dz = -\mathbb{E}\{\log p(Z)\}.$$

Example 12. (f-divergence) Let $Z = (A, Y)$ for $A \in \{0, 1\}$ a group indicator and Y a random variable with conditional density $p(y \mid a)$. Then the f-divergence of $p(y \mid a = 1)$ from $p(y \mid a = 0)$ is

$$\psi = \int f\left(\frac{p(y \mid a = 1)}{p(y \mid a = 0)}\right) p(y \mid a = 0)\, dy$$

for a known function f. Particular choices of f yield Kullback-Leibler, Hellinger, total variation, and χ^2 distances, for example (Kandasamy et al., 2015).

10.2.2 Model Assumptions

Recall from Section 10.1 that the distribution $\mathbb{P}$ from which we sample is assumed to lie in a model, i.e., a set of distributions $\mathcal{P}$. In this review we focus on nonparametric models; in Section 10.3 we typically take $\mathcal{P}$ to be the simplest nonparametric model, consisting of all probability distributions on the sample space, while in Section 10.4 we introduce models with smoothness or sparsity. We focus on nonparametric rather than semiparametric models mostly for simplicity; many ideas extend to the more restricted semiparametric case, and we refer to Bickel et al. (1993), van der Laan and Robins (2003), and Tsiatis (2006) for more details there. As noted in Remark 2, we only briefly mention identifying assumptions, despite their importance, since the focus of this review is on the statistical aspects of causal inference, post-identification.

10.3 Benchmarks: Nonparametric Efficiency Bounds

After having selected an appropriate target parameter ψ matching the scientific question of interest, identifying (or bounding) it under appropriate causal or other assumptions, and laying out a statistical model $\mathcal{P}$ (which in our case will be nonparametric), a next line of business is to understand *lower bounds* or *benchmarks* for estimation error. In other words, how well can we possibly hope to estimate the parameter ψ over the model $\mathcal{P}$? This is important both theoretically, as a fundamental measure of the statistical difficulty of estimating ψ, as well as practically, since it helps tell us whether a particular method is optimally efficient, making the best use of the data (if not, one may need to search for better, more efficient methods). Note there are two parts to showing optimality: (i) that no estimator can do better than some benchmark, and (ii) that a particular estimator does in fact attain that benchmark. Part (i) is discussed in this section, and part (ii) in the next section.

A classic benchmarking or lower bound result for smooth parametric models is the Cramer-Rao bound (Casella and Berger, 2001; van der Vaart, 2002). In its simplest form, this result states that for smooth parametric models $\mathcal{P} = \{P_\theta : \theta \in \mathbb{R}\}$ and smooth functionals (i.e., with P_θ and $\psi(\theta)$ differentiable in θ), the variance of *any* unbiased estimator $\widehat{\psi}$ must satisfy

$$\text{var}_\theta(\widehat{\psi}) \geq \frac{\psi'(\theta)^2}{\text{var}_\theta\{s_\theta(Z)\}}, \tag{10.1}$$

where $s_\theta(z) = \frac{\partial}{\partial\theta} \log p_\theta(z)$ is the score function, i.e., no unbiased estimator can have a smaller variance than the above ratio. A standard way to benchmark estimation error more generally is through minimax lower bounds of the form

$$\inf_{\widehat{\psi}} \sup_{P \in \mathcal{P}} \mathbb{E}_P\left[\{\widehat{\psi} - \psi(P)\}^2\right] \geq R_n. \tag{10.2}$$

These kinds of lower bounds say that the risk for estimating ψ (in this case, in terms of worst-case mean squared error), over the model $\mathcal{P}$, cannot be smaller than R_n. For example, when $\psi(P)$ is a density or regression function and $\mathcal{P}$ is the class of all s-smooth Hölder densities, then $R_n = Cn^{-1/(1+d/2s)}$ (Tsybakov, 2009).

Indeed the Cramer-Rao bound (10.1) also acts as a benchmark in a more general minimax sense. In fact, for smooth parametric models, one can go beyond the global lower bounds of the form (10.2) and say something about more nuanced local minimax behavior. This is illustrated in the following theorem.

Theorem 1 (Theorem 8.11, van der Vaart (2000)). Assume P_θ is differentiable in quadratic mean at θ with nonsingular Fisher information $I_\theta = \text{var}_\theta\{s_\theta(Z)\}$. If $\psi(\theta)$ is differentiable at θ, with $\psi'(\theta) = \frac{\partial}{\partial\theta}\psi(\theta)$, then for any estimator $\widehat{\psi}$ it follows that

$$\inf_{\delta>0} \liminf_{n\to\infty} \sup_{\|\theta'-\theta\|<\delta} n\, \mathbb{E}_{\theta'}\left[\{\widehat{\psi} - \psi(\theta')\}^2\right] \geq \psi'(\theta)\text{var}_\theta\{s_\theta(Z)\}^{-1}\psi'(\theta)^{\mathrm{T}}.$$

Intuitively, Theorem 1 says the (asymptotic, worst-case) mean squared error cannot be smaller than $\psi'(\theta)^2/n\text{var}_\theta\{s_\theta(Z)\}$, for any estimator $\widehat{\psi}$ in a smooth parametric model.

Thus optimality in the above local asymptotic minimax sense is somewhat settled for *smooth parametric models*. However, what if anything does this say about larger semi- or nonparametric models? Can the above Cramer-Rao bounds be exploited to construct lower bound benchmarks there as well? These questions will be answered in the following subsection.

10.3.1 Parametric Submodels

The standard way to connect classic Cramer-Rao bounds for parametric models to larger more complicated nonparametric models is through a technical device called the *parametric submodel* (Stein, 1956). We first give a definition, then describe high-level ideas and give some examples.

Definition 1. A *parametric submodel* is a smooth parametric model $\mathcal{P}_\epsilon = \{P_\epsilon : \epsilon \in \mathbb{R}\}$ that satisfies (i) $\mathcal{P}_\epsilon \subseteq \mathcal{P}$, and (ii) $P_{\epsilon=0} = \mathbb{P}$.

Thus, in other words, a parametric submodel is a parametric model that (i) is contained in the larger model $\mathcal{P}$ of interest, and (ii) equals the true distribution at $\epsilon = 0$, i.e., contains the truth $\mathbb{P}$. It is important to recognize that a parametric submodel is a technical device used to extend theory from parametric to nonparametric models, and not a tool for data analysis (Tsiatis, 2006); in particular, to ensure that property (ii) $P_{\epsilon=0} = \mathbb{P}$ holds, parametric submodels must depend on the true distribution $\mathbb{P}$, which is of course unknown.

The high-level idea behind using submodels is that it is never harder to estimate a parameter over a *smaller* model, relative to a larger one in which the smaller model is contained. So any lower bound for a submodel will also be a valid lower bound for the larger model $\mathcal{P}$. Of course, valid but vacuous lower bounds are easy to construct (e.g., the mean squared error can be no less than zero), so in the next section we will also have to show that these bounds are *relevant*, in the sense that they can actually be attained under some plausible conditions.

It turns out that, for the purposes of constructing lower-bound benchmarks for functional estimation, it often suffices to use one-dimensional parametric submodels. A common choice of submodel for nonparametric $\mathcal{P}$ is, for some mean-zero function $h : \mathcal{Z} \to \mathbb{R}$,

$$p_\epsilon(z) = d\mathbb{P}(z)\{1 + \epsilon h(z)\} \tag{10.3}$$

where $\|h\|_\infty \leq M < \infty$ and $\epsilon < 1/M$ so that $p_\epsilon(z) \geq 0$. Note for this submodel the score function is $\frac{\partial}{\partial\epsilon} \log p_\epsilon(z)|_{\epsilon=0} = \frac{\partial}{\partial\epsilon} \log\{1 + \epsilon h(z)\}|_{\epsilon=0} = h(z)$. Therefore the Cramer-Rao lower bound for some P_ϵ in the example one-dimensional submodel $\mathcal{P}_\epsilon$ above is given by

$$\frac{\psi'(P_\epsilon)^2}{\text{var}_{P_\epsilon}\{s_\epsilon(Z)\}} = \frac{\frac{\partial}{\partial\epsilon}\psi(P_\epsilon)|_{\epsilon=0}}{\mathbb{E}_{P_\epsilon}\{h(Z)^2\}}.$$

Other examples of submodels can be found in Section 4.2 of (Tsiatis, 2006), for example.

Since any lower bound for the submodel $\mathcal{P}_\epsilon$ is also a lower bound for $\mathcal{P}$, the best and most informative is the *greatest* such lower bound. Can we say anything about the best such as lower bound for generic functionals and/or submodels? The next two subsections consider this question.

10.3.2 Pathwise Differentiability

Recall the Cramer-Rao bound

$$\frac{\frac{\partial}{\partial\epsilon}\psi(P_\epsilon)|_{\epsilon=0}}{\mathbb{E}_{P_\epsilon}\{s_\epsilon(Z)^2\}} \tag{10.4}$$

for submodel $\mathcal{P}_\epsilon$ described in the previous subsection. To find the best such lower bound, we would like to optimize the above over all P_ϵ in some submodel. It is not a priori clear how generally this can be accomplished since different functionals ψ could yield very different numerators. Therefore let us first consider what we can say about the derivative in the numerator of (10.4), for a large class of *pathwise differentiable* functionals.

Namely, suppose the functional $\psi : \mathcal{P} \mapsto \mathbb{R}$ is smooth, as a map from distributions to the reals, in the sense that it admits a kind of *distributional Taylor expansion*

$$\psi(\overline{P}) - \psi(P) = \int \varphi(z;\overline{P})\, d(\overline{P} - P)(z) + R_2(\overline{P}, P) \tag{10.5}$$

for distributions $\overline{P}$ and P, often called a *von Mises expansion*, where $\varphi(z;P)$ is a mean-zero, finite-variance function satisfying $\int \varphi(z;P)\, dP(z) = 0$ and $\int \varphi(z;P)^2\, dP(z) < \infty$, and $R_2(\overline{P}, P)$ is a *second-order remainder* term (which means it only depends on *products* or *squares* of differences between $\overline{P}$ and P).

Intuitively, the von Mises expansion above is just an infinite-dimensional or distributional analog of a Taylor expansion, with $\varphi(z;Q)$ acting as a usual derivative term; it describes how the functional ψ changes locally when the distribution changes from P to $\overline{P}$. For example, when $Z \in \{1, ..., k\}$ is discrete and so $\overline{P}$ and P have k countable components, the von Mises expansion reduces to a standard multivariate Taylor expansion with

$$R_2(\overline{P}, P) = \psi(\overline{p}_1, ..., \overline{p}_k) - \psi(p_1, ..., p_k) - \sum_j \frac{\partial}{\partial t_j}\psi(t_1, ..., t_k)\Big|_{t=\overline{p}} (\overline{p}_j - p_j).$$

We refer to Fisher and Kennedy (2021) for more intuition and visual illustrations.

Remark 3. The von Mises terminology comes from, e.g., von Mises (1947), and has been used by Fernholz (1983), van der Vaart (2000), Robins et al. (2009), Kandasamy et al. (2015), among others. The function $\varphi(z;P)$ has been referred to as an influence function, pathwise derivative, gradient, and Neyman orthogonal score (Pfanzagl, 1982; Bickel et al., 1993; Newey, 1994; Tsiatis, 2006; van der Laan and Robins, 2003; Chernozhukov et al., 2018). However it can be important to distinguish between the influence function for a *parameter*, as in (10.5), and the influence function for an *estimator*; this point will be discussed in more detail in the next section. To distinguish between the two, we typically refer to the influence function for a parameter as in (10.5) as an *influence curve*. Note that for now, the expansion (10.5) is only a smoothness property of the functional $\psi : \mathcal{P} \mapsto \mathbb{R}$, and has nothing to do yet with any data or estimation procedure.

Many important functionals satisfy the expansion (10.5); we detail a few in the following examples.

Example 2 (continuing from p. 208). The average treatment effect or missing outcome functional

$$\psi(P) = \mathbb{E}_P\{\mathbb{E}_P(Y \mid X, A = 1)\}$$

satisfies (10.5) with

$$\varphi(Z;P) = \frac{\mathbb{1}(A=1)}{P(A=1 \mid X)}\Big\{Y - \mathbb{E}_P(Y \mid X, A=1)\Big\} + \mathbb{E}_P(Y \mid X, A=1) - \psi(P)$$

and

$$R_2(\overline{P}, P) = \int \left\{\frac{1}{\overline{\pi}(x)} - \frac{1}{\pi(x)}\right\}\Big\{\mu(x) - \overline{\mu}(x)\Big\}\pi(x)\, dP(x)$$

where $\pi(x) = P(A = 1 \mid X = x)$ and $\overline{\pi}(x) = \overline{P}(A = 1 \mid X = x)$, and similarly for $\mu(x) = \mathbb{E}_P(Y \mid X = x, A = 1)$.

Example 4 (continuing from p. 208). The expected conditional covariance functional

$$\psi(P) = \mathbb{E}_P\{\text{cov}_P(A, Y \mid X)\}$$

satisfies (10.5) with

$$\varphi(Z; P) = \Big\{A - \mathbb{E}_P(A \mid X)\Big\}\Big\{Y - \mathbb{E}_P(Y \mid X)\Big\} - \psi(P)$$

and

$$R_2(\overline{P}, P) = \int \Big\{\overline{\pi}(x) - \pi(x)\Big\}\Big\{\overline{\mu}(x) - \mu(x)\Big\}\, dP(x)$$

where $\pi(x) = \mathbb{E}_P(A \mid X = x)$ and $\mu(x) = \mathbb{E}_P(Y \mid X = x)$, with $\overline{\pi}$ and $\overline{\mu}$ corresponding versions under $\overline{P}$.

Example 10 (continuing from p. 210). The expected density functional

$$\psi(P) = \mathbb{E}_P\{p(Z)\} = \int p(z)^2\, dz$$

satisfies (10.5) with

$$\varphi(Z; P) = 2\Big\{p(Z) - \psi(P)\Big\}$$

and

$$R_2(\overline{P}, P) = -\int \Big\{\overline{p}(z) - p(z)\Big\}^2\, dz.$$

A related notion of smoothness is *pathwise differentiability*, i.e., that

$$\frac{\partial}{\partial \epsilon}\psi(P_\epsilon)\Big|_{\epsilon=0} = \int \varphi(z; \mathbb{P}) s_\epsilon(z)\, d\mathbb{P}(z) \tag{10.6}$$

for every smooth submodel P_ϵ. This is implied by the von Mises expansion (10.5), under regularity conditions, by taking $(P, Q) = (P_\epsilon, P)$, differentiating both sides and noting that R_2 being second-order means

$$\frac{\partial}{\partial \epsilon} R_2(P, P_\epsilon)\Big|_{\epsilon=0} = 0.$$

For more details, see for example Lemma 2 of Kennedy et al. (2021); the above condition is essentially equivalent to what Chernozhukov et al. (2018) refer to as Neyman orthogonality. Pathwise differentiability (10.6), and the von Mises expansion (10.5) more generally, play key roles in both deriving lower bound benchmarks (via the *efficient influence function*) and constructing estimators that attain the benchmark. We will continue exploring this first role in the following subsection.

10.3.3 The Best Lower Bound & Efficient Influence Function

Armed with the smoothness of our functional ψ, as characterized by the von Mises expansion (10.5) and related pathwise differentiability (10.6), we now have enough to characterize the greatest lower bound for generic smooth parametric submodels.

For simplicity consider the particular submodel in (10.3); it turns out this class of submodel is often sufficient to yield relevant (attainable) lower bounds. For this submodel, the score is $s_\epsilon(z) = h(z)$ and by pathwise differentiability we have

$$\frac{\partial}{\partial \epsilon}\psi(P_\epsilon)\Big|_{\epsilon=0} = \int \varphi(z; \mathbb{P}) h(z)\, d\mathbb{P}(z).$$

Therefore over all Cramer-Rao bounds at $\epsilon = 0$ we have

$$\sup_{P_\epsilon} \frac{\psi'(P_\epsilon)^2}{\text{var}\{s_\epsilon(Z)\}} = \sup_h \frac{\mathbb{E}\{\varphi(Z;\mathbb{P})h(Z)\}^2}{\mathbb{E}\{h(Z)^2\}} \leq \mathbb{E}\{\varphi(Z;\mathbb{P})^2\} = \text{var}\{\varphi(Z)\}$$

where the first equality followed by pathwise differentiability and the form of the submodel, and the inequality by Cauchy-Schwarz. The fact that the greatest lower bound is not just bounded above by $\mathbb{E}(\varphi^2) = \text{var}(\varphi)$, but that this upper bound is actually attained follows from the fact that, for one of the submodels we can take $h(z) = \varphi(z;\mathbb{P})$, as long as φ is in the tangent space (i.e., closure of submodel score space). We refer to Lemma 25.19 of van der Vaart (2000) for more details and discussion.

Remark 4. Recall in this review we are mostly focusing on proper nonparametric models, where the tangent space is the whole Hilbert space of mean-zero, finite-variance functions (see Theorem 4.4 of Tsiatis (2006)); in that case (10.5) only holds for at most one influence curve φ, which must also be a valid score. However, in proper semiparametric models with a restricted tangent space, the expansion (10.5) can hold for potentially many influence curves φ, and then the one that is also a valid score is called the *efficient influence function*. In contrast, in nonparametric models, there is only one influence curve, and that influence curve is also the efficient influence function.

Therefore the variance of the efficient influence function

$$\text{var}\{\varphi(Z;\mathbb{P})\} \tag{10.7}$$

acts as a nonparametric analog of the Cramer-Rao bound. This is critically important, as it implies no estimator can have a smaller mean squared error than (10.7), in a local asymptotic minimax sense. In particular, if we can show for a particular estimator $\widehat{\psi}$ that

$$\sqrt{n}(\widehat{\psi} - \psi) \rightsquigarrow N\Big(0, \text{var}\{\varphi(Z)\}\Big)$$

then we can say the estimator attains the nonparametric efficiency bound. This local asymptotic minimaxity can be formalized as in the following result, for example.

Theorem 2 (Corollary 2.6, van der Vaart (2002)). Let $\psi : \mathcal{P} \mapsto \mathbb{R}$ be pathwise differentiable with efficient influence function φ. Assume the model is nonparametric or the tangent space is a convex cone. Then

$$\inf_{\delta>0} \liminf_{n\to\infty} \sup_{\text{TV}(P,Q)<\delta} n\, \mathbb{E}_Q\Big[\{\widehat{\psi} - \psi(Q)\}^2\Big] \geq \text{var}\{\varphi(Z;P)\}$$

for any estimator sequence $\widehat{\psi} = \widehat{\psi}_n$.

10.3.4 Deriving Influence Functions

In the previous section we showed the crucial importance of the von Mises expansion (10.5), whose derivative term (i.e., influence curve) is the efficient influence function in nonparametric models, and thus the key component of local minimax lower bounds for functional estimation. Further, the efficient influence function not yields efficiency bounds, but also indicates how to construct efficient estimators and sheds light on the conditions required for such estimators to be efficient (these latter points will be discussed shortly, in the next section). In the last subsection we gave some examples of functionals for which the expansion holds, with particular influence curves and remainder terms, but it may not be clear how to derive these expansions from scratch. This is the main topic of this subsection.

There are several ways to derive influence curves. The most general approach is to explicitly compute the pathwise derivative $\psi'(P_\epsilon)$ for appropriate submodels, set this equal to the right-hand-side of the pathwise differentiability equation (10.6), and solve for the influence curve φ. In the following example we show how this works in two simple cases, for regression functions with discrete X and the expected density.

Example 1 (continuing from p. 208). Consider the regression function $\mathbb{E}(Y \mid X = x)$. Here we will show that

$$\varphi(z;P) = \frac{\mathbb{1}(X = x)}{P(X = x)}\Big\{Y - \mathbb{E}_P(Y \mid X = x)\Big\}$$

is the efficient influence function when X is discrete, by showing that (10.6) holds for this choice of φ. Let $s_\epsilon(z) = \frac{\partial}{\partial\epsilon}\log dP_\epsilon(z)|_{\epsilon=0}$ denote the submodel score, and note

$$\begin{aligned}
\mathbb{E}\{s(Z) \mid X = x\} &= \int \frac{\partial}{\partial\epsilon}\log dP_\epsilon(z)\Big|_{\epsilon=0} d\mathbb{P}(y \mid x) \\
&= \int \frac{\partial}{\partial\epsilon}\log\Big\{P_\epsilon(X = x)dP_\epsilon(y \mid x)\Big\}\Big|_{\epsilon=0} d\mathbb{P}(y \mid x) \\
&= \int \Big\{\frac{\partial}{\partial\epsilon}\log P_\epsilon(X = x)\Big|_{\epsilon=0} \\
&\qquad + \frac{\partial}{\partial\epsilon}\log dP_\epsilon(y \mid x)\Big|_{\epsilon=0}\Big\} d\mathbb{P}(y \mid x) \\
&= \frac{\partial}{\partial\epsilon}\log P_\epsilon(X = x)\Big|_{\epsilon=0}
\end{aligned}$$

where the last equality uses the facts that $\int d\mathbb{P}(y \mid x) = 1$ and that scores have mean zero, i.e.,

$$\begin{aligned}
\int \frac{\partial}{\partial\epsilon}\log dP_\epsilon(y \mid x)\Big|_{\epsilon=0} d\mathbb{P}(y \mid x) &= \int \frac{\frac{\partial}{\partial\epsilon}dP_\epsilon(y \mid x)\mid_{\epsilon=0}}{d\mathbb{P}(y \mid x)} d\mathbb{P}(y \mid x) \\
&= \int \frac{\partial}{\partial\epsilon}dP_\epsilon(y \mid x)\Big|_{\epsilon=0} \\
&= \frac{\partial}{\partial\epsilon}\int dP_\epsilon(y \mid x)\Big|_{\epsilon=0} = 0
\end{aligned}$$

where the first equality used the fact that $\frac{\partial}{\partial\epsilon}\log dP_\epsilon(y \mid x) = \frac{\partial}{\partial\epsilon}dP_\epsilon(y \mid x)/dP_\epsilon(y \mid x)$. Thus in this case the pathwise derivative on the left-hand side of (10.6) is

$$\begin{aligned}
\frac{\partial}{\partial\epsilon}\int y\, dP_\epsilon(y \mid x)\Big|_{\epsilon=0} &= \int y\Big\{\frac{\partial}{\partial\epsilon}\log dP_\epsilon(y \mid x)\Big\}\Big|_{\epsilon=0} d\mathbb{P}(y \mid x) \\
&= \int y\Big\{\frac{\partial}{\partial\epsilon}\log\frac{dP_\epsilon(z)}{P_\epsilon(X = x)}\Big\}\Big|_{\epsilon=0} d\mathbb{P}(y \mid x) \\
&= \int y\Big\{\frac{\partial}{\partial\epsilon}\log dP_\epsilon(z) \\
&\qquad - \frac{\partial}{\partial\epsilon}\log P_\epsilon(X = x)\Big\}\Big|_{\epsilon=0} dP_\epsilon(y \mid x) \\
&= \mathbb{E}\{Y s_\epsilon(Z) \mid X = x\} - \mathbb{E}\{s_\epsilon(Z) \mid X = x\} \\
&\qquad \times \mathbb{E}(Y \mid X = x).
\end{aligned}$$

where the first equality holds as long as we can exchange integrals and derivatives and since $P_{\epsilon=0} = \mathbb{P}$. Now for the right-hand side of (10.6) we have

$$\begin{aligned}\int \varphi(z;\mathbb{P}) s_\epsilon(z)\, d\mathbb{P}(z) &= \mathbb{E}\left[\frac{\mathbb{1}(X=x)}{\mathbb{P}(X=x)}\Big\{Y - \mathbb{E}(Y \mid X=x)\Big\} s_\epsilon(Z)\right] \\ &= \mathbb{E}\{Y s_\epsilon(Z) \mid X=x\} - \mathbb{E}\{s_\epsilon(Z) \mid X=x\} \\ &\qquad \times \mathbb{E}(Y \mid X=x)\end{aligned}$$

by iterated expectation. This yields the result.

Example 10 (continuing from p. 210). Let p_0 denote the density of $\mathbb{P}$. Under regularity conditions, the pathwise derivative for the expected density functional is given by

$$\begin{aligned}\frac{\partial}{\partial\epsilon}\int p_\epsilon(z)^2\, dz\,\Big|_{\epsilon=0} &= \int \frac{\partial}{\partial\epsilon} p_\epsilon(z)^2\, dz\,\Big|_{\epsilon=0} \\ &= \int 2p_\epsilon(z)\frac{\partial}{\partial\epsilon}p_\epsilon(z)\, dz\,\Big|_{\epsilon=0} \\ &= \int 2p_\epsilon(z)\left\{\frac{\partial}{\partial\epsilon}\log p_\epsilon(z)\right\} p_\epsilon(z)\, dz\,\Big|_{\epsilon=0} \\ &= \int \Big\{2p_0(z) - \psi(\mathbb{P})\Big\}\left\{\frac{\partial}{\partial\epsilon}\log p_\epsilon(z)\right\}\Big|_{\epsilon=0} p_0(z)\, dz\end{aligned}$$

where the first equality holds as long as we can exchange integrals and derivatives, the second by the chain rule, the third since $\frac{\partial}{\partial\epsilon}\log p_\epsilon(z) = \frac{\partial}{\partial\epsilon}p_\epsilon(z)/p_\epsilon(z)$, and the last since the score function $s_\epsilon(z) = \frac{\partial}{\partial\epsilon}\log p_\epsilon(z)|_{\epsilon=0}$ has mean zero so that subtracting ψ times the mean does not change the expression. Now equating the above with the right-hand side of (10.6) shows that $2p(z) - \psi$ is the efficient influence function for the expected density.

10.3.4.1 Two Simple Strategies

As was seen above, even for two very simple functionals, the previously described general approach is somewhat indirect and non-constructive. For the mean, we had a putative efficient influence function at our disposal, which may not always be the case, and for the expected density we had to solve an integral equation (which was straightforward in that case but can be complicated in general). Luckily there are some tricks for making influence function derivations easier and less time-consuming. We will give two strategies that build off of each other and can both be useful:

1. Compute Gateaux derivatives assuming data are discrete.
2. Use derivative rules with simple influence functions as building blocks.

The first strategy is somewhat commonplace and has been used and detailed for example in Kandasamy et al. (2015) and Hines et al. (2022), for example. We have not seen the second strategy described in the literature.

The first step in both strategies is to initially pretend that the data are discrete. This eases calculations and allows for direct computation rather than solving integral equations, while typically still leading to influence functions that are valid in the general continuous or mixed case. The latter can always be verified by checking the general integral version of the pathwise differentiability condition (10.6), for a putative influence function computed by potentially ad hoc means. Ichimura and Newey (2022) show that similar calculations can be used in the general case by replacing indicators with kernels indexed by a bandwidth converging to zero; however, dealing with indicators eases notation so we use that approach here.

10.3.4.2 Strategy 1

After reducing to discrete data, the first strategy is to compute the Gateax derivative of the parameter in the direction of a point mass contamination. Specifically, letting $\delta_z = \mathbb{1}(Z = z)$ denote the Dirac measure at $Z = z$, one computes the Gateaux derivative

$$\frac{\partial}{\partial \epsilon}\psi\{(1-\epsilon)d\mathbb{P}(z) + \epsilon\delta_{z'}\}\Big|_{\epsilon=0}$$

which equals the influence function $\varphi(z'; P)$. This approach is based on computing the pathwise derivative described in the previous section, but at a special submodel of the form $(1-\epsilon)d\mathbb{P}(z) + \epsilon\delta_{z'}$, for which the right-hand side of (10.6) happens to equal the influence function itself, rather than its covariance with the score. The reason the latter is true is because the score for this submodel is

$$\frac{\partial}{\partial \epsilon}\log\Big\{(1-\epsilon)d\mathbb{P}(z) + \epsilon\delta_{z'}\Big\}\Big|_{\epsilon=0} = \frac{\delta_{z'} - d\mathbb{P}(z)}{(1-\epsilon)d\mathbb{P}(z) + \epsilon\delta_{z'}}\Big|_{\epsilon=0} = \frac{\delta_{z'}}{d\mathbb{P}(z)} - 1$$

which implies

$$\int \varphi(z;\mathbb{P})s_\epsilon(z)\, d\mathbb{P}(z) = \varphi(z';\mathbb{P}).$$

Therefore this strategy can be described as choosing a clever submodel, so that the pathwise derivative immediately returns the influence function itself, at least in discrete models. (Though again, one can either use the approach of Ichimura and Newey (2022) to generalize, or else check that the pathwise differentiability condition (10.6) holds in the general case for the putative influence function that is derived.)

In what follows we show an example of using this strategy for the regression function parameter in the discrete case. We refer to Hines et al. (2022) for more examples, including the expected density and average treatment effect.

Example 1 (continuing from p. 208). Now we compute the influence function for $\mathbb{E}(Y \mid X = x)$ in the discrete case, using Strategy 1 via the Gateaux derivative. Let δ_z be the Dirac measure at $Z = z$, and note that for the submodel $\mathbb{P}_\epsilon(Z = z) = (1-\epsilon)\mathbb{P}(Z = z) + \epsilon\delta_{z'}$ we have

$$\mathbb{P}_\epsilon(Y = y \mid X = x) = \frac{\mathbb{P}_\epsilon(Z = z)}{\mathbb{P}_\epsilon(X = x)} = \frac{(1-\epsilon)\mathbb{P}(Z = z) + \epsilon\mathbb{1}(z = z')}{(1-\epsilon)\mathbb{P}(X = x) + \epsilon\mathbb{1}(x = x')}.$$

Therefore the Gateaux derivative is

$$\begin{aligned}
&\frac{d}{d\epsilon}\psi\{(1-\epsilon)\mathbb{P}(z) + \epsilon\delta_{z'}\}\Big|_{\epsilon=0} \\
&\quad = \frac{d}{d\epsilon}\sum_y y\frac{(1-\epsilon)\mathbb{P}(Z = z) + \epsilon\mathbb{1}(z = z')}{(1-\epsilon)\mathbb{P}(X = x) + \epsilon\mathbb{1}(x = x')}\Big|_{\epsilon=0} \\
&\quad = \sum_y y\frac{1}{\mathbb{P}(X = x)^2}\{\mathbb{1}(z = z') - \mathbb{P}(Z = z)\}\mathbb{P}(X = x) \\
&\qquad\qquad - \{\mathbb{1}(x = x') - \mathbb{P}(X = x)\}\mathbb{P}(Z = z) \\
&\quad = \sum_y y\Bigg\{\frac{\mathbb{1}(z = z') - \mathbb{P}(Z = z)}{\mathbb{P}(X = x)} \\
&\qquad\qquad - \frac{\mathbb{1}(x = x') - \mathbb{P}(X = x)}{\mathbb{P}(X = x)}\mathbb{P}(Y = y \mid X = x)\Bigg\}
\end{aligned}$$

$$
\begin{aligned}
&= \sum_y y\left\{\frac{\mathbb{1}(z=z') - \mathbb{1}(x=x')\mathbb{P}(Y=y \mid X=x)}{\mathbb{P}(X=x)}\right\} \\
&= \frac{y'\mathbb{1}(x=x')}{\mathbb{P}(X=x)} - \frac{\mathbb{1}(x=x')\mathbb{E}(Y \mid X=x)}{\mathbb{P}(X=x)} \\
&= \varphi(z';\mathbb{P})
\end{aligned}
$$

where the second equality follows from the quotient rule, and the rest by rearranging. This gives the result.

As illustrated above, the Gateaux derivative strategy is more constructive and direct, and only requires simple derivative calculations.

10.3.4.3 Strategy 2

Strategy 2 is similar in spirit to Strategy 1, but allows for extra shortcuts and can bypass unnecessary derivative calculations required in the standard Gateaux derivative approach. The main idea consists of the following tricks:

TRICK 1. Pretend the data are discrete.

TRICK 2. Treat influence functions as derivatives, allowing the use of differentiation rules.

TRICK 3. Use influence function building blocks, e.g., that the influence function of $\mathbb{E}(Y \mid X=x)$ is $\frac{\mathbb{1}(X=x)}{\mathbb{P}(X=x)}\{Y - \mathbb{E}(Y \mid X=x)\}$.

To help make ideas concrete, we introduce an operator $\mathbb{IF} : \Psi \to L_2(\mathbb{P})$ that maps functionals $\psi : \mathcal{P} \to \mathbb{R}$ to their influence functions $\varphi(z) \in L_2(\mathbb{P})$ in a nonparametric model. Then Trick 2 can for example include

TRICK 2a. *(product rule)* $\mathbb{IF}(\psi_1\psi_2) = \mathbb{IF}(\psi_1)\psi_2 + \psi_1\mathbb{IF}(\psi_2)$

TRICK 2b. *(chain rule)* $\mathbb{IF}(f(\psi)) = f'(\psi)\mathbb{IF}(\psi)$

and Trick 3 can be written as $\mathbb{IF}(\mathbb{E}(Y \mid X=x)) = \frac{\mathbb{1}(X=x)}{\mathbb{P}(X=x)}\{Y - \mathbb{E}(Y \mid X=x)\}$.

For comparison, we include derivations of the influence function for the average treatment effect using the general indirect approach and the Gateaux approach of Strategy 1 in the Appendix. The former requires about two pages of calculations, and the latter about one page. Contrast this with the following calculations, which only comprise *four lines* (in addition to not requiring explicit submodels or complicated derivative calculations).

Example 2 (continuing from p. 208). Let $\mu(x) = \mathbb{E}(Y \mid X=x, A=1)$, $\pi(x) = \mathbb{P}(A = 1 \mid X=x)$, and $p(x) = \mathbb{P}(X=x)$, and let $\psi = \mathbb{E}\{\mathbb{E}(Y \mid X, A=1)\}$ denote the average treatment effect functional. Then the influence function is given by

$$
\begin{aligned}
\mathbb{IF}(\psi) = \mathbb{IF}\left\{\sum_x \mu(x)p(x)\right\} &= \sum_x \Big[\mathbb{IF}\{\mu(x)\}p(x) + \mu(x)\mathbb{IF}\{p(x)\}\Big] \\
&= \sum_x \Big[\frac{\mathbb{1}(X=x, A=1)}{p(1,x)}\Big\{Y - \mu(x)\Big\}p(x) \\
&\qquad\qquad + \mu(x)\{\mathbb{1}(x=X) - p(x)\}\Big] \\
&= \frac{A}{\pi(X)}\Big\{Y - \mu(X)\Big\} + \mu(X) - \psi
\end{aligned}
$$

where the first equality followed by Trick 1, the second by Trick 2a, the third by Trick 3, and the fourth by rearranging.

Example 5 (continuing from p. 209). Let $\psi = \int\int \mu(x,a)dG(a \mid x)\; d\mathbb{P}(x)$ denote the stochastic intervention effect, where $\mu(x,a) = \mathbb{E}(Y \mid X = x, A = a)$ and $\pi(a \mid x) = \mathbb{P}(A = a \mid X = x)$ as usual. Then

$$\begin{aligned}
\mathbb{IF}(\psi) &= \mathbb{IF}\left\{\sum_{x,a} \mu(x,a)g(a \mid x)p(x)\right\} \\
&= \sum_{x,a}\Big[\mathbb{IF}\{\mu(x,a)\}g(a \mid x)p(x) + \mu(x,a)g(a \mid x)\mathbb{IF}\{p(x)\}\Big] \\
&= \sum_{x,a}\Bigg[\frac{\mathbb{1}(A = a, X = x)}{\pi(a \mid x)p(x)}\Big\{Y - \mu(x,a)\Big\}g(a \mid x)p(x) \\
&\qquad\qquad + \mu(x,a)g(a \mid x)\Big\{\mathbb{1}(X = x) - p(x)\Big\}\Bigg] \\
&= \frac{g(A \mid X)}{\pi(A \mid X)}\Big\{Y - \mu(X,A)\Big\} + \sum_a \mu(X,a)g(a \mid X) - \psi
\end{aligned}$$

where the first equality follows by Trick 1, the second by Trick 2a, the third by Trick 3, and the fourth by rearranging. In general when $A^* \sim dG(a \mid x)$ this influence function would be

$$\frac{g(A \mid X)}{\pi(A \mid X)}\Big\{Y - \mu(X,A)\Big\} + \int \mu(X,a)\; dG(a \mid X) - \psi.$$

Example 6 (continuing from p. 209). Let $\psi = \frac{\mathbb{E}\{\mathbb{E}(Y|X,R=1)-\mathbb{E}(Y|X,R=0)\}}{\mathbb{E}\{\mathbb{E}(A|X,R=1)-\mathbb{E}(A|X,R=0)\}} \equiv \frac{\mathbb{E}\{\mu(X,1)-\mu(X,0)\}}{\mathbb{E}\{\eta(X,1)-\eta(X,0)\}}$ denote the local average treatment effect with instrument R. First note that $\psi = \psi_{iv,num}/\psi_{iv,den}$ where $\psi_{iv,num} = \mathbb{E}(Y^{R=1} - Y^{R=0})$ and $\psi_{iv,den} = \mathbb{E}(A^{R=1} - A^{R=0})$, so that

$$\begin{aligned}
\varphi_{iv,num} \equiv \mathbb{IF}(\psi_{iv,num}) = &\frac{2R-1}{\varpi(R \mid X)}\Big\{Y - \mu(X,R)\Big\} \\
&+ \mu(X,1) - \mu(X,0) - \psi_{iv,num}
\end{aligned}$$

$$\begin{aligned}
\varphi_{iv,den} \equiv \mathbb{IF}(\psi_{iv,den}) = &\frac{2R-1}{\varpi(R \mid X)}\Big\{A - \eta(X,R)\Big\} \\
&+ \eta(X,1) - \eta(X,0) - \psi_{iv,den}
\end{aligned}$$

for $\varpi(r \mid x) = \mathbb{P}(R = r \mid X = x)$. Therefore

$$\begin{aligned}
\mathbb{IF}(\psi) = \mathbb{IF}\left(\frac{\psi_{iv,num}}{\psi_{iv,den}}\right) &= \frac{\mathbb{IF}(\psi_{iv,num})}{\psi_{iv,den}} - \left(\frac{\psi_{iv,num}}{\psi_{iv,den}}\right)\frac{\mathbb{IF}(\psi_{iv,den})}{\psi_{iv,den}} \\
&= \frac{1}{\psi_{iv,den}}\Bigg(\frac{2Z-1}{\varpi(Z \mid X)}\Big\{Y - \mu(X,Z)\Big\} + \mu(X,1) - \mu(X,0) \\
&\qquad - \psi\left[\frac{2Z-1}{\varpi(Z \mid X)}\Big\{A - \eta(X,Z)\Big\} + \eta(X,1) - \eta(X,0)\right]\Bigg)
\end{aligned}$$

where the second equality follows by Trick 2a, and the third by Trick 3.

Example 7 (continuing from p. 209). Let $\mu_{11}(x_2, x_1) = \mathbb{E}(Y \mid A_2 = 1, X_2 = x_2, A_1 = 1, X_1 = x_1)$, $\pi_t(h_t) = \mathbb{P}(A_t = 1 \mid H_t = h_t)$ for $H_t = (\overline{X}_t, \overline{A}_{t-1})$, and let

$$\psi \equiv \mathbb{E}(Y^{11}) = \int\int \mathbb{E}(Y \mid A_2 = 1, X_2, A_1 = 1, X_1) \, d\mathbb{P}(X_2 \mid A_1 = 1, X_1) \, d\mathbb{P}(X_1)$$

denote the g-formula functional. Then using the same logic as in previous examples, we have

$$\begin{aligned}
\mathbb{IF}(\psi) &= \mathbb{IF}\Bigg\{ \sum_{x_1,x_2} \mathbb{E}(Y \mid A_2 = 1, X_2 = x_2, A_1 = 1, X_1 = x_1) \\
&\qquad\qquad \times p(x_2 \mid a_1 = 1, x_1) p(x_1) \Bigg\} \\
&= \sum_{x_1,x_2} \Bigg[\mathbb{IF}\Big\{ \mathbb{E}(Y \mid A_2 = 1, X_2 = x_2, A_1 = 1, X_1 = x_1) \Big\} \\
&\qquad\qquad \times p(x_2 \mid a_1 = 1, x_1) p(x_1) \\
&\quad + \mathbb{E}(Y \mid A_2 = 1, X_2 = x_2, A_1 = 1, X_1 = x_1) \\
&\qquad\qquad \times \mathbb{IF}\Big\{ p(x_2 \mid a_1 = 1, x_1) \Big\} p(x_1) \\
&\quad + \mathbb{E}(Y \mid A_2 = 1, X_2 = x_2, A_1 = 1, X_1 = x_1) \\
&\qquad\qquad \times p(x_2 \mid a_1 = 1, x_1) \mathbb{IF}\Big\{ p(x_1) \Big\} \Bigg] \\
&= \sum_{x_1,x_2} \Bigg[\frac{A_2 A_1 \mathbb{1}(X_2 = x_2, X_1 = x_1)}{\pi_2(h_2)\pi_1(h_1)} \Big\{ Y - \mu_{11}(x_2, x_1) \Big\} \\
&\quad + \mu_{11}(x_2, x_1) \frac{A_1 \mathbb{1}(X_1 = x_1)}{\pi_1(h_1)} \\
&\qquad\qquad \times \Big\{ \mathbb{1}(X_2 = x_2) - p(x_2 \mid a_1 = 1, x_1) \Big\} \\
&\quad + \mu_{11}(x_2, x_1) p(x_2 \mid a_1 = 1, x_1) \Big\{ \mathbb{1}(X_1 = x_1) - p(x_1) \Big\} \Bigg] \\
&= \frac{A_2 A_1}{\pi_2(H_2)\pi_1(H_1)} \Big\{ Y - \mu_{11}(X_2, X_1) \Big\} \\
&\quad + \frac{A_1}{\pi_1(H_1)} \Big[\mu_{11}(X_2, X_1) - \mathbb{E}\{\mu(X_2, X_1) \mid A_1 = 1, X_1\} \Big] \\
&\quad + \mathbb{E}\{\mu(X_2, X_1) \mid A_1 = 1, X_1\} - \psi.
\end{aligned}$$

Example 10 (continuing from p. 210). For $\psi = \mathbb{E}\{p(Z)\}$ the expected density functional we have

$$\begin{aligned}
\mathbb{IF}(\psi) &= \mathbb{IF}\left\{ \sum_x p(x)^2 \right\} = \sum_x 2p(x) \mathbb{IF}\{p(x)\} \\
&= \sum_x 2p(x) \Big\{ \mathbb{1}(X = x) - p(x) \Big\} = 2 \Big\{ p(X) - \psi \Big\}
\end{aligned}$$

where the first equality follows by Trick 1, the second by Trick 2b, and the third by Trick 3.

10.4 Methods: Influence Function-Based Estimators

We now have a generic minimax lower bound, i.e., a benchmark for efficient estimation, in nonparametric models (e.g., Theorem 2). Further, we have some simple practical tools for deriving efficient influence functions, which are the key components in these minimax lower bounds. However, at this point, nothing has been said about whether these bounds are actually attainable in any generality with real estimators. This is the goal of the present section.

10.4.1 Using IFs to Correct Plug-In Estimators

Recall the von Mises (i.e., distributional Taylor) expansion (10.5), in which the functional $\psi : \mathcal{P} \mapsto \mathbb{R}$ satisfies

$$\psi(\overline{P}) - \psi(P) = \int \varphi(z; \overline{P}) \, d(\overline{P} - P)(z) + R_2(\overline{P}, P) \tag{10.8}$$

for distributions $\overline{P}$ and P, where $\varphi(z; P)$ is a mean-zero, finite-variance function satisfying $\int \varphi(z; P) \, dP(z) = 0$ and $\int \varphi(z; P)^2 \, dP(z) < \infty$, and $R_2(\overline{P}, P)$ is a *second-order remainder* term (which means it only depends on *products* or *squares* of differences between $\overline{P}$ and P). This expansion suggests that generic *plug-in estimators* of the form $\widehat{\psi}_{pi} = \psi(\widehat{\mathbb{P}})$ have a first-order bias, since evaluating the expansion at $(\widehat{\mathbb{P}}, \mathbb{P})$ gives

$$\psi(\widehat{\mathbb{P}}) - \psi(\mathbb{P}) = -\int \varphi(z; \widehat{\mathbb{P}}) \, d\mathbb{P}(z) + R_2(\widehat{\mathbb{P}}, \mathbb{P})$$

after noting that $\int \varphi(z; \widehat{\mathbb{P}}) \, d\widehat{\mathbb{P}}(z) = 0$ since the influence curve φ has mean zero. The following example illustrates the average treatment effect parameter.

Example 2 (continuing from p. 208). A plug-in estimator for the average treatment effect functional $\psi = \mathbb{E}\{\mathbb{E}(Y \mid X, A = 1)\}$ is given by $\widehat{\psi}_{pi} = \mathbb{P}_n\{\widehat{\mu}(X)\}$, for $\widehat{\mu}(x)$ an estimator of $\mu(x) = \mathbb{E}(Y \mid X = x, A = 1)$. Suppose for simplicity that $\widehat{\mu}$ is estimated on a separate sample independent of the sample on which $\mathbb{P}_n$ operates. Then the bias of this plug-in estimator is given by

$$\mathbb{E}(\widehat{\psi}_{pi} - \psi) = \int \mathbb{E}\{\widehat{\mu}(x) - \mu(x)\} \, d\mathbb{P}(x),$$

which is just the integrated bias of the regression estimator $\widehat{\mu}$ itself. For generic estimators $\widehat{\mu}$ this integrated bias would be expected to be of the same order as the say pointwise bias itself, and so in large nonparametric models with standard tuning (e.g., via cross-validation) would be larger than $1/\sqrt{n}$. Intuitively, this plug-in estimator (if used without special tuning) essentially makes the problem of parameter estimation as hard as regression estimation, whereas the results of the previous section suggest the former should be easier (e.g., in terms of smaller mean squared errors, of the order $1/\sqrt{n}$, being achievable).

Crucially, the expansion (10.5) also suggests how to correct or de-bias generic plug-in estimators, namely by estimating the bias term $-\int \varphi(z; \widehat{\mathbb{P}}) \, d\mathbb{P}(z)$ and subtracting it off. Since this expression is just a mean, a natural estimator is given by the corresponding sample average $-\mathbb{P}_n\{\varphi(Z; \widehat{\mathbb{P}})\}$, leading to the bias-corrected estimator

$$\widehat{\psi} = \psi(\widehat{\mathbb{P}}) + \mathbb{P}_n\{\varphi(Z; \widehat{\mathbb{P}})\}. \tag{10.9}$$

This estimator is also often called a *one-step estimator* and can be viewed as a generalization of Newton methods for mimicking maximum likelihood estimators in parametric models (Pfanzagl, 1982; Bickel et al., 1993).

Example 2 (continuing from p. 208). The one-step estimator for the average treatment effect functional $\psi = \mathbb{E}\{\mathbb{E}(Y \mid X, A = 1)\}$ is

$$\widehat{\psi} = \mathbb{P}_n \left[\widehat{\mu}(X) + \frac{A\{Y - \widehat{\mu}(X)\}}{\widehat{\pi}(X)} \right]$$

where $\widehat{\mu}$ and $\widehat{\pi}$ are estimators of $\mu(x) = \mathbb{E}(Y \mid X = x, A = 1)$ and $\pi(x) = \mathbb{P}(A = 1 \mid X = x)$.

Example 5 (continuing from p. 209). Let $\psi = \int \int \mu(x, a) dG(a \mid x)\ d\mathbb{P}(x)$ denote the stochastic intervention effect, where $\mu(x, a) = \mathbb{E}(Y \mid X = x, A = a)$ and $\pi(a \mid x) = \mathbb{P}(A = a \mid X = x)$. The one-step estimator is given by

$$\widehat{\psi} = \mathbb{P}_n \left[\sum_a \widehat{\mu}(X, a) g(a \mid X) + \frac{g(A \mid X)}{\widehat{\pi}(A \mid X)} \Big\{ Y - \widehat{\mu}(X, A) \Big\} \right].$$

Example 6 (continuing from p. 209). Let $\psi = \frac{\mathbb{E}\{\mathbb{E}(Y|X,R=1) - \mathbb{E}(Y|X,R=0)\}}{\mathbb{E}\{\mathbb{E}(A|X,R=1) - \mathbb{E}(A|X,R=0)\}} \equiv \frac{\mathbb{E}\{\mu(X,1) - \mu(X,0)\}}{\mathbb{E}\{\eta(X,1) - \eta(X,0)\}}$ denote the local average treatment effect with instrument R. The one-step estimator is given by

$$\widehat{\psi} = \frac{\mathbb{P}_n\{\widehat{\mu}(X,1) - \widehat{\mu}(X,0)\}}{\mathbb{P}_n\{\widehat{\eta}(X,1) - \widehat{\eta}(X,0)\}} \left[1 - \frac{\mathbb{P}_n\{\varphi_{den}(Z; \widehat{\mathbb{P}})\}}{\mathbb{P}_n\{\widehat{\eta}(X,1) - \widehat{\eta}(X,0)\}} \right] + \frac{\mathbb{P}_n\{\varphi_{num}(Z; \widehat{\mathbb{P}})\}}{\mathbb{P}_n\{\widehat{\eta}(X,1) - \widehat{\eta}(X,0)\}}$$

where

$$\varphi_{num}(z; \mathbb{P}) = \frac{2Z - 1}{\varpi(Z \mid X)} \Big\{ Y - \mu(X, Z) \Big\} + \mu(X,1) - \mu(X,0)$$
$$\varphi_{den}(z; \mathbb{P}) = \frac{2Z - 1}{\varpi(Z \mid X)} \Big\{ A - \eta(X, Z) \Big\} + \eta(X,1) - \eta(X,0).$$

Alternatively one could use the one-step estimators for the numerator and denominator separately, yielding $\widehat{\psi} = \mathbb{P}_n\{\varphi_{num}(Z; \widehat{\mathbb{P}})\} / \mathbb{P}_n\{\varphi_{den}(Z; \widehat{\mathbb{P}})\}$.

Example 7 (continuing from p. 209). Let $\mu_{11}(x_2, x_1) = \mathbb{E}(Y \mid A_2 = 1, X_2 = x_2, A_1 = 1, X_1 = x_1)$, $\pi_t(h_t) = \mathbb{P}(A_t = 1 \mid H_t = h_t)$ for $H_t = (\overline{X}_t, \overline{A}_{t-1})$, and let

$$\psi \equiv \mathbb{E}(Y^{11}) = \int \int \mathbb{E}(Y \mid A_2 = 1, X_2, A_1 = 1, X_1)\ d\mathbb{P}(X_2 \mid A_1 = 1, X_1)\ d\mathbb{P}(X_1)$$

denote the g-formula functional. The one-step estimator is given by

$$\widehat{\psi} = \mathbb{P}_n \bigg(\frac{A_2 A_1}{\widehat{\pi}_2(H_2)\widehat{\pi}_1(H_1)} \Big\{ Y - \widehat{\mu}_{11}(X_2, X_1) \Big\} + \frac{A_1}{\widehat{\pi}_1(H_1)} \Big[\widehat{\mu}_{11}(X_2, X_1) - \widehat{\mathbb{E}}\{\widehat{\mu}(X_2, X_1) \mid A_1 = 1, X_1\} \Big] + \widehat{\mathbb{E}}\{\widehat{\mu}(X_2, X_1) \mid A_1 = 1, X_1\} \bigg).$$

Example 10 (continuing from p. 210). The one-step estimator for the expected density functional $\psi = \mathbb{E}\{p(Z)\}$ is

$$\widehat{\psi} = 2\mathbb{P}_n\{\widehat{p}(Z)\} - \int \widehat{p}(z)^2 \, dz.$$

The one-step estimator (10.9) can be analyzed in some generality, as it is a simple average of an estimated function. By definition we have the important decomposition

$$\begin{aligned} \widehat{\psi} - \psi &= \psi(\widehat{\mathbb{P}}) + \mathbb{P}_n\{\varphi(Z;\widehat{\mathbb{P}})\} - \psi(\mathbb{P}) \\ &= (\mathbb{P}_n - \mathbb{P})\{\varphi(Z;\widehat{\mathbb{P}})\} + R_2(\widehat{\mathbb{P}},\mathbb{P}) \\ &= (\mathbb{P}_n - \mathbb{P})\{\varphi(Z;\mathbb{P})\} + (\mathbb{P}_n - \mathbb{P})\{\varphi(Z;\widehat{\mathbb{P}}) - \varphi(Z;\mathbb{P})\} + R_2(\widehat{\mathbb{P}},\mathbb{P}) \\ &\equiv S^* + T_1 + T_2 \end{aligned} \tag{10.10}$$

where the first line follows by definition of the one-step estimator $\widehat{\psi}$, the second by the expansion (10.5), and the third after adding and subtracting $(\mathbb{P}_n - \mathbb{P})\{\varphi(Z;\mathbb{P})\}$. The first term

$$S^* = (\mathbb{P}_n - \mathbb{P})\{\varphi(Z;\mathbb{P})\}$$

is a simple sample average of a fixed function, and so by the central limit theorem, for example, it behaves as a normally distributed random variable with variance $\text{var}(\varphi)/n$, up to error $o_{\mathbb{P}}(1/\sqrt{n})$. The second term

$$T_1 = (\mathbb{P}_n - \mathbb{P})\{\varphi(Z;\widehat{\mathbb{P}}) - \varphi(Z;\mathbb{P})\}$$

is often called an empirical process term, and is typically of smallest order since it is a sample average of a term with shrinking variance (as long as $\varphi(z;\widehat{\mathbb{P}})$ converges to $\varphi(z;\mathbb{P})$ in a sense to be made formal shortly). The third term

$$T_2 = R_2(\widehat{\mathbb{P}},\mathbb{P}) = \psi(\widehat{\mathbb{P}}) - \psi(\mathbb{P}) + \int \varphi(z;\widehat{\mathbb{P}}) \, d\mathbb{P}(z)$$

is the really crucial one. For non-bias-corrected plug-in estimators, this term will generally dominate, but for one-step estimators, it will generally involve second-order products of errors, which can be negligible under nonparametric conditions (such as sparsity or smoothness).

Remark 5 (Alternatives to One-Step Correction). Although the above one-step estimator is intuitive and relatively straightforward to analyze, it is not the only way to construct efficient estimators of pathwise differentiable functionals in nonparametric models. For example, one alternative (which sometimes reduces to one-step estimation) is to solve an *estimating equation* of the form

$$\mathbb{P}_n\{\varphi(z;\widehat{\mathbb{P}},\psi)\} = 0$$

in ψ, where we write the influence curve as $\varphi(z;\widehat{\mathbb{P}}) = \varphi(z;\widehat{\mathbb{P}},\psi)$ to stress that in general, it depends on the parameter of interest ψ. Of course if the influence curve is linear in the parameter, i.e., taking the form $\varphi(z;\mathbb{P}) = \phi(z;\mathbb{P}) - \psi(\mathbb{P})$, then the estimating equation approach is equivalent to the one-step correction; however in the general nonlinear case these could lead to distinct estimators. Another alternative to one-step correction is to use targeted maximum likelihood estimation (TMLE) (van der Laan and Rubin, 2006; van der Laan and Rose, 2011). TMLE does not correct bias on the parameter scale by adding an estimate of bias to the plug-in estimator; instead, it aims to correct bias on the distributional scale, by constructing a fluctuated estimate $\widehat{\mathbb{P}}^*$ for which $\mathbb{P}_n\{\varphi(Z;\widehat{\mathbb{P}}^*)\} \approx 0$, so that

$$\psi(\widehat{\mathbb{P}}^*) \approx \psi(\widehat{\mathbb{P}}^*) + \mathbb{P}_n\{\varphi(Z;\widehat{\mathbb{P}}^*)\},$$

i.e., a plug-in estimator based on the fluctuated distribution $\widehat{\mathbb{P}}^*$ solves the efficient influence curve estimating equation and behaves like a one-step estimator asymptotically. Despite its asymptotic equivalence to the one-step estimator, an argument for using TMLE is that it could give better finite-sample properties, for example if $\psi(\mathbb{P})$ and $\psi(\widehat{\mathbb{P}}^*)$ are bounded, e.g., in $[0,1]$. A simple one-step estimator can potentially lie outside such bounds on the parameter space depending on the behavior of the correction term $\mathbb{P}_n\{\varphi(z;\widehat{\mathbb{P}})\}$.

Based on the decomposition (10.10), the task of analyzing the one-step estimator $\widehat{\psi}$ (e.g., deriving its rate of convergence and limiting distribution, and determining if and when it attains the nonparametric efficiency bound of Theorem 2) boils down to understanding the behavior of the empirical process term T_1 and bias term T_2.

In particular, when the T_1 and T_2 terms are of the order $o_{\mathbb{P}}(1/\sqrt{n})$, then the sample average term S^* dominates the decomposition, and so

$$\sqrt{n}(\widehat{\psi}-\psi)=\sqrt{n}S^*+o_{\mathbb{P}}(1) \rightsquigarrow N\Big(0,\text{var}\{\varphi(Z;\mathbb{P})\}\Big)$$

by the central limit theorem and Slutsky's theorem. Such a conclusion would yield several crucial insights, including:

1. $\widehat{\psi}$ is root-n consistent,
2. $\widehat{\psi}$ is asymptotically normal, with asymptotically valid 95% confidence intervals for ψ given by the closed-form expression $\widehat{\psi}\pm 1.96\sqrt{\widehat{\text{var}}\{\varphi(Z;\widehat{\mathbb{P}})\}/n}$,
3. $\widehat{\psi}$ is efficient in the local asymptotic minimax sense of Theorem 2.

The next two subsections detail conditions under which the terms T_1 and T_2 can be negligible relative to S^*, even in large nonparametric models where one only assumes some smoothness or sparsity, for example.

10.4.2 Empirical Process Term T_1

There are two main approaches for arguing that the empirical process term

$$T_1=(\mathbb{P}_n-\mathbb{P})\{\varphi(Z;\widehat{\mathbb{P}})-\varphi(Z;\mathbb{P})\}$$

is of the order $o_{\mathbb{P}}(1/\sqrt{n})$: one is based on assuming the function class $\{\varphi(z;P):P\in\mathcal{P}\}$ and corresponding estimators are not too complex (e.g., Donsker), and the other is to use sample splitting. Both approaches can be viewed as ways to avoid a certain kind of overfitting, as will be discussed in detail shortly.

Regardless of which of these two approaches is used, at a minimum it is generally also required that $\varphi(Z;\widehat{\mathbb{P}})$ be converging to $\varphi(Z;\mathbb{P})$ in $L_2(\mathbb{P})$ norm, i.e., that

$$\|\varphi(;\widehat{\mathbb{P}})-\varphi(;\mathbb{P})\|^2\equiv\int\Big\{\varphi(z;\widehat{\mathbb{P}})-\varphi(z;\mathbb{P})\Big\}^2\,d\mathbb{P}(z)=o_{\mathbb{P}}(1). \tag{10.11}$$

Some intuition for this latter requirement is that if $\varphi(Z;\widehat{\mathbb{P}})$ is converging to $\varphi(Z;\mathbb{P})$, then T_1 is a sample average of a quantity tending to zero, and so would not only be bounded after scaling by $\sqrt{n}$ (i.e., of order $O_{\mathbb{P}}(1/\sqrt{n})$), but tending to zero in probability (i.e., of order $o_{\mathbb{P}}(1/\sqrt{n})$). In general, this would be satisfied if $\widehat{\mathbb{P}}$ converges to $\mathbb{P}$ (or for relevant estimated components appearing in φ) and if $\varphi(;P)$ is smooth in P. The next example illustrates with the average treatment effect functional.

Example 2 (continuing from p. 208). For the average treatment effect functional $\psi = \mathbb{E}\{\mathbb{E}(Y \mid X, A = 1)\}$ the one-step estimator is given by

$$\widehat{\psi} = \mathbb{P}_n \left[\widehat{\mu}(X) + \frac{A\{Y - \widehat{\mu}(X)\}}{\widehat{\pi}(X)} \right]$$

and we have

$$\begin{aligned} T_1 &= (\mathbb{P}_n - \mathbb{P}) \left[\widehat{\mu}(X) + \frac{A\{Y - \widehat{\mu}(X)\}}{\widehat{\pi}(X)} - \mu(X) - \frac{A\{Y - \mu(X)\}}{\pi(X)} \right] \\ &\equiv (\mathbb{P}_n - \mathbb{P})\{\widehat{f}(Z) - f(Z)\} \end{aligned}$$

since $(\mathbb{P}_n - \mathbb{P})(\widehat{\psi} - \psi) = (\widehat{\psi} - \psi)(\mathbb{P}_n - \mathbb{P})(1) = 0$. Now note that

$$\widehat{f} - f = \left(1 - \frac{A}{\pi}\right)(\widehat{\mu} - \mu) + \frac{A(Y - \widehat{\mu})}{\widehat{\pi}\pi}(\pi - \widehat{\pi})$$

and so one set of simple sufficient conditions for (10.11) to hold for $(\widehat{f} - f)$ is that

1. $\pi(x) \geq \epsilon$ and $\widehat{\pi}(x) \geq \epsilon$ with probability one, for some $\epsilon > 0$,
2. $|Y - \widehat{\mu}| \leq C$ with probability one, for some $C < \infty$, and
3. $\|\widehat{\mu} - \mu\| = o_{\mathbb{P}}(1)$ and $\|\widehat{\pi} - \pi\| = o_{\mathbb{P}}(1)$,

since under these conditions, it follows that

$$\|\widehat{f} - f\| \leq \left(1 + \frac{1}{\epsilon}\right)\|\widehat{\mu} - \mu\| + \left(\frac{C}{\epsilon^2}\right)\|\pi - \widehat{\pi}\|.$$

Note boundedness of $|Y - \widehat{\mu}|$ could be relaxed to bounded moment conditions, as usual (e.g., using Holder's inequality).

Remark 6. For so-called doubly robust influence functions, it can in some cases be enough to argue $\overline{T}_1 = o_{\mathbb{P}}(1/\sqrt{n})$ for $\overline{T}_1 = (\mathbb{P}_n - \mathbb{P})\{\varphi(Z; \widehat{\mathbb{P}}) - \varphi(Z; \overline{\mathbb{P}})\}$, where only some components of $\overline{\mathbb{P}}$ equal $\mathbb{P}$, while others can merely be set to whatever corresponding estimators converge to. For the average treatment effect functional, for example, one may only have consistency of $\widehat{\pi}$ but not $\widehat{\mu}$, in which case one could define $\varphi(Z; \overline{\mathbb{P}}) = \overline{\mu}(X) + \frac{A\{Y - \overline{\mu}(X)\}}{\pi(X)}$, where $\overline{\mu} \neq \mu$ is defined as the misspecified limit of $\widehat{\mu}$. However, in this case the influence function $\varphi(Z; \overline{\mathbb{P}})$ would not be the efficient one, and in general the T_2 term would be too large to be of order $o_{\mathbb{P}}(1/\sqrt{n})$, and so would contribute to the limiting distribution. If $\widehat{\pi}$ and $\widehat{\mu}$ were estimated with parametric models, the contribution from the T_2 term could behave like a sample average asymptotically, but for nonparametric estimators this would not hold in general, and so there the rate of convergence would in general degrade from $1/\sqrt{n}$ to something slower, depending on the rate at which π was estimated.

Now we briefly describe a first approach for analyzing the empirical process term T_1 in nonparametric models, which is based on assuming the function class $\{\varphi(z; P) : P \in \mathcal{P}\}$ and corresponding estimators are not too complex (e.g., Donsker). We only briefly describe this approach for two primary reasons: (i) as the more classical approach, there are already widely available references (Andrews, 1994; van der Vaart and Wellner, 1996; van der Vaart, 2000; van der Vaart, 2002; Kosorok, 2008; Kennedy, 2016), (ii) the second way to control the term T_1, using sample splitting, is much simpler and requires weaker assumptions. Nonetheless we give some intuition for the main idea here.

Intuitively, when not using sample splitting (i.e., when $\widehat{\mathbb{P}}$ is estimated on the same sample on which $\mathbb{P}_n$ operates), the bias correction in the one-step estimator (10.9) is using the same data twice, for two different tasks, in a kind of "double-dipping". One task is to construct relevant nuisance components in $\widehat{\mathbb{P}}$, and the other to estimate the bias term $\mathbb{P}_n\{\varphi(Z;\widehat{\mathbb{P}})\}$. This double-dipping introduces a threat of overfitting. A nice illustration of this overfitting can be found in Figure 2 of Chernozhukov et al. (2018), and the surrounding discussion. One natural way to avoid overfitting in general, is to not fit overly complex models; this is precisely what a Donsker-type assumption on the complexity of $\mathbb{P}$ and $\widehat{\mathbb{P}}$ achieves. In particular, Donsker classes include smooth parametric models, but also bounded monotone functions, smooth functions with bounded partial derivatives, Sobolev classes, functions with bounded sectional variation, etc. (van der Vaart (2000) has a nice review in Chapter 19).

However, Donsker assumptions can still be restrictive, as noted for example by Robins et al. (2008) (Remark 2.8), Zheng and van der Laan (2010), and Chernozhukov et al. (2018), and may require avoiding commonly used methods such as lasso or random forests. Chernozhukov et al. (2018) points out how high-dimensional models can fail to be Donsker, and more generally have large entropy unless one imposes potentially overly strict sparsity assumptions.

Luckily, there is a straightforward alternative to employing Donsker-type conditions, which is simpler to analyze despite requiring weaker assumptions: sample-splitting (and its swapped analog, now commonly referred to as cross-fitting). Sample-splitting allows one to completely avoid complexity restrictions (only requiring consistency (10.11)), but also greatly simplifies proofs. The latter advantage seems to have driven its initial use in functional estimation problems, as in, e.g., Hasminskii and Ibragimov (1978), Pfanzagl (1982), Schick (1986), Bickel and Ritov (1988), etc. It is important to note that although using sample-splitting and cross-fitting for handling terms like T_1 has become popular recently, it does have a long history, going back nearly half a century, at least.

Using sample splitting has some straightforward and simple intuition in this context: to avoid the overfitting that can come with the aforementioned "double-dipping" (i.e., using the data twice, once to estimate $\widehat{\mathbb{P}}$ and again to estimate the mean $\mathbb{P}_n\{\varphi(Z;\widehat{\mathbb{P}})\}$), just formally separate these two estimation tasks, performing them on different independent samples.

More specifically, cross-fitting works as follows. First randomly split observations $Z^n = (Z_1, ..., Z_n)$ into K disjoint folds. This can be formalized notationally via n realizations of a random variable $F \in \{1, ..., K\}$, drawn independently of the data Z^n, where $F_i = k$ means subject i is assigned to fold k. Then we can let $\widehat{\mathbb{P}}_{-k}$ denote an estimator of $\mathbb{P}$ (or its relevant components appearing in the influence curve φ) that only uses observations $F_i \neq k$, i.e., excludes fold k. Note that there will be K different such estimators, since there are K folds. Then, rather than constructing the estimator, in (10.9), where $\widehat{\mathbb{P}}$ and $\mathbb{P}_n$ are built from and operator on the same sample, instead one constructs the estimator

$$\widehat{\psi} = \sum_{k=1}^{K} \left(\frac{N_k}{n}\right) \widehat{\psi}_k \tag{10.12}$$

where $N_k = \sum_i \mathbb{1}(F_i = k)$ is the number of observations in the kth fold and

$$\widehat{\psi}_k = \psi(\widehat{\mathbb{P}}_{-k}) + \mathbb{P}_n^k\Big\{\varphi(Z;\widehat{\mathbb{P}}_{-k})\Big\} \tag{10.13}$$

is the usual one-step estimator in the kth fold, with $\mathbb{P}_n^k f(Z) = N_k^{-1} \sum_{F_i=k} f(Z_i)$ the empirical measure over the kth fold. Then for each $\widehat{\psi}_k$ the decomposition (10.10) becomes

$$\begin{aligned}
\widehat{\psi}_k - \psi &= \psi(\widehat{\mathbb{P}}_{-k}) + \mathbb{P}_n^k\Big\{\varphi(Z;\widehat{\mathbb{P}}_{-k})\Big\} - \psi(\mathbb{P}) \\
&= (\mathbb{P}_n^k - \mathbb{P})\{\varphi(Z;\widehat{\mathbb{P}}_{-k})\} + R_2(\widehat{\mathbb{P}}_{-k},\mathbb{P}) \\
&= (\mathbb{P}_n^k - \mathbb{P})\{\varphi(Z;\mathbb{P})\} + (\mathbb{P}_n^k - \mathbb{P})\{\varphi(Z;\widehat{\mathbb{P}}_{-k}) - \varphi(Z;\mathbb{P})\} \qquad (10.14)\\
&\qquad + R_2(\widehat{\mathbb{P}}_{-k},\mathbb{P}) \\
&\equiv S_k^* + T_{1k} + T_{2k} \qquad (10.15)
\end{aligned}$$

by the exact same logic as before, and similarly

$$\widehat{\psi} - \psi = S^* + \sum_{k=1}^{K}\left(\frac{N_k}{n}\right)\Big(T_{1k} + T_{2k}\Big) \equiv S^* + T_1 + T_2$$

which follows since $\sum_{k=1}^{K}\left(\frac{N_k}{n}\right)S_k^* = (\mathbb{P}_n - \mathbb{P})\{\varphi(Z;\mathbb{P})\} = S^*$. If the number of folds K is finite, then the order of the terms $\sum_{k=1}^{K}(N_k/n)(T_{1k}+T_{2k})$ is the same as $\max_k(T_{1k}+T_{2k})$, and one can just focus on T_{1k} and T_{2k} separately. Note the number of folds K would not be finite if it scaled with n, as in leave-one-out cross-validation, which requires a different analysis.

Remark 7. Typically one uses equally sized folds so that $N_k = n/K$, at least approximately, in which case $\widehat{\psi}$ is just an average of the fold-specific estimators $\widehat{\psi}_k$, and similarly T_1 and T_2 are averages of the T_{1k} and T_{2k} terms, respectively.

Here we assume a fixed number of folds K, and so can analyze the terms T_{1k} and T_{2k} on their own (the former here, and the latter in the next subsection). By virtue of the sample splitting, somewhat remarkably, a simple bias-variance analysis combined with Chebyshev's inequality is enough to control the T_{1k} terms. This is illustrated in the following lemma from Kennedy et al. (2020), though the same ideas are found in the aforementioned earlier work using sample splitting as well.

Lemma 1 (Kennedy et al. (2020)). Let $\widehat{f}(z)$ be a function estimated from a sample $Z^N = (Z_{n+1},\ldots,Z_N)$, and let $\mathbb{P}_n$ denote the empirical measure over $(Z_1,\ldots,Z_n)$, which is independent of Z^N. Then

$$(\mathbb{P}_n - \mathbb{P})(\widehat{f} - f) = O_{\mathbb{P}}\left(\frac{\|\widehat{f} - f\|}{\sqrt{n}}\right).$$

Proof. First note that, conditional on Z^N, the term in question has mean zero since

$$\mathbb{E}\Big\{\mathbb{P}_n(\widehat{f} - f) \Bigm| Z^N\Big\} = \mathbb{E}(\widehat{f} - f \mid Z^N) = \mathbb{P}(\widehat{f} - f).$$

The conditional variance is

$$\begin{aligned}
\text{var}\Big\{(\mathbb{P}_n - \mathbb{P})(\widehat{f} - f) \Bigm| Z^N\Big\} &= \text{var}\Big\{\mathbb{P}_n(\widehat{f} - f) \Bigm| Z^N\Big\} \\
&= \frac{1}{n}\text{var}(\widehat{f} - f \mid Z^N) \le \|\widehat{f} - f\|^2/n.
\end{aligned}$$

Therefore by iterated expectation and Chebyshev's inequality we have

$$\mathbb{P}\left\{\frac{|(\mathbb{P}_n - \mathbb{P})(\widehat{f} - f)|}{\|\widehat{f} - f\|/\sqrt{n}} \ge t\right\} = \mathbb{E}\left[\mathbb{P}\left\{\frac{|(\mathbb{P}_n - \mathbb{P})(\widehat{f} - f)|}{\|\widehat{f} - f\|/\sqrt{n}} \ge t \Bigm| Z^N\right\}\right] \le \frac{1}{t^2}.$$

Thus for any $\epsilon > 0$ we can pick $t = 1/\sqrt{\epsilon}$ so that the probability above is no more than ϵ, which yields the result. □

Thus the above lemma shows how, as long as $\varphi(z;\widehat{\mathbb{P}})$ is consistent for $\varphi(z;\mathbb{P})$ in $L_2(\mathbb{P})$ norm, and there are finitely many folds K, then sample-splitting/cross-fitting ensures that $T_1 = \sum_k (N_k/n)T_{1k} = o_{\mathbb{P}}(1/\sqrt{n})$, which is asymptotically negligible relative to the sample average term S^*. Importantly, no complexity-restricting conditions using Donsker classes or entropy bounds are required, which means arbitarily flexible methods can be accommodated (e.g., lasso, random forests), as long as they are consistent. Due to its simplicity, the sample-splitting-based approach is arguably also more transparent, as it only requires reasoning about means and variances, rather than Donsker classes and empirical processes.

We summarize the above results in the following proposition.

Proposition 10.4.1. *Let $\widehat{\psi}$ denote the cross-fit estimator in* (10.12)*. Assume $K \leq C < \infty$ is finite, and that $\|\varphi(z;\widehat{\mathbb{P}}_{-k}) - \varphi(z;\mathbb{P})\| = o_{\mathbb{P}}(1)$ for each k. Then*

$$\widehat{\psi} - \psi = (\mathbb{P}_n - \mathbb{P})\{\varphi(Z;\mathbb{P})\} + T_2 + o_{\mathbb{P}}(1/\sqrt{n})$$

for $T_2 = \sum_{k=1}^{K} \left(\frac{N_k}{n}\right) R_2(\widehat{\mathbb{P}}_{-k}, \mathbb{P})$ and $R_2(\overline{P}, P) = \psi(\overline{P}) - \psi(P) + \int \varphi(z;\overline{P})\, dP(z)$.

10.4.3 Remainder Bias Term T_2

We are now a step closer to obtaining estimators that are: (i) root-n consistent, (ii) asymptotically normal, and (iii) efficient in the local asymptotic minimax sense of Theorem 2. The last step is to analyze the bias term T_2, which typically needs to be studied on a case-by-case basis. This T_2 term is what makes bias-corrected estimators like (10.9) and (10.12) special, e.g., allows them to be asymptotically unaffected by nuisance estimation. For example, simple plug-in estimators would have similar decompositions as in Proposition 10.4.1, with similarly small T_1 terms, but the analog of the T_2 term would in general never be $o_{\mathbb{P}}(1/\sqrt{n})$. In contrast, for influence function-based estimators given above, the T_2 term just equals

$$T_2 = R_2(\widehat{\mathbb{P}}, \mathbb{P})$$

for $R_2(\overline{P}, P) = \psi(\overline{P}) - \psi(P) + \int \varphi(z;\overline{P})\, dP(z)$ the remainder of the distributional Taylor expansion (10.5) (or $T_2 = \sum_{k=1}^{K}(\frac{N_k}{n})R_2(\widehat{\mathbb{P}}_{-k}, \mathbb{P})$ in the cross-fitting case, which is basically the same, as we assume K is finite throughout). Therefore the bias term T_2 is essentially a byproduct of deriving and verifying the expansion (10.5), and in such cases will involve second-order *products* of differences between $\widehat{\mathbb{P}}$ and $\mathbb{P}$. Thus if each such error is of the order $n^{-1/4}$, the product will be of the order $1/\sqrt{n}$. In what follows we illustrate with several examples.

Example 2 (continuing from p. 208)**.** For the average treatment effect or missing outcome functional

$$\psi(P) = \mathbb{E}_P\{\mathbb{E}_P(Y \mid X, A = 1)\}$$

the remainder in (10.5) is given by

$$R_2(\overline{P}, P) = \int \left\{\frac{1}{\overline{\pi}(x)} - \frac{1}{\pi(x)}\right\} \left\{\mu(x) - \overline{\mu}(x)\right\} \pi(x)\, dP(x)$$

where $\pi(x) = P(A = 1 \mid X = x)$ and $\overline{\pi}(x) = \overline{P}(A = 1 \mid X = x)$, and similarly for $\mu(x) = \mathbb{E}_P(Y \mid X = x, A = 1)$. Therefore if $\widehat{\pi}(x) \geq \epsilon$ with probability one we have

$$\begin{aligned} |R_2(\widehat{\mathbb{P}}, \mathbb{P})| &\leq \left(\frac{1}{\epsilon}\right) \int |\pi(x) - \widehat{\pi}(x)||\mu(x) - \widehat{\mu}(x)|\, d\mathbb{P}(x) \\ &\leq \left(\frac{1}{\epsilon}\right) \|\widehat{\pi} - \pi\|\|\widehat{\mu} - \mu\| \end{aligned}$$

by Cauchy-Schwarz. Thus if $\|\widehat{\pi} - \pi\| = o_{\mathbb{P}}(n^{-1/4})$ and $\|\widehat{\mu} - \mu\| = o_{\mathbb{P}}(n^{-1/4})$, for example, then $T_2 = o_{\mathbb{P}}(1/\sqrt{n})$, as desired (though note that π and μ do not have to be estimated at the same rates for $T_2 = o_{\mathbb{P}}(1/\sqrt{n})$ to hold: any such combination whose product is $o_{\mathbb{P}}(1/\sqrt{n})$ would suffice). Conditions under which $L_2(\mathbb{P})$ errors satisfy, e.g., $\|\widehat{\pi} - \pi\| = o_{\mathbb{P}}(n^{-1/4})$ are available for many popular estimators. For example, if π is s-smooth (i.e., contained in a Hölder class with index s, so that all partial derivatives up to order $s-1$ are bounded and the highest order are continuous), and $\widehat{\pi}$ is a minimax optimal estimator (e.g., using local polynomials) then with appropriate tuning

$$\|\widehat{\pi} - \pi\| = O_{\mathbb{P}}\left(n^{-\frac{1}{2+d/s}}\right)$$

(Györfi et al., 2002; Tsybakov, 2009), and so for example the rate would be $o_{\mathbb{P}}(n^{-1/4})$ if $d/s < 2$, i.e., the smoothness was more than half the dimension. Similarly, if π is s-sparse and estimated say via lasso at a rate like

$$\|\widehat{\pi} - \pi\| = O_{\mathbb{P}}\left(\sqrt{\frac{s \log d}{n}}\right)$$

(Farrell, 2015; Chernozhukov et al., 2018; Bradic et al., 2019), then the rate would be $o_{\mathbb{P}}(n^{-1/4})$ if $s = o(\sqrt{n}/\log d)$, i.e., the sparsity s scales slower than $\sqrt{n}$ up to log factors. Similar results can be obtained for random forests, neural networks, etc., under appropriate conditions (Farrell et al., 2021).

Example 4 (continuing from p. 208). For the expected conditional covariance functional

$$\psi(P) = \mathbb{E}_P\{\text{cov}_P(A, Y \mid X)\}$$

the remainder in (10.5) is given by

$$R_2(\overline{P}, P) = \int \left\{\overline{\pi}(x) - \pi(x)\right\}\left\{\overline{\mu}(x) - \mu(x)\right\} dP(x)$$

where $\pi(x) = \mathbb{E}_P(A \mid X = x)$ and $\mu(x) = \mathbb{E}_P(Y \mid X = x)$. Therefore

$$|R_2(\widehat{\mathbb{P}}, \mathbb{P})| \leq \|\widehat{\pi} - \pi\| \|\widehat{\mu} - \mu\|$$

by Cauchy-Schwarz, and so this functional has the same kind of double robustness properties as the average treatment effect function in Example 2.

Example 10 (continuing from p. 210). For the expected density functional

$$\psi(P) = \mathbb{E}_P\{p(Z)\} = \int p(z)^2 \, dz$$

the remainder in (10.5) is given by $R_2(\overline{P}, P) = -\int\{\overline{p}(z) - p(z)\}^2 \, dz$, so that

$$|R_2(\widehat{\mathbb{P}}, \mathbb{P})| = \|\widehat{p} - p\|^2$$

where in a slight abuse of notation $\|\cdot\|$ above denotes the $L_2(\nu)$ norm for ν the uniform measure. Thus for the expected density, the standard one-step estimator is not doubly robust but still has nuisance errors that consist of a second-order product; therefore this estimator will still be root-n consistent, asymptotically normal, and efficient as long as the density is estimated at faster than $n^{-1/4}$ rates.

The above examples illustrate the kinds of arguments one can use to show the bias term T_2 is of order $o_{\mathbb{P}}(1/\sqrt{n})$. For some functionals, the remainder term in the expansion (10.5) can take multiple possible forms, some of which may be more or less useful depending on context (e.g., consider the expected conditional covariance in Example 4 and note that $\mu = \pi\mu_1 + (1-\pi)\mu_0$ for $\mu_a(x) = \mathbb{E}(Y \mid X = x, A = a)$), and in some cases the remainder terms can be quite complicated to derive (e.g., for longitudinal causal effects like Example 7 when there are more than two timepoints).

We summarize the above results in the following proposition.

Proposition 10.4.2. *Let $\widehat{\psi}$ denote the cross-fit estimator in* (10.12). *Assume $K \leq C < \infty$ is finite, $\|\varphi(z;\widehat{\mathbb{P}}_{-k}) - \varphi(z;\mathbb{P})\| = o_{\mathbb{P}}(1)$ for each k, and that $T_2 \equiv \sum_{k=1}^{K}\left(\frac{N_k}{n}\right) R_2(\widehat{\mathbb{P}}_{-k},\mathbb{P}) = o_{\mathbb{P}}(1/\sqrt{n})$, where $R_2(\overline{P},P) = \psi(\overline{P}) - \psi(P) + \int \varphi(z;\overline{P})\, dP(z)$. Then*

$$\widehat{\psi} - \psi = (\mathbb{P}_n - \mathbb{P})\{\varphi(Z;\mathbb{P})\} + o_{\mathbb{P}}(1/\sqrt{n})$$

and so $\widehat{\psi}$ is root-n consistent, asymptotically normal, and minimax optimal in the local asymptotic sense of Theorem 2 if φ is the efficient influence function.

10.5 Some Extensions & Open Problems

Although the theory sketched in previous sections has by now a relatively long history and is quite well-developed, there are many extensions and open problems still remaining, which will be important to further develop in the coming years. Here we briefly detail some recent examples.

10.5.1 New Functionals

First, every functional has a somewhat unique remainder term R_2 in the expansion (10.5), leading to corresponding unique bias term T_2 in the decomposition (10.10) (though see Rotnitzky et al. (2019) for some unifying properties). Thus, as new parameters are developed in causal inference and other fields, for example for newly defined causal effects (e.g., Díaz and van der Laan (2012); Young et al. (2014); Haneuse and Rotnitzky (2013); Kennedy (2019) for stochastic intervention effects), or with new data structures (e.g., Tchetgen Tchetgen and VanderWeele (2012); van der Laan (2014); Ogburn et al. (2017) for network data), or under new identifying assumptions (e.g., Tchetgen Tchetgen et al. (2020)), it will be crucial to understand the operating characteristics of these new quantities. This includes understanding terms like R_2 in (10.5) and T_2 in (10.10), even if this uses some already well-developed theoretical tools or arguments. One of the fascinating aspects of causal inference is that there are many different ways to characterize causal effects, each with its own nuances and subtleties.

10.5.2 High Complexity Regimes

In this review we focused on discussing conditions under which estimators are root-n consistent and asymptotically normal. However, when underlying nuisance functions are not smooth or sparse enough relative to the dimension, root-n consistency will be impossible to attain. For example, if a regression function is s-smooth with $s = 5$, but the dimension of the covariates is 50, then the minimax rate is $n^{-1/12}$, much slower than the $n^{-1/4}$ rates discussed in the previous section. This opens up several questions not addressed in this review: When influence function-based estimators like (10.9) and (10.12) are not root-n consistent, can any other estimator be? When are root-n rates achievable? What is the best possible rate that can be achieved when root-n rates are *not* achievable? Important progress along these lines has been made for complex causal effect-style functionals in the last decade by Robins et al. (2008, 2009, 2017), but many open problems remain, including: (i) minimax rates for other functionals beyond the average treatment effect and expected conditional covariance, and (ii) minimax rates for models with nuisances in non-Hölder function spaces (Bradic et al., 2019).

10.5.3 Non-Pathwise Differentiable Functionals

Throughout this review we have considered functionals that satisfy the von Mises/ distributional Taylor expansion (10.5). As explained and illustrated throughout, many important parameters in causal inference and other fields *do* satisfy this expansion; however, there are also many parameters that do not. These parameters are often referred to as non-pathwise differentiable. Non-pathwise differentiability arises in at least two prominent settings: (i) non-smooth finite-dimensional parameters, and (ii) infinite-dimensional parameters. By non-smooth finite-dimensional parameters, we mean parameters that resemble those studied in this review (e.g., take values in $\mathbb{R}$ and, e.g., can be represented as expectations over nuisance functions), but involve non-differentiable functions of nuisance quantities, such as indicators, maximums, absolute values, etc. These arise often, e.g., in the optimal treatment regime literature (Murphy, 2003; Hirano and Porter, 2012; Laber et al., 2014; Luedtke and van der Laan, 2016a). For example, under standard no unmeasured confounding and other assumptions, the value of the mean-optimal treatment regime is given by

$$\mathbb{E}\Big[\mu_1(X)\mathbb{1}\{\mu_1(X) \geq \mu_0(X)\} + \mu_0(X)\mathbb{1}\{\mu_1(X) < \mu_0(X)\}\Big]$$

where $\mu_a(x) = \mathbb{E}(Y \mid X = x, A = a)$. Since the nuisance functions μ_a appear inside non-smooth indicator functions, many arguments from the previous sections cannot be applied directly. Interestingly, though, it can be shown that the influence function for the value still exists under a margin condition (van der Laan, 2013; Luedtke and van der Laan, 2016a), but in general this is not the case.

A second place where pathwise differentiability fails is for parameters that are not simple expectations, but are instead given by infinite-dimensional curves or functions, like regression and density functions. These arise in many important and common settings in causal inference, for example: the effects of continuous treatments (Rubin and van der Laan, 2006; Díaz and van der Laan, 2013; Kennedy et al., 2017), counterfactual density estimation (Robins and Rotnitzky, 2001; Kim et al., 2018; Kennedy et al., 2021; Westling and Carone, 2020), heterogeneous effect estimation (Nie and Wager, 2021; Semenova and Chernozhukov, 2017; Foster and Syrgkanis, 2019; Kennedy, 2020; Kennedy et al., 2022), etc. Interestingly, although these quantities take values in infinite-dimensional function spaces like densities or regressions, they also involve structured combinations of nuisance quantities, and so are really regression/functional hybrids; it turns out that tools and concepts from standard functional estimation can therefore be adapted to these settings. For example, consider the conditional average treatment effect parameter

$$\tau(x) = \mathbb{E}(Y \mid X = x, A = 1) - \mathbb{E}(Y \mid X = x, A = 0);$$

the function $\tau(x)$ can be very smooth or sparse, even when the individual regression functions it differences are not. Exploiting such smoothness or sparsity when it exists requires adapting ideas described in this review to the infinite-dimensional context. We refer to Nie and Wager (2021); Semenova and Chernozhukov (2017); Foster and Syrgkanis (2019); Kennedy (2020); Kennedy et al. (2022) for some examples of such adaptation.

10.6 Appendix: Two Derivations of the Influence Function of the ATE

10.6.1 Integral Equation Approach

To derive the influence function via the pathwise differentiability condition, one needs to first calculate the derivative of the parameter

$$\frac{\partial}{\partial \epsilon} \psi(\mathbb{P}_\epsilon) \Big|_{\epsilon=0} \tag{10.16}$$

on any smooth parametric submodel $\mathbb{P}_\epsilon$ (satisfying $\mathbb{P}_0 = \mathbb{P}$), set it equal to the inner product (i.e., covariance)

$$\int \varphi(z) \left(\frac{\partial}{\partial \epsilon} \log d\mathbb{P}_\epsilon(z) \right) \Big|_{\epsilon=0} \, d\mathbb{P}(z) \tag{10.17}$$

and solve this integral equation for the influence function $\varphi(z)$. In what follows we tackle these two tasks separately, for the average treatment effect parameter.

Derivative of parameter

First, we will compute the derivative of the parameter in (10.16) for $\mathbb{P}_\epsilon$ a generic smooth parametric submodel satisfying $\mathbb{P}_0 = \mathbb{P}$. Note that the submodel score decomposes as a sum

$$\begin{aligned} s_\epsilon(z) &\equiv \frac{\partial}{\partial \epsilon} \log d\mathbb{P}_\epsilon(z) \\ &= \frac{\partial}{\partial \epsilon} \log d\mathbb{P}_\epsilon(y \mid x, a) + \frac{\partial}{\partial \epsilon} \log d\mathbb{P}_\epsilon(a \mid x) + \frac{\partial}{\partial \epsilon} \log d\mathbb{P}_\epsilon(x) \\ &\equiv s_\epsilon(y \mid x, a) + s_\epsilon(a \mid x) + s_\epsilon(x). \end{aligned}$$

Therefore, using the definition of the parameter, its derivative equals

$$\begin{aligned} \frac{\partial}{\partial \epsilon} \psi(\mathbb{P}_\epsilon) &= \frac{\partial}{\partial \epsilon} \int \int y \, d\mathbb{P}_\epsilon(y \mid x, 1) \, d\mathbb{P}_\epsilon(x) \\ &= \int \int y \, \frac{\partial}{\partial \epsilon} d\mathbb{P}_\epsilon(y \mid x, 1) \, d\mathbb{P}_\epsilon(x) \\ &\quad + \int \int y \, d\mathbb{P}_\epsilon(y \mid x, 1) \, \frac{\partial}{\partial \epsilon} d\mathbb{P}_\epsilon(x) \\ &= \int \int y \, s_\epsilon(y \mid x, 1) \, d\mathbb{P}_\epsilon(y \mid x, 1) \, d\mathbb{P}_\epsilon(x) \\ &\quad + \int \int y \, d\mathbb{P}_\epsilon(y \mid x, 1) \, s_\epsilon(x) \, d\mathbb{P}_\epsilon(x), \end{aligned}$$

where in the third equality we used the derivative of a logarithm, i.e., that $\frac{\partial}{\partial \epsilon} \log f_\epsilon(z) = \frac{\partial}{\partial \epsilon} f_\epsilon(z) / f_\epsilon(z)$. Therefore the derivative of the ATE on a submodel at $\epsilon = 0$ is given by

$$\frac{\partial}{\partial \epsilon} \psi(\mathbb{P}_\epsilon) \Big|_{\epsilon=0} = \int \int \Big\{ y \, s_0(y \mid x, 1) + \mu(x) s_0(x) \Big\} \, d\mathbb{P}(y \mid x, 1) \, d\mathbb{P}(x). \tag{10.18}$$

Now our task is to write this derivative in inner product form as in (10.17).

Expressing as inner product

Specifically here we aim to write the derivative (10.18) in the form

$$\int \varphi(z) \Big\{ s_0(y \mid x, a) + s_0(a \mid x) + s_0(x) \Big\} \, d\mathbb{P}(z)$$

for a mean zero function φ, i.e., we need to solve the integral equation

$$\int \left\{ \int y \; s_0(y \mid x, 1) \; d\mathbb{P}(y \mid x, 1) + \mu(x) s_0(x) \right\} \; d\mathbb{P}(x) = \int \varphi(z) s_0(z) \; d\mathbb{P}(z) \tag{10.19}$$

for φ. This does not have an obvious solution if the correct form for φ is not already known (in which case one can just check that the equation holds). A potentially time-consuming and error-bound path is to keep conjecturing candidates for φ, until one works.

Instead, it can be helpful to start by decomposing the influence function as $\varphi(z) = \varphi_y(y, x, a) + \varphi_a(a, x) + \varphi_x(x)$ where

$$\begin{aligned} \int \varphi_y(y, x, a) \; d\mathbb{P}(y \mid x, a) &= 0 \\ \int \varphi_a(a, x) \; d\mathbb{P}(a \mid x) &= 0 \\ \int \varphi_x(x) \; d\mathbb{P}(x) &= 0. \end{aligned} \tag{10.20}$$

Note that this decomposition holds for any random variable $\varphi = \varphi(Z)$ by simply centering appropriately, i.e., defining $\varphi_y(Y, X, A) = \varphi - \mathbb{E}(\varphi \mid X, A)$, $\varphi_a(A, X) = \mathbb{E}(\varphi \mid X, A) - \mathbb{E}(\varphi \mid X)$, and $\varphi_x(X) = \mathbb{E}(\varphi \mid X) - \mathbb{E}(\varphi)$. Importantly, with this decomposition, the inner product on the right-hand side of (10.19) simplifies to

$$\begin{aligned} &\int \left\{ \varphi_y(y, x, a) + \varphi_a(a, x) + \varphi_x(x) \right\} \\ &\qquad\qquad \times \left\{ s_0(y \mid x, a) + s_0(a \mid x) + s_0(x) \right\} d\mathbb{P}(z) \\ &= \int \left\{ \varphi_y(y, x, a) s_0(y \mid x, a) + \varphi_a(a, x) s_0(a \mid x) + \varphi_x(x) s_0(x) \right\} \; d\mathbb{P}(z) \end{aligned}$$

by virtue of the restrictions in (10.20), and the fact that $s_0(y \mid x, a)$, $s_0(a \mid x)$, and $s_0(x)$ are score functions and so similarly have conditional mean zero, i.e.,

$$\begin{aligned} \int s_0(y \mid x, a) \; d\mathbb{P}(y \mid x, a) &= 0 \\ \int s_0(a \mid x) \; d\mathbb{P}(a \mid x) &= 0 \\ \int s_0(x) \; d\mathbb{P}(x) &= 0. \end{aligned}$$

By using the decomposition (10.20) we have essentially transformed our problem from solving one big integral equation to solving three smaller and easier integral equations. Specifically, we now need to solve for $(\varphi_y, \varphi_a, \varphi_x)$ in

$$\begin{aligned} &\int \int \left\{ y \; s_0(y \mid x, 1) + \mu(x) s_0(x) \right\} \; d\mathbb{P}(y \mid x, 1) \; d\mathbb{P}(x) \\ &\quad = \int \left\{ \varphi_y(y, x, a) s_0(y \mid x, a) + \varphi_a(a, x) s_0(a \mid x) \right. \\ &\qquad\qquad\qquad \left. + \varphi_x(x) s_0(x) \right\} \; d\mathbb{P}(z). \end{aligned}$$

This immediately leads us to the choices $\varphi_a(a, x) = 0$ and $\varphi_x(x) = \mu(x) - \mathbb{E}\{\mu(X)\} = \mu(x) - \psi$.

The remaining task is to find $\varphi_y(y, x, a)$, which based on the above amounts to solving the integral equation

$$\int\int y\, s_0(y \mid x, 1)\; d\mathbb{P}(y \mid x, 1)\; d\mathbb{P}(x) = \int \varphi_y(y, x, a) s_0(y \mid x, a)\; d\mathbb{P}(z).$$

Note the derivative term on the left-hand side above equals

$$\begin{aligned}
&\int\int y\, s_0(y \mid x, 1)\; d\mathbb{P}(y \mid x, 1)\; d\mathbb{P}(x) \\
&= \int\int\int y\, s_0(y \mid x, 1)\; d\mathbb{P}(y \mid x, 1)\; d\mathbb{P}(a \mid x)\; d\mathbb{P}(x) \\
&= \int\int\int \frac{ay}{\pi(x)}\; s_0(y \mid x, a)\; d\mathbb{P}(y \mid x, a)\; d\mathbb{P}(a \mid x)\; d\mathbb{P}(x)
\end{aligned}$$

where in the first equality we simply introduced the treatment distribution $d\mathbb{P}(a \mid x) = a\pi(x) + (1 - a)(1 - \pi(x))$, and in the second we multiplied by the indicator a to pick out the required $s_0(y \mid x, 1)$ term, and then divided by $\pi(x)$ to cancel out the additional $\pi(x)$ term that appears due to averaging the indicator a. We note this logic is perhaps still a bit mysterious for those who have not used it before. The term $ay/\pi(x)$ has the right mean but needs to be centered so that it has conditional mean zero and thus satisfies the first line of (10.20). This leads to the choice

$$\varphi_y(y, a, x) = \frac{ay}{\pi(x)} - \int \frac{ay}{\pi(x)}\; d\mathbb{P}(y \mid x, a) = \frac{a}{\pi(x)}\Big\{y - \mu(x)\Big\}.$$

Combining with $\varphi_a(a, x)$ and $\varphi_x(x)$ above gives the overall influence function

$$\varphi(Z) = \frac{A}{\pi(X)}\Big\{Y - \mu(X)\Big\} + \mu(X) - \psi. \tag{10.21}$$

Since the work above shows that this satisfies the pathwise differentiability condition for any sufficiently smooth parametric submodel, it is the influence function.

10.6.2 Gateaux Derivative Approach

The Gateaux derivative approach can be viewed as a special case of the above, where one uses a particular choice of parametric submodel, for which the pathwise derivative is actually equal to the influence function, rather than an integral equation that needs to be solved. This is accomplished by using a submodel whose score is a point mass, as described in the main text.

One simple such submodel is given by $\mathbb{P}_\epsilon^*(z) = (1 - \epsilon)\mathbb{P}(z) + \epsilon\delta_Z$, where δ_Z is the Dirac measure at $z = Z$. Since z is discrete, we can just work with the mass function $p_\epsilon^*(z) = (1 - \epsilon)p(z) + \epsilon\mathbb{1}(z = Z)$. First note that for the submodel $p_\epsilon^*(z)$ we have

$$\begin{aligned}
p_\epsilon^*(y \mid x, a) &= \frac{p_\epsilon^*(z)}{p_\epsilon^*(a, x)} = \frac{(1 - \epsilon)p(z) + \epsilon\mathbb{1}(z = Z)}{(1 - \epsilon)p(a, x) + \epsilon\mathbb{1}(a = A, x = X)} \\
p_\epsilon^*(a \mid x) &= \frac{p_\epsilon^*(a, x)}{p_\epsilon^*(x)} = \frac{(1 - \epsilon)p(a, x) + \epsilon\mathbb{1}(a = A, x = X)}{(1 - \epsilon)p(x) + \epsilon\mathbb{1}(x = X)} \\
p_\epsilon^*(x) &= (1 - \epsilon)p(x) + \epsilon\mathbb{1}(x = X)
\end{aligned}$$

and

$$
\begin{aligned}
\frac{\partial}{\partial \epsilon} p_\epsilon^*(y \mid x, a) \Big|_{\epsilon=0} &= \frac{\mathbb{1}(z = Z) - p(z)}{(1-\epsilon)p(a,x) + \epsilon \mathbb{1}(a = A, x = X)} \Big|_{\epsilon=0} \\
&\quad - p_\epsilon^*(y \mid x, a) \frac{\mathbb{1}(a = A, x = X) - p(a,x)}{(1-\epsilon)p(a,x) + \epsilon \mathbb{1}(a = A, x = X)} \Big|_{\epsilon=0} \\
&= \frac{\mathbb{1}(z = Z) - p(z)}{p(a,x)} \\
&\qquad - p(y \mid x, a) \frac{\mathbb{1}(a = A, x = X) - p(a,x)}{p(a,x)} \\
&= \mathbb{1}(a = A, x = X) \left\{ \frac{\mathbb{1}(y = Y) - p(y \mid x, a)}{p(a,x)} \right\}
\end{aligned} \tag{10.22}
$$

where the first equality follows from the chain rule, and the rest by just rearranging.

Now we evaluate the parameter on the submodel, differentiate, and set $\epsilon = 0$, which gives

$$
\begin{aligned}
\frac{\partial}{\partial \epsilon} \psi(p_\epsilon^*) \Big|_{\epsilon=0} &= \frac{\partial}{\partial \epsilon} \sum_{x,y} y \, p_\epsilon^*(y \mid x, 1) \, p_\epsilon^*(x) \Big|_{\epsilon=0} \\
&= \sum_{x,y} y \left\{ \frac{\partial}{\partial \epsilon} p_\epsilon^*(y \mid x, 1) \, p_\epsilon^*(x) + p_\epsilon^*(y \mid x, 1) \, \frac{\partial}{\partial \epsilon} p_\epsilon^*(x) \right\} \Big|_{\epsilon=0} \\
&= \sum_{x,y} y \Big[\mathbb{1}(1 = A, x = X) \left\{ \frac{\mathbb{1}(y = Y) - p(y \mid x, 1)}{p(1,x)} \right\} p(x) \\
&\qquad + p(y \mid x, 1) \Big\{ \mathbb{1}(x = X) - p(x) \Big\} \Big] \\
&= \frac{A}{\pi(X)} \Big\{ Y - \mu(X) \Big\} + \mu(X) - \psi
\end{aligned}
$$

where the second equality follows by the chain rule, the third by substituting in the expression in (10.22), and the fourth rearranging.

Therefore the Gateaux derivative approach gives the same influence function as the more involved integral equation approach, though even the Gateaux derivative required more than a page of calculations, and some care with the submodel derivatives. Note also that the influence function we arrived at is perfectly well-defined outside of the discrete setup, as long as the regression functions π and μ are well-defined.

Acknowledgements

EK gratefully acknowledges support from NSF Grants DMS1810979 and CAREER Award 2047444, and NIH R01 Grant LM013361-01A1.

Chapter 11

Adversarial Monte Carlo Meta-Learning of Conditional Average Treatment Effects

Alex Luedtke, Incheoul Chung

11.1 Overview

Traditionally, statistical procedures have been derived via analytic calculations whose validity often relies on the sample size growing to infinity. In this chapter, we describe how to use deep adversarial learning to numerically construct a statistical procedure that performs well even in small samples. More concretely, we frame the meta-learning of conditional average treatment effect estimators as a search for an optimal strategy in a two-player game. In this game, Nature selects a prior over distributions that generate labeled data consisting of covariates, treatment, and an associated outcome, and the Estimator observes data sampled from a distribution drawn from this prior. The Estimator's objective is to learn a function that maps from a new feature to an estimate of the conditional average treatment effect. We argue that, under reasonable conditions, the Estimator has an optimal strategy that is equivariant to shifts and rescalings of the outcome, and is invariant to permutations of the observations and to shifts, rescalings, and permutations of the features. We introduce a neural network architecture that satisfies these properties.

11.2 Problem Formulation and Objective

Suppose we observe a dataset consisting of observations (X_i, A_i, Y_i), $i = 1, 2, \ldots, n$, drawn independently from a distribution P belonging to some known model $\mathcal{P}$, where X_i is a continuously distributed covariate with support contained in $\mathcal{X} := \mathbb{R}^p$, A_i is a treatment with support $\mathcal{A} := \{0, 1\}$, and Y_i is an outcome with support contained in $\mathcal{Y} := \mathbb{R}$. This dataset can be written as $\boldsymbol{D} := (\boldsymbol{X}, \boldsymbol{A}, \boldsymbol{Y})$, where $\boldsymbol{X}$ is the $n \times p$ matrix for which row i contains X_i and $\boldsymbol{A}$ and $\boldsymbol{Y}$ are the n-dimensional vectors for which entry i contains A_i and Y_i, respectively. The objective is to develop an estimator of the conditional average treatment effect function (CATE) θ_P that maps an evaluation point x_0 to $\mathbb{E}_P[Y|A = 1, X = x_0] - \mathbb{E}_P[Y|A = 0, X = x_0]$. An estimator T belongs to the collection $\mathcal{T}$ of operators that take as input a dataset $\boldsymbol{d} := (\boldsymbol{x}, \boldsymbol{a}, \boldsymbol{y})$ and output a prediction function $T(\boldsymbol{d}) : \mathcal{X} \to \mathbb{R}$, where, here and throughout, we use $\boldsymbol{d} = (\boldsymbol{x}, \boldsymbol{a}, \boldsymbol{y})$ to denote a possible realization of the random variable $\boldsymbol{D} = (\boldsymbol{X}, \boldsymbol{A}, \boldsymbol{Y})$. Examples of estimators include Bayesian additive regression trees (Hill, 2011), causal forests (Athey et al., 2019), and stacked ensemble learners (Luedtke and van der Laan, 2016b). We quantify the performance of an estimator T at a distribution P via its standardized mean-squared error (MSE), namely

$$R(T, P) := \mathbb{E}_P\left[\int \frac{[T(\boldsymbol{D})(x_0) - \theta_P(x_0)]^2}{\sigma_P^2} dP_X(x_0)\right], \tag{11.1}$$

where the expectation above is over the draw of $\boldsymbol{D}$ under sampling from P, P_X denotes the marginal distribution of X implied by P, and $\sigma_P^2 := \mathbb{E}_P[\mathrm{Var}_P(Y \mid A, X)/\pi_P(A \mid X)^2]$ with $\pi_P(a \mid x) := P(A = a \mid X = x)$ denoting the propensity to receive treatment a given

DOI: 10.1201/9781003216223-11

covariate value x. The standardization factor is chosen to scale with the semiparametric efficiency bound (Bickel et al., 1993) for estimating a smooth functional of θ_P, namely the marginal average treatment effect $q(\theta_P) := \int \theta_P(x) dP_X(x)$, in a model that is nonparametric up to the fact that P_X is known. The rationale for including this standardization factor is that, when estimating a smooth functional of θ_P is difficult (σ_P^2 is large), estimating θ_P itself must also be difficult. Consequently, there is little reason to disfavor an estimator for its performance at P if the estimation of $q(\theta_P)$ is inherently challenging.

Because P is not known in practice, $R(T, P)$ cannot be used to quantify the performance of an estimator T. Hence, another performance criterion must be sought. In this chapter, we focus on a general criterion known as the Γ-maximal risk (Berger, 1985). To define this notion, we let Γ denote a collection of priors Π with support on the statistical model $\mathcal{P}$. For a given prior Π, the Bayes risk of T is defined as $r(T, \Pi) := \int R(T, P)\Pi(dP)$, and the Γ-maximal risk is defined as $\sup_{\Pi \in \Gamma} r(T, \Pi)$. For a given prior Π, the Bayes risk expresses the expected performance of the estimator T under the prior assumptions encoded in Π. The Γ-maximal risk provides a means to avoid selecting a single prior and instead considers the worst-case performance, in terms of Bayes risk, over a collection of priors. At one extreme, when Γ is the singleton collection $\{\Pi\}$, the Γ-maximal risk and the Bayes risk coincide. At the other extreme, when Γ contains all priors with support on $\mathcal{P}$, the Γ-maximal risk instead coincides with the maximal risk $\sup_{P \in \mathcal{P}} R(T, P)$. Thus, the Γ-maximal risk provides a natural means to interpolate between adjudicating performance via a single set of prior beliefs, as is done by the Bayes risk, and via a worst-case analysis, as is done by the maximal risk.

An estimator $T^\star$ is called Γ-minimax if it achieves the minimal possible Γ-maximal risk, that is, if

$$\sup_{\Pi \in \Gamma} r(T^\star, \Pi) = \inf_{T \in \mathcal{T}} \sup_{\Pi \in \Gamma} r(T, \Pi).$$

Unfortunately, Γ-minimax estimators are rarely available in closed form, and so they have seen limited use in practice. In this chapter, we will describe how recently developed meta-learning techniques can be used to iteratively construct Γ-minimax estimators. Many of our arguments will allow for a general choice of Γ, and so, as special cases, the framework we describe can be used to iteratively approximate a Bayes estimator (when Γ is a singleton) or a minimax estimator (when Γ is large or unrestricted).

Regularity Conditions and Notation

For all $P \in \mathcal{P}$, we assume throughout that $\mathbb{E}_P[Y^2] < \infty$ and that $Y - \mathbb{E}_P[Y \mid A, X]$ is a continuous random variable. We also suppose that the strong positivity assumption holds, namely, that there exists a $\delta > 0$ such that, for all $P \in \mathcal{P}$, the following holds P-almost surely: $\min_{a \in \{0,1\}} P(A = a \mid X) \geq \delta$. Notably, these conditions imply that $\sigma_P^2 \in (0, \infty)$.

We now introduce the notation and conventions that we use. For any dataset $\boldsymbol{d} = (\boldsymbol{x}, \boldsymbol{a}, \boldsymbol{y})$ and mapping f with domain $\mathcal{D} := \mathcal{X}^n \times \mathcal{A}^n \times \mathcal{Y}^n$, we let $f(\boldsymbol{x}, \boldsymbol{a}, \boldsymbol{y}) := f(\boldsymbol{d})$. We take all vectors to be column vectors when they are involved in matrix operations. We write $\odot$ to mean the entrywise product and $b^{\odot 2}$ to mean $b \odot b$. For an $m_1 \times m_2$ matrix b, we let b_{i*} denote the ith row, b_{*j} denote the jth column, $\bar{b} := \frac{1}{m_1} \sum_{i=1}^{m_1} b_{i*}$ denote the column means, and $s(b)^{\odot 2} := \frac{1}{m_1} \sum_{i=1}^{m_1} (b_{i*} - \bar{b})^{\odot 2}$ denote the column standard variances. When we standardize a vector b as $[b - \bar{b}]/s(b)$, we always use the convention that $0/0 = 0$. We apply the same division-by-zero convention when standardizing the columns of an $m_1 \times m_2$ matrix b, where we write this standardization as $[b - \bar{b}]/s(b)$ to denote the $m_1 \times m_2$ matrix for which row i is equal to $[b_i - \bar{b}]/s(b)$. We write $[b \,|\, c]$ to denote the column concatenation of two matrices. For an $m_1 \times m_2 \times m_3$ array b, we let b_{i**} denote the $m_2 \times m_3$ matrix with entry (j, k) equal to b_{ijk}, b_{i*k} denote the m_2-dimensional vector with entry j equal to b_{ijk}, etc. For $b \in \mathbb{R}$ and $c \in \mathbb{R}^k$, we write $b + c$ to mean $b\mathbf{1}_k + c$.

11.3 Algorithm for Iteratively Constructing a CATE Estimator

We now present two algorithms for constructing a CATE estimator that performs well in terms of the Γ-maximal risk. These algorithms represent minimax optimization schemes that iteratively update the strategies of two players in a zero-sum game. One of these strategies corresponds to an estimator belonging to $\mathcal{T}$, and the other to a prior belonging to Γ. The estimator is repeatedly evaluated on simulated datasets and updated to perform as well as possible against the current prior, while the prior is also updated to be as unfavorable as possible for the current estimator. The proposed algorithms represent special cases of adversarial Monte Carlo meta-learning (AMC), which is a general approach for iteratively constructing (Γ-)minimax estimators introduced in Luedtke et al. (2020). This approach builds on earlier schemes developed by the statistics, econometrics, and machine learning communities — see the end of this chapter for a review.

The iterative schemes discussed in what follows will be easiest to implement when priors in Γ are easy to sample from. In this section, we focus on two types of collections Γ for which this is the case. In the first, the priors in Γ correspond to finite mixtures of m fixed priors $\Pi^{(1)}, \ldots, \Pi^{(m)}$, that is, is equal to $\Gamma_{\text{mix}} = \{\sum_{j=1}^{m} \alpha_j \Pi^{(j)} : \alpha \in \Delta_{m-1}\}$, where Δ_{m-1} denotes the $(m-1)$-simplex (Chamberlain, 2000). In the second, the priors in Γ are parameterized by a generator function G_g (Goodfellow et al., 2014), where g is a finite-dimensional index parameter that belongs to $\mathbb{R}^{\ell}$, $\ell < \infty$. Each G_g takes as input a source of noise U drawn from a user-specified distribution ν_u – such as a standard multivariate normal distribution – and outputs the parameters indexing a distribution in $\mathcal{P}$ (Luedtke et al., 2020). Though this form of sampling limits to parametric families $\mathcal{P}$, the number of parameters indexing this family may be much larger than the sample size n, which can, for all practical purposes, lead to a nonparametric estimation problem. For each g, we let Π_g denote the distribution of $G_g(U)$ when $U \sim \nu_u$. The collection Γ then takes the form $\Gamma_{\text{gen}} := \{\Pi_g : g \in \gamma\}$, where γ is a finite-dimensional index set.

The presented algorithms require that the class of estimators $\mathcal{T}$ is finite-dimensional, that is, that $\mathcal{T} = \{T_t : t \in \mathbb{R}^d\}$, where $d < \infty$. In our experiments, we focus on neural network classes for $\mathcal{T}$. More generally, we require that $t \mapsto T_t(\boldsymbol{d})(x_0)$ is differentiable for all datasets $\boldsymbol{d}$ and test points x_0. In the next section, we will describe a neural network architecture that satisfies certain group invariance properties that can be useful to impose on a class of CATE estimators.

Algorithm 11.1: Adversarially learn a CATE estimator when Γ consists of mixtures of m priors.

Requires step sizes η_1, η_2 and exploration probability $\epsilon \in (0, 1)$.
Initialize estimator T_t and mixture weights $\alpha = (\alpha_j)_{j=1}^{m} \in \Delta_{m-1}$.
for K iterations **do**
  Explore with probability ϵ.
  If exploring **then** draw $M \sim \text{Uniform}\{1, 2, \ldots, m\}$.
  else draw $M \sim \text{Categorical}(\alpha)$. ▷ returns j with probability α_j.
  Let $P \sim \Pi^{(M)}$, $(X_i, A_i, Y_i)_{i=0}^{n} \overset{\text{iid}}{\sim} P$, and $\boldsymbol{D}$ be the dataset containing $(X_i, A_i, Y_i)_{i=1}^{n}$.
  Let Loss $= [T_t(\boldsymbol{D})(X_0) - \theta_P(X_0)]^2/\sigma_P^2$.
  Update estimator: $t = t - \eta_1 \nabla_t \text{Loss}$. ▷ Loss depends on t through T_t.
  Update M-th entry of prior mixture weight: $\alpha_M = \alpha_M + \eta_2 \frac{1-\epsilon}{(1-\epsilon)\alpha_M + \epsilon/m} \text{Loss}$.
  Project back to simplex: Replace α by its Euclidean projection onto Δ_{m-1}.
end

Algorithm 11.1 provides an AMC scheme to adversarially construct a CATE estimator in cases where Γ consists of a finite mixture of m fixed priors ($\Gamma = \Gamma_{\text{mix}}$). This algorithm represents a variant of the stochastic gradient descent ascent (Lin et al., 2019) that iteratively updates the parameters t and α indexing the estimator and prior, respectively, via unbiased estimates of the gradients of the Bayes risk function $(t, \alpha) \mapsto r(T_t, \Pi_\alpha)$ with respect to t and α, where T_t and Π_α denote the current estimator and prior, respectively. To update the estimator, this unbiased gradient estimate is obtained by differentiating the standardized squared-error loss $[T_t(\boldsymbol{D})(X_0) - \theta_P(X_0)]^2/\sigma_P^2$ in the parameter t for a randomly drawn distribution P, dataset $\boldsymbol{D}$, and test point X_0. To update the prior, this unbiased gradient estimate is instead obtained via a variant of the likelihood ratio method (Glynn, 1987). To account for the fact that the mixture weights α must belong to the simplex, the gradient updates to α are projected to the simplex Δ_{m-1}, so that the update to α corresponds to a projected stochastic gradient ascent step (Nemirovski et al., 2009). All gradients used in this and the upcoming algorithm can be computed via backpropagation as implemented in standard software packages such as TensorFlow or Pytorch (Abadi et al., 2016; Paszke et al., 2019).

We now provide an algorithm for cases where the priors in Γ are parameterized via a generator function ($\Gamma = \Gamma_{\text{gen}}$). To simplify the presentation, we will suppose that the propensity function π_P is known when considering these cases, which makes it so that $\pi_P = \pi_{P'}$ for all possible distributions $P, P' \in \mathcal{P}$; such a condition is plausible, for example, in a randomized experiment. Algorithm 11.2 provides an implementation of AMC that iteratively updates the parameter g indexing the generator function G_g and the parameter t indexing the estimator T_t via stochastic gradient descent ascent (Lin et al., 2019). Implementing this algorithm requires the ability to differentiate realized datasets through the parameters indexing the prior. To ensure that this is possible, for each $P \in \mathcal{P}$, the algorithm requires access to a generator function $H_P : \mathcal{V} \to \mathcal{X} \times \mathcal{A} \times \mathcal{Y}$ such that $H_P(V)$ has the same distribution as $(X, A, Y) \sim P$ when noise V is drawn from a user-specified distribution ν_v with support on $\mathcal{V}$. The algorithm further requires that $g \mapsto H_{G_g(u)}(v)$ is differentiable at g_0 for all realizations of the noise u in the support of ν_u and v in the support of ν_v. An example of a setting where such a function H_P can be defined is provided at the end of this section. Note that there is no reason to expect that $g \mapsto H_{G_g(u)}(v)$ will be everywhere differentiable if the support of X or Y is discrete — consequently, Algorithm 11.2 will not apply in those settings. This problem can be avoided by modifying the algorithm to instead use the likelihood ratio method to obtain an unbiased gradient estimate (Glynn, 1987). The likelihood ratio method could similarly be used to obtain an unbiased gradient estimate in cases where the propensity function π_P is not known.

Algorithm 11.2: Adversarially learn a CATE estimator when prior is parameterized as a generator.

Requires step sizes η_1, η_2.
Initialize estimator T_t and generator G_g.
for K iterations **do**
  Independently draw $U \sim \nu_u$ and $V_0, V_1, \ldots, V_p \overset{\text{iid}}{\sim} \nu_v$.
  Let $P = G_g(U)$, $(X_i, A_i, Y_i) = H_P(V_i)$, $i = 0, 1, \ldots, n$, and $\boldsymbol{D} = (X_i, A_i, Y_i)_{i=1}^n$.
  Let Loss $= [T_t(\boldsymbol{D})(X_0) - \theta_P(X_0)]^2/\sigma_P^2$.
  Update estimator: $t = t - \eta_1 \nabla_t \text{Loss}$. ▷ Loss depends on t through T_t.
  Update prior: $g = g + \eta_2 \nabla_g \text{Loss}$. ▷ Loss depends on g through P, X_0, and $\boldsymbol{D}$.
end

Many variants of Algorithms 11.1 and 11.2 are possible. For example, rather than computing the loss on a single dataset, a batch of multiple datasets can be sampled, and the loss can correspond to the average loss across all datasets in this batch. As another example, two-timescale learning rates could be used so that η_1 and η_2 both converge to zero as the number of iterations increases, but η_2 converges to zero at a faster rate than does η_1, that is, $\eta_2/\eta_1 \to 0$ as the number of iterations increases. Such two-timescale learning rate strategies have proven to be effective in stabilizing the optimization problem pursued by generative adversarial networks (Heusel et al., 2017). As a final example, an alternative first-order minimax optimization scheme could be employed, such as a stochastic extragradient method (Mishchenko et al., 2020).

We now provide an example of a setting where the generator functions G_g and H_P needed to implement Algorithm 11.2 can be defined so that $g \mapsto H_{G_g(u)}(v)$ is differentiable. Suppose that the model $\mathcal{P}$ consists of all distributions P for which there exist $(\lambda_P, \beta_P) \in (0,\infty) \times \mathbb{R}^4$ such that $X \sim \text{Exponential}(\lambda_P)$, $A|X \sim \text{Bernoulli}(1/2)$, and $Y|A,X \sim N(\beta_P^\top(1, A, X, AX), 1)$. Further, suppose that the generator G_g is a multilayer perceptron with weights g mapping from $\mathbb{R}^k$ to $(0,\infty) \times \mathbb{R}^4$ and that the activation functions used to define this neural network are differentiable. Let ν_u be a $N(\mathbf{0}_k, \text{Id}_k)$ distribution. A draw from a prior Π_g can be obtained by sampling $U \sim \nu_u$ and letting $(\lambda_P, \beta_P) = G_g(U)$; the value of the parameters (λ_P, β_P) then fully determines the value of $P \in \mathcal{P}$. We now provide the form of a generator H_P and a noise distribution ν_v such that $H_P(V)$ has distribution P when $V \sim \nu_v$. In particular, let $V = (V_1, V_2, V_3)$ be a vectored-valued random variable whose three entries consist of mutually independent draws from a standard uniform distribution (V_1), Bernoulli distribution with success probability $1/2$ (V_2), and standard normal distribution (V_3). Let H_P be the function mapping from (v_1, v_2, v_3) to $(f_{P,1}(v_1), v_2, f_{P,3}(v_1, v_2, v_3))$, where $f_{P,1}(v_1) = -\log(1 - v_1)/\lambda_P$ is the inverse cumulative distribution function of an Exponential(λ) distribution evaluated at v_1 and $f_{P,3}(v_1, v_2, v_3) = \beta_P^\top(1, v_2, f_1(v_1), v_2 f_1(v_1)) + v_3$. By the chain rule, it can be verified that, for any $u \in \mathbb{R}^k$ and $v \in (0,1) \times \{0,1\} \times \mathbb{R}$, $g \mapsto H_{G_g(u)}(v)$ is a differentiable function.

11.4 Class of Estimators

11.4.1 Desired Invariance Properties

Before introducing the class of estimators that we propose using when implementing Algorithms 11.1 and 11.2, we describe several invariance properties that we will ensure that the estimators it contains satisfy. To do this, we will need to introduce some notation. For $k \in \mathbb{N}$, we let $\mathcal{B}_k$ denote the collection of all $k \times k$ permutation matrices and $\mathcal{D}_0 := \{(\boldsymbol{d}, x_0) \in \mathcal{D} \times \mathcal{X} : s(\boldsymbol{y}) \neq 0, s(\boldsymbol{x})_j \neq 0 \, \forall \, j = 1, 2, \dots, p\}$. When X and Y are continuous random variables under sampling from P, a dataset-test-point pair $(\boldsymbol{D}, X_0)$ that is sampled according to P belongs to $\mathcal{D}_0$ with probability one. With this notation in hand, we are now in a position to state the invariance properties that we would like all estimators in $\mathcal{T}$ to satisfy. In particular, we want that, for all $T \in \mathcal{T}$, the following properties are satisfied for all $(\boldsymbol{d}, x_0) \in \mathcal{D}_0$:

T1) *Invariant to permutations of the observations:* For all $B \in \mathcal{B}_n$, $T(B\boldsymbol{x}, B\boldsymbol{a}, B\boldsymbol{y})(x_0) = T(\boldsymbol{d})(x_0)$.

T2) *Invariant to permutations of the covariates:* For all $B \in \mathcal{B}_p$, $T(\boldsymbol{x}B, \boldsymbol{a}, \boldsymbol{y})(B^\top x_0) = T(\boldsymbol{d})(x_0)$.

T3) *Invariant to increasing affine transformations of the covariates:* For all $b \in \mathbb{R}^p$ and $c \in (0,\infty)^p$, $T(\boldsymbol{x}^{b,c}, \boldsymbol{a}, \boldsymbol{y})(b + c \odot x_0) = T(\boldsymbol{d})(x_0)$, where $\boldsymbol{x}^{a,b}$ is the $n \times p$ matrix with row i equal to $a + b \odot \boldsymbol{x}_{i*}$.

T4) *Invariant to shifts of the outcomes:* For all $b \in \mathbb{R}$, $T(\boldsymbol{x}, \boldsymbol{a}, b + \boldsymbol{y})(x_0) = T(\boldsymbol{d})(x_0)$.

T5) *Equivariant to increasing linear transformations of the outcomes:* For all $c > 0$, $T(\boldsymbol{x}, \boldsymbol{a}, c\boldsymbol{y})(x_0) = cT(\boldsymbol{d})(x_0)$.

In the context of regression problems, Luedtke et al. (2021) motivated similar conditions (Eqs. 4 and 5 from that work) by showing that the corresponding decision problem is invariant under the action of an appropriately defined group (Lemmas 10 and 11 from that work). They then derived a variant of the Hunt-Stein theorem (Hunt and Stein, 1946) to establish that, for many natural collections of priors Γ, there exists an invariant Γ-minimax regression estimator. Though these arguments could be directly modified to establish similar results in CATE estimation settings, doing so is beyond the scope of this work. Instead, a hybrid approach is pursued in what follows: the rationale for imposing 11.4.1 and 11.4.1 is formally justified via Jensen's inequality, while an informal, but intuitive, rationale is provided for imposing 11.4.1-11.4.1.

Our rationale for imposing 11.4.1-11.4.1 is based on several properties of conditional expectations. We begin by motivating 11.4.1 and 11.4.1. Fix $(b, c) \in \mathbb{R} \times (0, \infty)$. By the linearity of expectation, the CATE $\theta_P(x_0) := E_P[Y|A = 1, X = x_0] - E_P[Y|A = 0, X = x_0]$ of A on an outcome Y can be related to the CATE $\tilde{\theta}_P(x_0) := E_P[\tilde{Y}|A = 1, X = x_0] - E_P[\tilde{Y}|A = 0, X = x_0]$ of A on the linear transformation $\tilde{Y} := b + cY$ of this outcome as follows:

$$\begin{aligned}\tilde{\theta}_P(x_0) &= E_P[b + cY|A = 1, X = x_0] - E_P[b + cY|A = 0, X = x_0] \\ &= c(E_P[Y|A = 1, X = x_0] - E_P[Y|A = 0, X = x_0]) = c\,\theta_P(x_0).\end{aligned}$$

This suggests that an estimate $T(\boldsymbol{x}, \boldsymbol{a}, b + c\boldsymbol{y})$ of $\tilde{\theta}_P$ should be equal to c times the estimate $T(\boldsymbol{x}, \boldsymbol{a}, \boldsymbol{y})$ of θ_P, which is precisely what 11.4.1 and 11.4.1 require when taken in combination. In principle we could ask for even stronger version of 11.4.1, namely $T(\boldsymbol{x}, \boldsymbol{a}, c\boldsymbol{y}) = cT(\boldsymbol{x}, \boldsymbol{a}, \boldsymbol{y})$ for all $c \in \mathbb{R}$, rather than just for $c > 0$. Because the estimators that we present later in this work do not satisfy this stronger invariance property, we do not comment on it further here. We now motivate 11.4.1. Fix $(b, c) \in \mathbb{R}^p \times (0, \infty)^p$. By the injectivity of the map $x \mapsto b + c \odot x$, the CATE $\theta_P(x_0) := E_P[Y|A = 1, X = x_0] - E_P[Y|A = 0, X = x_0]$ of A on an outcome Y can be related to the CATE $\bar{\theta}_P(\bar{x}_0) := E_P[Y|A = 1, \bar{X} = \bar{x}_0] - E_P[Y|A = 0, \bar{X} = \bar{x}_0]$ of A based on the transformed covariates $\bar{X} := b + c \odot X$ being equal to $\bar{x}_0 := b + c \odot x_0$ as follows:

$$\begin{aligned}\bar{\theta}_P(\bar{x}_0) &= E_P[Y|A = 1, \bar{X} = \bar{x}_0] - E_P[Y|A = 0, \bar{X} = \bar{x}_0] \\ &= E_P[Y|A = 1, X = x_0] - E_P[Y|A = 0, X = x_0] = \theta_P(x_0).\end{aligned}$$

This suggests that estimates of $\bar{\theta}_P(\bar{x}_0)$ based on a given dataset should coincide with those of $\theta_P(x_0)$ based on that same dataset, which is exactly what 11.4.1 requires.

We now provide justification for imposing 11.4.1. This condition will be seen to be reasonable in light of the fact that the observations are independent and identically distributed, and therefore exchangeable. This exchangeability can be used to show that, for any estimator T, there exists an invariant estimator T_1 that uniformly performs at least as well as T in the sense that $R(T_1, P) \leq R(T, P)$ for all $P \in \mathcal{P}$. As a consequence of this, T_1 achieves a Γ-minimax risk that is at least as small as that of T. By Jensen's inequality and the convexity of $R(\,\cdot\,, P)$ for each P, T_1 can be chosen to be equal to $T_1(\boldsymbol{d})(x_0) = (n!)^{-1} \sum_{B \in \mathcal{B}_n} T(B\boldsymbol{x}, B\boldsymbol{a}, B\boldsymbol{y})(x_0)$, which corresponds to the average of the evaluations of T across permutations of the n observations in $\boldsymbol{d}$. In fact, under slightly stronger conditions that make it so that Jensen's inequality is strict (details omitted), T_1 can be shown to dominate T in the sense that $R(T_1, P)$ is strictly smaller than $R(T, P)$ for one or more $P \in \mathcal{P}$. Imposing that all estimators in $\mathcal{T}$ satisfy 11.4.1 makes it so that $T_1 = T$ for all $T \in \mathcal{T}$, so that there is no estimator in $\mathcal{T}$ that can be dominated by simply averaging across its evaluations on permutations of the observations.

In cases where nothing is known *a priori* about the ordering of the different entries of the covariate X, Jensen's inequality can similarly be used to justify 11.4.1. In particular, in what follows we consider cases where Γ is agnostic to the ordering of the covariates in the sense that $\Pi \in \Gamma$ implies that $\Pi \circ f_B^{-1} \in \Gamma$ for all $B \in \mathcal{B}_p$, where $f_B(P)$ is the pushforward measure $P \circ g_B^{-1}$ with $g_B(x,a,y) = (B^\top x, a, y)$. In such cases, for any $T \in \mathcal{T}$, it will be shown that there exists an estimator T_2 that performs at least as well as T in terms of Γ-maximal risk, in the sense that

$$\sup_{\Pi \in \Gamma} r(T_2, \Pi) \leq \sup_{\Pi \in \Gamma} r(T, \Pi). \tag{11.2}$$

The estimator T_2 can be evaluated by averaging the estimates obtained from T across permutations of the covariates. In particular, T_2 takes the form $T_2(\boldsymbol{d})(x_0) = (p!)^{-1} \sum_{B \in \mathcal{B}_p} T_B(\boldsymbol{d})(x_0)$, where $T_B(\boldsymbol{d})(x_0) = T(\boldsymbol{x}B, \boldsymbol{a}, \boldsymbol{y})(B^\top x_0)$. To see this, let $h_B(x) := B^\top x$ for $B \in \mathcal{B}_p$ and note that, for any $P \in \mathcal{P}$, Jensen's inequality and the change of variables formula for pushforward measures show that

$$\begin{aligned} R(T_2, P) &\leq \frac{1}{p!} \sum_{B \in \mathcal{B}_p} R(T_B, P) \\ &= \frac{1}{p!} \sum_{B \in \mathcal{B}_p} \mathbb{E}_{P \circ g_B^{-1}} \left[\int \tfrac{[T(\boldsymbol{D})(x_0) - \theta_P(Bx_0)]^2}{\sigma_P^2} dP_X \circ h_B^{-1}(x_0) \right]. \end{aligned}$$

Combining the above with the fact that $\theta_P(Bx_0) = \theta_{P \circ g_B^{-1}}(x_0)$, which holds since $E_P[Y|A = a, X = Bx_0] = E_P[Y|A = a, B^\top X = x_0]$ for $a \in \{0,1\}$, we see that $R(T_2, P) \leq (p!)^{-1} \sum_{B \in \mathcal{B}_p} R(T, P \circ g_B^{-1})$. Integrating P against Π on both sides and noting that $\int R(T, P \circ g_B^{-1}) \Pi(dP) = r(T, \Pi \circ f_B^{-1})$ then shows that

$$r(T_2, \Pi) \leq \frac{1}{p!} \sum_{B \in \mathcal{B}_p} r(T, \Pi \circ f_B^{-1}) \leq \max_{B \in \mathcal{B}_p} r(T, \Pi \circ f_B^{-1}) \leq \sup_{\Pi' \subset \Gamma} r(T, \Pi'),$$

where the final inequality used that $\Pi \circ f_B^{-1}$ is contained in Γ. As Π was an arbitrary element of Γ, taking a supremum in Π on the left-hand side shows that (11.2) holds. Imposing that all estimators in $\mathcal{T}$ satisfy 11.4.1 makes it so that $T_2 = T$ for all $T \in \mathcal{T}$, so that there is no estimator in $\mathcal{T}$ that can be dominated by simply averaging across its evaluations on permutations of the covariates.

11.4.2 Proposed Class of Estimators

Algorithm 11.3 presents the class of CATE estimators $\mathcal{T}$ that we propose to use when employing Algorithm 11.1 or 11.2. This class is the same as the one introduced in Luedtke et al. (2021) in the context of regression problems—namely, in the estimation of $x \mapsto E[Y \mid X = x]$—except has been adapted to include treatment assignments $A_1, \ldots, A_n$ as inputs to the estimator and to account for the fact that CATE estimators should be invariant, rather than equivariant, to shifts in the outcome. Algorithm 11.3 relies on four modules. Each module m_k, $k \in \{1,2,3,4\}$, can be represented by a function m_k belonging to a collection $\mathcal{M}_k$ of functions mapping from $\mathbb{R}^{b_k}$ to $\mathbb{R}^{c_k}$, where the values of b_k and c_k can be deduced from the statement of the algorithm. For given data $\boldsymbol{d}$, a prediction at a covariate x_0 can be obtained sequentially by calling the modules and, between calls, either mean pooling across one of the dimensions of the output or concatenating the evaluation point as a new column in the output matrix.

Algorithm 11.3: Use data $\boldsymbol{d}$ to obtain CATE estimate at x_0.

1 **Preprocess:** Let $x_0^0 := \frac{x_0 - \bar{\boldsymbol{x}}}{s(\boldsymbol{x})}$ and define $\boldsymbol{d}^0 \in \mathbb{R}^{n \times p \times 2}$ so that $\boldsymbol{d}^0_{i*1} = \frac{x_i - \bar{\boldsymbol{x}}}{s(\boldsymbol{x})}$ for all $i = 1, \ldots, n$ and, for all $j = 1, \ldots, p$, $\boldsymbol{d}^0_{*j2} = \boldsymbol{a}$ and $\boldsymbol{d}^0_{*j3} = \frac{\boldsymbol{y} - \bar{\boldsymbol{y}}}{s(\boldsymbol{y})}$. ▷ Process observed dataset $\boldsymbol{d}$.

2 **Module 1:** $\boldsymbol{d}^1 := m_1(\boldsymbol{d}^0)$. $\boldsymbol{d}^1 \in \mathbb{R}^{n \times p \times o_1}$

3 **Mean Pool:** $\bar{\boldsymbol{d}}^1 := n^{-1} \sum_{i=1}^n \boldsymbol{d}^1_{i**}$.

4 **Module 2:** $\boldsymbol{d}^2 := m_2(\bar{\boldsymbol{d}}^1)$. $\boldsymbol{d}^2 \in \mathbb{R}^{p \times o_2}$ ▷ Generate and return a CATE prediction at a test point x_0.

5 **Augment:** $\tilde{\boldsymbol{d}}^2 := [\boldsymbol{d}^2 \mid x_0^0]$. $\tilde{\boldsymbol{d}}^2 \in \mathbb{R}^{p \times (o_2+1)}$

6 **Module 3:** $\boldsymbol{d}^3 := m_3(\tilde{\boldsymbol{d}}^2)$. $\boldsymbol{d}^3 \in \mathbb{R}^{p \times o_3}$

7 **Mean Pool:** $\bar{\boldsymbol{d}}^3 := p^{-1} \sum_{j=1}^p \boldsymbol{d}^3_{j*}$. $\bar{\boldsymbol{d}}^3 \in \mathbb{R}^{o_3}$

8 **Module 4:** $\boldsymbol{d}^4 := m_4(\bar{\boldsymbol{d}}^3)$. $\boldsymbol{d}^4 \in \mathbb{R}$

9 **return** $s(\boldsymbol{y})\boldsymbol{d}^4$.

We let $\mathcal{T}_{\mathcal{M}}$ represent the collection of all CATE estimators described by Algorithm 11.3, where here $(m_k)_{k=1}^4$ varies over $\prod_{k=1}^4 \mathcal{M}_k$. Estimators in $\mathcal{T}_{\mathcal{M}}$ can be seen to automatically satisfy 11.4.1-11.4.1. Indeed, by virtue of the standardization of the covariates on line 1 of Algorithm 11.3, conditions 11.4.1 and 11.4.1 are satisfied. Furthermore, by this standardization along with the rescaling of the output by the empirical standard deviation on line 8, 11.4.1 is also satisfied. Provided the module classes $\mathcal{M}_1$, $\mathcal{M}_2$, and $\mathcal{M}_3$ satisfy certain sufficient conditions, estimators in $\mathcal{T}_{\mathcal{M}}$ also satisfy 11.4.1 and 11.4.1. These conditions are as follows:

M1) $m_1(BvC)_{**\ell} = B[m_1(v)_{**\ell}]C$ for all $m_1 \in \mathcal{M}_1$, $B \in \mathcal{B}_n$, $C \in \mathcal{B}_p$, $v \in \mathbb{R}^{n \times p \times 3}$, and $\ell \in \{1, \ldots, o_1\}$.

M2) $m_2(Bv) = Bm_2(v)$ for all $m_2 \in \mathcal{M}_2$, $B \in \mathcal{B}_p$, and $v \in \mathbb{R}^{p \times o_1}$.

M3) $m_3(Bv) = Bm_3(v)$ for all $m_3 \in \mathcal{M}_3$, $B \in \mathcal{B}_p$, and $v \in \mathbb{R}^{p \times (o_2+1)}$.

Many different choices of the module classes $\mathcal{M}_1$, $\mathcal{M}_2$, and $\mathcal{M}_3$ satisfy the above conditions. Here, we focus on a particular neural network classes that satisfy these properties.

There are several reasons that neural network classes provide appealing choices for these module classes. First, readily available software frameworks (e.g., Paszke et al., 2019; Abadi et al., 2016) make it easy to implement Algorithms 11.1 and 11.2 when the estimators are parameterized as a neural network class. Second, in a variety of settings, sufficiently wide or deep neural networks have been shown to be able to approximate any smooth function arbitrarily well (e.g., Cybenko, 1989; Hornik, 1991; Maron et al., 2019). Working over a rich class of estimators should, in principle, yield some estimators with better Γ-maximal risk than would be available within a smaller class. Third, there are well-established neural network architectures that can be used to parameterize the module classes $\mathcal{M}_1$, $\mathcal{M}_2$, and $\mathcal{M}_3$ so that they satisfy the invariance properties 9-9. One possible drawback to making these module classes neural network classes is that the resulting minimax optimization problems that Algorithms 11.1 and 11.2 seek to solve are not convex-concave. Nevertheless, in our experiments, we show that the proposed approach appears to yield high-performing estimators despite this difficulty. This is consistent with findings in other minimax optimization problems where neural networks are employed, such as those arising in the optimization of generative adversarial networks (Goodfellow et al., 2014; Arjovsky et al., 2017).

The neural network classes used for the modules are parameterized in the same way as was done for regression problems in Luedtke et al. (2021). To orient readers, their presentation is organized in the same way here. For each k, $\mathcal{M}_k$ contains the neural networks consisting of h_k hidden layers of widths $w_k^1, w_k^2, \ldots, w_k^{h_k}$, where the types of layers used depends on the module k. When $k = 1$, multi-input-output channel equivariant layers as defined in Hartford et al. (2018) are used. For $j = 1, \ldots, h_1 + 1$, $\mathcal{L}_1^j$ denotes the collection of all such layers that map from $\mathbb{R}^{n \times p \times w_1^{j-1}}$ to $\mathbb{R}^{n \times p \times w_1^j}$, where $w_1^0 = 3$ and $w_1^{h_1+1} = o_1$. For each j, each member L_1^j of $\mathcal{L}_1^j$ is equivariant in the sense that, for all $B \in \mathcal{B}_n$, $C \in \mathcal{B}_p$, and $v \in \mathbb{R}^{n \times p \times w_1^{j-1}}$, $L_1^j(BvC)_{**\ell} = BL_1^j(v)_{**\ell}C$ for all $\ell = 1, \ldots, o_1$. When $k = 2, 3$, multi-input-output channel equivariant layers as described in Eq. 22 of Zaheer et al. (2017) are used, except that the sum-pool term in that equation is replaced with a mean-pool term. For $j = 1, \ldots, h_k + 1$, the collection of all such equivariant layers that map from $\mathbb{R}^{p \times w_k^{j-1}}$ to $\mathbb{R}^{p \times w_k^j}$ is denoted by $\mathcal{L}_k^j$. For each j, each member L_k^j of $\mathcal{L}_k^j$ is equivariant in the sense that, for all $B \in \mathcal{B}_p$ and $v \in \mathbb{R}^{p \times w_k^{j-1}}$, $L_k^j(Bv) = BL_k^j(v)$. When $k = 4$, standard linear layers mapping from $\mathbb{R}^{w_4^{j-1}}$ to $\mathbb{R}^{w_4^j}$ are used for each $j = 1, \ldots, h_4 + 1$, where $w_4^0 = o_3$ and $w_4^{h_4+1} = 1$. For each j, the collection of all such layers is denoted by $\mathcal{L}_4^j$. For a user-specified activation function q, the module classes are defined as follows for $k = 1, 2, 3, 4$:

$$\begin{aligned}\mathcal{M}_k := \{v \mapsto q \circ L_k^{h_k+1} \circ q \circ L_k^{h_k} \circ \ldots \circ q \circ L_k^1(v) \\ : L_k^j \in \mathcal{L}_k^j, j = 1, 2, \ldots, h_k + 1\}.\end{aligned}$$

Notably, $\mathcal{M}_1$ satisfies 9 (Ravanbakhsh et al., 2017; Hartford et al., 2018), and $\mathcal{M}_2$ and $\mathcal{M}_3$ satisfy 9 and 9, respectively (Ravanbakhsh et al., 2016; Zaheer et al., 2017). Each element of $\mathcal{M}_4$ is a multilayer perceptron.

The proposed class of estimators satisfies several nice properties. The first is computational in nature. In particular, if the estimated CATE function will be evaluated at several different values of the test point x_0, then the computational cost can be amortized across these runs by only processing the data on lines 1-3 of Algorithm 11.3 a single time. A prediction at a new test point x_0 can then be evaluated by evaluating lines 4-8. When there are many test points at which to obtain CATE estimates, this can lead to meaningful savings in computational time relative to rerunning the entirety of Algorithm 11.3 for every new test point. Another advantage of the proposed class of estimators is that its members can be evaluated on datasets that have a different sample size than the datasets used during meta-training. In the notation of Eq. 4 from Hartford et al. (2018), this corresponds to noting that the weights from an $\mathbb{R}^{N \times M \times k} \to \mathbb{R}^{N \times M \times o}$ multi-input-output channel layer can be used to define an $\mathbb{R}^{N' \times M \times k} \to \mathbb{R}^{N' \times M \times o}$ layer for which the output $Y_{n,m}^{\langle o \rangle}$ is given by the same symbolic expression as that displayed in Eq. 4 from that work, but now with n ranging over $1, \ldots, N'$. In the context of regression, Luedtke et al. (2021) showed that estimators trained using 500 observations can perform well even when evaluated on datasets containing only 100 observations. It is similarly possible to evaluate the proposed architecture on datasets containing different numbers of covariates than did the datasets used during meta-training — again see Eq. 4 in Hartford et al. (2018), and also see Eq. 22 in Zaheer et al. (2017), but with the sum-pool term replaced by a mean-pool term. Taken together, these observations make it so that an estimator learned for a setting where n observations and p covariates are observed can be evaluated without modification on datasets with $n' \neq n$ observations and $p' \neq p$ covariates. When $n' \approx n$ and $p' \approx p$, it is reasonable to expect that the learned estimator will perform as well as would have an estimator constructed explicitly for the case where the sample size is n' and p' covariates are observed.

11.5 Numerical Experiments

The performance of the proposed AMC approach was evaluated via a numerical experiment similar to experiments that Luedtke et al. (2021) used to evaluate AMC in the context of regression problems. In these experiments, the model $\mathcal{P}$ consisted of distributions for which there exists a vector $v \in \mathbb{R}^p$, a positive definite matrix $\Sigma \in \mathbb{R}^{p \times p}$, a p-variate distribution

$Q_{\boldsymbol{v},\Sigma}$ with the same copula as a $N(\boldsymbol{v},\Sigma)$ distribution, a variance $\sigma^2>0$, and an outcome regression $\mu:\mathcal{A}\times\mathcal{X}\to\mathbb{R}$ belonging to a class $\mathcal{R}_{m,s}$ that will be defined shortly such that

$$X\sim Q_{\boldsymbol{v},\Sigma},\quad A\mid X\sim \text{Bernoulli}(1/2),\quad Y\mid A,X\sim N[\sigma\cdot\mu(A,X),\sigma^2].$$

The class $\mathcal{R}_{m,s}$ is indexed by $m\in(0,\infty)$ and $s\in\{1,2,\ldots,p\}$. The definition of this class relies on the notion of the total variation of a function. Recall that the total variation of $f:\mathbb{R}\to\mathbb{R}$, denoted by $V(f)$, is equal to the supremum of $\sum_{\ell=1}^{k}|f(b_{\ell+1})-f(b_\ell)|$ over all $(b_\ell)_{\ell=1}^{k+1}$ such that $k\in\mathbb{N}$ and $b_1<b_2<\ldots<b_{k+1}$ (Cohn, 2013). Writing x_j to denote the j-th covariate, the model we considered imposes that μ falls in

$$\mathcal{R}:=\left\{(a,x)\mapsto\sum_{j=1}^{p}\mu_j(a,x_j)\ :\ \max_{a'\in\mathcal{A}}\|v_{a'}(\mu)\|_1\le m,\ \|v_0(\mu)\odot v_1(\mu)\|_0\le s\right\},$$

where $v_{a'}(\mu):=(V(\mu_j(a',\cdot)))_{j=1}^{p}$, $\|\cdot\|_1$ denotes the ℓ^1 norm, and $\|\cdot\|_0$ returns the number of non-zero entries of its $\mathbb{R}^p$-valued argument. The above class $\mathcal{R}$ enforces that the treatment-specific outcome regressions $x\mapsto\sigma\cdot\mu(a,x)$, $a\in\mathcal{A}$, should belong to a variant of the fused lasso additive regression model (FLAM) and, together, these functions should rely on no more than s of the covariates (Petersen et al., 2016).

In our experiments, we fix $(n,p,m,s)=(500,10,10,4)$. The collection of priors Γ considered was the same as that presented in Appendices D.2.1 and D.2.3 of Luedtke et al. (2021) in the context of regression, but with two modifications to adapt to our CATE estimation setting. First, a draw from a distribution P in the support of Γ corresponded to a covariate-treatment-outcome tuple (X,A,Y), rather than a covariate-outcome tuple (X,Y). As specified by the model, all $P\in\mathcal{P}$ are such that $A\mid X\sim\text{Bernoulli}(1/2)$ for all $P\in\mathcal{P}$. Second, the generator network used to sample from a given prior returns two regression functions, corresponding to $x\mapsto E_P[Y|A=0,X=x]$ and $x\mapsto E_P[Y|A=1,X=x]$, from a given prior rather than only the single regression function $x\mapsto E_P[Y|X=x]$. These two regression functions were sampled independently of one another from the same generator network as described in Appendix D.2.3 of Luedtke et al. (2021). By setting $s=4$, we imitate the "dense" FLAM setting reported in Luedtke et al. (2021). Following Luedtke et al. (2021), we preprocessed the covariates before supplying them to the estimator. In particular, we replaced each entry with its rank statistic among the n observations so that, for each $i\in\{1,\ldots,n\}$ and $j\in\{1,\ldots,p\}$, we replaced $\boldsymbol{x}_{ij}$ by $\sum_{k=1}^{n}I\{\boldsymbol{x}_{ij}\ge\boldsymbol{x}_{kj}\}$ and x_{0j} by $\sum_{k=1}^{n}I\{x_{0j}\ge\boldsymbol{x}_{kj}\}$. As each prior in Γ is parameterized via a generator function, Algorithm 11.2 was used to construct the estimator. This estimator was constructed over approximately 3 million iterations, where each stochastic gradient update to the prior and estimator was based on 100 datasets. Consequently, the final constructed estimator, hereafter referred to as the AMC estimator, was iteratively updated based on its performance on approximately 300 million datasets. Further details of the implementation used in these experiments, along with the neural network weights used by the constructed estimator, can be found at the following GitHub repository: `https://github.com/alexluedtke12/amc-meta-learning-of-optimal-cate-estimators`.

The performance of the AMC estimator was evaluated using a simulation study. Four scenarios were considered. In all of these scenarios, X consists of covariates $X_1,X_2,\ldots,X_{10}$ that are independently drawn from a Uniform$[-1,1]$ distribution. The treatment A is generated independently of X according to a Bernoulli(1/2) distribution, and, conditionally on A and X, the outcome Y is normally distributed with mean $(2A-1)\theta(X)/2$ and variance 1, where the value of the CATE θ varies across the four scenarios. In particular, $\theta(x)=0.884(1-x_1-x_2)$ in scenario 1, $\theta(x)=2(x_2-0.25x_1^2-1)$ in scenario 2, $\theta(x)=2(0.5-x_1^2-x_2^2)(x_1^2+x_2^2-0.3)$ in scenario 3, and $\theta(x)=2(1-x_1^3+\exp[x_3^2+x_5]+0.6x_6-[x_7+x_8]^2)$ in scenario 4. The Performance of AMC was evaluated via Monte Carlo simulation and compared to that of three

Table 11.1 *MSEs of four estimators of the CATE across the four simulation scenarios.*

	Scenario			
	1	2	3	4
Linear Model	**0.092**	**0.117**	0.655	4.640
FLAM	0.403	0.423	0.545	**3.601**
Causal Forests	0.169	0.144	0.435	4.208
AMC (ours)	0.156	0.148	**0.316**	3.823

existing methods. The first comparator corresponds to causal forests (Athey et al., 2019) as implemented in the `grf` package in R (Tibshirani et al., 2022), where all tuning parameters were selected via cross-validation. The latter two comparators correspond to simple plug-in estimators of the treatment-specific outcome regressions $x \mapsto E_P[Y|A = 1, X = x]$ and $x \mapsto E_P[Y|A = 0, X = x]$ whose difference defines the CATE. Such plug-in approaches were referred to as T-learners in Künzel et al. (2019). The first of these approaches estimates each treatment-specific outcome regression with a main terms linear regression, whereas the second estimates each of them using the fused lasso additive model as implemented in the `flam` package in R with tuning parameters selected via cross-validation (Petersen, 2018). The performance of all approaches was evaluated using 1000 Monte Carlo repetitions.

Table 11.1 reports the performance of the four approaches. The linear-model-based T-learner outperformed all other approaches for scenario 1, which is unsurprising given that the outcome regressions were truly linear in that setting. The AMC estimator outperformed the remaining two comparators in this setting. In the second scenario, the AMC estimator was again outperformed by the linear model, was slightly outperformed by causal forests, and outperformed FLAM. The strong performance of the linear model in scenario 2 may be due to the fact that the CATE is nearly a linear function of the covariates in that setting. In scenario 3, the AMC estimator outperformed all comparators, with the next best estimator being causal forests and the worst-performing estimator being the linear model. Finally, in scenario 4, the AMC estimator was only outperformed by FLAM.

Overall, AMC demonstrated a reasonable level of adaptivity in these scenarios, being able to perform relatively well both in the simpler scenarios 1 and 2 and the more complex scenarios 3 and 4. In future work, it would be interesting to explore this adaptivity further by using cross-validation to select between several AMC estimators, each constructed to be Γ-minimax against a different collection of priors Γ. For example, these different collections of priors may be indexed by different bound m on the total variation of the outcome regression μ or sparsity levels s. Alternatively, some of these collections of priors may enforce parsimony of the CATE function (e.g., linearity) while others may allow for a much more complex form (e.g., via a collection of Bayesian additive regression tree priors; (Chipman et al., 2010; Hill, 2011)).

11.6 Notes and Further Reading

This chapter belongs to a recent body of literature introducing AMC schemes for general decision problems (Luedtke et al., 2020; Qiu and Luedtke, 2020) and in a special case, namely regression settings (Luedtke et al., 2021). Owing to the similarity between CATE estimation and regression estimation, the AMC approach proposed described in this chapter is most closely related to the approach described in Luedtke et al. (2021). Therefore, to facilitate comparisons, we have organized the presentation of the method and results similarly.

More broadly, the proposed approach is related to several prior works from the statistics, econometrics, and machine learning communities. We begin by describing those in the statistics and econometrics literature. In finite-dimensional models, early works showed that it is possible to numerically learn minimax rules (Nelson, 1966; Kempthorne, 1987) and, in settings where Γ consists of all priors that satisfy a finite number of generalized moment conditions, Γ-minimax rules (Noubiap and Seidel, 2001). Other works have studied the Γ-minimax case where Γ consists of priors that only place mass on a pre-specified finite set of distributions or priors, both for general decision problems (Chamberlain, 2000) and for constructing confidence intervals (Schafer and Stark, 2009). The collections Γ that we consider in Algorithm 11.1 are of this same form. In contrast to the earlier works that considered collections Γ of this type, we explicitly consider the equivariance properties that are desirable for an estimator to have in the context of CATE estimation. We moreover present a neural network class of estimators that has these properties and construct our estimator via a form of stochastic gradient descent ascent that is easy to implement efficiently using standard software.

The approach proposed in this work is also related to the meta-learning literature from the machine learning community (Schmidhuber, 1987; Thrun and Pratt, 1998; Hochreiter et al., 2001; Vilalta and Drissi, 2002). As noted in Luedtke et al. (2021), most existing works in that literature focus on the special case where $\Gamma = \{\Pi\}$ for some fixed, user-specified prior Π, so that the goal is to construct a Bayes estimator. To our knowledge, these works have not previously been developed in the context of CATE estimation. Nevertheless, there are a number of interesting meta-learning approaches that have been used in supervised learning settings (e.g., Vinyals et al., 2016; Ravi and Larochelle, 2017; Finn et al., 2017; Garnelo et al., 2018). Adapting these approaches to estimate the CATE for cases where $\Gamma = \{\Pi\}$ would be an interesting area for future work.

Acknowledgements

Generous support was provided by the National Institutes of Health (NIH) under award number DP2-LM013340. The content is solely the responsibility of the authors and does not necessarily represent the official views of the NIH.

Chapter 12

Personalized Policy Learning

Min Qian, Xinyu Hu, Bin Cheng

12.1 Introduction

Recent advances in mobile technologies have enabled the continuous monitoring of health-related information, such as environmental stressors and users' health behaviors, over an extended period of time. This has facilitated the development of mobile health applications for delivering interventions to improve users' self-care management of their health concerns (Heron and Smyth, 2010). For example, Mohr et al. (2013) implemented a mobile intervention platform to continuously evaluate the behavioral intervention technologies for depression and anxiety; Haapala et al. (2009) developed a mobile phone-operated weight-loss program to instruct a staggered reduction of food intake and daily weight reporting with immediate tailored feedback; and Depp et al. (2015) evaluated a mobile device delivered interactive psychosocial intervention linking patient-reported mood states with personalized self-management strategies for bipolar disorder.

Compared with a traditional in-person intervention, a mobile-delivered intervention has the advantages of being more accessible to the user and more responsive to user's momentary environmental, social, and health state changes (Riley et al., 2011). Most importantly, it can be tailored to individual users to achieve maximal treatment benefit. In this chapter, we introduce a personalized policy learning (PPL) framework to support implementing the delivery of such individualized interventions. Our goal is to devise decision support systems that optimize the decision quality of smartphone health applications tailored to user characteristics and usage history.

This work is motivated by the IntelliCare study (Mohr et al., 2017). IntelliCare is a suite of smartphone apps for users with depression or anxiety, designed on the notion that people are better served by a collection of simple apps, each with specific goals, psychological strategies, and simple interactive elements. The suite contains 12 individual apps that instantiate a variety of psychological strategies using several interactional styles to support the acquisition of a set of skills related to depression or anxiety, including goal setting and cognitive restructuring. In addition, each user's experience, including messages and notifications, weekly apply recommendations, and prompts to complete health surveys, are managed by a central Hub app. Each task orchestrated by the Hub app entails a set of decisions about treatments or interventions, such as which app to recommend or when to send a health survey, that are made over time for each user. The objective is to develop policies to support and improve the decision quality of smartphone health applications that are tailored to each user's characteristics and app usage patterns over time.

The chapter is organized as follows. In Section 12.2, we discuss the trade-off between long-term and short-term treatment benefits. In Section 12.3, we provide the rationale of a personalized policy. In Section 12.4, we establish the personalized policy learning framework and outline the batch mode learning approach to optimizing immediate outcomes. We discuss extensions of this approach to online mode learning and to long-term outcomes in Section 12.5 and Section 12.6, respectively. We conclude the chapter with a discussion of future directions in Section 12.7.

DOI: 10.1201/9781003216223-12

12.2 Long-Term versus Immediate Outcomes

In most mobile health apps studies, while the ultimate goal is to improve a patient's overall health status, decisions must be taken at various time points so that information can be collected without interruption. Such decisions will have both immediate and long-term impacts, thus one must decide upfront which outcome to optimize. In this section, we discuss the implications of this choice.

Many tasks in mobile health applications can be viewed as decision processes evolving in time. At each time point t, we use A_t to denote the decision, and Y_t the scalar outcome which immediately follows this decision. When designing an optimal policy, one needs to balance the immediate (short-term) outcome Y_t, and long-term outcome (e.g., $\sum_{s=0}^{\infty} \gamma^s Y_{t+s}$ for continuing tasks, where γ is a discount factor, or $\sum_{s=0}^{T-t} Y_{t+s}$ for episodic tasks; Sutton and Barto (1998)), and decide which one to optimize given a specific task.

In the IntelliCare example, a major feature of the Hub app is to make weekly recommendations to improve a user's overall engagement with the apps. Here, A_t would be the app(s) recommended in week t, and Y_t is a measure of app usage intensity in the week following the recommendation. The impact of a decision could be positive (e.g., the user likes the recommended app and wants to try other apps in the suite as well) or negative (e.g., the user sticks to the recommended app, and does not have the desire or time to explore other apps). It is possible that the impact of a decision only starts to manifest itself after a certain period of time. For example, a good decision leads to a favorable usage experience of the recommended app, which in turn enhances its adherence; or excessive usage of the recommended app generates boredom, leading to a subsequent reduction in usage. Because the objective of the IntelliCare study was to engage the users of the IntelliCare suite of apps as long as possible, and given the possibility of delayed effects in app recommendation, it makes sense to target some sort of long-term outcomes, as in the continuing or episodic tasks described in the previous paragraph.

While optimizing long-term outcomes (e.g., long-term app usage) seems fundamental, we argue that in mobile health applications, it is equally important, if not more so, to optimize short-term outcomes. First, because user engagement on mobile health systems often declines quickly over time (Christmann et al. 2009; Mohr et al. 2013), it is necessary to implement decisions that promote short-term engagement and boost immediate outcomes. In the IntelliCare example, one objective was to learn the best time to push a prompt, a factor that is known to impact mobile application usage (Bohmer et al., 2011). The rationale is that, through constant attention and prompt reminders, a user's engagement will be sustained and thus their behavior changes will gradually materialize. Second, when multiple outcomes are of interest, an immediate response in one outcome can be useful in recommending decisions for the other outcomes. In the IntelliCare example, one other function of Hub app is to send push notifications to prompt a user to complete a short four-item patient health questionnaire (PHQ-4), which measures the severity of depression and anxiety symptoms, repeatedly at 7-day intervals. Thus, a specific goal is to identify a daily prompt schedule (time) that maximizes response rate. This information can assist the Hub app to determine the best app(s) to recommend for the user in the following week, but this is not feasible for prompt non-responders. Third, while optimization based on the long-term outcome is arguably more fundamental, it is both theoretically more challenging and practically more onerous. In mobile health studies, aiming for immediate outcomes faces a minimal risk in practical implementation. Personalized policy learning in long-term outcomes will be further discussed in Section 12.6.

12.3 Personalized Medicine via Personalized Policy

The use of mobile apps and wearable devices provides real-time data that would help better monitor illness dynamics and thus facilitate the delivery of personalized care when it is most needed. One way to operationalize personalized treatment is to account for between user heterogeneity by mapping user-specific covariates to personalized interventions. In this approach, one assumes a population-level *nomothetic* model to capture between-user heterogeneity by incorporating individual characteristics in the model and estimating their effects by pooling data across individuals. There is a large amount of literature on learning methods in this direction, including contextual bandits methods for optimizing immediate outcomes (Woodroofe, 1979; Lei et al., 2017), reinforcement learning methods for optimizing long-term outcomes for episodic tasks (Murphy, 2003; Robins, 2004; Murphy, 2005b; Laber et al., 2014; Song et al., 2015b; Oh et al., 2022), and continuing tasks (Watkins, 1989; Sutton and Barto, 1998; Luckett et al., 2020; Ertefaie and Strawderman, 2018). This paradigm, henceforth termed *one-policy-for-all*, assumes that the between-user heterogeneity has been fully captured by the observed variables, and the policy is therefore fully tailored to all individuals in the population.

The above paradigm makes the important assumption that individualized treatment can be achieved by accounting for heterogeneity in a collection of observable covariates. Such an assumption is tenuous as unobserved covariates may also lead to heterogeneity. In this chapter, we define a *personalized policy* as one that depends on a user's up-to-date characteristics, observed or not. A personalized policy represents a paradigm shift from one-policy-for-all users delineated in the previous paragraph to an *ideographic* or completely individualized policy for each user. In this personalized policy framework, even the observed information at a given time point is the same for the users, the optimal interventions may still be different, due to potential unobserved moderators.

We illustrate the effects of unobserved moderators under a single-time decision setting, assuming there are no carryover or delayed intervention effects. At a given decision period, for each user, we have the pre-treatment variables $S \in \mathcal{S}$, treatment A, taking values in a finite, discrete treatment space $\mathcal{A}$, and a real-valued outcome Y, assuming large values are desirable. In this context, a deterministic policy π is a decision rule mapping $\mathcal{S}$ into the treatment space $\mathcal{A}$. Under the one-policy-for-all paradigm, personalized treatment can be realized by recommending treatment $a = \pi(s)$ based on a user's characteristics s. A policy is called optimal if the expected outcome is maximized when all patients in the study population follow the policy. That is, the optimal policy satisfies $\pi^o = \arg\max_\pi E_\pi(Y)$, where $E_\pi(Y)$ denotes the expected outcome Y when treatment is consistent with π (i.e., $A = \pi(S)$). In particular, it can be shown that the optimal policy π^o satisfies

$$\pi^o(S) = \arg\max_{a \in \mathcal{A}} E(Y|S, A = a).$$

This policy, once developed, can be applied to the whole study population to achieve personalized treatment.

Suppose there is an additional unobserved pre-treatment covariate U that moderates the effect of intervention A on Y. Were U observed, then personalized treatment would be further improved by setting optimal policy

$$\pi^u(S, U) = \arg\max_{a \in \mathcal{A}} E(Y|S, U, A = a),$$

and using π^u as a population policy to assign treatment for each user. Note that $E_{\pi^u}(Y) \geq E_{\pi^o}Y$. In an optimal personalized policy, instead of viewing U as an argument in the policy function π^u, we incorporate U in the policy function itself, namely, $\pi^o(S) = \pi^u(S, U)$. The optimal personalized policy π^o may vary from user to user due to unobserved moderators U.

12.4 Personalized Policies via Mixed Effects Model Framework

To develop personalized policies, an ideographic approach is to estimate a person's best intervention decision using the person's own data only. For example, in "N-of-1" trials, a person's longitudinal data is viewed as a multi-period crossover study, and time series methods are used to estimate individual treatment effects on immediate outcome, thereby identifying the optimal treatment for the individual (Lillie et al., 2011; Kravitz R.L., 2014). Alternatively, reinforcement learning methods can be applied to each individual's data to develop a policy (Lei et al., 2017). The "N-of-1" approach in principle allows for insights about individuals without assumptions about any reference population. However, the quality of the estimated decision and its practicality rely on how much data can be obtained from this user. In general, the efficiency of this approach may suffer, especially in situations where user-level data is sparse or an action exhibits similar effects on all individuals.

In this section, we introduce personalized policy learning via generalized linear mixed effects models (GLMM) to optimize the immediate outcome. In such a model, the immediate outcome at each time point is the dependent variable and time-varying covariates, treatment, and their interactions are the predictors. The estimated policy would recommend the treatment that optimizes the predicted outcome based on each user's information at a given time point. Note that each user in the data set would yield a different policy due to the presence of random effects. The fixed effects part of the model represents the population effect, and the random effects part captures individual departure from the population due to unobserved heterogeneity.

Suppose we have collected data from n mobile app users. For each user $i = 1, \ldots, n$, the observed data can be represented as repeated measures of the same set of variables over time, denoted by $(S_{it}, A_{it}, Y_{it})_{t=1}^{m_i}$, where m_i is the number of observed time points for subject i. For each time point $t = 1, \ldots, m_i$, $S_{it} \in \mathcal{S}$ is a vector of covariates observed prior to the t-th time point, A_{it} is the action-taking values in the pre-specified set $\mathcal{A}$ of action space, and Y_{it} is the scalar outcome of interest observed after each action, with the convention that prefers larger values. As noted in Qian et al. (2020), a covariate process S_{it} is called *exogenous* if $S_{i,t+1}$ is independent of prior outcome and decision $(\bar{A}_{it}, \bar{Y}_{it})$ conditional on $\bar{S}_{i,t}$, where an overbar denotes the history of the random variable; otherwise, S_{it} is *endogenous*. In this chapter, S_{it} may include exogenous covariates, such as baseline variables, functions of time t, and weekday/weekend indicator, as well as endogenous covariates that may depend on prior outcome and decision, such as app usage at each time point.

We assume that the unobserved individual heterogeneity can be summarized in the form of random effects $\boldsymbol{\alpha}_{0i\cdot}$, a q-dimensional mean 0 random vector. In addition, suppose for each user i, the conditional mean of Y_{it} given past history is *Markovian* and *stationary* over time. That is,

$$\begin{aligned} E(Y_{it}|S_{i1}, A_{i1}, Y_{i1}, \ldots, S_{it}, A_{it}, \boldsymbol{\alpha}_{0i\cdot}) =& E(Y_{it}|S_{it}, A_{it}, \boldsymbol{\alpha}_{0i\cdot}) \\ \triangleq& Q_0(S_{it}, A_{it}; \boldsymbol{\alpha}_{0i\cdot}) \end{aligned} \tag{12.1}$$

where Q_0 is the time-invariant conditional mean function of Y_{it} given $(S_{it}, A_{it}, \boldsymbol{\alpha}_{0i\cdot})$. The first equality in (12.1) is the result of the Markovian condition, and the second equality in (12.1) is implied by the stationary condition so that the conditional mean function depends on time t only through S_{it}, A_{it}, and $\boldsymbol{\alpha}_{0i\cdot}$. For each mobile app user $i = 1, \ldots, n$, we operationalize the personalized decision problem via a personalized policy, π_i, that takes covariates S_{it} as input, and outputs a decision A_{it} at each time point. Our goal is to develop a policy π_i, that when implemented, will result in the maximal expected conditional outcome, $E_{\pi_i}(Y_{it}|S_{it}, A_{it}, \boldsymbol{\alpha}_{0i\cdot})$, where the expectation is taken with respect to Y_{it} conditional on the past history S_{it}, assuming π_i is used to select an action at decision point t. This policy is called the optimal *myopic* policy for user i, and denoted by π_{0i}. Once developed, the policy can be used to guide decision making for the user in the future. It is easy to see that the optimal myopic policy satisfies $\pi_{0i}(s) = \arg\max_{a\in\mathcal{A}} E(Y_{it}|S_{it} = s, A_{it} = a, \boldsymbol{\alpha}_{0i\cdot}) = \arg\max_{a\in\mathcal{A}} Q_0(s, a, \boldsymbol{\alpha}_{0i\cdot})$. So the key is to estimate the conditional mean model $Q_0(s, a, \boldsymbol{\alpha}_{0i\cdot})$.

We approach the problem using a generalized linear mixed models framework. Specifically, we assume

$$g(Q_0(S_{it}, A_{it}; \boldsymbol{\alpha}_{0i\cdot})) = h_1(S_{it}, A_{it})^{\mathrm{T}}\boldsymbol{\beta}_0 + h_2(S_{it}, A_{it})^{\mathrm{T}}\boldsymbol{\alpha}_{0i\cdot}^{\mathrm{T}}, \tag{12.2}$$

for $i = 1, \ldots, n$ and $t = 1, \ldots, m_i$, where $g(\cdot)$ is a known strictly monotone increasing link function. For example, $g(\cdot)$ could be an identity function for a continuous outcome, logit function for a binary outcome, and log function for a count outcome. Here $\boldsymbol{\beta}_0$ is a p-dimensional vector of unknown parameters, and $h_1(S_{it}, A_{it}) \in \mathbb{R}^p$ is a pre-specified vector function of (S_{it}, A_{it}) so that $h_1(S_{it}, A_{it})^{\mathrm{T}}\boldsymbol{\beta}_0$ is the mean effect (i.e., the fixed effects part), e.g., $h_1(S_{it}, A_{it})^{\mathrm{T}}\boldsymbol{\beta} = \beta_0 + \beta_1 S_{it} + \beta_2 A_{it} + \beta_3 S_{it} A_{it}$; $\boldsymbol{\alpha}_0$ is the $n \times q$ $(q \le p)$ matrix of random effects with the i-th row, $\boldsymbol{\alpha}_{0i\cdot}$, being the random effects parameters for the i-th user, and $h_2(S_{it}, A_{it}) \in \mathbb{R}^q$ is a sub-vector of $h_1(S_{it}, A_{it})$ chosen so that $h_2(S_{it}, A_{it})^{\mathrm{T}}\boldsymbol{\alpha}_{0i\cdot}^{\mathrm{T}}$ models subject-specific deviations from the mean model. Under model (12.2) and the monotone increasing property of $g(\cdot)$, the optimal myopic policy π_{0i} for subject i is

$$\pi_{0i}(S_{it}) = \arg\max_{a\in\mathcal{A}} \left(h_1(S_{it}, a)^{\mathrm{T}}\boldsymbol{\beta}_0 + h_2(S_{it}, a)^{\mathrm{T}}\boldsymbol{\alpha}_{0i\cdot}^{\mathrm{T}}\right). \tag{12.3}$$

Note that $\boldsymbol{\alpha}_{0i\cdot}$ has dual roles. On one hand, it characterizes the unobserved deviation of the i-th user from the mean model. Thus, when a user is specified, $\boldsymbol{\alpha}_{0i\cdot}$ is viewed as a fixed parameter. On the other hand, since users i for $i = 1, \ldots, n$, are randomly selected from the population, $\boldsymbol{\alpha}_{0i\cdot}$'s can also be viewed as independent and identically distributed (i.i.d.) latent random vectors from the population point of view.

Parameter Estimation

GLMM is one of the most popular methods to handle longitudinal data (Laird and Ware, 1982). The fixed effects parameter in the GLMM has a conditional interpretation in the sense that it measures the effects of a covariate conditional on the random effects. This interpretation is consistent with the scientific interest in the prediction of person-specific effects to guide personalized decision making. Standard GLMM-based estimation methods are designed for settings where covariates are exogenous with respect to the outcome process. When covariates are endogenous, estimates of the fixed effects parameters based on Generalized Estimating Equations (GEE) or other likelihood-based methods are likely to be biased (i.e. the estimate does not have a conditional interpretation, see (Pepe and Anderson, 1994; Diggle et al., 2002)). Qian et al. (2020) studied the causal treatment effects in longitudinal studies under the linear mixed models (LMM) framework. They showed that when endogenous covariates are present, standard LMM software can still be used to obtain a valid estimate of the fixed effects parameter (with conditional interpretation) under an additional assumption that the time-varying covariates are independent of random effects parameters conditional on past history.

We mention some previous work on studying personalized treatment effects using the mixed effects model framework. Diaz et al. (2007) applied random intercept linear models to determine individualized optimal drug dosage for producing a desired drug plasma concentration level. This was the first attempt to provide random-effects model interpretation in the personalized medicine literature. Cho et al. (2017) used GLMM to predict individual outcomes under each treatment arm with a random slope on the treatment indicator, and built a random forest model to predict random slopes using patients' baseline covariates. The fixed and random effects parameters were estimated using a GEE type of method to accommodate potential correlation in longitudinal outcome observations. Personalized treatment can then be implemented by selecting the treatment with the maximal estimated random effects. These methods are also developed for exogenous covariate processes.

In Hu et al. (2021), we proposed a novel algorithm that jointly estimates the fixed effects and the random effects by maximizing a penalized pseudo-log-likelihood type objective function. A ridge-type penalty on the random effects terms is used to shrink and stabilize the estimation of the random effects. In addition, to avoid unnecessary parameterization of individual departure, we impose a group lasso penalty (Yuan and Lin, 2006) on the random effects. Intuitively, we view the random effects coefficient of a covariate as a way to accommodate potential interaction between unobserved confounders and the covariate in the model. If such interaction does not exist, then we expect the corresponding random effect coefficients for all users to shrink to zero; otherwise, the random effects term remains active and yields heterogeneous policies across users.

Specifically, let $\{\ell(Y_{it}, S_{it}, A_{it}; \boldsymbol{\beta}, \boldsymbol{\alpha}_{i\cdot}, \phi) : \boldsymbol{\beta} \in \mathbb{R}^p, \boldsymbol{\alpha}_{i\cdot}^{\mathrm{T}} \in \mathbb{R}^q\}$ denote the working conditional log-likelihood of Y_{it} under a fully specified GLMM with the systematic component (12.2). For example, with a continuous Y_{it}, we may set $\ell(\cdot)$ to be the Gaussian log-likelihood with mean $Q(S_{it}, A_{it}; \boldsymbol{\beta}, \boldsymbol{\alpha}_{i\cdot})$, variance σ^2, and an identity link. When Y_{it} is binary, we may choose $\ell(\cdot)$ to be the Bernoulli log-likelihood with probability $Q(S_{it}, A_{it}; \boldsymbol{\beta}, \boldsymbol{\alpha}_{i\cdot})$ and a logit link. Correspondingly, we define the penalized pseudo-log-likelihood

$$\begin{aligned} L_{ppl}(\boldsymbol{\beta}, \boldsymbol{\alpha}) = &\sum_{i=1}^{n} \sum_{t=1}^{m_i} \ell(Y_{it}, S_{it}, A_{it}; \boldsymbol{\beta}, \boldsymbol{\alpha}_{i\cdot}, \phi) \\ &- \frac{1}{2} \sum_{i=1}^{n} \boldsymbol{\alpha}_{i\cdot} \boldsymbol{D}^{-} \boldsymbol{\alpha}_{i\cdot}^{\mathrm{T}} - \lambda \sum_{l=1}^{q} w_l \|\boldsymbol{\alpha}_{\cdot l}\|, \end{aligned} \tag{12.4}$$

where $\boldsymbol{D} \in \mathbb{R}^{q \times q}$ is a symmetric positive semi-definite matrix, $\boldsymbol{D}^{-}$ is the Moore-Penrose generalized inverse of $\boldsymbol{D}$ and $\lambda \geq 0$ is a tuning parameter.

We propose to estimate $\boldsymbol{\beta}_0$ and $\boldsymbol{\alpha}_0$ by maximizing (12.4). The maximum penalized-pseudo-likelihood estimator is denoted by

$$(\hat{\boldsymbol{\beta}}, \hat{\boldsymbol{\alpha}}) = \arg \max_{\boldsymbol{\beta} \in \mathbb{R}^p, \boldsymbol{\alpha} \in \mathbb{R}^{n \times q}} L_{ppl}(\boldsymbol{\beta}.\boldsymbol{\alpha}), \tag{12.5}$$

and the corresponding personalized policy for user i is estimated by

$$\hat{\pi}_i(s) \in \arg \max_{a \in \mathcal{A}} \left(h_1(s, a)^{\mathrm{T}} \hat{\boldsymbol{\beta}} + h_2(s, a)^{\mathrm{T}} \hat{\boldsymbol{\alpha}}_{i\cdot}^{\mathrm{T}} \right),$$

analogously to π_{0i} in (12.3).

Under the viewpoint that $\{\boldsymbol{\alpha}\}$ is a random sample of a population, it is natural to choose $\boldsymbol{D}$ in the second term of (12.4) to reflect the variance-covariance matrix of $\boldsymbol{\alpha}_{0i\cdot}^{\mathrm{T}}$, although it is not required for the asymptotic properties to hold. Similarly, since group l in the third term of (12.4) contains the random effects parameter of the l-th term in $h_2(S_{it}, A_{it})$ for all n users, it is intuitive to set the group-specific weight $w_l \geq 0$ to be inversely proportional to the variance of $\boldsymbol{\alpha}_{\cdot l}$.

In practice, we propose to update $\boldsymbol{D}$, ϕ and w_l's iteratively, in conjunction with the trust region newton (TRON) algorithm in the estimation of $\boldsymbol{\beta}$ and $\boldsymbol{\alpha}$. Briefly, the TRON algorithm combines the trust region method (Steihaug, 1983) and the truncated newton method (Nash, 2000) to solve an unconstrained convex optimization problem. At each iteration, TRON defines a trust region and approximates the objective function using a quadratic model within the region. If a pre-specified change of the objective function is achieved in the current iteration, the updated direction is accepted and the region is expanded; the region will be shrunk otherwise. The approximation sub-problem is solved via the conjugate gradient method. Since TRON solves the inverse of a potentially large Hessian matrix by iteratively updating the parameters, convergence can be achieved quickly with a large and dense Hessian. Overall, the computational cost per iteration is of the order of the number of nonzero elements in the design matrix. See Section S1 in Supplementary Material of Hu et al. (2021) for the detailed description of the TRON algorithm. and the selection of tuning parameter λ.

Connection and Comparison to traditional GLMM estimation methods

The traditional GLMM estimation methods assume three conditions:

(i) a distributional assumption on the random effects parameters;

(ii) $\ell(\cdot)$ is the true log-likelihood of Y_{it} given $(S_{it}, A_{it}, \boldsymbol{\alpha}_{0i})$; and

(iii) S_{it} is an exogenous process; that is,

$$S_{it} \perp \{(Y_{is}, A_{is}) : s = 1, \ldots, t-1\} \Big| \{S_{is} : s = 1, \ldots, t-1\},$$

where $A \perp B | C$ means that A is independent of B conditional on C.

For example, assume $\{\boldsymbol{\alpha}_{i\cdot} : i = 1, \ldots, n\}$ to be i.i.d. mean zero normal random vectors. In the LMM setting, a conventional method is to estimate $\boldsymbol{\beta}$ first by maximizing the marginal density of observations Y_{it}'s (with $\boldsymbol{\alpha}_i$'s integrated out), and then estimate $\boldsymbol{\alpha}_i$ using empirical Bayes (Laird and Ware, 1982). This, however, could be computationally challenging for GLMM since the marginal likelihood usually has no closed form and approximating the marginal likelihood is challenging especially with high-dimensional random effects. Breslow and Clayton (1993) proposed a penalized quasi-likelihood (PQL) approach by maximizing the joint density of the observations and random effects. Specifically, the PQL criterion is equivalent to the sum of the first two terms of L_{ppl} defined in (12.4) (without the group lasso penalty). In the setting of normal densities with identity link, PQL and the conventional method are equivalent and lead to the BLUE (best linear unbiased estimate) and BLUP (best linear unbiased predictor) of $\boldsymbol{\beta}$ and $\boldsymbol{\alpha}_{i\cdot}$'s, respectively. They are approximately identical in other general settings, such as with binary or count outcomes. From this point of view, the objective function $L_{ppl}(\boldsymbol{\beta}, \boldsymbol{\alpha})$ can be viewed as a penalized PQL.

In Hu et al. (2021), we examined conditions under which the proposed method yields consistent estimators of the fixed and random effects parameters. In contrast to conditions (i)-(iii) mentioned above, we relaxed the assumptions to:

(i') The latent random effects $\boldsymbol{\alpha}_{0i\cdot}, i = 1, \ldots, n$, are independent and identically distributed with mean $\mathbf{0}$ and finite variance $\boldsymbol{\Sigma}$.

(ii') $\ell(Y_{it}, S_{it}, A_{it}; \boldsymbol{\beta}, \boldsymbol{\alpha}_{i\cdot}, \phi)$ is a pseudo-log-likelihood that is concave in $(\boldsymbol{\beta}, \boldsymbol{\alpha})$, satisfies

$$E\Big[\sum_{i=1}^{n}\sum_{t=1}^{m_i} \nabla_{\boldsymbol{\beta}}\ell(Y_{it}, S_{it}, A_{it}; \boldsymbol{\beta}, \boldsymbol{\alpha}_{i\cdot}, \phi)\big|_{\boldsymbol{\beta}=\boldsymbol{\beta}_0, \boldsymbol{\alpha}=\boldsymbol{\alpha}_0}\Big] = \mathbf{0}$$

$$\text{and } E\Big[\sum_{t=1}^{m_i} \nabla_{\boldsymbol{\alpha}_{i\cdot}}\ell(Y_{it}, S_{it}, A_{it}; \boldsymbol{\beta}, \boldsymbol{\alpha}_{i\cdot}, \phi)\big|_{\boldsymbol{\beta}=\boldsymbol{\beta}_0, \boldsymbol{\alpha}=\boldsymbol{\alpha}_0}\Big] = \mathbf{0}$$

$$\text{for } i = 1, \ldots, n, \tag{12.6}$$

and its expected second-order derivative is continuous in $(\boldsymbol{\beta}, \boldsymbol{\alpha})$, where $\boldsymbol{\alpha}_{i\cdot}$ is the i-th row of $\boldsymbol{\alpha}$, and $\nabla_{\boldsymbol{\beta}}\ell$ and $\nabla_{\boldsymbol{\alpha}_{i\cdot}}\ell$ denote the partial derivatives of ℓ with respect to $\boldsymbol{\beta}$ and $\boldsymbol{\alpha}_{i\cdot}$, respectively.

(iii') Denote $\ell_1(\boldsymbol{\beta}, \boldsymbol{\alpha}) = \sum_{i=1}^{n}\sum_{t=1}^{m_i} \ell(Y_{it}, S_{it}, A_{it}; \boldsymbol{\beta}, \boldsymbol{\alpha}_{i\cdot}, \phi)$. We assume the following regularity conditions:

(a) As $N := \sum_{i=1}^{n} m_i \to \infty$, $\boldsymbol{\beta}_0$ satisfies

$$N^{-1}E\left\{\left[\nabla_{\beta}\ell_1(\beta_0,\alpha_0)\right]^{\mathrm{T}}\nabla_{\beta}\ell_1(\beta_0,\alpha_0)\right\}=O(1);$$
$$\sup_{(\beta,\alpha)\in\Omega}\left\|N^{-1}\nabla_{\beta}^{\mathrm{T}}\nabla_{\beta}\ell_1(\beta,\alpha)-E\left\{N^{-1}\nabla_{\beta}^{\mathrm{T}}\nabla_{\beta}\ell_1(\beta,\alpha)|\alpha_0\right\}\right\|_{\mathrm{F}}$$
$$=o_P(1)$$

P_{α_0}-almost surely, where $\|\cdot\|_{\mathrm{F}}$ denotes the Frobenius norm;
and $M_{\beta\beta}\triangleq-\liminf_{N\to\infty}E\left\{N^{-1}\nabla_{\beta}^{\mathrm{T}}\nabla_{\beta}\ell_1(\beta_0,\alpha_0)\right\}$ is positive definite with all eigenvalues greater than $\delta_0>0$.

(b) $\sup_i m_i^{-1}E\{\nabla_{\alpha_{i\cdot}}\ell_1(\beta_0,\alpha_0)^{\mathrm{T}}\nabla_{\alpha_{i\cdot}}\ell_1(\beta_0,\alpha_0)\}=O(1)$.

(c) For $i=1,\ldots,n$, as $m_i\to\infty$, $\alpha_{0i\cdot}$ satisfies

$$\sup_{(\beta,\alpha)\in\Omega}\left\|m_i^{-1}\nabla_{\alpha_{i\cdot}}^{\mathrm{T}}\nabla_{\alpha_{i\cdot}}\ell_1(\beta,\alpha)-E\left\{m_i^{-1}\nabla_{\alpha_{i\cdot}}^{\mathrm{T}}\nabla_{\alpha_{i\cdot}}\ell_1(\beta,\alpha)|\alpha_0\right\}\right\|_{\mathrm{F}}$$
$$=o_P(1)$$

P_{α_0}-almost surely;
and $M_{\alpha_{i\cdot}\alpha_{i\cdot}}\triangleq-\liminf_{m_i}E\{m_i^{-1}\nabla_{\alpha_{i\cdot}}^{\mathrm{T}}\nabla_{\alpha_{i\cdot}}\ell_1(\beta_0,\alpha_0)\}$ is positive definite with all eigenvalues greater than $\delta_0>0$.

It is easy to see that conditions (i')-(iii') are relaxed versions of (i)-(iii). In particular, condition (ii') can be viewed as first-order condition. Under model (12.2), we can verify that the Gaussian and the Bernoulli log-likelihoods satisfy (12.6); and since they are often the practical choices for continuous and binary outcomes, they may be used as pseudo-log-likelihood in many applications. Condition (iii') is similar to the regularity conditions required in maximum likelihood estimation. Under condition (iii) of exogenous covariate process S_{it}, (iii') holds under the regularity conditions used in GLMM. In addition, Condition (iii') also holds under many situations when S_{it}'s are endogenous. In Hu et al. (2021), we verify this condition in two illustrative examples: one containing covariates that depend on the latent random effects, and one containing a covariate that depends on the outcome in previous time points.

Properties of the Derived Personalized Policies

As we aim to consistently estimate the fixed and random effects parameters, we would expect that the estimated policies behave similar to π_{0i} defined in (12.3). The quality of a policy $\pi:\mathcal{S}\to\mathcal{A}$ can be evaluated by the expected outcome if the subject follows the policy. In particular, for user i, $E_{\pi}(Y_{it}|S_{it}=s_t,\alpha_{0i\cdot})$ is the conditional expected outcome at time t if treatment assignment A_{it} is consistent with π given $S_{it}=s_t$, and $E_{\pi}(Y_{it}|\alpha_{0i\cdot})$ is the marginal expected outcome at time t if treatment assignment A_{is} is consistent with π for all time points $1\le s\le t$. Note that under model (12.2), π_{0i} satisfies

$$\pi_{0i}(S_{it})=\arg\max_{a\in\mathcal{A}}E(Y_{it}|S_{it}=s_t,A_{it}=a,\alpha_{0i\cdot})$$
$$=\arg\max_{\pi}E_{\pi}(Y_{it}|S_{it}=s_t,\alpha_{0i\cdot})$$

That is, π_{0i} is optimal in the conditional sense. However, π_{0i} may not necessarily be optimal in a marginal sense after integrating out S_{it}, because the distribution of S_{it} may depend on previous treatment assignments.

In Hu et al. (2021), we showed the convergence of the estimated personalized policies to $\pi_{0i},i=1,\ldots,n$ in both conditional and marginal expected outcomes (in sample average). This implies that the estimated policies are conditionally optimal but not marginally optimal.

12.5 Online Personalized Policy Learning

So far, we have described batch mode learning of personalized policies for existing users. That is, one single analysis is performed after data is collected. A key element in creating an evidence-based mobile app intervention delivery system is to keep users engaged by improving user experience and decision quality over time (Mohr et al., 2013). That means one would like to learn the personalized policies in an online mode, i.e., updating the personalized policies for existing users in an incremental manner by continuously feeding in data as it arrives individually or in small groups, as well as designing and updating policies for new users.

Among the online learning methods of decision policies for optimizing immediate outcomes, contextual bandits is one of the most popular approaches to developing personalized interventions in mobile health applications (Tewari and Murphy, 2017a). Contextual bandits aim to develop policies that minimize the difference between the maximal possible rewards and the rewards from a given policy under a finite, but possibly unknown, time horizon based on current contextual information. There are two types of contextual bandit problems. Stochastic contextual bandits assume that the contexts are stochastic, independent and identically distributed, or more generally, that future contexts are independent of current actions. In an adversarial contextual bandit setting, the contexts are determined by an adversary that has access to the accrued history. The majority of contextual bandit methods considered one policy for all individuals or one policy for each user based on the user's own data. Tomkins et al. (2021) proposed an Intelligent Pooling approach to generate personalized policies by pooling data from different users. In particular, they considered mixed effects models similar to (12.2), and used Thompson Sampling methods to estimate parameters and select treatments in an online manner.

The online learning procedure often involves repeated iterations of model/parameter estimation based on batch data and an adaptive treatment selection rule based on the model. Our proposed PPL algorithm coupled with the adaptive randomization (AR), may be used to build an online decision support system. Specifically, we may use the proposed PPL algorithm to construct an initial personalized policy for each existing user, and tilts the allocation of empirically superior interventions (actions) to the user with high probabilities using ϵ-greedy or other types of adaptive randomization schemes. The policy can be further updated using the PPL algorithm as more data are collected.

Below we briefly describe an alternative adaptive randomization approach for online treatment updating. In clinical trials, adaptive randomization (AR) tilts the allocation of future subjects so that they will receive empirically superior interventions (actions) with high probabilities. This idea can be adapted to the online learning setting by choosing an action with probability that is proportional to the predicted outcome at each time point. For example, for an existing user i at time $t+1$ with observed covariate $S_{i,t+1}$, based on current model parameter estimates $(\hat{\boldsymbol{\beta}}, \hat{\boldsymbol{\alpha}})$, a soft-max AR scheme assigns the user to action a^* with probability

$$P(a^*|S_{i,t+1}) = \frac{\exp\left[\kappa g^{-1}(h_1(S_{i,t+1}, a^*)^{\mathrm{T}}\hat{\boldsymbol{\beta}} + h_2(S_{i,t+1}, a^*)^{\mathrm{T}}\hat{\boldsymbol{\alpha}}_{i\cdot}^{\mathrm{T}})\right]}{\sum_{a \in \mathcal{A}} \exp\left[\kappa g^{-1}(h_1(S_{i,t+1}, a)^{\mathrm{T}}\hat{\boldsymbol{\beta}} + h_2(S_{i,t+1}, a)^{\mathrm{T}}\hat{\boldsymbol{\alpha}}_{i\cdot}^{\mathrm{T}})\right]}. \tag{12.7}$$

For a new user, we first draw randomly $\boldsymbol{\alpha}_{new}$ from the existing $\{\hat{\boldsymbol{\alpha}}_{i\cdot} : i = 1, \ldots, n\}$. Then the treatment allocation probability can be devised similarly to (12.7) with $\hat{\boldsymbol{\alpha}}_{i\cdot}$ replaced by $\boldsymbol{\alpha}_{new}$ and $S_{i,t+1}$ replaced by the new user's observed covariate at the time point. Here $\kappa \geq 0$ is a tuning parameter. The above AR reduces to non-adaptive balanced randomization when $\kappa = 0$, and to the "play-the-winner" type allocation when $\kappa \to \infty$. The choice of κ can be made by simulation conducted under an ensemble of realistic scenarios based on prior data.

An important element of implementing AR in practice is that we need to keep track and model the enrollment time of mobile app users. Cheung et al. (2015) introduced the implementation of real-time AR in a population multi-stage policy setting. A future research direction is to incorporate the real-time AR in the PPL framework in the mobile decision support system.

12.6 Personalized Policy Learning for Long-Term Outcomes

As noted earlier, maximizing the long-term outcomes are often more appealing, particularly when it is feasible to follow a subject for a long period time. In this section, we describe how to apply the PPL idea to optimize long-term decision making.

For easy explanation, we expand the covariate space $\mathcal{S}$ as $\mathcal{S} \cup \{c\}$, where c denotes an absorbing state, such as dropping out of the study. We adopt the convention that if $S_{it} = c$ for some t, then $S_{is} = c$ for all $s > t$, $A_{is} = u$ and $Y_{is} = 0$ for all $s \geq t$, where u denotes "undefined". With the above convention, the data trajectory for user i can be written as $\{(S_{it}, A_{it}, Y_{it}) : t = 1, 2, \ldots\}$. Let $\gamma \in [0, 1)$ be a discount factor. At a given time point t, the cumulative discounted reward for user i is defined as $G_{it} = \sum_{k=0}^{\infty} \gamma^k Y_{i,t+k}$. The goal is to develop a personalized policy to optimize the expected cumulative reward.

For theoretical simplicity, we assume the covariate process is Markovian, namely, $S_{i,t+1} \perp (\bar{S}_{i,t-1}, \bar{A}_{i,t-1}) | (S_{it}, A_{it})$ for $t \geq 1$, and the conditional density of $S_{i,t+1}$ given (S_{it}, A_{it}) is time-homogeneous. Under this assumption, the optimal policy would also be Markovian and time-homogeneous. That is, we only need to consider function mappings $\pi : \mathcal{S} \cup \{c\} \to \mathcal{A}$. For a given policy $\pi : \mathcal{S} \cup \{c\} \to \mathcal{A}$, define the Q-function as

$$Q_i^{\pi}(s, a) = E\left[\sum_{k=0}^{\infty} \gamma^k Y_{i,t+k} \middle| S_{i,t} = s, A_{i,t} = a\right].$$

The optimal Q-function is $Q^*(s, a) = \max_{\pi} Q_i^{\pi}(s, a)$ and the optimal policy satisfies $\pi_i^*(s) = \arg\max_a Q_i^*(s, a)$.

It is easy to verify that the optimal Q-function satisfies Bellman's equation

$$Q_i^*(s, a) = E\left[Y_{i,t+1} + \gamma \max_{a'} Q^*(S_{i,t+1}, a') \middle| S_{it} = s, A_{it} = a\right].$$

Thus, the problem boils down to the estimation of $Q_i^*(s, a)$. Note that as a conditional mean function $Q_i^*(s, a)$ can be modeled similarly to (12.2).

Methods have been proposed to estimate the optimal Q-functions, such as fitted Q-interaction (Ernst et al., 2005), greedy gradient Q-learning (Maei et al., 2010; Ertefaie and Strawderman, 2018). However, constructing personalized policies in this setting necessitates the inclusion of random effects in defining the optimal Q-function. New methods need to be developed to estimate the optimal Q-functions in the presence of random effects.

12.7 Discussion

With the increasing utilization of mobile devices, behavioral intervention via mobile applications has become a viable option for delivering personalized treatment to patients who would otherwise not have access to traditional treatments. On the other hand, the absence of a suitable method for evaluating behavioral intervention technologies has been widely acknowledged (Mohr et al., 2015). With the rising focus on improving personal health and fitness using smart devices and wearables, it is crucial to create a mobile clinical decision support system.

In this chapter, we proposed a personalized policy learning framework for delivering mobile health interventions under the GLMM setting. The advantage of using GLMM is that when data from each user are limited, it allows for the estimation of the shared features (i.e., fixed effects) as well as the individual features (i.e., random effects), which are both indispensable components of a personalized policy. In addition to batched learning from existing data with restrictions to the immediate outcome, we also discussed how to incorporate adaptive randomization to achieve online learning and how to extend the proposed methods to long-term outcome optimization. This is an active area of research with many new ideas to be investigated.

The proposed research provides analytical tools to build toward our eventual goal of a deeply personalized mobile decision support system for health management. As more data are collected, the statistical models used in the analysis can be enriched to include more patient covariates, more decision options, and more stages. As a result, a dynamic decision support system can be developed over time in a patient-centric manner. A future direction is to incorporate more flexible modeling techniques in order to develop an enhanced decision support program through model enrichment.

Chapter 13

Bandit Algorithms for Precision Medicine

Yangyi Lu, Ziping Xu, Ambuj Tewari

13.1 Introduction

The Oxford English Dictionary defines precision medicine as "medical care designed to optimize efficiency or therapeutic benefit for particular groups of patients, especially by using genetic or molecular profiling." It is not an entirely new idea: physicians from ancient times have recognized that medical treatment needs to consider individual variations in patient characteristics (Konstantinidou et al., 2017). However, the modern precision medicine movement has been enabled by a confluence of events: scientific advances in fields such as genetics and pharmacology, technological advances in mobile devices and wearable sensors, and methodological advances in computing and data sciences.

This chapter is about bandit algorithms: an area of data science of special relevance to precision medicine. With their roots in the seminal work of Bellman, Robbins, Lai and others, bandit algorithms have come to occupy a central place in modern data science (see the book by Lattimore and Szepesvári (2020) for an up-to-date treatment). Bandit algorithms can be used in any situation where treatment decisions need to be made to optimize some health outcome. Since precision medicine focuses on the use of patient characteristics to guide treatment, *contextual* bandit algorithms are especially useful since they are designed to take such information into account.

The role of bandit algorithms in areas of precision medicine such as mobile health and digital phenotyping has been reviewed before (Tewari and Murphy, 2017b; Rabbi et al., 2019). Since these reviews were published, bandit algorithms have continued to find uses in mobile health and several new topics have emerged in the research on bandit algorithms. This chapter is written for quantitative researchers in fields such as statistics, machine learning, and operations research who might be interested in knowing more about the algorithmic and mathematical details of bandit algorithms that have been used in mobile health.

We have organized this chapter to meet two goals. First, we want to provide a concise exposition of basic topics in bandit algorithms. Section 13.2 will help the reader become familiar with basic problem setups and algorithms that appear frequently in applied work in precision medicine and mobile health (see, for example, Paredes et al. (2014); Piette et al. (2015); Rabbi et al. (2015); Piette et al. (2016); Yom-Tov et al. (2017); Rindtorff et al. (2019); Forman et al. (2019); Liao et al. (2020); Ameko et al. (2020); Aguilera et al. (2020); Tomkins et al. (2021)). Second, we want to highlight a few advanced topics that are important for mobile health and precision medicine applications but whose full potential remains to be realized. Section 13.3 will provide the reader with helpful entry points into the bandit literature on non-stationarity, robustness to corrupted rewards, satisfying additional constraints, algorithmic fairness, and causality.

13.2 Basic Topics

In this section, we begin by introducing the most simple of all bandit problems: the multi-armed bandit. Then we discuss a more advanced variant called contextual bandit that is

DOI: 10.1201/9781003216223-13

especially suitable for precision medicine applications. The last topic we discuss in this section is offline learning which deals with algorithms that can use already collected data. The offline learning setting is to be contrasted with the online learning setting where the bandit algorithm has control over the data it collects.

13.2.1 Multi-armed Bandit

In recent years, the multi-armed bandit (MAB) framework has attracted a lot of attention in many application areas such as healthcare, marketing, and recommendation systems. MAB is a simple model that describes the interaction between an *agent*[1] and an *environment*. At every time step, the agent makes a choice from an action[2] set and receives a reward. The agent may have different goals, such as maximizing the (discounted) cumulative reward within a time horizon, identifying the best arm, or competing with the arm with the best risk-return trade-off etc. In this section, we focus on maximizing the cumulative rewards for simplicity. An important observation is that the agent needs to balance between *exploration* and *exploitation* to achieve its goal of receiving high cumulative reward. That is, both under-explored arms as well as tested-and-tried arms with high rewards should be selected often but for different reasons: the former have the potential to achieve high rewards and the latter are already confirmed to be good based on past experience.

To formally define the bandit framework, we start with introducing some notation. Suppose the agent interacts with the environment for T time steps, where T is called the horizon. In each round $t \in [T]$, the learner chooses an action A_t from the action set $\mathcal{A}$ and receives a corresponding reward $R_t \in \mathbb{R}$. We denote the cardinality of $\mathcal{A}$ by K. The choice of A_t depends on the action/reward history up to time $t-1$: $H_{t-1} = (A_1, R_1, \ldots, A_{t-1}, R_{t-1})$. A policy π_t is defined as a mapping from the history up to time $t-1$ to the actions. For short, we use π as the sequence of policies $(\pi_0, \ldots, \pi_{T-1})$.

In a healthcare setting, the fundamental pattern that often occurs is the following. Of course, this simple pattern fails to capture the full complexity of decision-making in healthcare, but it is a reasonable starting point, especially for theoretical analysis.

Algorithm 13.1: Bandit Framework in Healthcare

```
Input: Available treatment options, treatment period length T.
for t = 1, ..., T do
    A treatment option (action) is selected and delivered to the patient
    Patient's health outcome (reward) following the treatment is recorded
end
```

In the remainder of this section, we will review bandit algorithms that learn good decision policies over time. We focus on the two key settings: *stochastic bandit* and *adversarial bandit*. In both settings, the algorithms aim at minimizing their regret, which measures the difference between the maximal reward one can get, and the reward obtained by the algorithm. We will formally define regret in each setting.

13.2.1.1 Stochastic Multi-armed Bandit

A stochastic bandit is a set of distributions $\nu = (P_a : a \in \mathcal{A})$ and we define the environment class $\mathcal{E}$ as a set of such distributions

$$\mathcal{E} = \{\nu = (P_a : a \in \mathcal{A}) : P_a \in \mathcal{M}_a \text{ for all } a \in \mathcal{A}\},$$

[1]Also referred to as a *learner*, *statistician*, or *decision maker*.

[2]Since the historical roots of probability theory lie in gambling and casinos, it is not surprising that the MAB terminology comes from imagining a slot machine in a casino. A slot machine is also called a "one-armed bandit" as it robs you of your money. Therefore, we will use *actions* and *arms* interchangeably.

where for each a, $\mathcal{M}_a$ is a set of distributions. For unstructured bandits, playing one action cannot help the agent deduce anything about other actions. Environment classes that are not unstructured are called structured, such as linear bandits (Abbasi-Yadkori et al., 2011), low-rank bandits (Lu et al., 2021b) and combinatorial bandits (Cesa-Bianchi and Lugosi, 2012) etc. Throughout this chapter, we assume all bandit instances are $\mathcal{E}_{\text{SG}}^K(1)$, which means the reward distribution for all K arms is 1-subgaussian.

Definition 1 (Subgaussianity). A random variable X is σ-subgaussian if for all $\lambda \in \mathbb{R}$, $\mathbb{E}\left[e^{\lambda X}\right] \leq e^{\lambda^2\sigma^2/2}$.

It is not hard to see from the definition that many well-known distributions are subgaussian, e.g., any bounded-domain distribution, Bernoulli distribution and Gaussian distributions. Intuitively, a subgaussian distribution has tails no heavier than a Gaussian distribution. Many nice concentration inequalities have been developed for subgaussian variables and are widely used in the proofs of bandit algorithms.

In the process of interactions, once the agent performs action a_t following a particular policy, the environment samples a reward R_t from the distribution P_{a_t}. The combination of an environment and agent policy induces a probability measure on the sequence of outcomes $a_1, R_1, \ldots, a_T, R_T$. A standard stochastic MAB protocol is following. At every time step $t = 1, \ldots, T$, the learning agent

1. picks an action $a_t \in \mathcal{A}$ following policy π_{t-1},
2. receives reward $R_t \sim P_{a_t}$,
3. updates its policy to π_t.

We note that P_{a_t} is the conditional reward distribution of R_t given $\{H_{t-1}, a_t\}$ and π_t is a function from H_{t-1} to $\mathcal{A}$. The expected reward of action a is defined by $\mu_a(\nu) \stackrel{\text{def}}{=} \mathbb{E}_\nu[R|a] = \int_{-\infty}^{\infty} r dP_a(r)$, where R is used as the reward variable. Then the maximum expected reward and the optimal actions are given by

$$\mu^*(\nu) = \max_{a\in\mathcal{A}} \mu_a(\nu) \text{ and } a^*(\nu) \in \arg\max_{a\in\mathcal{A}} \mu_a(\nu).$$

According to the above definition, more than one optimal action can exist and the optimal policy is to select an optimal action at every round. For actions whose expected rewards are less than optimal actions, we call them sub-optimal actions and define the reward gap between actions a and $a^*(\nu)$ by $\Delta_a := \mu^*(\nu) - \mu_a(\nu)$.

As mentioned earlier, the learner's goal is to maximize the cumulative reward $S_T = \sum_{t=1}^T R_t$. We now define a performance metric called *regret* which is the difference between the expected reward that $\pi^*(\nu)$ can obtain and $\mathbb{E}[S_T]$. Minimizing the regret is equivalent to maximizing the reward. The reason why we do not directly optimize S_T is that the cumulative rewards depend on the environment and it is hard to tell whether a policy is good or not by merely looking at the cumulative rewards unless it is compared to a good policy. So we define the problem-dependent regret of a policy π on bandit instance ν by

$$\text{Reg}_T(\pi, \nu) = T\mu^*(\nu) - \mathbb{E}[S_T],$$

where the expectation is taken over actions and rewards up to time T. The worst-case regret of a policy π is defined by

$$\text{Reg}_T(\pi) = \sup_{\nu\in\mathcal{E}} \text{Reg}_T(\pi, \nu).$$

We will drop π and ν from the regret when they are clear from the context.

Remark about Pure Exploration. Throughout this chapter, we focus on minimizing regret by balancing exploration and exploitation. We also want to point out that in a different setting, the exploration cost may not be a concern and the agent just wants to output a final recommendation for the best arm after an exploration phase. Problems of this type are called pure exploration problems. In such cases, algorithms are usually evaluated by sample complexity or simple regret (Bubeck et al., 2009). Pure exploration is also related to randomized controlled trials (RCTs) including modern variants that involve sequential randomization such as sequential multiple assignment randomized trials (SMARTs) (Lei et al., 2012) and micro-randomized trials (MRTs) (Klasnja et al., 2015). Randomized trials are typically designed to enable the estimation of treatment effects with sufficient statistical power. Since the concerns of pure exploration and randomized controlled trials are different from those of bandit algorithms, we do not discuss them further in this chapter. However, note that in an actual application, methodology from bandits and randomized trials may need to be integrated. Researchers may start off with a randomized trial and follow it up with a bandit algorithm in the next iteration of their health app. They can also decide to run a randomized trial for one health outcome while simultaneously running a bandit for a different outcome (e.g., an outcome related to user engagement with the health app) in the same study. There is also ongoing work (Yao et al., 2020; Zhang et al., 2021) on enabling the kind of statistical analysis done after randomized trials on data collected via online bandit algorithms.

Explore-then-Commit (ETC). We start with a simple two-stage algorithm: Explore-then-Commit (ETC). In the first stage of ETC, the learner plays every arm for a fixed number of times (m) and obtains estimates of the expected rewards. In the second stage, the learner commits to the best arm according to the estimates in the first stage. For every arm a, let $\hat{\mu}_a(t)$ denote the estimated expected reward up to time t:

$$\hat{\mu}_a(t) = \frac{1}{T_a(t)} \sum_{s=1}^{t} \mathbb{1}_{\{A_s=a\}} R_s,$$

where $T_a(t) = \sum_{s=1}^{t} \mathbb{1}_{\{A_s=a\}}$ is the number of times action a has been performed up to round t.

Algorithm 13.2: Explore-then-Commit (ETC)

Input: action space $\mathcal{A}$, where $K = |\mathcal{A}|$, number of exploration steps, m, horizon T.

for $t = 1, \ldots, T$ **do**
  if $t \leq mK$ **then**
    play $A_t = (t \mod K) + 1$
  else
    play $A_t = \arg\max_a \hat{\mu}_a(mK)$
  end
  receive R_t
end

With the above definitions, we are ready to present the ETC in Algorithm 8. The overall performance of ETC crucially depends on the parameter m. If m is too small, the algorithm cannot estimate the performance of every arm accurately, so it is likely to exploit a sub-optimal arm in the second stage, which leads to high regret. If m is too big, the first stage (explore step) plays with sub-optimal arms for too many times, so that the regret can be large again. The art is to choose an optimal value for m in order to minimize the total regret incurred in both stages. Specifically, ETC achieves $O(T^{2/3})$ worst-case regret[3] by choosing $m = O(T^{2/3})$ (Lattimore and Szepesvári, 2020). Sub-linear regret $O(T^{2/3})$ performance is good as a starting point. Next, we will introduce another two classic algorithms which incur even less regret.

[3]Ignoring parameters other than T.

Upper Confidence Bound (UCB). There are several types of exploration strategies to select actions such as greedy, Boltzmann, optimism and pessimism. Suppose the agent has reward estimates $\hat{\mu}_a$ for all actions. A greedy exploration strategy simply selects the action with the highest $\hat{\mu}_a$. A Boltzmann exploration strategy picks each action with probability proportional to $\exp(\eta\hat{\mu}_a)$, where η is a tuning parameter. Boltzmann becomes greedy as η goes to infinity. For an optimism strategy, one picks the action with the highest reward estimate plus some bonus term, i.e. $\arg\max_a \hat{\mu}_a + \text{bonus}_a$. In contrast, a pessimism strategy would pick the action: $\arg\max_a \hat{\mu}_a - \text{bonus}_a$.

Out of these strategies, UCB algorithm follows the optimism strategy, in particular, a famous principle called *optimism in the face of uncertainty (OFU)*, which means that one should act as if the environment is the best possible one among those that are *plausible* given current experience. The reason OFU works is that misplaced optimism gets corrected when under-explored actions are tried and low rewards are observed. In contrast, pessimism does not work (at least in the online setting; for the offline setting things can be different (Jin et al., 2021)) since wrong beliefs about low performance of under-explored actions do not get a chance to get revised by collecting more data from those actions.

At every step t, the UCB algorithm updates a value called the *upper confidence bound* defined for each action $a \in \mathcal{A}$ and confidence level $\delta \in [0, 1]$ as follows.

$$\text{UCB}_a(t-1,\delta) = \begin{cases} \infty, & \text{if } T_a(t-1) = 0 \\ \hat{\mu}_a(t-1) + \sqrt{\frac{2\log(1/\delta)}{T_a(t-1)\vee 1}}, & \text{otherwise.} \end{cases} \tag{13.1}$$

The learner chooses the action with the highest UCB value at each step. Overall, UCB (Algorithm 4) guarantees a $\tilde{O}(\sqrt{T})$ worst-case regret (where the informal $\tilde{O}(\cdot)$ notation hides constants and logarithmic factors).

Algorithm 13.3: Upper Confidence Bound (UCB)

Input: δ, $\mathcal{A}$ where $K = |\mathcal{A}|$.
for $t = 1, \ldots, T$ **do**
    play $A_t = \arg\max_{a\in\mathcal{A}} \text{UCB}_a(t-1,\delta)$
    receive reward R_t and update the upper confidence bound terms according to (13.1)
end

According to the construction of upper confidence bounds, an action will be selected under two circumstances: under-explored ($T_a(t-1)$ small) or well-explored with good performance ($\hat{\mu}_a(t-1)$ large). The upper confidence bound for an action gets close to its true mean after being selected for enough times. A sub-optimal action will only be played if its upper confidence bound is larger than that of the optimal arm. However, this is unlikely to happen too often. The upper confidence bound for the sub-optimal action will eventually fall below that of the optimal action as we play the sub-optimal actions more times. We present the regret guarantee for UCB (Algorithm 4) in Theorem 13.2.1.

Theorem 13.2.1 (Regret for UCB Algorithm). *If $\delta = 1/T$, then the problem-dependent regret of UCB, as defined in Algorithm 4, on any 1-subgaussian bandit ν is bounded by*

$$\text{Reg}_T(\text{UCB},\nu) \le 3\sum_{a\in\mathcal{A}} \Delta_a + \sum_{a:\Delta_a>0} \frac{16\log T}{\Delta_a}, \tag{13.2}$$

where $\Delta_a := \mu^*(\nu) - \mu_a(\nu)$ represents the corresponding gap term. The worst-case regret bound of UCB is:

$$\text{Reg}_T(\text{UCB}) = O(\sqrt{KT\log T}). \tag{13.3}$$

Proof. We only present the worst-case regret for simplicity. For the problem-dependent regret proof, we refer the reader to Chapter 7 in Lattimore and Szepesvári (2020).

We define a good event E as follows:

$$E := \left\{ |\hat{\mu}_a(t-1) - \mu_a| \le \sqrt{\frac{2\log(1/\delta)}{T_a(t-1) \vee 1}}, \forall t \in [T], a \in \mathcal{A} \right\}.$$

By Hoeffding inequality and union bound, one can show that $\mathbb{P}(E^c) \le 2TK\delta^4$. Next, we decompose the regret.

$$\begin{aligned}
\text{Reg}_T(\text{UCB}) &= \mathbb{E}\Bigg[\sum_{t=1}^{T} \mu^* - \text{UCB}_{a^*}(t-1,\delta) + \text{UCB}_{a^*}(t-1,\delta) \\
&\qquad - \text{UCB}_{A_t}(t-1,\delta) + \text{UCB}_{A_t}(t-1,\delta) - \mu_{A_t}\Bigg] \\
&\le \mathbb{E}\left[\sum_{t=1}^{T} \mu^* - \text{UCB}_{a^*}(t-1,\delta) + \text{UCB}_{A_t}(t-1,\delta) - \mu_{A_t}\right].
\end{aligned}$$

The inequality in the above expression is due to the action selection criterion in UCB algorithm. Condition on event E, we have $\mu^* - \text{UCB}_{a^*}(t-1,\delta) \le 0$ for all $t \in [T]$; otherwise, the regret can be bounded by $2T$. Combining these arguments, we have

$$\begin{aligned}
\text{Reg}_T(\text{UCB}) &\le \mathbb{P}(E^c) \cdot 2T + \mathbb{P}(E) \cdot \mathbb{E}\left[\sum_{t=1}^{T} \text{UCB}_{A_t}(t-1,\delta) - \mu_{A_t} \mid E\right] \\
&\le 4T^2K\delta^4 + 2\mathbb{E}\left[\sum_{t=1}^{T} \sqrt{\frac{2\log(1/\delta)}{T_{A_t}(t-1) \vee 1}}\right] \quad \text{(By definition of event } E\text{)} \\
&\le 4T^2K\delta^4 + \sqrt{8\log(1/\delta)} \sum_{a \in \mathcal{A}} \sum_{t=1}^{T} \mathbb{E}\left[\sqrt{\frac{1}{T_{A_t}(t-1) \vee 1}} \mathbb{1}_{\{A_t = a\}}\right] \\
&\le 4T^2K\delta^4 + \sqrt{8\log(1/\delta)} \sum_{a \in \mathcal{A}} \int_1^{T_a(T)} \sqrt{1/s}\, \mathrm{d}s \\
&\le 4T^2K\delta^4 + \sqrt{8\log(1/\delta)}\sqrt{KT} = O(\sqrt{KT\log T}) \ (\text{Set } \delta = 1/T).
\end{aligned}$$

The last inequality in above is by Cauchy-Schwarz inequality. □

The UCB family has many variants, one of which is to replace the upper confidence bound for every action by $\hat{\mu}_a(t-1) + \sqrt{2\log\left(1 + t\log^2(t)\right)/T_a(t-1)}$. Even though the regret dominant terms ($\sqrt{KT\log T}$ and $\sum_{a:\Delta_a>0} \frac{\log T}{\Delta_a}$) for this version has the same order as those of Algorithm 4, the leading constants for the two dominant terms become smaller.

Then one may ask the question: is it possible to further improve the regret bound of UCB and above variant? The answer is yes. Audibert et al. (2009) proposed an algorithm called *MOSS* (Minimax Optimal Strategy in the Stochastic case). *MOSS* replaces the upper confidence bounds in Algorithm 4 by

$$\hat{\mu}_a(t-1) + \sqrt{\frac{\max\left\{\log\left(\frac{T}{KT_a(t-1)}\right), 0\right\}}{T_a(t-1)}}.$$

Under this construction, the worst-case regret of *MOSS* is guaranteed to be only $O(\sqrt{KT})$.

However, *MOSS* is not always good. One can easily construct regimes where the problem-dependent regret of MOSS is worse than UCB (Lattimore, 2015). On the other hand, the improved UCB algorithm proposed by Auer and Ortner (2010) satisfies a problem-dependent regret that is similar to (13.1), but the worst-case regret is $O(\sqrt{KT\log K})$. Later on, by carefully constructing the upper confidence bounds, Optimally Confidence UCB algorithm (Lattimore, 2015) and AdaUCB algorithm (Lattimore, 2018) are shown to achieve $O(\sqrt{KT})$ worst-case regret and their problem-dependent regret bounds are also not worse than that of the UCB algorithm. There are many more UCB variants in the literature that we do not cover in this chapter. The reader may refer to Table 2 in Lattimore (2018) for a comprehensive summary.

Successive Elimination (SE). We now describe the SE algorithm that also relies on the upper confidence bound calculations. The idea is similar to UCB such that a sub-optimal arm is very unlikely to have large a upper confidence bound if it has been selected for enough times. At every round, SE maintains a confidence interval for the mean reward of every arm and removes all arms whose reward upper bound is smaller than the lower bound of the biggest estimated reward arm. The procedure ends when there is only one arm remained. We describe the SE algorithm in Algorithm 4 and define the UCB terms as (13.1) and LCB terms as

$$\mathrm{LCB}_a(t-1,\delta)=\begin{cases}\infty, & \text{if } T_a(t-1)=0\\ \hat{\mu}_a(t-1)-\sqrt{\frac{2\log(1/\delta)}{T_a(t-1)\vee 1}}, & \text{otherwise.}\end{cases} \tag{13.4}$$

Algorithm 13.4: Successive Elimination (SE)

```
Input: δ, A where K = |A|.
while A contains more than one arm do
    play every arm in A once and update the UCBs and LCBs using (13.1) and
      (13.4)
    Eliminate all arms a s.t. ∃a' ∈ A with UCB_a(t − 1, δ) < LCB_a'(t − 1, δ)
end
```

SE was first proposed in Even-Dar et al. (2006) along with a similar action elimination-based algorithm: Median Elimination (ME). They studied the probably approximately correct (PAC) setting (Haussler and Warmuth, 2018). In particular, Even-Dar et al. (2006) shows that for given K arms, it suffices to pull the arms for $O(\frac{K}{\varepsilon^2}\log(1/\delta)$ times to find an ε-optimal arm with probability at least $1-\delta$. It is not hard to prove that SE also satisfies the following regret bound.

Theorem 13.2.2 (Regret for SE Algorithm)**.** *If $\delta = 1/T$, the worst-case regret of SE over 1-subgaussian bandit environments is bounded by*

$$\mathrm{Reg}_T(\mathrm{SE}) = O(\sqrt{KT\log T}). \tag{13.5}$$

Proof. Without loss of generality, we assume the optimal arm a^* is unique. Define the event E by $\{|\hat{\mu}_a(t)-\mu_a|\le c_a(t,\delta),\forall a,t\}$, where $c_a(t,\delta)=\sqrt{\frac{2\log(1/\delta)}{T_a(t)\vee 1}}$ denotes the confidence set width. By Hoeffding inequality and union bound, one can show that $\mathbb{P}(E^c)\le 2\delta^4 TK$.

Define t as the last round when arm a is not eliminated yet. According to the elimination criterion in SE, the reward gap term can be bounded as:

$$\Delta_a := \mu^* - \mu_a \le 2(c_{a^*}(t,\delta)+c_a(t,\delta)) = O(c_a(t,\delta)).$$

The last equality holds as $T_a(t)$ and $T_{a^*}(t)$ differ at most by 1 by construction. Since t is the last round a being played, we have $T_a(t) = T_a(T)$ and $c_a(t) = c_a(T)$, which implies below property for all non-optimal arms a:

$$\Delta_a \leq O\left(\sqrt{\frac{\log(1/\delta)}{T_a(T)}}\right).$$

We thus obtain that under event E,

$$\begin{aligned}\sum_{t=1}^{T} \mathbb{E}[\mu^* - \mu_{a_t}|E] &\leq \sum_{a \in \mathcal{A}\setminus\{a^*\}} T_a(T)\Delta_a \\ &\leq O(\sqrt{\log(1/\delta)}) \sum_{a \in \mathcal{A}} \sqrt{T_a(T)} \leq O(\sqrt{KT\log(1/\delta)}),\end{aligned}$$

where the last inequality is by Cauchy-Schwarz inequality. Take $\delta = 1/T$, $\text{Reg}_T(\text{SE}) = O(\sqrt{KT\log T})$ by conditional expectation calculations. □

Thompson Sampling (TS). All of the methods we have mentioned so far select their actions based on a frequentist view. TS uses one of the oldest heuristic (Thompson, 1933) for choosing actions and addresses the exploration-exploitation dilemma based on a Bayesian philosophy of learning. The idea is simple. Before the game starts, the agent chooses a prior distribution over a set of possible bandit environments. At every round, the agent samples an environment from the posterior and acts according to the optimal action in that environment. The exploration in TS comes from the randomization over bandit environments. In the beginning, the posterior is usually poorly concentrated, then the policy will likely explore. As more data being collected, the posterior tends to concentrate towards the true environment and the rate of exploration decreases. We present the TS algorithm in Algorithm 4.

To formally describe how TS works, we start with several definitions related to Bayesian bandits.

Definition 2 (K-armed Bayesian bandit environment). A K-armed Bayesian bandit environment is a tuple $(\mathcal{E}, \mathcal{G}, Q, P)$ where $(\mathcal{E}, \mathcal{G})$ is a measurable space and Q is a probability measure on $(\mathcal{E}, \mathcal{G})$ called the prior. $P = (P_{\nu a} : \nu \in \mathcal{E}, a \in \mathcal{A})$ is the reward distribution for arms in bandit ν, where $|\mathcal{A}| = K$.

Given a K-armed Bayesian bandit environment $(\mathcal{E}, \mathcal{G}, Q, P)$ and a policy π, the Bayesian regret is defined as:

$$\text{BReg}_T(\pi, Q) = \int_{\mathcal{E}} \text{Reg}_T(\pi, \nu) dQ(\nu).$$

Algorithm 13.5: Thompson Sampling (TS)

Input: Bayesian bandit environment $(\mathcal{E}, \mathcal{B}(\mathcal{E}), Q, P)$ ($\mathcal{B}(\cdot)$ is the Borel set), action set $\mathcal{A}$ with $|\mathcal{A}| = K$.

for $t = 1, \ldots, T$ **do**
  Sample $\nu_t \sim Q(\cdot|A_1, R_1, \ldots, A_{t-1}, R_{t-1})$
  Play $A_t = \arg\max_{i \in [K]} \mu_i(\nu_t)$
end

TS has been analyzed in both of the frequentist and the Bayesian settings and we will start with the Bayesian results.

Theorem 13.2.3 (Bayesian Regret for TS Algorithm). *For a K-armed Bayesian bandit environment $(\mathcal{E}, \mathcal{G}, Q, P)$ such that $P_{\nu a}$ is 1-subgaussian for all $\nu \in \mathcal{E}$ and $a \in [K]$ with mean in $[0,1]$. Then the policy π of TS satisfies*

$$\text{BReg}_T(\pi, Q) = O(\sqrt{KT \log T}). \tag{13.6}$$

Proof. The proof is quite similar to that of UCB. We abbreviate $\mu_a = \mu_a(\nu)$ and let $a^* = \arg\max_{a \in [K]} \mu_a$ be the optimal arm. Note that a^* is a random variable depending on ν. For every $a \in [K]$, we define a clipped upper bound term

$$\text{UCB}_a(t-1) = \hat{\mu}_a(t-1) + \sqrt{\frac{2\log(1/\delta)}{1 \vee T_a(t-1)}},$$

where $\hat{\mu}_a(t-1)$ and $T_a(t-1)$ are defined in the same way as those in UCB. We define event E such that for all $t \in [T]$ and $a \in \mathcal{A}$,

$$|\hat{\mu}_a(t-1) - \mu_a| < \sqrt{\frac{2\log(1/\delta)}{1 \vee T_a(t-1)}}.$$

By Hoeffding inequality and union bound, one can show that $\mathbb{P}(E^c) \le 2TK\delta^4$. This result will be used in later steps.

Let $\mathcal{F}_t = \sigma(A_1, R_1, \ldots, A_t, R_t)$ be the σ-algebra generated by the interaction sequence up to time t. The key insight for the whole proof is to observe below property from the definition of TS:

$$\mathbb{P}(a^*|\mathcal{F}_{t-1}) = \mathbb{P}(A_t|\mathcal{F}_{t-1}) \text{ a.s.} \tag{13.7}$$

Using above property and $\text{BReg}_T = \mathbb{E}\left[\sum_{t=1}^T (\mu_{a^*} - \mu_{A_t})\right] = \mathbb{E}\left[\sum_{t=1}^T \mathbb{E}\left[(\mu_{a^*} - \mu_{A_t}) \mid \mathcal{F}_{t-1}\right]\right]$, we have

$$\mathbb{E}\left[\mu_{a^*} - \mu_{A_t} \mid \mathcal{F}_{t-1}\right] = \mathbb{E}\left[\mu_{a^*} - \text{UCB}_{a^*}(t-1) + \text{UCB}_{A_t}(t-1) - \mu_{A_t} \mid \mathcal{F}_{t-1}\right],$$

and thus

$$\text{BReg}_T = \mathbb{E}\left[\sum_{t=1}^T (\mu_{a^*} - \text{UCB}_{a^*}(t-1)) + \sum_{t=1}^T (\text{UCB}_{A_t}(t-1) - \mu_{A_t})\right].$$

Conditioning on the high-probability event E, the first sum is negative and the second sum is of the order $O(\sqrt{KT\log(1/\delta)})$, while $\text{BReg}_T \le 2T$ if conditioning on E^c. Take $\delta = 1/T$, one can verify that $\text{BReg}_T = O(\sqrt{KT \log T})$.

□

Compared to the analysis for Bayesian regret, frequentist (worst-case) regret analysis for TS gets a lot more technical. The key reason behind this is that the worst-case regret does not have an expectation with respect to the prior and therefore the property in (13.7) cannot be used. Even though TS was well-known to be easy to implement and competitive with state of the art methods, it lacked worst-case regret analysis for a long time. Significant progress was made by Agrawal and Goyal (2012) and Kaufmann et al. (2012). In Agrawal and Goyal (2012), the first logarithmic bound on the frequentist regret of TS was proven. Kaufmann et al. (2012) provided a bound that matches the asymptotic lower bound of Lai and Robbins (1985). However, both of these bounds were problem-dependent. The first near-optimal worst-case regret $O(\sqrt{KT \log T})$ was proved by Agrawal and Goyal (2013a) for Bernoulli bandits with Beta prior, where the reward is either zero or one. For TS that uses Gaussian prior, the same work proved a $O(\sqrt{KT \log K})$ worst-case regret. Jin et al. (2020) proposed a variant of TS called MOTS (Minimax Optimal TS) that achieves $O(\sqrt{KT})$ regret.

13.2.1.2 Adversarial Multi-armed Bandit

In stochastic bandit models, the rewards are assumed to be strictly i.i.d. given actions. This assumption can be violated easily in practice. For example, the health feedback for a patient after certain treatments may vary slightly across times and the way it varies is usually unknown. In such scenarios, the best action that maximizes the total reward still exists, but algorithms designed for stochastic bandit environments are no longer guaranteed to work. As a more robust counterpart to the stochastic model, we study the adversarial bandit model in this section, in which the assumption that a single action is good in hindsight is retained but the rewards are allowed to be chosen adversarially.

The adversarial bandit environment is often called as the adversary. In an adversarial bandit problem, the adversary secretly chooses reward vectors $r := \{r_t\}_{t=1}^T$ where $r_t \in [0,1]^K$ corresponds to the rewards over all actions at time t. In every round, the agent chooses a distribution over the actions P_t. An action $A_t \in [K]$ is sampled from P_t and the agent receives the reward r_{tA_t}. A policy π in this setting maps the history sequences to distributions over actions. We evaluate the performance of policy π by the expected regret, which is the cumulative reward difference between the best fixed action and the agent's selections:

$$\mathrm{Reg}_T(\pi, r) = \max_{a\in\mathcal{A}} \sum_{t=1}^T r_{ta} - \mathbb{E}\left[\sum_{t=1}^T r_{tA_t}\right] \tag{13.8}$$

The worst-case regret of policy π is defined by

$$\mathrm{Reg}_T(\pi) = \sup_{r\in[0,1]^{T\times K}} \mathrm{Reg}_T(\pi, r). \tag{13.9}$$

It may not be very clear at the beginning that why we define the regret by comparing to the fixed best action instead of the best action at every round. In the later case, the regret should be $\mathrm{Reg}'_T(\pi, x) = \mathbb{E}\left[\sum_{t=1}^T \max_{a\in\mathcal{A}} r_{ta} - \sum_{t=1}^T r_{tA_t}\right]$. However, this definition provides the adversary too much power so that for any policy, one can show $\mathrm{Reg}'_T(\pi, r)$ can be $\Omega(T)$ for certain reward vectors $r \in [0,1]^{K\times T}$.

Remark on randomized policy: In stochastic bandit models, the optimal action is deterministic and the optimal policy is simply to select the optimal action at every round. However, in adversarial bandit setting, the adversary has great power in designing the reward. It may know the agent's policy and design the rewards accordingly, so that a deterministic policy can incur linear regret. For example, we consider there are two actions, whose reward is either 0 or 1 at any time. For a deterministic policy, the agent decides to choose an action at time t. Then the adversary knows it and can set the reward of that action at time t to be 0 and the reward of the unselected action to be 1. The cumulative regret will be T after T rounds. However, one can improve the performance by a randomized policy, e.g., choosing either action with probability 0.5, then the adversary cannot make you incur regret 1 at every round by manipulating the reward values for both actions.

Exponential-weight algorithm for Exploration and Exploitation (EXP3). We now study one of the most famous adversarial bandit algorithms called EXP3. Before describing the algorithm, we define some related terms below. In a randomized policy, the conditional probability of the action a being played is denoted by

$$P_{ta} = \mathbb{P}(A_t = a \mid A_1, R_1, \ldots, A_{t-1}, R_{t-1}).$$

Assuming $P_{ta} > 0$ almost surely for all policies, a natural way to define the importance-weighted estimator of r_{ta} is

$$\hat{R}_{ta} = \frac{\mathbb{1}_{\{A_t=a\}} R_t}{P_{ta}}. \tag{13.10}$$

Let $\mathbb{E}_t[\cdot] = \mathbb{E}[\cdot \mid A_1, R_1, \ldots, A_{t-1}, R_{t-1}]$. A simple calculation shows that $\hat{R}_{ta}$ is conditionally unbiased, i.e. $\mathbb{E}_t[\hat{R}_{ta}] = r_{ta}$. However, the variance of estimator $\hat{R}_{ta}$ can be extremely large when P_{ta} is small and r_{ta} is non-zero. Let $A_{ta} := \mathbb{1}_{\{A_t=a\}}$, then the variance of the estimator is:

$$\mathbb{V}_t[\hat{R}_{ta}] = \mathbb{E}_t[\hat{R}_{ta}^2] - r_{ta}^2 = \mathbb{E}_t\left[\frac{A_{ta} r_{ta}^2}{P_{ta}^2}\right] - r_{ta}^2 = \frac{r_{ta}^2(1 - P_{ta})}{P_{ta}}.$$

An alternative estimator is:

$$\hat{R}_{ta} = 1 - \frac{\mathbb{1}_{\{A_t=a\}}}{P_{ta}}(1 - R_t). \tag{13.11}$$

This estimator is still unbiased and its variance is

$$\mathbb{V}_t[\hat{R}_{ta}] = y_{ta}^2 \frac{1 - P_{ta}}{P_{ta}},$$

where we define $y_{ta} = 1 - r_{ta}$.

The best choice of the estimator $\hat{R}_{ta}$ depends on the actual rewards. One should use (13.10) for small rewards and (13.11) for large rewards. So far we have learned how to construct reward estimators for given sampling distributions P_{ta}. EXP3 algorithm provides a way to design the P_{ta} terms. Let $\hat{S}_{t,a} = \sum_{s=1}^{t} \hat{R}_{sa}$ be the total estimated reward until the end of round t, where $\hat{R}_{si}$ is defined in (13.11). We present EXP3 in Algorithm 6.

Algorithm 13.6: Exponential-weight Algorithm for Exploration and Exploitation (Exp3)

Input: T, K, η

Set $\hat{S}_{0,a} = 0$ for all a

for $t = 1, \ldots, T$ **do**

  Calculate $P_{ta} \leftarrow \frac{\exp(\eta \hat{S}_{t-1,a})}{\sum_{a' \in \mathcal{A}} \exp(\eta \hat{S}_{t-1,a'})}$ for all $a \in [K]$

  Sample A_t from P_t and receive reward R_t

  Calculate $\hat{S}_{t,a} \leftarrow \hat{S}_{t-1,a} + 1 - \frac{\mathbb{1}_{\{A_t=a\}}(1-R_t)}{P_{ta}}$

end

Surprisingly, even though adversarial bandit problems look more difficult than stochastic bandit problems due to the strong power of the adversary, one can show that the adversarial regret for EXP3 algorithm has the same order as before, i.e., $O(\sqrt{KT \log T})$.

Theorem 13.2.4 (Regret for EXP3 Algorithm)**.** *Let $r \in [0,1]^{T \times K}$. With learning rate $\eta = \sqrt{\log K/(KT)}$, we have*

$$\text{Reg}_T(\text{EXP3}, r) \leq 2\sqrt{KT \log K}. \tag{13.12}$$

Proof. The proof for EXP3 is different than those for the stochastic bandit algorithms. We first define the expected regret relative to using action a in T rounds:

$$\text{Reg}_{Ta} = \sum_{t=1}^{T} r_{ta} - \mathbb{E}\left[\sum_{t=1}^{T} R_t\right].$$

According to the definition of the adversarial bandit regret, the final result will follow if we can upper bound R_{Ta} for every $a \in \mathcal{A}$. It's not hard to show $\mathbb{E}[\hat{S}_{T,a}] = \sum_{t=1}^{T} r_{ta}$ and $\mathbb{E}_t[R_t] = \sum_{a \in \mathcal{A}} P_{ta} r_{ta} = \sum_{i=1}^{K} P_{ta} \mathbb{E}[\hat{R}_{ta}]$ hold using the definition of $\hat{R}_{ta}$. Then we can rewrite R_{Ta} as $\mathbb{E}\left[\hat{S}_{T,a} - \hat{S}_T\right]$, where $\hat{S}_T = \sum_{t=1}^{T} \sum_{a \in \mathcal{A}} P_{ta} \hat{R}_{ta}$. Let $W_t = \sum_{a \in \mathcal{A}} \exp\left(\eta \hat{S}_{t,a}\right)$,

$\hat{S}_{0,a} = 0$ and $W_0 = K$, then one can show that

$$\exp\left(\eta \hat{S}_{T,a}\right) \le \sum_{a' \in \mathcal{A}} \exp\left(\eta \hat{S}_{T,a'}\right) = W_T = K \prod_{t=1}^{T} \frac{W_t}{W_{t-1}}$$
$$= K \prod_{t=1}^{T} \sum_{a' \in \mathcal{A}} P_{ta'} \exp\left(\eta \hat{R}_{ta'}\right).$$

We next bound the ratio term

$$\frac{W_t}{W_{t-1}} \le 1 + \eta \sum_{a' \in \mathcal{A}} P_{ta'} \hat{R}_{ta'} + \eta^2 \sum_{a \in \mathcal{A}} P_{ta'} \hat{R}_{ta'}^2$$
$$\le \exp\left(\eta \sum_{a' \in \mathcal{A}} P_{ta'} \hat{R}_{ta'} + \eta^2 \sum_{a' \in \mathcal{A}} P_{ta'} \hat{R}_{ta'}^2\right),$$

using inequalities $e^x \le 1 + x + x^2$ for $x \le 1$ and $1 + x \le e^x$ for $x \in \mathbb{R}$.

Combining with previous results, we have

$$\exp\left(\eta \hat{S}_{T,a}\right) \le K \exp\left(\eta \hat{S}_T + \eta^2 \sum_{t=1}^{T} \sum_{a' \in \mathcal{A}} P_{ta'} \hat{R}_{ta'}^2\right).$$

Taking logarithm on both sides and rearranging give us

$$\hat{S}_{T,a} - \hat{S}_T \le \frac{\log K}{\eta} + \eta \sum_{t=1}^{T} \sum_{a' \in \mathcal{A}} P_{ta'} \hat{R}_{ta'}^2. \tag{13.13}$$

To upper bound R_{Ta}, we only need to upper bound the expectation of the second term in the above. By standard (conditional) expectation calculations, one can get

$$\mathbb{E}\left[\sum_{t=1}^{T} \sum_{a' \in \mathcal{A}} P_{ta'} \hat{R}_{ta'}^2\right] \le TK.$$

By substituting above inequality into (13.13), we get

$$\mathrm{Reg}_{Ta} \le \frac{\log K}{\eta} + \eta TK = 2\sqrt{KT \log K}, \tag{13.14}$$

where we choose $\eta = \sqrt{\log K/(TK)}$. By definition, the overall regret $\mathrm{Reg}_T(\mathrm{EXP3}, r)$ has the same upper bound as above. □

We just proved the expected regret of EXP3. However, if we consider the distribution of the random regret, EXP3 is not good enough. Define the random regret as $\widehat{\mathrm{Reg}}_T = \max_{a \in \mathcal{A}} \sum_{t=1}^{T} r_{ta} - \sum_{t=1}^{T} R_t$. One can show that for all large enough T and reasonable choices of η, there exists a bandit such that the random regret of EXP3 satisfies $\mathbb{P}(\widehat{\mathrm{Reg}}_T \ge T/4) \ge c > 0$, where c is a constant. That means EXP3 sometimes can incur linear regret with non-trivial probability, which makes EXP3 unsuitable for practical problems. This phenomenon is caused by the high variance of the regret distribution. In next section, we will discuss how to resolve this problem by slightly modifying EXP3.

EXP3-IX (EXP3 with Implicit eXploration). We have learned that small P_{ta} terms can cause enormous variance on the reward estimator, which then leads to high variance on the regret distribution. Thus, EXP3-IX (Neu, 2015) redefines the loss-estimator as

$$\hat{Y}_{ta} = \frac{\mathbb{1}_{\{A_t=a\}} Y_t}{P_{ta} + \gamma}, \tag{13.15}$$

where $Y_t = 1 - R_t$ denotes the loss at round t and $\gamma > 0$. $\hat{Y}_{ta}$ is a biased estimator for $y_{ta} = 1 - r_{ta}$ due to γ, but the variance can be reduced. An optimal choice for γ needs to balance the bias and variance. Other than this slight change in the loss estimator, the remaining procedures remain the same as EXP3. The name of 'IX' (Implicit eXploration) can be justified by the following argument:

$$\mathbb{E}_t[\hat{Y}_{ta}] = \frac{P_{ta} y_{ta}}{P_{ta} + \gamma} \leq y_{ta}.$$

The effect of adding a γ to the denominator is that EXP3-IX tries to decrease the large losses for some actions so that such actions can still be chosen occasionally. As a result, EXP3-IX explores more than EXP3. Neu (2015) has proved the following high probability regret bound for EXP3-IX.

Theorem 13.2.5 (Regret for EXP3-IX Algorithm). *With* $\eta = 2\gamma = \sqrt{\frac{2\log K}{KT}}$, *EXP3-IX guarantees that*

$$\widehat{\text{Reg}}_T(\textit{EXP3-IX}) \leq 2\sqrt{2KT\log K} + \left(\sqrt{\frac{2KT}{\log K}} + 1\right)\log(2/\delta) \tag{13.16}$$

with probability at least $1 - \delta$.

13.2.1.3 Lower Bound for MAB Problems

We have discussed two types of bandit models and their corresponding algorithms in regret minimization. Then a natural question is: what is the minimal regret bound we can hope for? To answer this question, we will introduce two types of lower bound results: minimax lower bound and instance-dependent lower bound. Both of them are useful for describing the hardness of a class of bandit problems and are often used to evaluate the optimality of an existing algorithm. For example, suppose the worst-case regret of a policy π matches the minimax lower bound up to a universal constant, we say that the policy π is minimax-optimal.

Minimax Lower Bounds. We consider a Gaussian bandit environment, in which the reward for every arm is Gaussian-distributed. We denote the class of Gaussian bandits with unit variance by $\mathcal{E}_{\mathcal{N}}^K(1)$ and use $\mu \in \mathbb{R}^K$ as the reward mean vector. In particular, $\nu_\mu \in \mathcal{E}_{\mathcal{N}}^K(1)$ is a Gaussian bandit for which the ith arm has reward distribution $\mathcal{N}(\mu_i, 1)$. The following result provides a minimax lower bound for the Gaussian bandit class $\mathcal{E}_{\mathcal{N}}^K(1)$.

Theorem 13.2.6 (Minimax Lower Bound for Gaussian Bandit Class). *Let* $K > 1$ *and* $T \geq K - 1$. *For any policy* π, *there exists a mean vector* $\mu \in [0,1]^K$ *such that*

$$\text{Reg}_T(\pi, \nu_\mu) = \Omega(\sqrt{KT}). \tag{13.17}$$

Proof. To prove the lower bound, we start with constructing two bandit instances that are very similar to each other and hard to distinguish. Let $\mu = (\Delta, 0, 0, \ldots, 0)$ denote the mean vector for the first unit variance Gaussian bandit. We use $\mathbb{P}_\mu$ and $\mathbb{E}_\mu$ to denote the probability and expectation induced by environment ν_μ and policy π up to time T. To choose the second environment, let

$$i = \arg\min_{j>1} \mathbb{E}_\mu[T_j(T)].$$

Define the reward mean vector for the second bandit as $\mu' = (\Delta, 0, \ldots, 0, 2\Delta, 0, \ldots, 0)$, where $\mu'_i = 2\Delta$. Decomposing the regret leads to

$$\text{Reg}_T(\pi, \nu_\mu) \geq \mathbb{P}_\mu(T_1(T) \leq T/2)\frac{T\Delta}{2},$$
$$\text{Reg}_T(\pi, \nu_{\mu'}) > \mathbb{P}_{\mu'}(T_1(T) > T/2)\frac{T\Delta}{2}.$$

Then, applying the Bretagnolle-Huber inequality, we get

$$\text{Reg}_T(\pi, \nu_\mu) + \text{Reg}_T(\pi, \nu_{\mu'}) \geq \frac{T\Delta}{4}\exp(-\text{KL}(\mathbb{P}_\mu, \mathbb{P}_{\mu'})).$$

It remains to upper bound the KL-divergence term in above. By divergence decomposition, one can show that

$$\begin{aligned}\text{KL}(\mathbb{P}_\mu, \mathbb{P}_{\mu'}) = \sum_{i=1}^{K} \mathbb{E}_\mu[T_i(T)]\text{KL}(\mathbb{P}_i, \mathbb{P}'_i) &= \mathbb{E}_\mu[T_i(T)]\text{KL}(\mathcal{N}(0,1), \mathcal{N}(2\Delta, 1)) \\ &= \mathbb{E}_\mu[T_i(T)]\frac{(2\Delta)^2}{2} \leq \frac{2T\Delta^2}{K-1}.\end{aligned}$$

In above, we use $\mathbb{P}_i$ and $\mathbb{P}'_i$ denote the reward distribution of the ith arm in ν_μ and $\nu_{\mu'}$, respectively. For the last inequality, since $\sum_{j=1}^{K} \mathbb{E}_\mu[T_j(T)] = T$, it holds that $\mathbb{E}_\mu[T_i(T)] \leq \frac{T}{K-1}$. Combining with previous results, we know that

$$\text{Reg}_T(\pi, \nu_\mu) + \text{Reg}_T(\pi, \nu_{\mu'}) \geq \frac{T\Delta}{4}\exp\left(-\frac{2T\Delta^2}{K-1}\right).$$

Choosing $\Delta = \sqrt{(K-1)/4T} \leq 1/2$, the result follows. □

An algorithm is called minimax-optimal if its worst-case regret matches with the minimax lower bound.

Instance Dependent Lower Bounds. An algorithm with nearly minimax-optimal regret is not always preferred, since it may fail to take advantage of environments that are not the worst case. In practice, what is more desirable is to have algorithms that are near minimax-optimal, while their performance gets better on "easier" instances Lattimore and Szepesvári (2020). This motivates the study of instance-dependent regret. In this section, we present two types of lower bound for instance dependent regret: one is asymptotic, and the other is finite-time.

We first define consistent policy and present the asymptotic instance-dependent lower bound result.

Definition 3 (Consistent Policy). A policy π is consistent if over bandit environment $\mathcal{E}$ if for all bandits $\nu \in \mathcal{E}$ and for all $p > 0$ it holds that

$$\text{Reg}_T(\pi, \nu) = O(T^p) \text{ as } n \to \infty.$$

Theorem 13.2.7 (Asymptotic Instance Dependent Lower Bound for Gaussian Bandits (Lattimore and Szepesvári, 2020)). *For any policy π consistent over K-armed unit-variance Gaussian environments $\mathcal{E}_{\mathcal{N}}^K(1)$ and any $\nu \in \mathcal{E}_{\mathcal{N}}^K(1)$, it holds that*

$$\liminf_{T\to\infty} \frac{\text{Reg}_T(\pi, \nu)}{\log T} \geq \sum_{i:\Delta_i>0} \frac{2}{\Delta_i}.$$

A policy is called asymptotically optimal if the equality in the above theorem holds. Interestingly, building on the similar idea of Theorem 13.2.7, one can also develop a finite-time instance-dependent lower bound result.

Theorem 13.2.8 (Instance Dependent Lower Bound for Gaussian Bandits (Lattimore and Szepesvári, 2020)). *Let $\nu \in \mathcal{E}_{\mathcal{N}}^K(1)$ be a K-armed Gaussian bandit with mean vector $\mu \in \mathbb{R}^K$ and suboptimality gaps $\Delta \in [0, \infty)^K$. Define a bandit environment:*

$$\mathcal{E}(\nu) = \{\nu' \in \mathcal{E}_{\mathcal{N}}^K(1) : \mu_i(\nu') \in [\mu_i, \mu_i + 2\Delta_i]\}.$$

Suppose $C > 0$ and $p \in (0,1)$ are constants and π is a policy such that $\mathrm{Reg}_T(\pi, \nu') \le CT^p$ for all T and $\nu' \in \mathcal{E}(\nu)$. Then the regret for instance ν is lower bounded by

$$\mathrm{Reg}_T(\pi, \nu) \ge \frac{2}{(1+\varepsilon)^2} \sum_{i:\Delta_i > 0} \left(\frac{(1-p)\log T + \log\left(\frac{\varepsilon \Delta_i}{8C}\right)}{\Delta_i} \right)^+, \tag{13.18}$$

where $(x)^+ := \max\{x, 0\}$.

The proof for above two instance-dependent lower bounds are too technical that we do not want to go beyond. Interested readers are referred to Chapter 16 in Lattimore and Szepesvári (2020) for details.

13.2.2 Contextual Bandit

In many real-world applications, some side information is available to facilitate decision making. For instance, in healthcare applications, it is important to make decisions based on contextual information such as the person's demographic information, genetic information, life history, biomarkers, and environmental exposures. Ignoring such contextual information may lead to suboptimal decision making. To this end, the contextual bandits setting was introduced to model the side information that determines the reward distribution. The term "contextual bandit" is due to Langford and Zhang (2007) but similar settings have been considered earlier under the names "bandit problems with covariates" (Clayton, 1989; Sarkar, 1991; Yang et al., 2002) and "bandit problems with side information" (Wang et al., 2005; Goldenshluger and Zeevi, 2011). Let $\mathcal{C}$ be a context space for the side information. The contextual bandits setting considered in this section is the same as the MAB described in Section 13.2.1 except for an extra contextual information $C_t \in \mathcal{C}$ at each step t, respectively. We extend our modeling of the environment from $\nu = (P_a : a \in \mathcal{A})$ to $\nu = (P_{a,c} : a \in \mathcal{A}, c \in \mathcal{C})$, i.e. the distribution of rewards depends on both action and context. The trajectory is extended to a sequence of triples, (A_t, R_t, C_t), which represents the action, rewards and context at step t. An instantiation of the contextual bandit protocol in the healthcare setting is given in Algorithm 5. Contextual bandits enable precision medicine by taking appropriate actions for particular patients rather than the same action for a variety of patients. Many papers, like Rindtorff et al. (2019) on precision oncology with *in vitro* data and Zhou et al. (2019) on cancer treatment with genetic data, have effectively applied contextual bandits to precision medicine. Other applications can be found in Shrestha and Jain (2021).

Throughout the section, we discuss the setting where C_t is presented adversarially, rather than assuming C_t is sampled stochastically from an underlying distribution. For the stochastic setting, Goldenshluger and Zeevi (2013) give an algorithm with some parametric assumptions and Yang et al. (2002) with non-parametric algorithm. In fact, the stronger stochastic assumption does not improve the worst-case regret bound over the adversarial setting in linear contextual bandit that we will introduce later. The stochastic setting does help when the instance-dependent regret bound is considered.

Algorithm 13.7: Contextual Bandit Framework in Healthcare

Input: Available treatment options ($\mathcal{A}$), treatment period length T.

for $t = 1, \ldots, T$ **do**

  Agent receives the context information (C_t) for the current patient

  A treatment decision (A_t) is made based on the history and the context information

  Record the post-treatment health outcome (R_t) for the patient

end

In this section, we review the online learning literature on bandit problems with an adversarial context. We will first see a naive one bandit per context approach, which does not make any assumption on the data generating process. We will also introduce the linear contextual bandit setting with linear assumption on the reward distribution. In the end, we introduce some variants of the standard contextual bandits that address sparsity or different types of outputs.

13.2.2.1 One bandit per context

The simplest solution for contextual bandits is possibly one bandit per context (OBPC), which solves the MAB for each context separately. Given any algorithm that solves MAB, OBPC maintains a trajectory for each context. On each step t, if $C_t = c$, the agent applies the algorithm on the trajectory corresponding to c and selects an action. Combined with the EXP3 algorithms, which we call EXP3 per Context, OBPC achieves a regret bound of $\sqrt{K \log(K)|\mathcal{C}|T}$. OBPC does not make any further assumption on the data-generating process ν, so it only works when $\mathcal{C}$ is finite and small. As pointed out in Lattimore and Szepesvári (2020), the awareness of the context information improves the performance over the non-contextual algorithm only when the context actually leads to a non-stationary environment and causes a large gap between the best context-aware policy $\sum_{c \in \mathcal{C}} \max_{a \in [K]} \sum_{t \in [n]: X_t = c} R_{t,a}$ and non-context policy $\max_{a \in [K]} \sum_{t=1}^{n} R_{t,a}$.

13.2.2.2 Bandits with expert advice

OBPC fails when the context space is large and each context does not receive enough samples. In practice, context space has some internal structure that allows information sharing among different contexts. For instance, there can be thousands of categorical variables in precision health applications and many of them may be irrelevant to the reward distribution. Thus, grouping context based on these variables can reduce the context space while keeping the same performance.

Let $\mathcal{P} \subset 2^{\mathcal{C}}$ be a partition over context space, i.e. any $P, P' \in \mathcal{P}$, $P \cap P' = \emptyset$ and $\cup_{P \in \mathcal{P}} P = \mathcal{C}$. The above structural information can be seen as restricting the policy space within

$$\Pi(\mathcal{P}) = \{\pi : \mathcal{C} \rightarrow [K]; \forall c, c' \in \mathcal{C} \text{ s.t. } c, c' \in P \text{ for some } P \in \mathcal{P}, \pi(c) = \pi(c')\}.$$

In other words, we represent the structural information as a restricted policy space that is expected to be essentially smaller than the whole policy space. To allow more flexibility in structural information, we study the general restricted policy space $\Pi \subset \{\pi : \mathcal{C} \mapsto [K]\}$. The aim of agent is now to compete against a fixed class of policies, instead of competing against a set of actions which is a special case of the former.

The recommendations of the policies in the restricted set can be thought of as "expert advice". We can therefore design an algorithm to use such advice by extending the EXP3 algorithm. The extended algorithm EXP4 (Exponential weighting for Exploration and Exploitation with Experts) is given in Algorithm 9. Following the idea of EXP3, EXP4 first uses the same importance-weighted estimator for each action, i.e. $\hat{R}_{t,i} = 1 - \mathbb{1}_{\{A_t=i\}}(1-R_t)/P_{ti}$. Then EXP4 estimates the reward for each expert (policy)

$$\tilde{R}_{t,\pi} = \sum_{i\in[K]} \mathbb{1}\{\pi(C_t) = i\} \hat{R}_{t,i},$$

and keeps a distribution $Q_{t,\pi}$ over the policy space. The distribution is updated using exponentially weighting of the rewards:

$$Q_{t+1,\pi} = \exp(\eta R_{t,\pi}) Q_{t,\pi} / \sum_{\pi'\in\Pi} \exp(\eta R_{t,\pi'}) Q_{t,\pi},$$

where $\eta \in (0,1]$ is the learning rate.

Algorithm 13.8: Exponential-weight Algorithm for Exploration and Exploitation with Experts (Exp4)

Input: T, K, hyper-parameter $\eta \in (0,1]$ and policy space Π
Set the distribution $Q_{1,\pi} = 1/|\Pi|$ for all $\pi \in \Pi$
for $t = 1, \ldots, T$ **do**
  Receive context C_t
  For all $i \in [K]$, compute $P_{t,i} = \sum_{\pi\in\Pi} Q_{t,\pi}\mathbb{1}\{\pi(C_t) = i\}$
  Sample A_t from P_t and receive reward R_t
  Set $\hat{R}_{t,i} = 1 - \frac{\mathbb{1}\{A_t=i\}}{P_{t,i}}(1-R_t)$
  Propagate the rewards to the experts: $\tilde{R}_{t,\pi} = \sum_{i\in[K]} \mathbb{1}\{\pi(C_t) = i\}\hat{R}_{t,i}$ for all $\pi \in \Pi$
  Update $Q_{t+1,\pi} = \frac{\exp(\eta\tilde{R}_{t,\pi})Q_{t,\pi}}{\sum_{\pi'\in\Pi}\exp(\eta\tilde{R}_{t,\pi'})Q_{t,\pi}}$ for all $\pi \in \Pi$
end

We define regret not with respect to the best action but with respect to the best expert:

$$\text{Reg}_T = \mathbb{E}\left[\max_{\pi\in\Pi} \sum_{t=1}^{T} \boldsymbol{r}_t^T \pi(C_t) - \sum_{t=1}^{n} R_t\right],$$

where $\boldsymbol{r}_t = (r_{t,i})_i$ is the K-dimensional vector of rewards of the individual actions and $\pi(C_t)$ is the K-dimensional vector of the probability of selecting each action using policy π under context C_t.

Theorem 13.2.9. *Let $\eta = \sqrt{2\log(|\Pi|/(TK))}$. The regret of EXP4 satisfies*

$$\text{Reg}_T(\text{EXP4}) \leq \sqrt{2\log(|\Pi|)KT}.$$

Proof. Similarly to the way we show (13.13) in the proof in Theorem 13.2.4, we can also show that the for any $\pi^* \in \Pi$:

$$\sum_{t=1}^{T} \tilde{R}_{t,\pi^*} - \sum_{t=1}^{T}\sum_{\pi\in\Pi} Q_{t,\pi}\tilde{R}_{t,\pi} \leq \frac{\log(|\Pi|)}{\eta} + \frac{\eta}{2}\sum_{t=1}^{T}\sum_{\pi\in\Pi} Q_{t,\pi}\left(1 - \tilde{R}_{t,\pi}\right)^2. \tag{13.19}$$

Let $\hat{\boldsymbol{R}}_t = (\hat{R}_{t,i})_{i=1}^K$ and $\tilde{\boldsymbol{R}}_t = (\tilde{R}_{t,\pi})_{\pi\in\Pi}$ denote the vector of $R_{t,i}$'s and $\tilde{R}_{t,\pi}$'s. Since the estimator is unbiased, $\mathbb{E}_t[\hat{R}_t] = \boldsymbol{r}_t$ and letting $\boldsymbol{E}^{(t)}$ be the $|\Pi| \times K$ matrix with each row corresponding to a $\pi \in \Pi$ that gives the row vector $(\mathbb{1}\{\pi(C_t) = i\})_{i=1}^K$, we have

$$\mathbb{E}_t[\tilde{\boldsymbol{R}}_t] = \mathbb{E}_t[\boldsymbol{E}^{(t)}\hat{\boldsymbol{R}}_t] = \boldsymbol{E}^{(t)}\mathbb{E}_t[\hat{\boldsymbol{R}}_t] = \boldsymbol{E}^{(t)}\boldsymbol{r}_t.$$

Taking expectation over both side of Eq. (13.19) and using the fact that $Q_{t,\pi}$ is $\mathcal{F}_t$-measurable leads to

$$\text{Reg}_T \le \frac{\log(|\Pi|)}{\eta} + \frac{\eta}{2}\sum_{t=1}^{T}\sum_{\pi\in\Pi}\mathbb{E}Q_{t,\pi}\left(1-\tilde{R}_{t,\pi}\right)^2. \tag{13.20}$$

Let $\hat{Y}_{t,i} = 1 - \hat{R}_{t,i}$, $y_{t,i} = 1 - r_{t,i}$ and $\tilde{Y}_{t,\pi} = 1 - \tilde{R}_{t,\pi}$ for all $i \in [K]$ and $\pi \in \Pi$. Define vectors $\tilde{\boldsymbol{Y}}_t$ and $\hat{\boldsymbol{Y}}_t$ similarly. Note that $\tilde{\boldsymbol{Y}}_t = \boldsymbol{E}^{(t)}\hat{\boldsymbol{Y}}_t$ and let $A_{t,i} = \mathbb{1}\{A_t = i\}$, which gives us $\hat{Y}_{t,i} = A_{t,i}y_{t,i}/P_{t,i}$ and

$$\mathbb{E}_t\left[\tilde{Y}_{t,\pi}^2\right] = \mathbb{E}_t\left[\left(\frac{E^{(t)}_{\pi,A_t}y_{t,A_t}}{P_{t,A_t}}\right)^2\right] = \sum_{i=1}^{K}\frac{\left(E^{(t)}_{\pi,i}y_{t,i}\right)^2}{P_{t,i}} \le \sum_{i=1}^{K}\frac{E^{(t)}_{\pi,i}}{P_{t,i}}.$$

Thus, by the definition of $P_{t,i}$,

$$\mathbb{E}[\sum_{\pi\in\Pi}Q_{t,\pi}(1-\tilde{R}_{t,\pi})] \le \left[\sum_{\pi\in\Pi}Q_{t,\pi}\sum_{i=1}^{K}\frac{E^{(t)}_{\pi,i}}{P_{t,i}}\right] = K.$$

Substituting into Eq. (13.20) gives us

$$\text{Reg}_T \le \frac{\log(|\Pi|)}{\eta} + \frac{\eta TK}{2} \le \sqrt{2TK\log(|\Pi|)},$$

when $\eta = \sqrt{2\log(|\Pi|)/(TK)}$. □

Now we take a look at the context space partition example introduced before. Assume we have a M-partition of the context space $\mathcal{C}$. The regret bound is reduced from $\sqrt{2|\mathcal{C}|\log(K)KT}$ to $\sqrt{2M\log(K)KT}$ with the structural information.

13.2.2.3 Linear bandits and contextual linear bandits

One bandit per context method learns a distinct environment for each context, which fails when the context space is large or even infinite. Many healthcare applications, especially in mobile health, have continuous context including heart rate, sleeping time, etc. To model such applications with efficient algorithms, we need to assume some nice relationship between the context and environment. The simplest and most frequently used model of this kind is the contextual linear bandit.

Before we introduce the setting for contextual linear bandit, we first define linear bandit. In linear bandit, we do not directly model contexts but assume that the action space $\mathcal{A}_t \subset \mathbb{R}^d$ (we will soon reveal the reason behind choosing a time-varying action space) for some positive integer d, the reward on step t is sampled from a linear model:

$$R_t = \langle\theta^*, A_t\rangle + \eta_t, \text{ for some } \theta^* \in \mathbb{R}^d, \tag{13.21}$$

and the noise η_t is usually assumed to be subgaussian. Note that, depending on the choice of $\mathcal{A}_t$, linear bandits can subsume other bandit problems. For example, to capture the standard stochastic bandit environment with d actions, we set $\mathcal{A}_t = \{e_1, \ldots, e_d\}$ for unit vectors $(e_i)_i$. Note that this choice of action set is not time varying. The flexibility to choose time-varying action sets is critical to capture contextual bandits. We simply let $\mathcal{A}_t = \{\psi(C_t, i) \in \mathbb{R}^d : i \in [K]\}$, for some known function $\psi : \mathcal{C}\times[K] \mapsto \mathbb{R}^d$. A common setup (Li et al., 2010) considers one context per arm, where $\mathcal{C} \subset \mathbb{R}^{d\times K}$ and the function $\psi(c, i)$ extracts the i-th column of the matrix c. Another formulation assumes the same context $c_t \in \mathbb{R}^d$ for every arm but assumes each arm i has a parameter $\theta_i^* \in \mathbb{R}^d$: $R_t = \langle\theta_i^*, c_t\rangle + \eta_t$, when arm i is chosen. Note that this is a special case of the general formulation in (13.21). We can write $\theta^* = (\theta_1^{*T}, \ldots, \theta_K^{*T})^T$ and $\mathcal{A}_t = \{(\mathbf{0}_{d(i-1)}, C_t^T, \mathbf{0}_{d(K-i)})\}_{i=1}^K \subset \mathbb{R}^{dK}$, where $\mathbf{0}_n$ is the all-zero row vector of dimension n.

Linear Upper Confidence Bound (LinUCB). The regret for linear bandit is defined as

$$\mathrm{Reg}_T = \mathbb{E}[\sum_{t=1}^{T} \max_{a_t \in \mathcal{A}_t} \langle \theta^*, a_t \rangle - \sum_{t=1}^{T} R_t].$$

We have seen UCB for the regular bandit environment as a powerful algorithm to balance the exploration and exploitation. In this section, we introduce a new UCB algorithm called LinUCB for linear bandit setting (Auer, 2002; Dani et al., 2008; Rusmevichientong and Tsitsiklis, 2010).

As the case in UCB, we follow the principle *optimism in the face of uncertainty (OFU)*. Instead of directly building confidence set over the mean function μ_a, we build confidence set $\Theta_t \subset \mathbb{R}^d$ over the linear coefficient θ^* that satisfies the following two properties: 1) Θ_t contains the optimal θ^* with a high probability; 2) the set Θ_t should be as small as possible.

For that purpose, we consider the regularized least-square estimator up to step t,

$$\hat{\theta}_t = \mathrm{argmin}_{\theta \in \mathbb{R}^d} \left(\sum_{s=1}^{t} (R_s - \langle \theta, A_s \rangle)^2 + \lambda \|\theta\|_2^2 \right), \tag{13.22}$$

where $\lambda > 0$ is the penalty factor. Equ. (13.22) gives

$$\hat{\theta}_t = V_t^{-1} \sum_{s=1}^{t} A_s R_s, \quad \text{where } V_0 = \lambda I_d \text{ and } V_t = V_0 + \sum_{s=1}^{t} A_s A_s^\top. \tag{13.23}$$

Then the confidence set centering at $\hat{\theta}_t$ is defined by

$$\Theta_{t+1} = \{\theta \in \mathbb{R}^d : \|\theta - \hat{\theta}_t\|_{V_t}^2 \leq \beta_{t+1}\}, \tag{13.24}$$

where $(\beta_t)_t$ is an increasing sequence of constants that controls the level of confidence with $\beta_1 \geq 1$ as $(V_t)_t$ also have increasing eigenvalues. Lemma 2 shows the correctness of the confidence set defined in (13.24). LinUCB chooses actions that maximize the expected reward over all the possible θ's in the confidence set. Details are given in Algorithm 6.

Algorithm 13.9: Linear Upper Confidence Bound (LinUCB)

Input: δ, d, $(\mathcal{A}_t)_t \subset \mathbb{R}^d$, $(\beta_t)_t$, λ.
for $t = 1, \ldots, T$ **do**
  Calculate $\hat{\theta}_t$ using (13.22)
  Compute the confidence set $\Theta_t = \{\theta \in \mathbb{R}^d : \|\theta - \hat{\theta}_{t-1}\|_{V_{t-1}}^2 \leq \beta_t\}$
  Play $A_t = \arg\max_{a \in \mathcal{A}_t} \max_{\theta \in \Theta_t} \langle \theta, a \rangle$
  Receive reward R_t and update V_t using (13.23)
end

Lemma 2. Let $\delta \in (0, 1)$. Then, with a probability at least $1 - \delta$, it holds that for all $t \in \mathbb{N}$, $\theta^* \in \Theta_t$ defined in (13.24) with any sequence $(\beta_t)_t$ satisfying

$$\beta_t \leq \sqrt{\lambda} \|\theta^*\|_2 + \sqrt{2 \log\left(\frac{1}{\delta}\right) + d \log\left(\frac{\det V_t}{\lambda^d}\right)}.$$

Now using the confidence set in Lemma 2, we can show the following regret bound under some mild assumption on the boundedness of the action space. We refer reader to Part V of Lattimore and Szepesvári (2020) for the proof of Lemma 2.

Theorem 13.2.10. *Assuming* $\max_{t\in[n]}\sup_{a,b\in\mathcal{A}_t}\langle\theta^*, a-b\rangle \leq 1$ *and* $\|a\|_2 \leq L$ *for all* $a \in \bigcup_{t=1}^n \mathcal{A}_t$, *using the confidence set defined in Lemma 2, we have with a probability at least* $1-\delta$, *the expected regret of LinUCB is bounded by*

$$\mathrm{Reg}_T(LinUCB, \nu) \leq Cd\sqrt{T}\log(L/\delta), \text{ for some } C > 0.$$

Proof. We first analyze the regret on each step. Let $\theta_t \in \Theta_t$ be the parameter that maximize the expected reward. Let A_t^* be the optimal action given context C_t. Then, using the fact that $\theta^* \in \Theta_t$, we have $\langle\theta^*, A_t^*\rangle \leq \langle\theta, A_t\rangle$. Using Cauchy-Schwarz inequality, we have

$$r_t = \langle\theta_*, A_t^* - A_t\rangle \leq \langle\theta_t - \theta_*, A_t\rangle \leq \|A_t\|_{V_{t-1}^{-1}}\|\tilde{\theta}_t - \theta_*\|_{V_{t-1}} \leq 2\|A_t\|_{V_{t-1}^{-1}}\sqrt{\beta_t}.$$

Then the total regret is given by

$$\mathrm{Reg}_T \leq \sum_{t=1}^T 2\|A_t\|_{V_{t-1}^{-1}}\sqrt{\beta_t} \leq \sqrt{T\sum_{t=1}^T r_t^2} \leq \sqrt{T\beta_T\sum_{t=1}^{}\|A_t\|^2_{V_{t-1}^{-1}}}. \tag{13.25}$$

Using the elliptical potential lemma (Carpentier et al., 2020), $\sum_{t=1}^T\left(1 \wedge \|A_t\|^2_{V_{t-1}^{-1}}\right) \leq 2\log\left(\det V_T/\det V_0\right)$. The results follow by plugging this into (13.25) with the chosen β_T and the fact that

$$\det\left(V_T\right) = \prod_{i=1}^d \lambda_i \leq \left(\frac{1}{d}\operatorname{trace} V_T\right)^d \leq \left(\frac{\operatorname{trace} V_0 + TL^2}{d}\right)^d,$$

where $\lambda_1, \ldots, \lambda_d$ are eigenvalues of V_t.

□

LinUCB gives a regret bound that scales with d. However, this is not the optimal rate when the action set is finite. Auer (2002) proposed SupLinUCB which maintains a master algorithm that achieves a regret bound of $\sqrt{dT\log(TK)}$ when the action space is finite.

LinUCB for contextual bandits. Chu et al. (2011) applied the LinUCB to the contextual bandit problems. To be specific, they assume a context and an unknown parameter θ for each arm a and the reward is generated by

$$R_t = C_{t,A_t}^\top\theta_{A_t}^* + \eta_t, \text{ where } C_{t,a}, \theta_a^* \in \mathbb{R}^d.$$

Applying Theorem 13.2.10 gives us the regret bound of $Kd\sqrt{T}$. Li et al. (2010) showed a good performance of the contextual bandit with LinUCB on News Article Recommendation task.

13.2.2.4 Sparse LinUCB

So far we have achieved the regret bound of $d\sqrt{T\log(T)}$, which scales linearly with d. However, the bound can be vacuous for high-dimensional context ($d \gg T$). Such high dimensional problems can occur in healthcare applications. For example, Bastani and Bayati (2020) incorporates the high-dimensional genetic profile and medical records with contextual bandits to design patient's optimal medication dosage. Following the idea of UCB, the key is to construct a confidence set that accounts for the sparsity. To tackle the problem, we introduce a powerful tool that converts online prediction problem to confidence set estimation, with which a UCB-style algorithm can be designed using any online predicting method and we can analyze its regret in a unified way.

Online to Confidence Set Conversion. There is a conversion from the online prediction to confidence sets. We consider online linear regression problem with a squared loss, which has been well-explored in the past decade (Huang et al., 2008; Javanmard and Montanari, 2014). The agent interacts with the environment in the following manner where in each round t:

1. The environment chooses a context $C_t \in \mathbb{R}$ and $A_t \in \mathbb{R}^d$ in an arbitrary way.
2. The value of A_t is revealed to the agent.
3. The agent generate a prediction $\hat{R}_t$.
4. The environment reveals R_t to the agent as well as the loss $(R_t - \hat{R}_t)^2$.

The regret of an agent with respective to the best linear predictor is given by

$$\rho_T = \sum_{t=1}^{T} (R_t - \hat{R}_t)^2 - \inf_{\theta \subset \mathbb{R}^d} \sum_{t=1}^{T} (R_t - \langle \theta, A_t \rangle)^2.$$

Theorem 13.2.11 (Online-to-Confidence-Set Conversion (Abbasi-Yadkori et al., 2012)). *Let $\delta \in (0, 1)$ and assume that $\theta^* \in \Theta$, noise η_t's are R-sub-Gaussian and $\rho_t \leq B_t$. Let*

$$\beta_t(\delta) = 1 + 2B_t + 32R^2 \log\left(\frac{R\sqrt{8} + \sqrt{1 + B_t}}{\delta}\right).$$

Then

$$\Theta_{t+1} = \left\{\theta \in \mathbb{R}^d : \sum_{s=1}^{t} (\hat{R}_s - \langle \theta, A_s \rangle)^2 \leq \beta_t(\delta)\right\}, \tag{13.26}$$

satisfies $\mathbb{P}(\theta^* \in \Theta_{t+1} \forall t \in \mathbb{N}) \geq 1 - \delta$.

Algorithm 13.10: Online linear predictor UCB

Input: $\delta \in (0, 1)$, an online predictor with a regret bound B_t

for $t = 1, \ldots, T$ **do**
- Receive action set $\mathcal{A}_t$
- Compute the confidence set Θ_t using (13.26)
- Play $A_t = \arg\max_{a \in \mathcal{A}_t} \max_{\theta \in \Theta_t} \langle \theta, a \rangle$ and receive reward R_t
- Feed A_t to the online linear predictor and obtain prediction $\hat{R}_t$
- Feed R_t and loss to the linear predictor as feedback

end

Theorem 13.2.11 provides a tool for constructing a confidence set for the prediction of any online learning algorithm with a regret guarantee. One can develop the Online linear predictor UCB (OLR-UCB) as shown in Algorithm 7.

Let $\|\theta^*\|_2 \leq m_2$. Using Theorem 13.2.11 and the standard regret decomposition for UCB-style algorithm, one can show the following regret bound:

$$R_T \leq \sqrt{8dT\left(m_2^2 + \beta_{T-1}(\delta)\right) \log\left(1 + \frac{T}{d}\right)}.$$

Application to sparse online linear prediction. Note that our goal is to derive a regret bound with a lower dependency on the ambient dimension d. In the standard regression problem, learnability of high-dimensional data relies on the sparsity assumption which assumes the number of non-zero dimensions is less or equal to a positive integer s.

Assumption 1. (sparse parameter) The true parameter θ^* satisfies $\|\theta^*\|_0 \leq s$ for some $s > 0$.

To this end, we adopt SeqSEW (Gerchinovitz, 2011) as the online linear prediction algorithm, which achieves the online learning regret $\rho_T = \mathcal{O}(s\log(T))$. Combined with Theorem 13.2.11, we have the following result:

Theorem 13.2.12. *With a high probability, the we bound the regret of OLR-UCB with SeqSEW as the online predictor by*

$$\mathrm{Reg}_T = \tilde{\mathcal{O}}(\sqrt{dsT}). \tag{13.27}$$

This improves over the $d\sqrt{T}$ by LinUCB in the previous section when $s \ll d$. As pointed out by Lattimore and Szepesvári (2020), for any algorithm, there exists an infinite action space such that $\mathrm{Reg}_T = \Omega(\sqrt{dsT})$. Thus, the bound in (13.27) is minimax optimal. Despite its optimality, our result still has the unavoidable dependence of $\sqrt{d}$. Bastani and Bayati (2020) derived a regret bound of $\mathcal{O}(K(s\log(d)\log(T))^2)$, when the action set is finite. More variants of high-dimensional sparse linear bandits are discussed in Hao et al. (2020).

13.2.3 Offline Learning

So far we have been discussing bandit problems in the *online learning* setting, where we are free to choose actions while collecting the dataset. In many real applications, collecting data in an online manner can be expensive and can cost a lot of time. In such situations, we might want to evaluate a target policy using a large but fixed dataset that has been collected for years by a different policy. This setting is called *offline learning*.

Given a fixed contextual bandit environment, the value of a policy is defined as $v_\pi = \mathbb{E}_{a_t\sim\pi(c_t)} r_t$ Formally, offline bandits, also referred as *off-policy evaluation* aims at evaluating the value v_π of a new policy using a sequence of interactions $S_T = (c_t, a_t, r_t)_{t=1}^T$, where c_t, a_t and r_t are the context, action and reward respectively at step t. The actions are chosen by the data-generating policy π_D, which is also referred as *behavior policy* or *logging policy*. In this section,

One solution is to learn the reward and context distribution using a parametric or non-parametric method and then evaluate the new policy with the simulator by sampling context and rewards from the learned distribution. Although this approach is straightforward, the modeling step is often very expensive and difficult, and more importantly, it often introduces modeling bias to the simulator, making it hard to justify reliability of the obtained evaluation results.

Li et al. (2011) proposed a simple algorithm (Algorithm 8) that uses an unbiased estimator of the policy value when the behavior policy picks arms uniformly at random. The method is to simply use all the interactions in the dataset that coincide with the action that the policy being evaluated would have taken. They show that $\hat{v}_\pi$ is an unbiased estimator of v_π and with a high probability $(\hat{v}_\pi - v_\pi)^2 = \tilde{\mathcal{O}}\left(Kv_\pi/n\right)$, where v_π is the true expected value of the policy as defined above. They also successfully applied the off-policy evaluation to the News Article Recommendation system. Mary et al. (2014) improved upon Algorithm 8 via bootstrapping techniques. They give a bootstrapped estimator for any quantile of the distribution of the estimated value $\hat{v}_\pi$ that allows some evaluation of the uncertainty.

Algorithm 13.11: Policy Evaluator

Input: a policy π; stream of interactions S_T of length T

$h_0 \leftarrow \emptyset$, $\hat{V}_\pi \leftarrow 0$ and $N \leftarrow 0$
for $t = 1, \ldots, T$ **do**
  Get the i-th interaction (c_i, a_i, r_t) from S_T
  if $\pi(h_{t-1}, c_t) = a_t$ **then**
    $h_t \leftarrow h_{t-1} \cup (c_t, a_t, r_t)$
    $\hat{V}_\pi \leftarrow \hat{V}_\pi + r_t$ and $N \leftarrow N + 1$
  end
end

Output: $\hat{v}_\pi = \hat{V}_\pi / N$

Minimax rate lower bound. To understand how good our algorithms perform, we start with establishing a minimax lower bound that characterizes the inherent hardness of the off-policy value estimation problem. Let $R_{\max}, \sigma \in \mathbb{R}^+$. Define the class of reward distributions $\mathcal{V}(\sigma, R_{\max})$ with bounded mean and variance as

$$\mathcal{V}(\sigma, R_{\max}) := \{\nu = (P_{a,c})_{a,c \in \mathcal{A}\times\mathcal{C}} : 0 \le \mathbb{E}_{R\sim P_{a,c}}[R] \le R_{\max} \text{ and } \mathrm{Var}[R \mid a, c] \le \sigma^2,\ \forall a, c \in \mathcal{A} \times \mathcal{C}\}.$$

Any estimator $\hat{v}$ is a function that maps (π, π_D, S_T) to an estimate of v_π. Let the context $C \sim \lambda$ with a density relative to the Lebesgue measure. The minimax rate is defined as

$$M_n(\pi, \lambda, \pi_D, \sigma, R_{\max}) := \inf_{\hat{v}} \sup_{\nu \in \mathcal{V}(\sigma, R_{\max})} \mathbb{E}[(\hat{v}(\pi, \pi_D, S_T) - v_\pi)^2],$$

where the expectation is taken over the distribution of the dataset S_T that depends on (π, λ, π_D).

A critical value that determines the hardness of the problem is

$$V_1 := \mathbb{E}_{C\sim\lambda, A\sim\pi_D(\cdot, C)}\left[\pi^2(A, C)/\pi_D^2(A, C)\right].$$

Wang et al. (2017) (Corollary 1) gives the following lower bound for R_n:

$$M_n(\pi, \lambda, \pi_D, \sigma, R_{\max}) \ge \frac{V_1(\sigma^2 + R_{\max}^2)}{700T}. \tag{13.28}$$

Importance sampling estimator. Wang et al. (2017) give some analysis on the minimax rate of the off-policy evaluation given a known data-generating policy, denoted by π_D. We slightly abuse the notation and let $\pi(a, c)$ denote the probability of choosing a using policy π under the context c. They consider the Importance Sampling (IS) estimator (Charles et al., 2013) and the Weighted Importance Sampling (WIS) estimator given by

$$\hat{v}_{\mathrm{IS},\pi} = \frac{1}{T}\sum_{t=1}^{T} \frac{\pi(a_t, c_t)}{\pi_D(a_t, c_t)} r_t \quad \text{and}$$

$$\hat{v}_{\mathrm{WIS},\pi} = \sum_{t=1}^{T} \frac{\frac{\pi(a_t,c_t)}{\pi_D(a_t,c_t)}}{\sum_{t'=1}^{T} \frac{\pi(a_{t'},c_t)}{\pi_D(a_{t'},c_t)}} r_t, \text{ respectively.}$$

It is shown in Dudík et al. (2014) that the IS estimator is unbiased and it achieves the minimax rate in (13.28) when n is sufficiently large. The WIS estimator is biased with a lower variance. It also enjoys the minimax optimality up to a logarithmic constant.

Regression estimator. Another common method, so-called regression estimator or plug-in estimator, simply learns the reward distribution and plugs it in. Let $\hat{r} : \mathcal{A} \times \mathcal{C} \mapsto \mathbb{R}$ is an estimator for the mean reward. The regression estimator is given by

$$\hat{v}_{\text{Reg},\pi} := \frac{1}{T} \sum_{t=1}^{T} \sum_{a} \pi(a, c_t) \hat{r}(a, c_t).$$

When the context space and action space are finite. One can use the simple sample average estimator $\hat{r}(a, c) = (\sum_{t=1}^{T} \mathbb{1}(a_t = a, c_t = c) r_i) / (\sum_{t=1}^{T} \mathbb{1}(a_t = a, c_t = c))$. Interestingly, one can write the regression estimator using sample average as

$$\hat{v}_{\text{Reg}} = \frac{1}{T} \sum_{t=1}^{T} \frac{\pi(a_t, c_t)}{\hat{\pi}_D(a_t, c_t)} r_t, \text{ where } \hat{\pi}_D(a, c) = \frac{\sum_t \mathbb{1}(a_t = a, c_t = c)}{T}.$$

There is a strong connection between IS and regression estimators. That is regression estimator simply replaces the π_D with its empirical estimator. Regression estimator is biased while its variance is normally lower than IS (Dudík et al., 2011; Li et al., 2015). Regression estimator is also shown to be minimax optimal when n is sufficiently large. The simple plugin method using sample average is not applicable when context space is infinite. When more information on how rewards depend on contexts and actions, we can posit a parametric or non-parametric model of $\mathbb{E}[R \mid C, A]$ and fit it to obtain an estimator. Due to the difficulties of having a good estimation $\hat{x}$, which may suffer model-misspecification or high variance, a pure regression estimator only works well in problems with finite actions. For more details, we refer the reader to a more recent paper (Kim et al., 2021).

Doubly robust estimator. Based on the above discussions about IS and Regression Estimator, it is natural to combine both. Doubly Robust (DR) (Bang and Robins, 2005; Dudík et al., 2011; Jiang and Li, 2016) which is a combination of regression and IS estimator, and can achieve the low variance of regression and no (or low) bias of IS. The method is named by Doubly Robust because it is accurate if at least one of the estimator is accurate. DR estimator is defined as

$$\hat{v}_{DR} = \frac{1}{T} \sum_{t} \left[\frac{\pi(a_t, c_t)}{\pi_D(a_t, c_t)} (r_t - \hat{r}(a_t, c_t)) + \sum_{a} \pi(a, c_t) \hat{r}(a, c_t) \right].$$

Informally, the estimator uses $\hat{r}(a, c)$ as a baseline and corrects the baseline when the action is more likely to be sampled from the target policy. DR enjoys both the low variance of Regression estimator and the low bias of the IS estimator and also matches the minimax lower bound in 13.28. Wang et al. (2017) further introduce the SWITCH estimator that takes account into the scale of the importance weight. When the importance weight is large, it switches to the regression estimator, which significantly reduces the variance while introducing only a little bias. It performs better in the numerical experiments.

Non-asymptotic regime. All of the above estimators achieve minimax optimality when n is sufficiently large. Ma et al. (2021) discussed a regime when the sample size is not large. They showed that there is a fundamental statistical gap between algorithms with and without the knowledge of the behavior policy in this regime. They proposed a *competitive ratio* that measures the MSE of an algorithm with an unknown behavior policy relative to the lower bound of all algorithms with a known behavior policy. Competitive ratio is always greater than 1. A competitive ratio closer to 1 indicates that the algorithm can performance as good as the algorithm with a known behavior policy. Ma et al. (2021) showed that the regression estimator has a minimax optimal competitive ratio of the rate is $\mathcal{O}(K)$, where K is the number of actions. That means an algorithm without the knowledge of the behavior policy has to pay a multiplicative factor of K compared to that with the knowledge.

13.3 Advanced Topics

We now review a selection of advanced topics in bandit algorithms that are relevant to applications in healthcare.

13.3.1 Non-stationarity

We have discussed two basic and extreme cases of bandit theory: stochastic bandit models and adversarial bandit models. In the former, the reward distribution for every arm is static whereas in the latter, it can change arbitrarily over time. In this section, we describe a more practical setting that sits in the "middle" of the above two extreme models: non-stationary bandits. Specifically, the reward distributions change over time, but the amount of changes cannot be as arbitrary as the adversarial setting.

For a non-stationary multi-armed bandit environment ν, we define the reward mean for arm a at time t by $\mu_{a,t}(\nu)$ or $\mu_{a,t}$ for simplicity. Then the dynamic regret is

$$\mathrm{Reg}_T = \sum_{t=1}^{T} \max_a \mu_{a,t} - \mathbb{E}\left[\sum_{t=1}^{T} \mu_{A_t,t}\right].$$

Unlike the regret definition for the adversarial setting that is with respect to the best single arm, dynamic regret is defined with respect to the sequence of best arms at each time step. There are two popular constraints that quantify the reward changes. One is the total count of changes in the mean reward that occur before time T:

$$S_T = 1 + \sum_{t=2}^{T} \mathbb{1}\{\mu_{a,t-1} \neq \mu_{a,t}, \text{ for some } a\}.$$

Settings where the above quantity is assumed to be small are also called piece-wise stationary. Another constraint quantifies the total variation for the reward mean:

$$B_T = \sum_{t=2}^{T} \max_a |\mu_{a,t} - \mu_{a,t-1}|.$$

Piecewise Stationary Setting. The first algorithm designed for the non-stationary MAB under a finite number of reward mean changes is Exp3.S (Auer et al., 2002), which is a variant of the Exp3 algorithm. The expected regret of Exp3.S is $O(S_T\sqrt{KT\log(KT)})$ in general, but can be improved to $O(\sqrt{S_T KT\log(KT)})$ if S_T is used to tune the algorithm parameters. Later on, Garivier and Moulines (2011) proved that no policy can achieve problem-dependent regret smaller than $O(\sqrt{T})$ in the non-stationary case, and Exp3.S is thus optimal up to logarithmic factors of T. Garivier and Moulines (2011) also studied two UCB-based algorithms: discounted UCB (D-UCB) which was first proposed by Kocsis and Szepesvári (2006) and sliding-window UCB (SW-UCB). Their main idea is to encourage using more recent data in UCB reward estimations. When S is given, both algorithms achieve $O(K\sqrt{ST}\log T)$ regret. Another body of works explores the idea of monitoring the reward distributions by change-detection methods and reset the bandit algorithm accordingly. Using this idea, Monitored-UCB (M-UCB) (Cao et al., 2019) combines the UCB algorithm with a change-point detection component based on running sample means over a sliding window and achieves $O(\sqrt{KST\log T})$ regret under certain assumptions on the reward mean change. In the same year, Auer et al. (2019) proposed an action elimination algorithm ADSWITCH that again detects changes in the mean reward and restarts the learning algorithm accordingly. Without knowing S nor making other assumptions, ADSWITCH achieves $O(\sqrt{KST\log T})$ regret.

Bounded Total Variation Setting. Comparing with piecewise stationary setting, bounded total variation is a softer constraint. Here nature has the power to change the reward at every round but only up to a total amount limit B_T. Besbes et al. (2014) proposed the Rexp3 policy that uses the famous Exp3 algorithm as a subroutine and restarts it at every batch. Rexp3 with a batch size tuned by B_T has $O((B_T K \log K)^{1/3} T^{2/3})$ regret that nearly matches the lower bound of $\Omega(KB_T)^{1/3}T^{2/3})$ in this setting (Besbes et al., 2014).

The non-stationary setup has also been studied in linear bandits and contextual bandits. We briefly describe the latter one as an example. Define the distribution of the context-reward pairs $\mathcal{C} \times [0,1]^K$ by $\mathcal{D}_1, \ldots, \mathcal{D}_T$. At each round, the environment samples (c_t, x_t) and reveals c_t to the agent, then the agent picks an arm $A_t \in [K]$ and observes $x_t(A_t)$. For a fixed set of policies Π that contains mappings: $\mathcal{C} \to [K]$, the dynamic regret is defined as:

$$\mathrm{Reg}_T = \sum_{t=1}^{T} \max_{\pi \in \Pi} \mathbb{E}_{(c,x)\sim \mathcal{D}_t}[x(\pi(c))] - \sum_{t=1}^{T} x_t(A_t).$$

Similar to the MAB setting, there are two ways to measure the non-stationary of the environment: total number of changes and the total variation in below.

$$S = 1 + \sum_{t=2}^{T} \mathbb{1}\{\mathcal{D}_t \neq \mathcal{D}_{t-1}\},$$

$$B_T = \sum_{t=2}^{T} \|\mathcal{D}_t - \mathcal{D}_{t-1}\|_{TV}.$$

Chen et al. (2019) proposed ADA-ILTCB$^+$ algorithm that is parameter-free, efficient and achieves optimal regret $\widetilde{O}(\min\{\sqrt{K(\log|\Pi|)ST}, \sqrt{K(\log|\Pi|)T} + (K\log|\Pi|B_T)^{1/3}T^{2/3}\})$ by randomly entering replay phases to detect non-stationarity. More recently, a generic reduction has been studied that allows one to convert certain algorithms for the stationary setting into algorithms for the non-stationary setting (Wei and Luo, 2021). What is nice about this work is that the resulting algorithms often *simultaneously* achieve optimal guarantees in terms of both S and B_T *without* prior knowledge of any of these parameters.

13.3.2 Robustness

So far, we have discussed stochastic and adversarial bandits. Stochastic bandit is an ideal setting, since it assumes a fixed reward distribution. Adversarial, on the other hand, consider a too extreme scenario. In real-world applications, some of the observed rewards may be corrupted resulting in a deviation from purely stochastic behavior. For instance, there might be clerical errors while creating electronic health records or sensor errors in recording health status from wearable devices. If the reward is self-reported by patients, there can be corruption due to mistakes, lack of attention, boredom, etc. In this section, we consider algorithms that are *robust* to possible corruption. Note that this setting is between the purely stochastic and the adversarial settings but in a different way than the non-stationary bandit discussed in Section 13.3.1.

Fraction corruption model. The fraction corruption model limits the fraction of the total number of rounds that an adversarial corruption can happen. Assume corruptions happen with a probability $\eta \in [0,1]$. The adversary closely follows the progress of arm pulling and reward generation. At each time step t, after the algorithm has decided to pull an arm A_t, the adversary first decides whether to corrupt this arm pull or not by performing a Bernoulli trail $Z_t \in \{0,1\}$ with a mean $\eta \in [0,1]$. Then it generates a corruption ζ arbitrarily. After this, the "clean reward" R_t^* is generated by the environment. The reward a player receives at step t is

$$R_t = \mathbb{1}\{Z_t = 0\}R_t^* + \mathbb{1}\{Z_t = 1\}\zeta_t.$$

Since the rewards may be contaminated, directly running the algorithms built for stochastic bandits can result in degraded performance. Several papers have proposed variants of UCB that use a more robust estimate. Kapoor et al. (2019) proposed RUCB-TUNE (Robust UCB) which makes two crucial changes to the classical UCB: RUCB-TUNE uses the median and a tuned variance estimate instead of the simple sample mean and variance to construct its upper bound. The algorithm requires an upper bound η_0 on the corruption rate η. Their analyses are built on the environment with Gaussian reward distributions and they have a regret bound of $\mathcal{O}((1-\eta)\sqrt{KT\log(T)} + \eta_0(\mu^* + B)T)$, where B is an upper bound on the scales of corruptions $|\zeta_t|$ and μ^* is the maximum expected reward of all the arms. They provide another algorithm RUCB with a similar result. RUCB does not require the knowledge of η_0 but it requires an upper bound on the variance of rewards for all the arms.

Niss and Tewari (2020) consider a stronger requirement that all the arms have no more than η-fraction of corruption. They proposed crUCB (contamination robust-UCB), which mimics RUCB in the general framework. The only difference is that they allow a variety of robust mean estimates including α-trimmed mean, mean estimates that ignore the largest $(1-\alpha)$-fraction of data, α-shorth mean. Their algorithms are evaluated by uncontaminated regrets, the regret between true rewards of the best possible actions and the algorithm-chosen actions:

$$\text{Reg}_T = \max_{a\in\mathcal{A}} \mathbb{E}[\sum_{t=1}^{T} R_a^*(t) - R_{A_t}^*(t)],$$

If the contamination fraction is small enough, both crUCB using α-shorth mean and α-trimmed mean achieve uncontaminated regret of $\sqrt{KT\log(T)} + \sum_a \Delta_a$, where Δ_a is the gap between the expected reward of a and the optimal action.

Budget-bounded corruption model. In budget-bounded corruption model (Lykouris et al., 2018), all the rounds can be possibly corrupted but the total deviation between the "clean rewards" and the corrupted rewards is bounded. We define the total corruption budget as

$$B_T = \sum_{t=1}^{T} \|R_t^* - R_t\|.$$

Gupta et al. (2019) proposed BARBAR (Bandit Algorithm with Robustness: Bad Arms get Recourse) based on the arm elimination algorithm discussed in Section 13.2 with some crucial modifications that make it robust to corruptions. Gupta et al. (2019) show that their algorithm achieves a gap-dependent regret bound of

$$\text{Reg}_T = \mathcal{O}\left(KB_T + \sum_{a\neq a^*} \frac{\log T}{\Delta_a} \log\left(\frac{K}{\delta}\log T\right)\right).$$

without knowing the value of C.

13.3.3 Dealing with Constraints

In standard bandit settings, the only criterion to evaluate the performance of an algorithm is the regret (either cumulative or simple regret). In this section, we introduce constrained bandit problems, where the agent also needs to satisfy certain constraints while minimizing its regret. Depending on the actual problem's demands, different types of constraints have been considered. For healthcare applications, two types of constraints frequently arise in practice. First, delivering an intervention might consume resources such as doctor's time, patient's attention, phone battery and power, etc. We might therefore want to maximize rewards subject to a budget on resource consumption. Second, we might be worried that uncontrolled exploration might yield performance that is substantially worse than an existing standard of care. With these concerns in mind, in this section we consider the following two settings: bandits with knapsacks and conservative bandits.

Bandits with Knapsacks (BwK). The name of *bandits with knapsacks* comes from the well-known knapsack problem in combinatorial optimization that studies packing items into a fixed-size knapsack. In a knapsack problem, each item has its value and size. Its ultimate goal is to fill the knapsack with as large value as possible. The *bandits with knapsacks* then focus on a stochastic online version of the knapsack problem. Many practical scenarios can be captured by this framework. For example, in medical trials, physicians may be limited by the cost of treatment materials while optimizing the health condition of the patients. In online recommendations, the website designer may be constrained by the advertisers' budgets while maximizing its profit. We follow the terminologies and notations in Badanidiyuru et al. (2018) to formally describe this setting and their proposed algorithms.

An agent is given an action set $\mathcal{A}$ and there are d resources being consumed. At every round, the agent selects an action $A_t \in \mathcal{A}$ and observes a reward X_t along with a d-dimensional resource consumption vector $\mathbf{c}_t$. For each resource $i \in [d]$, the total consumption should not exceed the pre-specified budget B_i at any round. The agent stops immediately when the total consumption of certain resources exceeds its budget. Denote the stopping time by τ, the goal is to maximize the total reward until time τ. The worst-case regret for an algorithm is defined as the difference between the benchmark total reward OPT[4] and the algorithm's expected total reward until τ.

To solve the problem, Badanidiyuru et al. (2018) proposed two algorithms. The first one is a primal-dual algorithm called PrimalDualBwK. At every round, it estimates the upper confidence bound for the expected reward and the lower confidence bound for the resource consumption for each arm. Then PrimalDualBwK plays the most "cost-effective" arm, i.e., the one with highest ratio of the expected reward's upper bound to the expected cost. The regret of PrimalDualBwK is proved to be $\widetilde{O}\left(\sqrt{|\mathcal{A}|\mathrm{OPT}} + \mathrm{OPT}\sqrt{|\mathcal{A}|/B}\right)$, where $B := \min_i B_i$. Note that without the resource constraints, the regret bound becomes $\widetilde{O}\left(\sqrt{|\mathcal{A}|\mathrm{OPT}}\right) = \widetilde{O}\left(\sqrt{|\mathcal{A}|T}\right)$ that is optimal up to logarithmic factors since the only constraint is the time horizon T and we can simply set $B = T$ in the general regret formula. The second algorithm is called BalancedExploration. Its design principle is to explore as much as possible while avoiding obviously sub-optimal strategies. They show that the regret of BalancedExploration is $\widetilde{O}\left(\sqrt{d|\mathcal{A}|\mathrm{OPT}} + \mathrm{OPT}\sqrt{d|\mathcal{A}|/B}\right)$. Even though its regret has worse dependence on d comparing with PrimalDualBwK, BalancedExploration performs better in some special cases.

Comparing with the general constraint in the above knapsack framework, researchers have also considered more specific settings. For example, other than the time horizon, there is a single resource with deterministic consumption and different arms consume the resource at different rates (Tran-Thanh et al., 2010, 2012; Ding et al., 2013; Xia et al., 2015; Zhou and Tomlin, 2018). Such problems are often called *budgeted bandits*. Agrawal and Devanur (2014) generalized the BwK model by allowing arbitrary concave rewards and convex constraints. Furthermore, similar constrained bandit problems are also studied in settings that include contextual bandits (Agrawal and Devanur, 2014; Wu et al., 2015; Agrawal and Devanur, 2016) and even adversarial bandits (Sun et al., 2017; Immorlica et al., 2019).

[4]An optimal dynamic policy that maximizes the expected total reward given prior knowledge on all latent distributions such as the reward distribution and the cost consumption for each action.

Conservative Bandits. It is well-known that standard bandit algorithms often explore wildly in their early stages, so their regret over initial rounds can be very high. However, safety is one of the crucial concerns for designing adaptive experiments, so the early stage of high regret cannot be tolerated in some high-stakes scenarios. For instance, the UCB algorithm can assign treatments almost randomly to a patient during the first several rounds, which may cause severe problems for the patient's overall health. A company may also not be able to withstand the extremely low revenue initially if its operation is in great need of cash flow. In these examples, the real situation is that the physician or the company already has their favorite policies that operate well. They would like to explore new strategies to optimize their treatment performance or revenue while maintaining their performance to not be significantly worse than a baseline, uniformly over time. *Conservative bandits* (Wu et al., 2016) exactly model this problem. We follow their terminology and notation to describe the problem framework.

We use $\{0, 1, \ldots, K\}$ as the indices of actions, in which the arm indexed by 0 corresponds to the default action (the agent's typical strategy) and the other arms are the alternatives to be explored. The agent selects an arm $A_t \in \{0, 1, \ldots, K\}$ in round t. Denote $R_{t,i}$ as the random reward received at time t after playing arm i, then the regret and pseudo-regret are defined as $\text{Reg}_T = \max_{i\in\{0,1,\ldots,K\}} \sum_{t=1}^{T} R_{t,i} - R_{t,A_t}$ and $\widetilde{\text{Reg}}_T = \max_{i\in\{0,1,\ldots,K\}} \sum_{t=1}^{T} \mu_i - \mu_{A_t}$. To ensure that the agent performs as good as his or her usual strategy, the algorithm needs to satisfy:

$$\sum_{s=1}^{t} R_{s,A_s} \geq (1-\alpha)\sum_{s=1}^{t} R_{s,0}, \tag{13.29}$$

where $0 < \alpha \leq 1$. The above constraint guarantees that the reward collected by the agent is at least $(1-\alpha)$ fraction of the reward from simply playing arm 0. The objective of conservative bandits algorithms is to minimize regret while satisfying (13.29) for all t. To solve the problem, (Wu et al., 2016) proposed a novel algorithm called conservative UCB which is based on UCB with the novel twist of maintaining (13.29) being satisfied. Basically, the agent follows the UCB suggestion if (13.29) can be satisfied from their estimation, otherwise, the agent switches to the conservative arm 0. They show that conservative UCB achieves pseudo-regret $\widetilde{\text{Reg}}_T = \widetilde{O}(\sqrt{KT} + \frac{K}{\alpha\mu_0})$, where μ_0 denotes the expected reward for arm 0. For more details, including gap-dependent regret and regret analysis for the adversarial setting, we refer the reader to Wu et al. (2016).

The concept of conservative bandits, namely performing as well as a baseline uniformly over time, is quite general. Recently, it has been generalized to more settings, e.g., conservative contextual bandits (Kazerouni et al., 2016; Garcelon et al., 2020b) and conservative reinforcement learning (Garcelon et al., 2020a).

13.3.4 Fairness

Algorithmic fairness has become an increasingly important topic in machine learning research (Barocas et al., 2021). Fairness is also a concern in healthcare applications due to the biases in data collection and algorithmic design (Paulus and Kent, 2020). Using healthcare cost as a proxy for healthcare needs leads to biased risk scores that hurt Black patients (Obermeyer et al., 2019). Using genetic datasets collected mostly from patients of European ancestry leads to biased genetic risk scores on patients with non-European ancestries (Martin et al., 2019). Unfairness can also be rooted in algorithmic design. Algorithms that simply maximize user responses can be unfair in how they allocate exposure to the items in recommendation systems (Singh and Joachims, 2018). In this section, we review several popular definitions of fairness in bandit literature and discuss how to calibrate unfairness.

Two types of fairness. Though there remains little agreement about what "fairness" should mean in different contexts, the literature can be divided into two broad families: those that target *group* fairness and those that target *individual* fairness. Group fairness requires the algorithm to maintain fairness across different demographic groups (say by race or gender) that are supposed to be treated equally. As we mentioned above, biased healthcare algorithms may hurt patients from certain demographic groups due to low representation. Individual fairness, on the other hand, asks for some constraints on the individual level, including two slightly different types: fairness through awareness, which requires that similar individuals be treated similarly, and meritocratic fairness, which requires that less qualified individuals not be favored over more qualified individuals. Individual fairness in healthcare is also important: for two patients with similar demographic information or physical conditions, we shall not develop an algorithm that performs much better for one patient while useless (or even harmful) for the other.

In the context of bandits, the literature can be further divided into those that model individuals as arms in the MAB setting and those that models individuals as contexts in the contextual bandits setting. We give some examples of fairness definitions from each category.

Individual fairness. We start from individual fairness in the MAB setting with each arm representing an individual. Joseph et al. (2016) proposed the use of meritocratic fairness. Formally, an algorithm is said to be δ-fair if over T time steps, for any pair of arms a, a', and any round t,

$$\pi_t(a) > \pi_t(a') \text{ only if } \mu_a > \mu_{a'}$$

with probability at least $1 - \delta$. This requires the algorithm to give equal probability to choose two arms unless one there is strong evidence that $\mu_a > \mu_{a'}$. Joseph et al. (2016) developed an algorithm that is δ-fair based on the traditional UCB algorithm. In specific, they maintain a set of arms that chains to the arm with highest UCB. All the arms in the set are given the same probability to be selected. Their regret bound is $\mathcal{O}(\sqrt{K^3 T \ln \frac{TK}{\delta}})$, with a higher cubic dependence on K, which is the price they pay to give equal probability to all the arms in the set. More generally, Liu et al. (2017) considers a fairness through awareness. An algorithm is said to be $(\epsilon_1, \epsilon_2, \delta)$-smooth fair [5], if for any pair of arms a, a' and any t, with a probability at least $1 - \delta$,

$$|\pi_t(a) - \pi_t(a')| \leq \epsilon_1 |\mu_a - \mu_{a'}| + \epsilon_2.$$

They introduced a fairness regret to quantify the violation that occurs when the arm with the highest reward realization at a given time is not selected with the highest probability. Formally, they have

$$\text{Reg}_T = \sum_{t=1}^{T} \mathbb{E}\left[\sum_{i=1}^{K} \max\{P^*(i) - \pi_t(i), 0\}\right],$$

where $P^*(i)$ is the probability that arm i has the highest regret. They developed a modified Thompson Sampling algorithm with an initial uniform exploration phase that achieves fairness regret of $\mathcal{O}((KT)^{2/3})$. Wang et al. (2021) also aim at fairness through awareness by comparing to the optimal fair policy π^*,

$$\frac{\pi^*(a)}{\pi^*(a')} = \frac{f(\mu_a)}{f(\mu_{a'})} \text{ for some metric function } f.$$

[5] Note that Liu et al. (2017) consider a general divergence function for the distribution of action selection and rewards, we introduce a special case here for a cleaner form.

They in turn target at the fairness regret, the cumulative L_0 norm of $\pi^* - \pi_t$. Other individual fairness definition that simply requires a minimum number of pulls for each arms is considered by Patil et al. (2020) and Chen et al. (2020).

Group fairness. For group fairness, one may divide arms into n groups $G_1, \ldots, G_n$. Schumann et al. (2019) proposed an algorithm ensuring that the probability of pulling an arm does not change based on group membership:

$$\mathrm{P}(\text{pull } a \mid a \in G_i) = \mathrm{P}(\text{pull } a \mid a \in G_j), \forall i, j < n \text{ and } a \in \mathcal{A}.$$

In other words, one cannot prefer one arm over the other one based on the group information.

Some literature treats each context c_t as an individual and aims at fairness among different contexts. (Huang et al., 2020) divides the context space into two groups, a privileged group G^+, and a protected group G^-. A group-level cumulative mean reward is defined as

$$\bar{R}^G = \frac{1}{|T_G|} \sum_{t \in T_G} R_t, \text{ where } T_G \text{ is the set of all rounds with } g_t \text{ in group } G.$$

Their group fairness requires that $|\mathbb{E}[\bar{R}^{G^+} - \bar{R}^{G^-}]| \leq \tau$, where $\tau \in \mathbb{R}^+$ reflects the tolerance degree of unfairness. Assuming a linear bandit setting, they proposed a Fair-LinUCB algorithm, that penalize the arms that are unfair by decreasing the corresponding UCB values.

Counterfactual fairness. Another line of work (Kusner et al., 2017) models fairness through causal inference. Their fairness definition is normally referred to as Counterfactual Fairness. In group fairness, we require the distributions of the value of interest to be the same across different demographic groups. However, what we really want is that the demographic group information does not cause unfairness, which can not be fully inferred from the group fairness definition. Counterfactual fairness, on the other hand, requires the distribution of the value of interest not to change when the demographic group is changed from one to the other while keeping all the other context variables unchanged.

General fairness metric. All the above methods require certain fairness definitions, it is natural to ask whether there is an universal algorithm that adapts to various fairness definitions. In real applications, we may not know the exact form of fairness metric. Instead, we may know whether certain policy violates fairness conditions. Instead of studying a specific fairness metric, Gillen et al. (2018) developed an algorithm that achieves fairness through a fairness oracle, which tells the algorithm whether fairness is violated. This also allows great flexibility in the choice of fairness metric. At each round, each arm $i \in [K]$ is given a context $C_{t,i} \in \mathbb{R}^d$. The probability of selecting action i at step t is denoted by $\pi_{t,i}$, which is a vector denoting the probability of selecting . We denote the vector of context (policy) at round t by c_t (π_t). The fairness oracle is defined as follows. Intuitively, it tells the algorithm, which pairs of actions violate the fairness metric.

Definition 4. Let $\Delta([K])$ be the set of all distributions over $[K]$. Given a user-specified distance function d, a fairness oracle O_d is a function $O_d : \mathbb{R}^{d \times K} \times \Delta([K]) \to 2^{[K] \times [K]}$, defined such that

$$O_d(c_t, \pi_t) = \{(i, j) : |\pi_{t,i} - \pi_{t,j}| > d(C_{t,i}, C_{t,j})\}.$$

They developed an algorithm that only has access to the fairness oracle. The algorithm has the number of fairness violations depending only logarithmically on T and a regret bound of the optimal rate $\mathcal{O}(\sqrt{T})$ with respect to the best fair policy.

13.3.5 Benefiting from Causal Knowledge

Causal bandit is an example of a structured bandit problem where actions are composed of interventions on variables of a causal graph. According to the underlying causal dynamics, performing an intervention can help learn another intervention's reward distribution. Algorithms for causal bandit problems exploit the causal dependency among interventions to reduce the regret or sample complexity.

Bareinboim et al. (2015) were the first to connect bandit problems with causal models. One of the main issues that make causal inference hard is the existence of confounders defined below, which can confuse correlation and causation. Bareinboim et al. (2015) pointed out the importance of capturing the confounders before actually performing actions. In particular, they proposed a new criterion for choosing actions called the regret decision criterion (RDC). Under the RDC rule, the agent collects her *intention* (includes information on confounders) on selecting actions and re-thinks based on the estimated reward statistics for the current *intention* and then decides which action to play. Since the actual selected action can be different than the agent's *intention*, the agent decides in a counterfactual way.

Definition 5 (Confounder). A confounder is a variable that influences both the dependent variable and independent variable.

Later on, Lattimore et al. (2016) formally proposed the causal bandit framework via causal graphs. A causal model consists of a directed acyclic graph G over a set of random variables $\mathcal{V} = \{V_1, \ldots, V_n\}$ and a joint distribution P that factorizes over G. A size m hard intervention (action) is denoted by $\mathrm{do}(\mathbf{V} = \mathbf{v})$, which assigns the values $\mathbf{v} = \{v_1, \ldots, v_m\} \subset \mathcal{V}$ to the corresponding variables $\mathbf{V} = \{V_1, \ldots, V_m\}$. In causal bandits, the action set is defined as

$$\mathcal{A} := \{\mathrm{do}(\mathbf{V} = \mathbf{v}) | \mathbf{V} \subset \mathcal{V}, \mathbf{v} \in \mathrm{Dom}(\mathbf{V})\},$$

or its subset and the optimal intervention is $a^* := \arg\max_{a \in \mathcal{A}} \mathbb{E}[R|a]$.

Many practical problems can be modeled via above framework. For example, in healthcare applications, the physician adjusts several features such as dose levels on different medicines or life-style advice to achieve some desirable clinical outcomes (Liu et al., 2020). Genetic engineering also involves direct manipulation of genes using biotechnology to produce improved organisms. In these problems, the number of interventions can be exponentially large in the number of manipulable variables so that standard MAB algorithms cannot work efficiently. To address this issue, recent work on causal bandits has developed methods that exploit causal information to achieve simple or cumulative regret that does not scale with the number of interventions (Lattimore et al., 2016; Sen et al., 2017; Lee and Bareinboim, 2018; Lu et al., 2020, 2021a). We summarize existing methodologies below.

Refining the Policy Space. Assuming the causal graph is known (confounders may also exist), Lee and Bareinboim (2018) proposed an intervention set reduction algorithm. They showed that not all interventions are worthwhile to be played because there are equivalences among interventions and some interventions can be proved to be no better than others. Their algorithm filters out redundant interventions using the causal graph structure before applying any standard MAB algorithm on the reduced intervention set, also called *possibly-optimal minimal intervention set* (POMIS). Since the size of POMIS is usually much smaller than $|\mathcal{A}|$, the corresponding regret can be reduced. Follow-up work in Lee and Bareinboim (2019) further showed that the expected reward for interventions in a POMIS can be estimated from each other in certain cases. Their method also works well when some variables are non-manipulable. We remark that the step of finding the POMIS solely relies on the given causal graph structure and does not involve performing any intervention.

Accelerating Using Causal Graph Side Information in Standard MAB Algorithms. Recall that a key step in bandit algorithm is estimating the expected reward for each arm $\hat{\mu}_a$.

Intuitively speaking, one needs to play each arm for enough number of times in order to get accurate estimations if interventions are independent. But in causal bandits, interventions are correlated with each other so that performing one intervention can help with estimating others according to the shared causal model. Lattimore et al. (2016) studied the best arm identification problem via importance weighting. Their algorithm achieves simple regret $O(\sqrt{m/T})$, where m can be smaller than $|\mathcal{A}|$ in many scenarios. Sen et al. (2017) further generalized the algorithm in Lattimore et al. (2016) to a soft intervention setting and proved gap-dependent regret guarantees. In soft interventions, the agent does not directly set values to specific variables, but instead change their conditional probabilities given their direct parents. Lu et al. (2020) proposed causal UCB and causal TS algorithms that achieve $\tilde{O}(\sqrt{ZT})$ cumulative regret, where Z is a graph-dependent number and can be exponentially smaller than $|\mathcal{A}|$. A causal linear bandit framework and its efficient algorithms were also well studied. Furthermore, gap-dependent worst-case regret bound and a budgeted causal bandit setting were also considered in follow-up works (Nair et al., 2021).

13.3.6 Multi-task Learning

Multitask learning is the learning paradigm in machine learning that aims at leveraging information in multiple tasks to achieve a better sample efficiency by solving them jointly rather than separately (Zhang and Yang, 2021). Multitask learning algorithms usually assume some similarity between tasks that allows information sharing. In the context of multitask bandit, each bandit is called a task and various similarity assumptions on the reward distribution can be made. This can model many interesting scenarios. For instance, a group of patients with the same disease can be seen as multiple tasks. We can not directly use the same policy, as a personalized treatment should be applied to each patient. However, some patients' responses may be similar to the others such that one can transfer the information across patients. Recall that we use $\nu = (P_a, a \in \mathcal{A})$ to denote a bandit instance. A general multitask bandit framework can be summarized below:

$$\begin{aligned}&\text{Given a set of bandits } \nu_1, \ldots, \nu_n,\ \text{Discrepancy}(\nu_i, \nu_j)\\ &\text{is small for some } i, j \in [n],\end{aligned}$$

for some discrepancy measure on bandit instances.

In this subsection, we will review some interesting works on multitask bandit and compare their assumptions on discrepancy and the corresponding regret bounds. We will also cover the potential applications of multitask bandits.

Parametric Model. Early work on multitask bandit was done by Cesa-Bianchi et al. (2013) who considered a gang of contextual bandits connected with a graph $\{V, E\}$, where $V = \{1, \ldots, n\}$ is the node set and E is the edge set. Each node i is assumed to be a linear bandit with rewards generated by $R_i(c) = \theta_i^T c + \epsilon_i(c)$ given a context c, where $\epsilon_i(c)$ is a conditionally zero-mean noise. Any two nodes that are adjacent on the graph have low discrepancy compared to the total scale: $\sum_{i \in V} \|\theta_i\|^2 \gg \sum_{(i,j) \in E} \|\theta_i - \theta_j\|^2$. Their discrepancy measure is simply the L_2 distance on the unknown parameters. However, their analysis only shows a benefit of a factor n in the logarithmic term. In the literature of supervised multitask learning, the benefit could be a factor of $n^{1/2}$ outside the logarithmic term (Maurer et al., 2016). Another property makes it hard for their algorithm to generalize to other settings is that the discrepancy information on tasks similarities is partially known to the agent through the graph structure. Generally speaking, the agent does not know which tasks are similar and has to adaptively learn the information.

As an improvement, Gentile et al. (2014); Li et al. (2016) consider an *unknown* graph with a clustered structure, and all the bandits within the same cluster share a common reward distribution, which is also from a linear model. The algorithm is to simply cluster the bandits based on the feedback and pool the data from all the bandits from the same cluster. Instead of having a dependency of n as for the baseline algorithm that learns all the bandit separately, their regret is $\tilde{\mathcal{O}}(dm\sqrt{T})$, where $m \ll n$ is the number of clusters.

Non-parametric Model. Despite the encouraging results by Gentile et al. (2014); Li et al. (2016), the clustered structure and linear payoffs are strong assumptions. Deshmukh et al. (2017) proposed a kernel regression model that allows general similarities. Formally, they assume the reward is generated by mean function $f : \mathcal{Z} \times \mathcal{C} \mapsto \mathbb{R}$, where $\mathcal{Z}$ is called the task similarity space, $\mathcal{C}$ is the context from the context space $\mathcal{C}$. Let $\tilde{k}$ be a SPD (semi-positive definite) kernel on $\mathcal{Z} \times \mathcal{C}$ with the form

$$\tilde{k}\left((z, c), (z', c')\right) = k_{\mathcal{Z}}\left(z, z'\right) k_{\mathcal{C}}\left(c, c'\right),$$

where $k_{\mathcal{Z}}$ and $k_{\mathcal{C}}$ are SPD kernels on $\mathcal{Z} = \{1, \ldots, n\}$ representing n tasks and $\mathcal{C}$. They assume that f is from the RKHS, $\mathcal{H}_{\tilde{k}}$ corresponding to $\tilde{k}$. Kernel $k_{\mathcal{Z}}$ characterized the similarity between different bandits, for instance:

1. Independent: $k_{\mathcal{Z}}(z, z') = \mathbb{1}_{z=z'}$, i.e. observations from different tasks are not sharing any information.
2. Pooled: $k_{\mathcal{Z}} \equiv 1$, i.e all the observations from different tasks are treated the same.
3. Multi-task: $k_{\mathcal{Z}}$ is a PDS matrix reflecting task similarity.

Their algorithm **KMTL-UCB** gives a regret bound of $\tilde{\mathcal{O}}(\sqrt{Tr_z r_c})$, where r_z is the rank of the $n \times n$ matrix $K_Z = \left[k_{\mathcal{Z}}\left(z_i, z_i\right)\right]_{i=1}^{n}$ and r_c is the rank of $K_{C_T} := \left[k_{\mathcal{C}}(c_{a_t,t}, c_{a_{t'},t'})\right]_{t,t'=1}^{T}$. To compare, the regular regret bound of learning one task independently is $\tilde{\mathcal{O}}(\sqrt{Tr_c})$ and learning all tasks independently gives $\tilde{\mathcal{O}}(n\sqrt{Tr_c})$. The scaling of r_z determines the benefits of multitask learning: $r_z = n$ corresponds to the first case above with $k_{\mathcal{Z}}(z, z') = \mathbb{1}_{z=z'}$ and $r_z = 1$ corresponds to the second case with $k_{\mathcal{Z}} \equiv 1$. Though Deshmukh et al. (2017) gives a general way to characterize the multitask bandit benefits, their algorithm still relies on the knowledge of the similarity kernel $k_{\mathcal{Z}}$. In practice, one can learn a kernel, but little theory has been established to justify this practice.

Adaptive Learning. Tomkins et al. (2021) proposed Intelligent Pooling, a generalization of a Thompson sampling contextual bandit for learning personalized treatment policies. They assume the reward for user $i \in [n]$ is generated by

$$R_i = \phi(C_i, A_i)^T \theta_i + \epsilon_i,$$

where $\phi : \mathcal{C} \times \mathcal{A} \mapsto \mathbb{R}^d$ is the pre-specified mapping from contexts and actions and $\theta_i \in \mathbb{R}^d$ is the personalized parameter to learn. IntelligentPooling imposes each w_i as a random-effects upon a population-level parameter w_{pop}, i.e. $w_i = w_{pop} + u_i$ with u_i the Gaussian random effect. Prior distribution of w_{pop} is also assumed to be Gaussian. IntelligentPooling runs by sampling $w_{i,t}$ from the posterior distribution of w_i. The algorithm uses random effects to adaptively pool users' data based on the degree to which users exhibit heterogeneous rewards that is away from the population behavior (w_{pop}). They showed a regret bound of $\tilde{\mathcal{O}}(dn\sqrt{T})$.

13.4 Conclusion

We reviewed basic topics in bandit algorithms that are helpful in understanding their increasing role in mobile health, and more broadly, precision medicine. We also discussed a selection of advanced topics that might inform the design of the next generation of bandit-driven mobile health applications. We hope that the reader has gained an appreciation of the beauty and power of bandit algorithms and of their relevance to mobile health and precision medicine. However, like any methodology, bandit algorithms do have their limitations. First, bandit algorithms assume that an appropriate reward is available upfront. In practice, especially in healthcare applications, the design of rewards to be optimized is a difficult problem with no easy solution. The issues involved in specified a reward function that is aligned with the goals of various human stakeholders have been brought into focus more recently under the term "the alignment problem" (Christian, 2020). Second, bandit algorithms do not take into account the delayed impacts of the agent's actions. When actions have delayed impacts, it might be beneficial to take an action with low immediate reward if it increases the probability of higher rewards later on. The full treatment of this problem of delayed impact of actions requires techniques from reinforcement learning (Sutton and Barto, 2018). In fact, bandit problems can be thought of as the simplest of reinforcement learning problems.

Part III

Precision Medicine in High Dimensions

Chapter 14

Tailoring Variable Selection and Ranking for Optimal Treatment Decisions

Zeyu Bian, Erica E.M. Moodie, Susan M. Shortreed, Sylvie Lambert, Sahir Bhatnagar

14.1 Introduction

Regression-based methods and value search methods (policy search or classification-based approaches) are two popular estimation approaches in the field of dynamic treatment regimes (DTRs). Consider, for instance, the one-interval setting of an individualized treatment rule (ITR). In regression-based methods such as A-learning (Robins, 2004; Murphy, 2003) and Q-learning (Watkins, 1989), the expected mean outcome model is decomposed into the baseline mean model and the blip function (throughout this paper, we denote observed variables with lower case and their random counterparts with uppercase):

$$\mathbb{E}\left[Y^*(a)|X=x;\beta,\psi\right] = \underbrace{\mu\left(x;\beta\right)}_{\text{baseline mean model}} + \underbrace{c\left(x,a;\psi\right)}_{\text{blip function}},$$

where Y is the observed outcome, $Y^*(a)$ is the potential outcome under the binary treatment a, x represents baseline covariates, μ is the baseline mean model with parameter β, which is irrelevant for making optimal treatment decisions (i.e., it can be considered a nuisance parameter), and c is the blip function with parameter ψ. The blip function (or contrast function) is defined as the difference in expected potential outcome between a population of patients when treated with a and that same population of patients when treated with a reference treatment, $a = 0$, modeled as a function of some covariates x: $c(x,a) = \mathbb{E}\left[Y^*(a) - Y^*(0)|X=x\right]$. Since μ does not involve the treatment variable and hence will not affect treatment decisions, ψ is the parameter of interest, and, given an estimator $\widehat{\psi}$ of ψ, the estimated optimal decision rule is given by $\widehat{a}^{opt} = \arg\max_a c\left(x,a;\widehat{\psi}\right)$. For example, if the blip function is assumed to be linear, say $c(x,a;\psi) = a(\psi_0 + \sum_{j=1}^{p}\psi_j x_j)$, then the estimated optimal treatment rule is $\widehat{a}^{opt} = I(\widehat{\psi}_0 + \sum_{j=1}^{p}\widehat{\psi}_j x_j > 0)$, where $I(\cdot)$ is the indicator function.

In contrast, value search methods specify a class of candidate regimes, and for each regime in the class estimate its value function (marginal mean outcome under the regime). The estimated optimal treatment regime is then chosen to be that which maximizes the estimated value function. Some examples of value search methods include dynamic marginal structural models (Orellana et al., 2010; van der Laan and Petersen, 2007), outcome weighted learning (Zhao et al., 2012), residual weighted learning (Zhou et al., 2017), and the inverse probability weighted estimator proposed in (Zhang et al., 2012). Given a class of decision rules, $\{d(x;\xi) : \xi \in \mathcal{E}\}$, let $V(\xi)$ denote the value function of the rule $d(x;\xi)$. The value function $V(\xi)$ can be modelled as a function of ξ non-parametrically, semi-parametrically, e.g., via restricted cubic splines (Cain et al., 2010), or parametrically, e.g., via a quadratic function (van der Laan and Petersen, 2007; Shortreed and Moodie, 2012). The optimal

DOI: 10.1201/9781003216223-14

treatment regime $\widehat{d}^{opt}(x; \widehat{\xi}^{opt})$ and the estimator $\widehat{\xi}^{opt}$ are selected such that the corresponding estimated value $\widehat{V}(\widehat{\xi}^{opt})$ is maximized.

However, in the current era of high computer memory and computational power, more and more patient information is collected in medical studies and electronic health records. This recording of many covariates brings challenges for the analytic approaches described above. First, the existing methods often suffer from the curse of dimensionality. For example, regression-based methods fail in the case where the number of variables exceeds the sample size ($p > n$). Second, even in the $n > p$ setting, in the presence of many covariates, it is difficult to know which prognostic factors are relevant for selecting an optimal treatment. Including all covariates in the analytic model can result in a loss of statistical efficiency and needlessly complex treatment decisions. Thus, applying variable selection to precision medicine becomes critical as the number of available covariates increases, since this can improve the treatment decision rules and simplify models to enhance interpretability and ease of implementation in clinical practice.

In this Chapter, we review a penalization approach to variable selection embedded within a regression-based method to ITR estimation–penalized dynamic weighted ordinary least squares (pdWOLS, Bian et al., 2021) and a variable ranking method (Wu et al., 2021) which ranks tailoring variables according to the estimated value function associated with an ITR based on each variable alone. A confounder selection method, outcome adaptive lasso (Shortreed and Ertefaie, 2017), will be incorporated into the implementation of pdWOLS. The rest of this chapter is organized as follows. In Section 14.2, we provide background on commonly used estimation, variable selection, and ranking methods for DTRs. We present the extension of dynamic weighted ordinary least squares (dWOLS) to its penalized counterpart, pdWOLS, in Section 14.3. We then provide some numerical results in the form of a simulation study in Section 14.4 and a case study in Section 14.5, applying tailoring variable selection to a pilot sequential multiple assignment randomized trial (SMART) of a web-based stress management approach.

14.2 Background

In Section 14.2.1, we first briefly review two regression-based methods and a value search method, then in Sections 14.2.2 and 14.2.3 we discuss how to select and rank the tailoring variables based on these methods.

14.2.1 Some Estimation Methods for DTRs

14.2.1.1 A-Learning

We begin this Section with a regression-based method A-learning (or G-estimation) (Robins, 2004; Murphy, 2003), a method which is doubly robust. That is, the approach yields consistent estimators of ψ while only requiring one of two nuisance models, either the baseline mean model $\mu(x; \beta)$ or the propensity score model $P(A = 1|X = x; \alpha) = \pi(x; \alpha)$, to be correctly specified. The blip parameter can be obtained by solving the following A-learning estimating equation:

$$n^{-1}X^T \text{diag}(A - \widehat{\pi})(Y - \mu(X; \widehat{\beta}) - c(X, a; \psi)) = 0,$$

where the plug-in estimators $\widehat{\pi}$ and $\mu(X; \widehat{\beta})$ can be estimated using (generalized) linear regression or other machine learning approaches, and α parameterizes the treatment model. When π or μ is correctly specified,

$$\begin{aligned} &\mathbb{E}\{\text{diag}(A - \pi)X^T(Y - \mu(X; \beta) - c(X, a; \psi))\} \\ &= \mathbb{E}_X \mathbb{E}\{\text{diag}(A - \pi)X^T(Y - \mu(X; \beta) - c(X, a; \psi))|X\} = 0, \end{aligned}$$

hence ψ is consistently estimated, under the assumption that the blip model is correctly specified.

While A-learning's robustness against model misspecification is appealing, its implementation can be somewhat complex. In the next subsection, we introduce a method offering easier implementation, while retaining the the double robustness property.

14.2.1.2 Dynamic Weighted Ordinary Least Squares

Dynamic weighted ordinary least squares (dWOLS) employs a weighted regression approach (Wallace and Moodie, 2015). If we assume that the blip function is correctly specified, the stable unit treatment value assumption (Rubin, 1980), and ignorability (Robins, 1997) assumptions hold, and the main effects for all covariates in the blip model are included in the baseline mean model, then the resulting blip parameter estimators of dWOLS are consistent if either the treatment model or the baseline mean model is correct, and so dWOLS enjoys the attractive double robustness property. The requirement that the baseline mean model include the main effects for covariates in the blip model is essential for dWOLS to consistently estimate ψ, unlike A-learning which imposes no restrictions on the nuisance model and can even simply assume an intercept-only baseline mean model.

Consider the following model with both a linear baseline mean model and linear blip function

$$Y = \psi_0 A + \sum_{j=1}^{p} X_j\beta_j + \sum_{j=1}^{p} \psi_j(A \circ X_j) + \varepsilon,$$

where $Y \in \mathbb{R}^n$ is a continuous response; A is the binary treatment; $X_j \in \mathbb{R}^n$ are the j-th covariates; $\beta_j \in \mathbb{R}$ are the corresponding parameters for the main effects of covariates; $\psi_j \in \mathbb{R}$ are the blip parameters for $j = 0, 1, \ldots, p$, "$\circ$" is the element-wise vector multiplication, and $\varepsilon \in \mathbb{R}^n$ is a vector of independent error terms, each with mean zero and finite variance. Estimation for dWOLS is accomplished using the weighted squared-error loss:

$$\mathcal{L}(Y;\theta) = \frac{1}{2n}\|\sqrt{W}(Y - \psi_0 A - \sum_{j=1}^{p} X_j\beta_j - \sum_{j=1}^{p} \psi_j(A \circ X_j))\|_2^2, \tag{14.1}$$

where $\theta = (\beta_1, \ldots, \beta_p, \psi_0, \ldots, \psi_p)$, and $W = \text{diag}(w_1(a, x), \ldots, w_n(a, x))$ is an $n \times n$ diagonal matrix of *balancing weights* used to address confounding (see below).

We now discuss the double robustness property of dWOLS. Consider the scenario that the propensity score is correctly specified, thus the weights are all consistently estimated. In this case, estimating the blip parameters from model $\mu(x;\beta) + \psi_0 a + a\psi^T x$ is equivalent to estimate the causal effect from a conditional structural model $\mathbb{E}(Y^*(a)) = \widetilde{\beta}^T x + \psi_0 a + a\psi^T x$ where $\widetilde{\beta}$ is the coefficient of the baseline covariates in the structural model (not necessarily identical to the underlying true parameter β^*). Wallace and Moodie (2015) showed that a weighted least square estimator of model $\widetilde{\beta}^T x + a\psi^T x$ with weights satisfied $\pi(x)w(1, x) = (1 - \pi(x))w(0, x)$ yield consistent estimators of the blip parameters ψ.

Now assuming that the baseline mean model is correct and the estimated weights converge to $\widetilde{w}$, dWOLS yields $\widehat{\theta} = (\widehat{\beta}, \widehat{\psi}) = \left(\phi(x, a)^T \widetilde{w} \phi(x, a)\right)^{-1} \phi(x, a)^T \widetilde{w} y$, where ϕ is the Jacobian matrix of the design matrix $\Phi(x, a)$. Let $\theta^* = (\beta^*, \psi^*)^T$, where θ^* is the true parameter of the model; by some simple algebra, it can be shown that $\mathbb{E}(\widehat{\theta}) = \theta^*$. Moreover, we have $Var(\widehat{\theta}) = \sigma^2 C \left(\phi(x, a)^T \widetilde{w}^{-1} w^* \widetilde{w}^{-1} \phi(x, a)\right)^{-1} C$ which is $O(n^{-1})$ under mild conditions, where $C = \left(\phi(x, a)^T \widetilde{w}^{-1} \phi(x, a)\right)^{-1}$. Hence, $P(|\widehat{\theta} - \theta^*| > \epsilon) \to 0$ and thus the blip parameters ψ are consistently estimated.

The choice of weights for dWOLS is an open but intriguing problem. Wallace and Moodie (2015) proposed to use the weights, $w(a, X) = |a - \mathbb{E}[A|X = x]|$, as they empirically found these to offer better efficiency than other alternatives such as inverse probability weights.

14.2.1.3 A Simple Value Search Method

We conclude this subsection by introducing a value search method that can be employed in settings where the decision rule is a simple threshold rule: for a tailoring variable X_j, we aim to find the optimal threshold value η_j^{opt} such that the decision rule is of the form $\widehat{a}^{opt} = I(X_j < \eta_j^{opt})$ or $I(X_j > \eta_j^{opt})$. In such value search methods, constructing an augmented data set is often a critical step in the estimation procedure. The augmented data set is created such that for each treatment regime $d(x;\xi)$ in the set of candidate regimes $\mathcal{A}$, and each observation i is repeated. If individual i's observed treatment a_i equals the recommended treatment under $d(x_i;\xi)$, then subject i's information is copied into the augmented data set, which also contains an extra column which represents the value of ξ. Once the augmented data set is created, it is used to model the value function $V(\xi)$ as a function of ξ. The optimal treatment regime $\widehat{d}^{opt}(x;\widehat{\xi}^{opt})$ and the estimator $\widehat{\xi}^{opt}$ are selected such that the corresponding value $\widehat{V}(\widehat{\xi}^{opt})$ is maximized. In this chapter, we only consider decision rules of the type, $\widehat{a}^{opt} = I(X_j < \eta_j^{opt})$ for convenience. Considering both directions does not involve any extra difficulty, and should be done in real data settings whenever there is any uncertainty about the direction of the threshold rule. In Section 14.2.3, we give a more detailed description of how to rank the tailoring variables based on this framework.

14.2.2 Review of Tailoring Variable Selection Techniques

Among the earliest work on selecting tailoring variables in the context of a regression-based method for DTR estimation, Lu et al. (2013) adopted an adaptive LASSO (Zou, 2006) approach within the A-learning framework. These authors thus adopted a method that allowed the misspecification of the baseline mean model μ, but only considered a randomized design in which the propensity score is correctly specified and the number of predictors p is fixed. Lu et al. (2013) proposed that the blip parameter vector be estimated by minimizing the objective function

$$n^{-1}\|Y - \mu(X;\widehat{\beta}) - \text{diag}(A - \widehat{\pi})X\psi\|_2^2 + \lambda_n \sum_{j=1}^{p} \rho(|\psi_j|),$$

where λ_n is a tuning parameter and $\rho(|\cdot|)$ is a penalty function. To see how this approach allows the misspecification of the baseline mean model μ, take the derivative of the loss function (the first term in the above equation) with respect to ψ and set it to zero to obtain

$$X^T\text{diag}(A - \widehat{\pi})\{Y - \mu(X;\widehat{\beta}) - \text{diag}(A - \widehat{\pi})X\psi\} = 0,$$

which is an unbiased estimating equation under the assumption that the posited propensity score model is correct. Hence, with a suitable choice of tuning parameter, the blip parameter estimators are approximately unbiased in the penalized framework.

Jeng et al. (2018) extended the work of Lu et al. (2013) to the case where p is allowed to grow with the sample size n using debiased LASSO (Zhang and Zhang, 2014), and Shi et al. (2016) generalized it to the situation where p is of non-polynomial order in n, i.e., $log\, p = O(n^b)$ for some $b < 1$.

Bian et al. (2021) proposed penalized dynamic weighted ordinary least squares (pdWOLS), a doubly robust method which can conduct estimation and selection of the tailoring variables simultaneously; we will review this method in detail in Section 14.3.

In singly-robust settings, Song et al. (2015a) added the smoothly clipped absolute deviation (SCAD, Fan and Li, 2001) penalty to the value search method of outcome weighted learning to incorporate sparsity and estimate the optimal treatment decision, where the treatment rule can be viewed as a classification problem. Zhu et al. (2019) combined Q-learning with SCAD penalty to select the important tailoring variables and conducted the hard-thresholding method proposed in Moodie and Richardson (2010) to tackle the challenge of nonregularity.

With the exception of the outcome weighted learning approach, the loss functions of the methods described above were all likelihood-based. In contrast to these methods, Shi et al. (2018) used the Dantzig selector (Candes and Tao, 2007) to directly penalize the estimating equations of A-learning instead of penalizing the likelihood: $\widehat{\psi} = \text{argmin}_{\psi} \|\psi\|_1$, subject to $\|X^T \text{diag}(A - \widehat{\pi})\{Y - \mu(X; \widehat{\beta}) - c(X, a; \psi)\}\|_\infty \leq n\lambda_{pal}$ where λ_{pal} is the tuning parameter. In this way, the double robustness property of A-learning was inherited, and sparsity can also be introduced to the model through the use of the Dantzig selector.

All the variable selection methods outlined above are designed for use in DTR estimation. The differences between these approaches and the variable selection methods in the prediction setting are twofold. First, the goal differs: variable selection for DTRs aims to improve the estimated decision rules rather than enhance the predictive power of the outcome (of course, both emphasize the interpretability of the model). Second, in DTRs, interest is primarily in effect modification, and hence the selection tends to be focused on the terms in the blip model. In contrast, variable selection approaches in the prediction setting usually seek to choose from among all variables with no special status given to effect modifiers.

14.2.3 Tailoring Variable Ranking

Ranking variables can be viewed as an indirect method of choosing among covariates, or selecting among several potentially useful tailoring variables to focus on a simpler, low-dimensional treatment rule. The earliest work in this domain is that of Gunter et al. (2011), who proposed a score-based method that can rank the tailoring variables based on the expected increase of the estimated value due to the inclusion of a variable, calling this the "S-score." This approach was primarily used to rank each potential tailoring variable individually, but was also extended to account for multiple tailoring variables in an iterative variable selection process. Fan et al. (2016) extended this work to take into account variables already in the model and determine whether to include a new variable by the additional improvement of the score.

Wu et al. (2021) considered ranking variables for their tailoring ability in single-variable decision rules of the form $a^{opt}(X_j) = I(X_j < \eta_j^{opt})$ or $I(X_j > \eta_j^{opt})$. They used linear splines to flexibly model the value function and potential tailoring variables were then ranked according to their estimated value. The approach considers the effect of each variable individually, focusing on simple and interpretable rules. While the approach could, in principle, be used repeatedly to consider a "value added" rank (e.g., select the most useful variable, then rank the remaining variables to see which–if any–improve the value in a two-variable rule, and so on), however this has not yet been explored numerically. We now give a brief overview of variable ranking approach in Wu et al. (2021).

Instead of modeling the relationship between the outcome and covariates, Wu et al. (2021) model the value function $V(\eta_j) = m(\eta_j; \nu)$, where $m(\cdot)$ is some function with parameter ν. We omit the subscript j from here for notational convenience when there is no confusion. Recall from Section 14.2.1.3, that value search estimators often rely on the construction of an augmented data set. Denote by N the number of rows in the augmented data, and by r the number of threshold candidate. Wu et al. (2021) used linear splines to flexibly model $V(\eta)$, with each candidate for η in the augmented data chosen as a potential knot. They employed penalization to shrink some of the coefficients to zero so that only the important thresholds (knots) were selected.

For a potential tailoring variable with the candidate threshold sequence $(\eta^1, \ldots, \eta^r)$, the coefficients were obtained by minimizing the following function:

$$\sum_{l=1}^{N} w_l \{Y_l - \nu_0 - \nu' \eta^l - \sum_{s=1}^{r} \nu_s (\eta^l - \eta^s)_+\}^2 + \sum_{s=1}^{r} \lambda_s |\nu_s|,$$

where w_l is the corresponding inverse probability of treatment weight for l-th observations), ν_0 is the intercept, ν' is the coefficient of η, ν_s is the coefficient of the s-th knot, and λ_s is a tuning parameter (which need not be the same for all s). After variable selection, the coefficients are re-calculated by solving the unpenalized weighted least squares with the selected variables. Then we could use inverse probability weighting to estimate the value function of a particular regime $I(X < \eta^s)$: $\widehat{V}(\eta^s) = \frac{\sum_{l=1}^{N} I(\eta^l = \eta^s) \widehat{Y}_l w_l}{\sum_{l=1}^{N} I(\eta^l = \eta^s) w_l}$, where $\widehat{Y}_l$ is the fitted outcome from the linear spline model. The optimal threshold η^{opt} is chosen such that $\widehat{V}(\eta^{opt}) = max_{1 \le s \le r} \widehat{V}(\eta^s)$. This procedure is carried out for each potential tailoring variable, and we rank all the variables by their fitted optimal value function $\widehat{V}(\eta_j^{opt})$ for $j = 1, \ldots p$. A limitation of this ranking method is that it only considers a single variable at a time.

As we shall detail in the next section, we posit that the penalized method outlined in Section 14.2.2 can also be used to rank the tailoring variables. This could be accomplished in a variety of ways. For example, we could rank them by the magnitude of the absolute value of the coefficient, or by the selected frequency among a sequence of tuning parameters. In the simulation studies, we will show how to rank the tailoring variables using the latter strategy.

14.3 Variable Selection and Ranking in DTRs

In this section, we review the tailoring variable selection method penalized dynamic weighted ordinary least squares, based on the dWOLS approach discussed in Section 14.2.1.2. We then discuss how to incorporate *confounder* selection into pdWOLS, and conclude this section with a proposal for using pdWOLS as a means of ranking variables in terms of their utility for tailoring.

14.3.1 Penalized Dynamic Weighted Ordinary Least Squares

We can extend dWOLS to penalized estimation for variable selection and estimating the optimal treatment regimes simultaneously (Bian et al., 2021). One can consider the following objective function that includes the ℓ_1 penalty for variable selection:

$$Q(\theta) = \mathcal{L}(Y; \theta) + \lambda(1 - \delta)(\|\beta\|_1 + |\psi_0|) + \lambda\delta\|\psi\|_1, \tag{14.2}$$

where $\mathcal{L}(Y; \theta)$ is the dWOLS loss function shown in equation (14.1), $\beta = (\beta_1, \ldots, \beta_p)$, $\psi = (\psi_1, \ldots, \psi_p)$, and $\lambda > 0$, $\delta \in (0, 1)$ are tuning parameters. In a slightly similar manner to elastic net regularization (Zou and Hastie, 2005), δ controls the relative penalties between the main effects and the interaction effects; for example, a δ that is less than 0.5 would tend to penalize the main effects more than the interaction effects. However, there is an issue with (14.2) in its current form. Recall that an important assumption required by dWOLS is that the baseline mean model includes the main effects for all covariates in the blip function. In a penalized model such as equation (14.2), this assumption can be violated, e.g., it is possible that an estimated interaction term is nonzero while the corresponding main effects are shrunk to zero by the penalization. This can lead to a bias induced by the violation of dWOLS assumptions (rather than bias induced by the penalization itself).

To remedy this, pdWOLS adds a constraint to (14.2), requiring the *strong heredity assumption* in the penalized model: an interaction term can be estimated to be non-zero if and only if its corresponding main effects are estimated to be non-zero, whereas a non-zero main effect does not necessarily imply a non-zero interaction term. This can be achieved by introducing a new set of parameters $\tau = (\tau_1, \tau_2, \ldots, \tau_p)$ and reparametrizing the coefficients for the interaction terms ψ_j as the product of τ_j, β_j and ψ_0 such that $\psi_j = \psi_0 \tau_j \beta_j$. In this way, strong heredity is assured and the following model is considered instead:

$$\mathcal{L}^*(Y;\theta) = \frac{1}{2n} \| \sqrt{W} \left(Y - \psi_0 A - \sum_{j=1}^{p} X_j \beta_j - \sum_{j=1}^{p} \underbrace{\psi_0 \tau_j \beta_j}_{\psi_j} (A \circ X_j) \right) \|_2^2,$$

where now the objective function is:

$$Q(\theta) = \mathcal{L}^*(Y;\theta) + \lambda(1-\delta)(\|\beta\|_1 + |\psi_0|) + \lambda\delta\|\tau\|_1. \quad (14.3)$$

It has been shown that pdWOLS inherits the double robustness property from dWOLS; the method relies on a model that includes adaptive weights, an efficient algorithm using cyclic coordinate descent to minimize Equation (14.3), and can be generalized from the one-stage setting to a multi-stage setting (Bian et al., 2021). Here we emphasize that pdWOLS is based on prediction: the solution to the estimating equation is solved by minimizing the objective function, and thus the method will select any variables that can improve the predictive ability of the model. In this way, pdWOLS may underestimate important tailoring variables that have small predictive ability.

14.3.2 Incorporating Confounder Selection into pdWOLS

Here we introduce a variable selection method for confounders in the propensity score model, called outcome-adaptive LASSO, which was proposed by Shortreed and Ertefaie (2017). This method considers both the treatment-covariate relationship and the outcome-covariates association, and hence avoids prioritizing possibly instrumental variables. The key to the approach is to apply data-adaptive weights to a penalized propensity score model, where the adaptive weights are estimates from a fit of an unpenalized outcome model. For example, we could posit a logit model $\pi(x;\alpha)$ for the propensity score, and $\widehat{\alpha}$ is obtained by solving the adaptive penalized logistic regression:

$$\widehat{\alpha}_{oal} = n^{-1} \sum_{i=1}^{n} \{log(1 + x_i^T \alpha) - A_i x_i^T \alpha\} + \lambda_{oal} \sum_{j=1}^{p} \widetilde{w}_j \alpha_j,$$

where λ_{oal} is the tuning parameter, $\widetilde{w}_j = |\widehat{\beta}_j|^{-q}$ for some $q > 0$, and $\widehat{\beta}$ is the estimated parameter of the baseline mean model $\mu(x;\beta)$. Shortreed and Ertefaie (2017) proposed to select the tuning parameter λ_{oal} such that the weighted absolute mean difference between the exposure groups

$$\sum_{j=1}^{p} |\widehat{\beta}_j| \left| \frac{\sum_{i=1}^{n} \widehat{\zeta}_i X_{ij} A_i}{\sum_{i=1}^{n} \widehat{\zeta}_i A_i} - \frac{\sum_{i=1}^{n} \widehat{\zeta}_i X_{ij}(1-A_i)}{\sum_{i=1}^{n} \widehat{\zeta}_i (1-A_i)} \right|$$

is minimized, where $\widehat{\zeta}_i = A_i \widehat{\pi}(X_i;\widehat{\alpha}_{oal})^{-1} + (1-A_i)(1-\widehat{\pi}(X_i;\widehat{\alpha}_{oal}))^{-1}$. This approach to confounder selection for inclusion in the propensity score can be incorporated into pdWOLS in a straightforward manner.

14.3.3 Tailoring Variables Ranking Using pdWOLS

As mentioned in Section 14.2.3, we could rank the tailoring variables by the selected frequency among a sequence of tuning parameters $\lambda_1, \ldots, \lambda_k$, using pdWOLS, as the solution is calculated over this sequence, we have k different solutions in total. For each variable X_j, the selected frequency is calculated as $\sum_{t=1}^{k} I(\widehat{\psi}_{jt} \neq 0)/k$, and we can rank the tailoring variables accordingly.

With these new additions (confounder selection and variable ranking) to the pdWOLS approach, the method can be made even more parsimonious while offering additional insights into the importance of the tailoring variables when used jointly in a multivariate linear decision rule.

14.4 Numerical Studies

We now evaluate the performance of pdWOLS using two different tuning parameter selection approaches for the variable selection rate, and the resulting error rate in the estimated treatment decision as well as the value function of the estimated decision rules. We also demonstrate its use as a method of ranking tailoring variables. All simulations use sample sizes of 200 and 500. Further, we consider pdWOLS both with and without the use of confounder selection in the propensity score.

Step 1: Generate 10 covariates, $X_1, \ldots, X_{10}$, where X_1 and X_{10} are Bernoulli random variables which take the value 1 with probability 0.5, and $X_2, \ldots, X_9$ are multivariate normal with zero mean, unit variance and correlation $\text{Corr}(X_j, X_{j'}) = 0.15^{|j-j'|}$ for $j, j' = 2, \ldots, 9$.

Step 2: Generate treatment such that $P(A_i = 1|x_1, x_2, x_3, x_4, x_5) = expit(1 + \sum_{j=1}^{5} x_j)$.

Step 3: Set the blip function as $c(x, a; \psi) = a(\psi_0 + \sum_{j=1}^{3} \psi_j x_j)$ for $\psi_0 = 0.5, \psi_1 = -0.8, \psi_2 = -0.5$ and $\psi_3 = -0.5$. Hence, the optimal treatment strategy depends only on X_1, X_2, and X_3.

Step 4: Set the baseline mean model to $\mu(x; \beta) = 0.5 - 0.6e^{x_1} - 2x_1 - 2x_2 + x_3 + 2x_6$.

Step 5: Generate the outcome $Y \sim N(\mu(x; \beta) + c(x, a; \psi), 1)$.

In the data generating process, X_1–X_3 are confounders, and X_4 and X_5 are instrumental variables. As argued in (Greenland, 2008; De Luna et al., 2011), the ideal propensity score model should include all the confounders and the predictors of outcome while excluding predictors of exposure not associated with outcome as well as all noise variables (covariates that are unrelated to both exposure and outcome). In our case, X_4 and X_5 were only used to generate the treatment, while X_6 is a predictor only of the outcome, hence we hope our propensity score model does not include X_4 and X_5 but does select X_6.

The estimation procedure proceeds as follows:
(a) Use OLS to regress y on $(1, x, ax)$ to obtain $\widehat{\beta}$.
(b) Construct the penalty factors (adaptive weights): $\widetilde{w}_j = |\widehat{\beta}_j|^{-q}$ for some $q > 0$; solve the adaptive penalized logistic regression to select the confounders to include in the propensity score. The choice of q can be arbitrary, and in this simulation we set it to be 3.
(c) Refit the propensity score model using the selected variables; this will yield the balancing weights in the pdWOLS. Here, we used weights of the form $w(a, x) = |a - \widehat{\mathbb{E}}[A|X = x]|$ as proposed in Wallace and Moodie (2015).
(d) Apply pdWOLS: regress Y on $(1, X, A, AX)$ using the weights obtained in step (c). Even though the baseline mean model is misspecified, the blip parameters can still be consistently estimated due to the double robustness property of pdWOLS.

The choices of tuning parameters in step (b) and step (d) are important. We adopt the ideas of Shortreed and Ertefaie (2017) to select the tuning parameter for outcome-adaptive LASSO such that the weighted absolute mean difference between the exposure groups is minimized. For pdWOLS, we set δ to be 0.5, and evaluate two different approaches, the

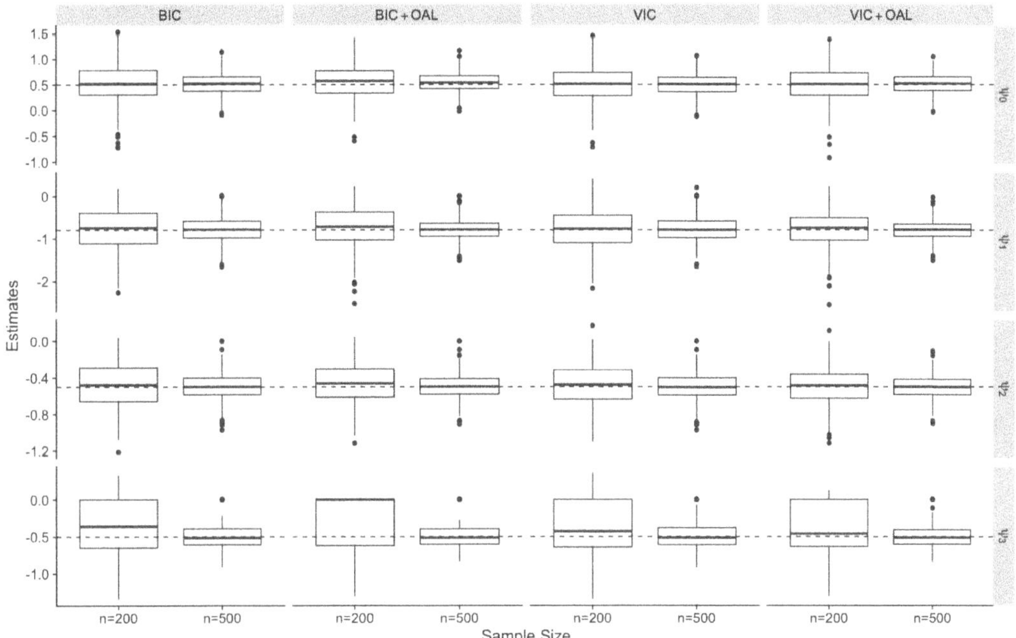

Figure 14.1 *Estimates of blip parameters using pdWOLS with and without applying OAL to select the propensity score model with n =200 and 500; 500 simulations. The tuning parameter of pdWOLS was selected by BIC and VIC. The true value is represented by the dotted line.*

value information criterion (VIC) (Shi et al., 2021) and the Bayesian information criterion (BIC) (Schwarz, 1978) to choose the λ such that either the VIC or the BIC is maximized. Analogous to the likelihood-based information criteria, VIC $= n\widehat{V}(\psi) - \kappa_n \|\psi\|_0$ where

$$\widehat{V}(\psi) = \frac{1}{n}\sum_{i=1}^{n} Y_i \frac{A_i \widehat{a}^{opt}(x_i;\psi) + (1-A_i)(1-\widehat{a}^{opt}(x_i;\psi))}{A_i\widehat{\pi}(x_i) + (1-A_i)(1-\widehat{\pi}(x_i))}$$

and κ_n is a positive sequence. Here we choose $\kappa_n = n^{1/3}\log(p)^{2/3}\log\log(n)$ as this can achieve model selection consistency under certain conditions (Shi et al., 2021).

Figure 14.1 summarizes the estimates of blip parameters using pdWOLS. When $n =$ 500, all four blip parameters were nearly unbiased, regardless of the method to select the tuning parameter and whether we use OAL, which showed that pdWOLS is robust to the misspecification of the baseline mean model. Nevertheless, using OAL can reduce the variance of the estimators. Table 14.3 presents the standard error of the pdWOLS estimators using VIC and BIC with and without applying OAL when the sample size is 200; we can see that the standard errors of the estimators obtained with OAL are uniformly smaller than those obtained without applying OAL, regardless using BIC or VIC to select the tuning parameter. When $n = 200$, the median of the estimator of ψ_3 obtained by BIC+OAL is about 0 as the coefficient is often shrunk to 0, while other estimators were similar to the case when $n = 500$.

Table 14.1 shows the variable selection results of pdWOLS with sample sizes of 200 and 500. In general, VIC has a lower false negative rate (i.e., excluding variables that are truly important) and a higher false positive rate (i.e., including variables that should be excluded) compared to BIC; OAL appears to improve the variable selection rate slightly. The irrelevant interaction AX_6 was frequently selected by all the methods, possibly due to the large main effect of X_6. When $n = 200$, the selection rate of the truly important

Table 14.1 *Variable selection rate (%) for pdWOLS using VIC and BIC with and without applying OAL (n =200 and 500; 500 simulations). The main effect of treatment is not penalized in the pdWOLS procedure. Variables with * are the truly important variables, the rest are noise variables* $(AX_3 - AX_{10})$.

	$n = 200$				$n = 500$			
	VIC+OAL	BIC+OAL	VIC	BIC	VIC+OAL	BIC+OAL	VIC	BIC
AX_1*	97	85	95	86	100	98	99	98
AX_2*	97	86	95	86	100	98	99	99
AX_3*	75	46	71	55	93	84	91	86
AX_4	8	2	10	6	8	1	14	2
AX_5	10	3	8	4	8	1	10	3
AX_6	78	54	72	60	85	64	83	68
AX_7	9	3	11	6	9	2	10	2
AX_8	10	3	10	5	8	1	10	3
AX_9	10	1	8	4	8	1	10	3
AX_{10}	11	2	11	5	7	1	11	2

Table 14.2 *Error rate (ER) and value (standard error in parentheses) for pdWOLS using VIC and BIC with and without applying OAL (sample size 500 and 200, 500 simulations, and test size 10,000). For comparison, the value function of the true optimal regime, always treated and never treated group are -1.15, -1.45, and -1.56, respectively.*

	VIC+OAL	BIC+OAL	VIC	BIC
ER ($n = 200$)	0.18	0.23	0.20	0.23
ER ($n = 500$)	0.10	0.11	0.12	0.12
Value ($n = 200$)	-1.22 (0.07)	-1.25 (0.10)	-1.23 (0.08)	-1.25 (0.09)
Value ($n = 500$)	-1.17 (0.02)	-1.18 (0.05)	-1.18 (0.03)	-1.18 (0.04)

interaction AX_3 was only 46% using BIC+OAL. Table 14.2 presents the error rate and the value function under the estimated rules of pdWOLS computed over a testing set of size 10,000. Despite small differences between the four methods, VIC+OAL has the smallest error rate as well as the largest and most accurate (smallest SE) value function.

Table 14.4 shows the variable selection rate for the propensity score using OAL. Note that the OAL selection is the same for both the BIC- and VIC-selected penalty in pdWOLS since the confounder selection is a first step in a multi-step estimation procedure. All the truly important variables were correctly picked with a high selection rate, even in the smaller sample size of $n = 200$.

Table 14.3 *Standard error of the pdWOLS estimators using BIC and VIC with and without applying OAL (sample size 200, 500 simulations).*

	VIC+OAL	BIC+OAL	VIC	BIC
ψ_0	0.33	0.31	0.35	0.34
ψ_1	0.40	0.47	0.47	0.51
ψ_2	0.21	0.25	0.25	0.28
ψ_3	0.30	0.35	0.33	0.36

Table 14.4 *Confounder selection rate using OAL. The variables with * are the truly important variables for the propensity score model*

	$n = 200$	$n = 500$
X_1*	100	100
X_2*	100	100
X_3*	99	100
X_4	7	1
X_5	8	1
X_6*	97	98
X_7	3	0
X_8	1	0
X_9	2	0
X_{10}	13	0

Table 14.5 *The proportion of times that tailoring variables are ranked over 500 replications using pdWOLS (n =200), which is based on the selected frequency among a sequence of tuning parameters.*

Ranking	1	2	3	4	5	6	7	8	9	10
X_1	88.2	9.8	1.2	0.6	0.2	0.0	0.0	0.0	0.0	0.0
X_2	11.2	87.2	0.6	0.8	0.0	0.2	0.0	0.0	0.0	0.0
X_3	0.0	1.0	38.0	59.0	1.2	0.4	0.0	0.0	0.2	0.2
X_4	0.0	0.0	0.0	2.0	19.6	18.8	16.6	12.0	17.4	13.6
X_5	0.0	0.0	0.0	1.8	15.2	16.8	14.6	16.6	17.0	18.0
X_6	0.6	2.0	60.2	32.4	2.4	1.8	0.4	0.0	0.0	0.2
X_7	0.0	0.0	0.0	0.6	17.0	15.8	15.2	17.4	17.4	16.6
X_8	0.0	0.0	0.0	1.2	15.0	17.0	18.0	15.0	18.6	15.2
X_9	0.0	0.0	0.0	0.4	14.8	14.8	19.4	19.0	15.0	16.6
X_{10}	0.0	0.0	0.0	1.2	14.6	14.4	15.8	20.0	14.4	19.6

Our simulations suggest that pdWOLS achieves the best performance when combined with VIC and OAL, as it had lowest false negative rate, lowest error rate, and the highest value function. Moreover, applying OAL can improve the efficiency of the estimators.

The second focus of our simulations was to investigate pdWOLS as a tool for ranking tailoring variables. We do so according to the selected frequency among a sequence of tuning parameters, although as noted above, other approaches to ranking could also be used. Tables 14.5 and 14.6 summarize the proportion of times that tailoring variables are ranked over 500 replications using pdWOLS for n =200 and 500, respectively. From Tables 14.5 and 14.6, we see that pdWOLS ranked the three truly important tailoring variables in the top three with high frequency, however, the variable X_6 – which predicts the outcome but is not a tailoring variable (i.e., does not interact with treatment) was also ranked as third 49% of the time when sample size was equal to 500. This result follows the same pattern as Table 14.1, where X_6 was incorrectly selected into the model with high probability.

14.5 Application to the Study of an Adaptive Web-Based Stress Management

In this section, we apply pdWOLS to data from a study of an adaptive web-based stress management tool. In this study, a pilot sequential multiple assignment randomized trial (SMART) was undertaken to assess the feasibility and potential effect size of a web-based,

Table 14.6 *The proportion of times that tailoring variables are ranked over 500 replications using pdWOLS (n =500), which is based on the selected frequency among a sequence of tuning parameters.*

Ranking	1	2	3	4	5	6	7	8	9	10
X_1	94.4	5.4	0.2	0.0	0.0	0.0	0.0	0.0	0.0	0.0
X_2	5.4	94.4	0.2	0.0	0.0	0.0	0.0	0.0	0.0	0.0
X_3	0.0	0.0	50.2	49.8	0.0	0.0	0.0	0.0	0.0	0.0
X_4	0.0	0.0	0.0	1.2	21.4	20.8	16.0	13.8	12.8	14.0
X_5	0.0	0.0	0.0	0.2	17.2	15.4	16.8	15.0	17.6	17.8
X_6	0.2	0.2	49.4	48.0	1.8	0.4	0.0	0.0	0.0	0.0
X_7	0.0	0.0	0.0	0.0	15.6	15.8	17.8	19.6	17.8	13.4
X_8	0.0	0.0	0.0	0.2	15.6	17.8	17.2	17.6	16.2	15.4
X_9	0.0	0.0	0.0	0.6	16.6	13.8	15.4	16.4	20.8	16.4
X_{10}	0.0	0.0	0.0	0.0	11.8	16.0	16.8	17.6	14.8	23.0

stress management intervention adapted over time based on a stepped-care approach for patients with a cardiovascular disease (CVD) (Lambert et al., 2022).

A two-stage SMART was piloted: at the first stage, 59 patients with CVD were randomized into two treatment groups with randomization stratified by recruitment source (clinical setting or community organization) and stress level (low or high). The randomization arms at the first stage were a website only group, and a website plus weekly telephone coaching group, each with probability of 0.5. Stage two followed after six weeks: patients who did not derive the anticipated benefits (non-responders) were re-randomized to either continue with their first stage intervention or to switch to the use of the website plus motivational interviewing (MI) for another six weeks (again, randomization with probability of 0.5 to each option); responders maintained their initial intervention from stage one. Responders were those participants whose stress scores improved by at least 50% or who were below the threshold of 16 on the stress subscale of the Depression Anxiety Stress Scales (DASS) (Lovibond and Lovibond, 1996).

We restrict our analysis to the first stage only (and limit ourselves to the 50 of 59 participants with complete data at 6 weeks), and hence a binary treatment is considered: $A = 0$ for the website only group and $A = 1$ for the website plus weekly telephone coaching group. The outcome of interest is the negative of the DASS measured at 6 weeks after stage 1 randomization; we target an individualized treatment rule that minimizes the DASS (conversely, maximizes the negative DASS) since this suggests the presence of fewer symptoms of stress. The aims of our analysis are to determine the potential tailoring variables that can improve the decision rule, and then estimate the optimal treatment regime of the adaptive web-based stress management study based on these tailoring variables.

Table 14.7 summarizes the baseline covariates of the 50 participants, including the standardized mean difference (SMD). Study groups were for the most part comparable with the exceptions of sex, employment, having a chronic vision condition, chronic back pain and chronic obesity, where SMDs all exceeded 0.25. These differences in baseline characteristics are likely a reflection of the relatively small sample size. For this stratified randomization, logistic regression was used to estimate the treatment model (adjusting for recruitment source and stress level), as estimation and use of a parametric propensity score model can improve the efficiency of the estimator compared with using the known propensity score (Henmi and Eguchi, 2004); further, covariate adjustment can remove any potential bias due to chance imbalances between randomization groups. The minimum, median, mean and maximum values of the estimated propensity score are 0.42, 0.48, 0.49 and 0.58 respectively. There are 16 potential tailoring variables: DASS at baseline, age, sex as well as

Table 14.7 *Characteristics of the adaptive web-based stress management study population stratified by stage 1 treatment; covariate (im)balance is measured by the standardized mean difference (SMD).*

	Website-only	Website+coach	SMD
n	25	25	
Age (mean (SD))	61.0 (13.4)	61.3 (10.7)	0.03
DASS Score at baseline (mean (SD))	19.2 (6.7)	18.9 (7.7)	0.03
Physical Component Score (mean (SD))	42.9 (12.2)	45.4 (11.6)	0.20
Mental Component Score (mean (SD))	40.4 (8.6)	40.9 (10.9)	0.04
Sex = Male (%)	13 (52.0)	9 (36.0)	0.33
Marital = Married / Common law (%)	14 (56.0)	15 (60.0)	0.08
Education = University degree (%)	13 (52.0)	16 (64.0)	0.25
Employment = Full time (%)	4 (16.0)	9 (36.0)	0.47
Chronic cardiac condition = Yes (%)	18 (72.0)	16 (64.0)	0.17
Chronic hypertension = Yes (%)	12 (48.0)	10 (40.0)	0.16
Chronic stomach condition = Yes (%)	10 (40.0)	12 (48.0)	0.16
Chronic vision condition = Yes (%)	11 (44.0)	7 (28.0)	0.34
Chronic backpain = Yes (%)	10 (40.0)	14 (56.0)	0.32
Chronic cholesterol condition = Yes (%)	9 (36.0)	11 (44.0)	0.16
Chronic obesity = Yes (%)	7 (28.0)	13 (52.0)	0.50
Chronic osteoarthritis = Yes (%)	9 (36.0)	8 (32.0)	0.09

several other measures of physical health (see Table 14.7). We also include three sociodemographic variables – education, employment, and marital status – which could potentially alter the impact of treatment.

Applying pdWOLS with the tuning parameter selected using VIC to this study, we find that eight variables are useful for tailoring treatment according to the pdWOLS variable ranking approach outlined in Section 14.3.3 (in decreasing order): mental component score (MCS), age, DASS at baseline, sex, marital status, diagnosis of a stomach condition, physical component score (PCS), and diagnosis of a chronic vision condition. The estimated treatment rule is $\widehat{a}_1^{opt} = I\{38.3 + 0.2\text{age} - 4.5I(\text{male}) - 15.4I(\text{unmarried}) - 1.0\text{DASS} + 0.2\text{PCS} - 0.7\text{MCS} - 9.9I(\text{stomach=yes}) + 2.5I(\text{vision=yes}) > 0\}$. The estimated value of DASS and the 95% confidence interval (CI) are $13.8\,(10.6, 17.0)$ where the CI is calculated using 4,000 nonparametric bootstrap (Efron, 1992) resamples. For comparison, the estimated value of DASS under the untailored approaches of the website+coach and the website are 15.0 and 18.5, respectively. No minimally important clinical difference has been established for the DASS, however, a value of 18.5 is well above our targeted threshold of 16 points, which would suggest a meaningful difference between the tailored strategy and offering website only to all. The difference of 1.2 points on the DASS between the tailored strategy and the website with coaching is less striking, however, it is worth noting that the tailored strategy is less resource intensive, offering the coaching to only a subset of the population while still potentially leading to reduced symptoms on average as compared to offering it to all under the untailored, website+coach strategy.

Since the sample size is relatively small, there can still be imbalances even if it is a randomized study. Thus we also apply OAL+pdWOLS to the study, with recruitment source, stress level and all the variables in Table 14.7 contained in the initial propensity score model. We find that seven variables are useful for tailoring treatment (listed in decreasing order according to the pdWOLS ranking): age, DASS at baseline, PCS, MCS, vision, sex, and employment status. Compared to the pdWOLS without applying OAL, the selection approach removes marital status and diagnosis of a stomach condition, and includes an extra tailoring variable employment status. The estimated treatment rule is $\widehat{a}_2^{opt} = I\{16.7 + 0.4\text{age} - 0.6\text{DASS} - 0.1\text{PCS} - 0.5\text{MCS} - 4.7I(\text{vision=yes}) - 5.2I(\text{male}) - 7.1I(\text{employed}) > 0\}$. The estimated value of DASS and the 95% confidence interval (CI) are 14.8 (11.8, 17.9). This yields a larger DASS score than the pdWOLS without applying the OAL approach.

The results above suggest that a linear decision rule of eight tailoring variables (pdWOLS) is better than a "one size fits all" approach. Due to the large CIs of these estimated values and the small size of the pilot study, we cannot make any definitive conclusions regarding the benefit of tailoring compared with the only website+coach strategy, nevertheless, these estimated values hint at clinically meaningful benefits and the potential for cost-savings since not all patients need a more costly or intensive treatment.

14.6 Discussion

In this chapter, we reviewed a penalized likelihood-based variable selection method, pdWOLS, which inherits the double robustness property from the regression-based dWOLS. Numerical studies indicated that VIC is a better tuning parameter selection method than BIC for pdWOLS. Additionally, it was demonstrated that a data-driven confounder selection approach for propensity score model construction can reduce the variance of the pdWOLS estimator. Further, pdWOLS functions well as a means of variable ranking, even with modest sample sizes.

Our analysis of adaptive web-based stress management pilot study data suggests that up to eight tailoring variables may be useful for the optimal treatment decisions, yielding a better clinical outcome than the untailored website+coach for all, or the only web for all approach (a DASS score of 13.4, 15.0, and 18.5, respectively). While the confidence intervals surrounding these estimated value functions were large and the pilot's size precludes making any definitive conclusions of benefit, these estimated values suggest clinically meaningful benefits and provide cost savings, as not all individuals need more expensive treatment options, including non-professional guidance. These results also underline the importance of considering comorbidities and social support in treating CVD patients' stress, and in collecting detailed information on these and related conditions in any subsequent full-scale SMART.

As shown here, OAL in combination with pdWOLS selects confounders for the propensity score model in a way that is decoupled from the selection of the tailoring variables, and ensures that instruments are unlikely to be included in the propensity score. The choice of q in OAL is an open and important question. In the simulations, we fixed it to be 3; alternatively, q can be selected using cross-validation. Many of the variable selection methods for DTRs are based on a penalized likelihood to screen out unneeded tailoring variables. However, DTRs are often estimated using estimating equations, and hence a quasi-likelihood framework is needed. Variable selection techniques in the context of estimating equations should be further studied, see, for example, (Fu, 2003) and (Candes and Tao, 2007).

There are several limitations and future directions for the methods discussed in this chapter. The pdWOLS method implemented in this chapter has been implemented only in the continuous outcome case; how to extend it to a more general setting such that the outcome is discrete is an interesting topic requiring further exploration. Post-selection inference should also be addressed; Zhao et al. (2017) proposed a valid tool to study the selective inference for effect modification using LASSO, which may be able to shed some light on how to combine the selection inferential tools with pdWOLS, and indeed with pdWOLS used in combination with OAL confounder selection.

Chapter 15

Selecting Optimal Subgroups for Treatment Using Many Covariates[1]

Tyler J. Vander, Alex R. Leudtke, Mark van der Laan, Ronald C. Kessler

15.1 Introduction

Biomedical researchers and social scientists are often interested in identifying the subgroups that would benefit most from a particular treatment or intervention. In randomized trials, subgroup analyses are often used to compare the effect of treatment across subgroups defined by various pre-treatment covariates (Yusuf et al., 1991; Assmann et al., 2000; Pocock et al., 2002; Rothwell, 1995; Lagakos et al., 2006; Wang et al., 2007). Such analyses can help give insight into whether a treatment might be more effective for men versus women, or for younger versus older persons, or for any other characteristic or variable defined prior to receipt of treatment. These types of analyses are relevant if the effect of treatment might vary across individuals in a population, a phenomenon often referred to as "effect heterogeneity". Such analyses can be useful in deciding who to treat, or who to treat first if resources are limited. They can also be useful when deciding which of two treatments to give to whom.

While well-established methodology has been used for decades to carry out such subgroup analyses across strata defined by a single covariate (Yusuf et al., 1991; Rothman et al., 1980, 2008; Hosmer and Lemeshow, 1992; Li and Chambless, 2007; VanderWeele and Knol, 2014), in actual practice it would be more desirable to make use of data on numerous covariates. Viewed from the individual perspective, we are interested in knowing how to best choose the appropriate treatment for an individual with a particular set of characteristics. This task is sometimes now described as "personalized medicine" or "precision medicine". It is the optimal selection of treatment for the individual (Murphy, 2003; Robins, 2004; Chakraborty and Moodie, 2013). However, viewed from the perspective of a population, if we optimize the treatment for each individual, we are also optimizing the outcomes for the population and are thus interested in which subgroups to give which treatment in order to maximize the outcomes within a population of interest, possibly subject to resource constraints.

To make progress with multiple covariates for this task, it is not uncommon in the biomedical or social sciences to form a "prognostic score (Rothwell, 1995; Hayward et al., 2006; Kent and Hayward, 2007; Pocock and Lubsen, 2008; Abadie et al., 2018). In a randomized trial with treatment and control, this prognostic score is defined as the predicted value of the outcome, conditional on an individual's covariates, if that person were not given treatment. The prognostic score is often obtained by first fitting a regression model of the outcome on the pre-treatment covariates among the control arm of the randomized trial. Using the estimates of the regression parameters of this model, one can then obtain predicted outcomes under the absence of treatment for each individual in the study to give the

[1]The text originally appeared as an article in: VanderWeele, T. J., Luedtke, A. R., van der Laan, M. J., & Kessler, R. C. (2019). Selecting optimal subgroups for treatment using many covariates. Epidemiology, 30(3), 334-341. Under a Creative Commons license and has been edited and adapted for inclusion in this handbook.

DOI: 10.1201/9781003216223-15

prognostic score. The prognostic score itself is then typically taken as the variable by which subgroups are formed. An analyst might for example, subsequently analyze the data within tertiles, quartiles, or quintiles of the prognostic score. If those with low prognostic scores would benefit most from treatment then this might be the group for which it would be best to target treatment. This approach is used with some frequency in the biomedical and social sciences (Abadie et al., 2018; Kent et al., 2002; Fox et al., 2005; Rothwell, 2005; Pane et al., 2014). It is sometimes also referred to as "risk stratification" (Kent and Hayward, 2007) or "endogenous stratification" (Abadie et al., 2018). While such procedures theoretically are effective with very large sample sizes, recent evidence suggests that in most practical settings, even with thousands of study participants (Abadie et al., 2018), biases from this sort of approach result from overfitting if the same data are used to form the prognostic score and to run the subgroup analyses (Abadie et al., 2018; Peck, 2003; Hansen, 2008). Various techniques, using cross-validation, have been proposed to address these biases (Abadie et al., 2018).

However, a more fundamental problem with the approach is that even if such biases were absent, using the prognostic score or individual-covariate subgroup analysis, does not in fact identify the optimal treatment allocation rule. There are better ways to use the covariate data available to optimize an individual's outcome and the mean outcomes for the population. A growing literature has begun to explore statistical approaches for more effective treatment selection rules (Cai et al., 2011; Zhao et al., 2013; van der Laan and Luedtke, 2015; Luedtke and van der Laan, 2016a; Luedtke and van der Laan, 2016c). In fact, what such an optimal rule depends subtly on precisely what question the analysis is intended to address.

In this paper we will present four settings in which optimal subgroup selection is of interest. We will describe these settings and the optimal treatment rule in each. We will discuss how the approaches in this paper relate to what is typically done in practice and how might be best to proceed in subsequent research when selecting optimal subgroups for treatment is of interest. New randomized trial designs are further proposed so as to implement and make use of optimal treatment selection rules in practice. The focus of this paper is conceptual. Our goal here is to more clearly consider the types of questions that arise with subgroup selection and to relate that to how subgroups are to be optimally formed. We then compare this to what is done in practice. The focus of the paper will not be statistical methods. Statistical methods are available to carry out some of this work and are described elsewhere (Cai et al., 2011; Zhao et al., 2013; van der Laan and Luedtke, 2015; Luedtke and van der Laan, 2016a; Luedtke and van der Laan, 2016c) and one approach developed by Luedtke and van der Laan (van der Laan and Luedtke, 2015; Luedtke and van der Laan, 2016a; Luedtke and van der Laan, 2016c) is summarized in the Appendix; but our focus here is on concepts and how we ought to think about subgroup selection within epidemiology and within the biomedical and social sciences more generally.

15.2 Notation

We will let A denote a treatment or intervention under study. We will assume that receipt of treatment has been randomized with probability $1/2$ but we will comment later in the paper on how the methodology described here is also potentially applicable to more general and to observational studies. We will let Y denote an outcome of interest. Finally, we will let C denote a set of pre-treatment covariates that are available for each individual in the study. We will let Y_1 denote the potential outcome (Rubin, 1974) that would have occurred for each individual if they had received treatment and we will let Y_0 denote the potential outcome that would have occurred under control. We only get to observe one of Y_1 and Y_0: we observe Y_1 for those who actually received treatment and Y_0 for those who were actually in the control arm. We do not in general know the potential outcome if an individual had been in the other arm of the trial.

In what follows, the task of treatment selection will essentially be to partition the population into two groups, which we will call "T" and "S", those receiving the treatment, and those not receiving the treatment, respectively. The goal will be, in each setting, to decide on how to partition the population into those who do versus do not receive treatment in order to maximize mean outcomes. We will refer to this partition of individuals who do and do not receive treatment as the optimal treatment rule.

We will, for simplicity, here assume that treatment A is binary with 1 denoting treatment and 0 denoting control. However, the ideas that are developed below are also applicable if we are comparing two different treatments so that $A = 1$ denotes one treatment and $A = 0$ denotes another. Although we will generally use of "treatment" and "control", the same methods and ideas described below are applicable also in the setting of comparing two treatments with "selecting who gets treatment" simply interpreted as "selecting who gets the first treatment" and "control" interpreted as "those receiving the second treatment." In the discussion section, we will also comment on how the ideas potentially extend to settings when more than two treatments are being considered.

In what follows we will provide an overview of the relevant concepts and methods. We will state results that are precise under some technical conditions. More formal statements and proofs are given in the Appendix (van der Laan and Luedtke, 2015; Luedtke and van der Laan, 2016a; Luedtke and van der Laan, 2016c).

15.3 Four Questions Relevant to Optimal Subgroup Selection

We will consider four settings that may be of interest in selecting optimal subgroups for treatment. Stated intuitively, these settings are:

1. Who do we treat if resources are limited so that we can only treat q% of the population?
2. Who do we treat if resources are not limited so that we could potentially treat everyone and are simply deciding who would benefit from treatment?
3. Who do we treat if resources are not limited, but are subject to costs or side effects?
4. How do we select subgroups to maximize the "effect heterogeneity" across subgroups?

We will address each question in turn.

15.3.1 Setting 1. Subgroup Selection Under Resource Constraints

First let us suppose that due to some form of resource constraints (e.g. costs, doses available, etc.), we are only able to treat at most q% of the population. We have data from a randomized trial of treatment A where we have collected outcome Y and pretreatment covariates C. We want to use the covariates C, and the outcome data from our randomized trial to determine a treatment rule in order to partition the population into those that we should treat so as to maximize the expected outcome for the population, subject to the constraint that we can only treat q% of the population. Once we decide on these two sets, T, the treated, and S, the untreated, then the expected outcome for the population under this treatment rule is:

$$\frac{q}{100}\mathbb{E}[Y|A=1,T] + \left(1-\frac{q}{100}\right)\mathbb{E}[Y|A=0,S]. \tag{15.1}$$

In other words, for q% of the population we get the average outcome under treatment for the subgroup T that we selected for treatment and for $(100-q)$% of the population, we get the average outcome under control for the subgroup S that we selected not to receive treatment.

It is shown in the Appendix that if we knew the potential outcomes, Y_1 and Y_0, for each individual in the population then the optimal treatment rule to maximize the expected outcome for the population would simply be to treat those for whom $\{Y_1 - Y_0 > k\}$ where k is determined so that exactly $q\%$ are treated. In other words, if we knew the potential outcomes for each individual so that we knew the actual effect, $Y_1 - Y_0$, of treatment for each individual, we would simply treat the $q\%$ for which the effect of treatment itself was largest. In actual fact, however, we do not know both potential outcomes for every individual in the population. We only have our randomized trial data, our outcomes Y, and our covariate C. So we want to use C to partition individuals into those who we do or do not treat to maximize outcomes. It is again shown in the Appendix that to maximize outcomes, using covariates C, the optimal treatment rule is to treat those with covariate values c such that

$$\{E[Y|A = 1, C = c] - E[Y|A = 0, C = c] > k\}$$

where the cut-off k is again determined so that exactly $q\%$ are treated. In other words, the optimal treatment rule is to treat the $q\%$ with the highest expected treatment effect conditional on their covariates. The expected treatment effect for each individual conditional on their covariates is something that can be estimated from the data in a randomized trial and thus this treatment rule can be implemented in practice. We could, for example, fit regression models for the expected outcome under treatment $E[Y|A = 1, C = c]$ and under control $E[Y|A = 0, C = c]$, (or, more directly, their difference) conditional on covariates, to obtain estimates. However, again, it can be shown, that the best we can do in terms of maximizing outcomes for the population using just the covariates C is to treat those with the highest expected treatment effect, $E[Y|A = 1, C = c] - E[Y|A = 0, C = c]$, conditional on their covariates. With this treatment rule, the expected outcome for the population is again then $\frac{q}{100}E[Y|A = 1, T] + (1 - \frac{q}{100})E[Y|A = 0, S]$.

The expected outcome under the treatment rule will not be as high as we could have obtained had we known both potential outcomes for all individuals, but again this is the best we can do with the measured covariates C. We could compare the expected outcome 15.1 under the treatment rule to what we would obtain if we simply randomly selected $q\%$ of the population for treatment, in which case we would have an expected outcome of:

$$\frac{q}{100}E[Y|A = 1] + \left(1 - \frac{q}{100}\right)E[Y|A = 0]. \tag{15.2}$$

How much better we do under the treatment rule using the covariates C will depend in part on how predictive the measured covariates are of the association between treatment and the outcome of interest, and also how well we statistically model the expected outcomes $E[Y|A = 1, C = c]$ and $E[Y|A = 0, C = c]$, or, more directly, their difference. We could compare the expected population outcomes in 15.1 under different estimates of the optimal treatment rule using different modeling techniques. Intuitively, how well we improve on the outcomes by selecting subgroups for treatment using covariates C, instead of randomly allocating treatment, will effectively depend on how well we can use the covariates C and statistical modeling to predict the potential outcomes. i.e. how well we estimate the true $E[Y|A = 1, C] - E[Y|A = 0, C]$.

15.3.2 Setting 2. Subgroup Selection Under Unconstrained Resources

We will now turn to a different setting in which resources are not constrained so that we could potentially treat anyone who might benefit from treatment. Once again our objective is to determine the treatment rule that partitions individuals into two sets: T, those who do receive treatment, and S, those who do not; so as to maximize the average outcome for the population, which is then:

$$E[Y|A = 1, T]P(T) + E[Y|A = 0, S]P(S). \tag{15.3}$$

It is shown in the Appendix that if we knew the potential outcomes, Y_1 and Y_0, for each individual in the population then the optimal treatment rule to maximize the expected outcome for the population would simply be treat those for whom $\{Y_1 - Y_0 > 0\}$. In other words, if we knew the potential outcomes for each individual, we would simply treat those for whom the effect of treatment itself was positive. This is, of course, relatively intuitive. In actual fact, we do not, of course, know both potential outcomes for every individual; we only have our covariates C. With covariates C, it shown in the Appendix that to maximize outcomes, using covariates C, the optimal treatment rule is to treat those with covariate values c such that

$$\{E[Y|A = 1, C = c] - E[Y|A = 0, C = c] > 0\}. \tag{15.4}$$

In other words, we treat those who have, conditional on their covariates, a positive expected treatment effect. We can again estimate this from the data from our randomized trial. Under this treatment rule, the expected outcome will simply be $E[Y|A = 1, T]P(T) + E[Y|A = 0, S]P(S)$. We could compare this expected outcome under the optimal treatment rule, to the expected outcome if we treated everyone in the population, $E[Y|A = 1]$, or if we treated no one, $E[Y|A = 0]$. Once again, how well we could optimize outcomes would depend on how predictive the covariate C were of the association between treatment and outcome.

An interesting feature of this second setting of unconstrained optimal treatment selection is that the tasks of individual decision-making and maximizing population outcomes in fact coincide. The approach to maximize population outcomes is simply to assign treatment to anyone who would benefit from it. The perspectives of the individual and the policy-maker coincide. This was not the case in the first setting wherein an individual might have a positive expected treatment effect and therefore, from an individual perspective, have expected benefit from treatment, whereas a policy-maker, to maximize population outcomes, might choose not to treat that individual because others have higher expected treatment effects and resources are limited.

15.3.3 Setting 3. Subgroup Selection Under Costs and Side-Effects

Now let us turn to a setting in which resources are not constrained so that we could once again, in principle, treat everyone but now suppose the treatment itself has a cost that we want to take into account, and/or has side-effects that we want to weigh against the potentially beneficial effects on our outcome of interest Y. Because of costs or side effects we might, for example, only want to treat those with treatment effects larger than some level δ. Or more generally, that level might depend on a person's covariates c so that we only want to treat those with treatment effects greater than some level $\delta(c)$. The optimal rule (see Appendix) if we knew both potential outcomes for all individuals would then simply be to treat those with $\{Y_1 - Y_0 > \delta(c)\}$ and the optimal rule with the actual trial data and measured covariates C would be to treat those with $\{E[Y|A = 1, C = c] - E[Y|A = 0, C = c] > \delta(c)\}$. Once again, how well we could optimize outcomes would depend on how predictive the covariate C were of the association between treatment and outcome.

15.3.4 Setting 4. Maximizing Effect Heterogeneity

When one reads through the subgroup analyses of many randomized trials, in which subgroup analyses are undertaken one covariate at a time, it often seems that the goal is to find a covariate, often dichotomous or dichotomized, such that the effect heterogeneity across subgroups defined by the covariate is as large as possible. When the effect estimate in one subgroup is much larger than that of the other, then the subgroup analysis is considered a success and that covariate defining the subgroups is subsequently considered important. In fact, we could carry out a similar exercise using data on multiple covariates. In this case, we would want to use covariates C to partition the population into two subsets, T and S, such that the effect in the subgroup T, $E[Y|A=1,T]-E[Y|A=0,T]$, was much larger than the effect in subgroup S, $E[Y|A=1,S]-E[Y|A=0,S]$. In other words, we would want to maximize effect heterogeneity by maximizing the difference between the effects in these two subgroups:

$$\{E[Y|A=1,T]-E[Y|A=0,T]\}-\{E[Y|A=1,S]-E[Y|A=0,S]\}$$

This is in some sense a generalization of what seems to be the traditional subgroup task but extended to multiple covariates simultaneously. It is shown in the Appendix that once again the solution to this maximization takes the form of selecting T to be those with an actual treatment effect, Y_1-Y_0 (if the potential outcomes were known), or expected treatment effect conditional covariates C, $E[Y|A=1,C=c]-E[Y|A=0,C=c]$, above some threshold k', where k' can be determined numerically as described in the Appendix. But once again, it is the expected conditional treatment effect, $E[Y|A=1,C=c]-E[Y|A=0,C=c]$, that is utilized in the criterion by which treatment decisions are to be made in this setting as well. Note, however, that although this treatment rule maximizes effect heterogeneity, the average outcome under this treatment rule will generally be worse than that selected by the treatment rule that maximizes the outcome itself as in Setting 2. It is thus not clear that this treatment rule that maximizes effect heterogeneity is of particular use in decision-making, unlike those in contexts 1, 2 and 3 above. We will return to this point in the discussion.

15.3.5 Extensions to Observational Studies

Our discussion thus far has been within the context of a randomized trial. However, as discussed further in the Appendix, all of the discussion above pertains also to optimal subgroup selection and treatment decisions from data arising from an observational study as well, provided that the covariates C suffice to control for confounding of the effect of treatment A on outcome Y, though the formulae for the optimized outcome need to be modified (see Appendix). With data from observational studies, an additional context that may be of interest is if, in data from the study, there are available covariates C that suffice to control for confounding for the effect of treatment A on outcomes Y, but if, when treatment decisions are made subsequently, only data on some subset W of the covariates C will be available. Methodology for this setting has been developed and is described elsewhere (van der Laan and Luedtke, 2015; Luedtke and van der Laan, 2016a; Luedtke and van der Laan, 2016c; van der Laan et al., 2007). Further discussion of statistical approaches is given in the Appendix.

15.4 Implications for Current Practices

We have shown that under a wide range of different goals and settings, including making treatment decisions with or without resource constraints, and with or without side effects, or even when trying to maximize effect heterogeneity, the correct approach to finding the optimal treatment rule is to estimate expected treatment effects for each individual conditional on the covariates. In each of the settings described above, the optimal treatment rule involved treating those above some threshold of the conditional expected treatment effect. The threshold differed according to whether there were or were not resource constraints,

Table 15.1 *Summary of Optimal Subgroup Selection Settings and Optimal Treatment Selection Rules.*

Setting	Optimal Treatment Rule	Threshold
Resource Constraints (can only treat $q\%$)	$E[Y\|A=1, C=c] - E[Y\|A=0, C=c] > k$	k is selected so $q\%$ are treated
Unconstrained Resources	$E[Y\|A=1, C=c] - E[Y\|A=0, C=c] > 0$	Treat all with positive expected treatment effect
Unconstrained Resource with costs or side effects	$E[Y\|A=1, C=c] - E[Y\|A=0, C=c] > \delta(c)$	Treat all with expected treatment effect above costs
Maximizing Effect Heterogeneity	$E[Y\|A=1, C=c] - E[Y\|A=0, C=c] > k'$	k' is determined by numerical optimization

or whether there were or were not costs or side effects, or whether we wanted to maximize effect heterogeneity, but the form of the treatment rule did not vary across these contexts. In each case, the form of the optimal treatment rule was simply to treat those with conditional expected treatment effects above a specific threshold. The results are summarized in Table 15.1. This has a number of important implications for the actual practice of subgroup analysis, treatment selection, precision medicine, and the modeling of interactions.

15.4.1 Subgroup Analysis

One fundamental insight from our discussion above is that for treatment selection and decisions, our discussion suggests a need to move away from subgroup analyses conducted one covariate at a time. The problems with this approach are numerous. First, subgroups may come into conflict: if subgroup analyses indicate that treatment A is better for women and treatment B is better for men, and also indicate that A is better for aged and B better for younger persons, and we want make treatment decisions for a younger woman, the subgroup analyses conflict. Second, the subgroup analyses often fail to answer the scientific question of interest. As they are typically carried out, they tend to be aimed at maximizing effect heterogeneity, whereas what is actually of interest is maximizing population outcomes or individual treatment decision making. The optimal treatment rule for maximizing population outcomes or individual treatment decision-making is not the same as for maximizing effect heterogeneity. Finally, compared to individual covariate subgroup analyses, we can in fact do better at maximizing mean outcomes by making simultaneous use of all covariates, rather than running analyses one covariate at a time. It is conceivable, of course, that the optimal treatment selection in some rare cases might involve only a single dichotomous covariate, or in some settings a single dichotomous covariate may constitute the decision to be made (e.g. resources are limited so we can only intervene in city 1 or city 2), but in general, the optimal decision-making rule will make fuller use of covariate data.

The need to move away from one-covariate-at-a-time approaches in optimizing population outcomes or individual treatment decision-making is relevant not just to traditional subgroup analyses when we are looking at whether the treatment effect is larger in one group versus another, but this same point is also relevant to the analysis of so-called "qualitative" or "cross-over" interactions (Gail and Simon, 1985; Piantadosi and Gail, 1993; Pan and Wolfe, 1997; Silvapulle, 2001; Li and Chan, 2006), in which the treatment has a positive effect in one subgroup and a harmful effect in another. The analysis of such cross-over interactions is again often done one covariate at a time, but for the purposes of decision-making, it ought to be done using all available relevant covariate data. In actual fact, the methodology described in Setting 2 above is doing precisely that.

15.4.2 Prognostic Scores

A second important implication of the discussion in this paper is that, for optimizing population outcomes or individual treatment decision making, we should move away from the "prognostic score", that is often employed in both the biomedical and social sciences (Kent and Hayward, 2007; Pocock and Lubsen, 2008; Abadie et al., 2018; Kent et al., 2002; Fox et al., 2005; Rothwell, 2005; Pane et al., 2014). The practice of stratifying on prognostic scores in small or medium-sized trials has numerous statistical problems with "overfitting" documented elsewhere (Abadie et al., 2018). At a more fundamental level, though, it gets the objective wrong because the patients at greatest risk of bad outcomes in the absence of treatment are not necessarily the same patients who will profit most from intervention. While stratifying the results of randomized trials using the predicted outcome under control can provide some insight into who might be considered to have greatest need for treatment, it is not the correct approach to optimize population outcomes or individual treatment decision-making. To optimize population outcomes or individual treatment decision-making, one stratifies, not by predicted outcome under control, but by the expected effect of treatment; that is, the difference between the predicted outcome under treatment and the predicted outcome under control, conditional on covariates. It is this stratification that gives one insight into optimal treatment decisions either with or without resource constraints.

15.4.3 Interaction Analysis

A third important implication, related somewhat to the first, concerns the modeling of interactions. In reading the literature, one is often left with the impression that the principal goal of interaction analysis is to determine whether, in a given statistical model, a product term involving two variables is "statistically significant" or non-zero. Methodology to detect "interactions" or non-zero product terms has become increasingly advanced (Moore et al., 2006; Green and Kern, 2012; Imai and Ratkovic, 2013; Berger et al., 2014). However, once again, if the purpose of the analysis is optimizing population outcomes or individual decision-making, the question as to whether a specific product term in a particular statistical model is present is, in fact, secondary. All that matters for the task of optimizing population outcomes or individual decision-making is having predictive covariates and having statistical models that give good predictions of expected outcomes conditional on those covariates. If the product terms help in a particular model, they can be included; if not, they can be omitted. In either case, though, their presence or absence is secondary to having a good predictive model so as to make optimal treatment decisions. Indeed using models both with and without product terms and, more generally, numerous models and machine learning algorithms, to generate predicted outcomes, and possibly ensemble methods to average over, or choose among them, as suggested above, is a preferable way to proceed.

It might be thought that subgroup analyses one-covariate-at-a-time or the analysis of individual product terms in statistical models may still be of interest for the purposes of understanding or explanation. While this may be true to some degree, it is important to clarify the goal of such understanding or the form of explanation that is in view. If what is thought to be of importance is to understand which covariates in fact are most relevant in decision-making (e.g., because it was thought undesirable to measure all of the covariates subsequently in treatment decision-making), then one could instead consider the result of optimal treatment rules on the maximized population outcome when only certain subsets of the covariates C are considered. On the other hand, if one simply wanted to assess which covariates in some sense seemed most "responsible" for the effect heterogeneity, one might instead still model the outcome with all covariates simultaneously, and then consider, for example, what a one-unit shift in any given covariate for all individuals would have in changing expected treatment effects. In linear models for the expected outcomes in each treatment arm, this would simply be the difference between the covariate coefficient in the model under treatment $E[Y|A = 1, C = c]$ and the covariate coefficient in the model under control $E[Y|A = 0, C = c]$. But the approach of considering a one-unit shift in a particular covariate across all individual could also be employed in non-linear models as well. Other metrics could also potentially be developed. Finally, sometimes analyses of interactions are undertaken for the purpose of understanding the joint effects of the treatment and a particular covariate, or to gain mechanistic insight (VanderWeele and Robins, 2007; VanderWeele, 2009, 2015). In this case, it may be appropriate to assess the joint effects of one covariate at a time, but in this case, if the effect of the covariate is in view, then confounding control must be made not only for the association of the treatment and outcome but also for the association between that covariate and the outcome (VanderWeele, 2009, 2015; VanderWeele and Knol, 2011) and what additional variables are needed to control for such confounding will vary depending on which covariate is in view. This is no longer simply a question of effect heterogeneity but of joint effects (VanderWeele and Knol, 2014; VanderWeele, 2009). A model which includes all of the covariates C available will not in general be adequate to provide appropriate control in addressing this type of question if the covariates themselves affect one another.

15.4.4 Heuristics and Multiple Treatments

Yet another argument that might be put forward for doing one-by-one subgroup analyses may involve trying to generate heuristics. A physician cannot remember the functional form of two conditional expectations but can remember that treatment A is better for women and treatment B is better for men. While such treatment heuristics can be of some value, they can, as already discussed above, come into conflict with one another. Moreover, the use of such heuristics in decision-making becomes even more complex when there are more than two potential options to choose among, which brings us to another topic of our discussion: extensions to multiple treatments.

The setting of multiple treatment options is important in general and especially so in an era of personalized or precision medicine. Full discussion of the issue is beyond the scope of the present chapter, but many of the points discussed above do generalize to the multiple treatments setting. Specifically, in the task of optimizing treatment decisions without resource constraints, the solution to maximizing the population outcome, which is itself identical, in this setting, to maximizing the outcome for each individual involves a very similar form to what has already been discussed above. The optimal treatment rule in this setting with measured covariates C simply involves obtaining the expected outcome given an individual's covariates C under each possible treatment, $E[Y|A = a, C = c]$, $a = 0, 1, 2, \ldots, N$, and then assigning to each individual the treatment that gives the highest predicted outcome. Likewise, for the same reasons as those given above, in this setting, if the goal is to maximize population outcomes or individual decision-making, there is little reason to carry out one-by-one-covariate subgroup analyses or to consider which product terms in statistical models are statistically significant.

15.4.5 Clinical Judgement and New Randomized Trial Designs

In the clinical setting, one might also wonder about the role of expert judgment. Are there perhaps aspects of a patient's profile that are not, or even cannot be, adequately captured by a variable that we can use in a statistical model? This of course remains a possibility. Are we to abandon clinical judgment and simply rely on statistical models to make such predictions? Are we to pit clinical judgment and modeling against one another? We would like to close this chapter by attempting to tackle this question head-on with a compromise, to allow both clinical judgment and predictive models, by proposing a new type of study design.

A possible design – what we will refer to as an "Expected Outcomes Trial" – is to first use either prior randomized trial data, and/or observational data, with a relatively rich set of covariates C to build models for the expected outcomes with and without treatment. With such models, for each study participant in the Expected Outcomes Trial, the clinician (or patient) is randomized either to receive no further information, or to receive information on the expected outcome given their covariates under each treatment scenario. This could include outcomes under multiple treatment options. The clinician (or patient) then decides, based on the information available and their own judgments and preferences, which treatment to select. Outcomes are measured after a suitable follow-up period to determine whether the information provided by the predictive outcome models is useful in such decision-making. A trial of this sort will allow decision-makers to make use of both individually-oriented outcome predictions under statistical models, and also personal judgments, in making treatment decisions. It would also preserve decision-maker autonomy, and be more likely to be palatable to clinicians, and therefore more likely also to be scalable. The trials themselves would determine the additional utility of the information provided by the predictive models. A variation that added an additional arm in which treatment always followed the predicted maximum outcome could also be used to evaluate the role of clinical judgement, whether beneficial or harmful, above and beyond reliance on predicted probabilities. We believe that such trials will be of use in determining the utility of prediction models for personalized or precision medicine in actual practical settings.

15.5 Conclusion

In summary, we believe that careful thought as to what the correct question is in individual treatment decision-making, and careful selection of the correct optimization question and statistical method corresponding to the question of interest, will result in better patient outcomes. Current practices of one-covariate-at-a-time subgroup analysis, the use of prognostic scores, and the detection of significant interactions are simply not optimal for decision-making. We hope this chapter will help change these practices.

15.6 Appendix: Statistical Analysis

In this Appendix we describe methods and formal statistical inference for estimating the optimal treatment rule and the outcome under it, as well as software to do so. While there are many ways to go about estimation, the methods described in the Appendix flexibly model the difference in observed outcomes across treatment groups conditional on the covariates and use an ensemble technique called "super-learner" (van der Laan et al., 2007) that considers numerous different possible models or algorithms for the conditional outcome differences and then weights these according to their mean square error predictive value using cross-validation. Statistical inference for the optimal treatment rule and for the outcome under it is challenging because the same data are being used to estimate the treatment rule and the expected outcome under it. Sample-splitting can potentially be used but is not efficient, and averaging across split samples does not yield valid inference (van der Laan and Luedtke, 2015). The Appendix describes a cross-validated targeted minimum loss-based approach to estimate the optimal treatment rule and the outcome under it. While the approach described in the Appendix has some desirable theoretical properties, considerable work remains to be done in assessing the sample sizes that are needed for these techniques to be useful and how the various methods that have been proposed in the literature compare to one another in actual practice. While the theoretical methodological development has come a long way in the past decade, much remains to be learned about the application of these methods.

15.6.1 *Parameter Definitions*

Notation

Let A denote a binary treatment of interest, Y an outcome and C a set of measured baseline covariates. Let Y_1 and Y_0 denote the potential outcomes for each individual under treatment levels 1 and 0 respectively. Let the population of individuals be denoted by Ω. We first assume treatment A is randomized and then consider treatment that may arise from an observational study. For simplicity in the next several section, in order to give intuitive proofs, we will assume a finite population of individuals with no ties at the cut-off for the optimal treatment rule. See Luedtke and van der Laan (2016c); Luedtke and van der Laan (2016a) for further discussion of these cases without these conditions.

Context 1: Treatment Subgroup Selection Under Limited Resources

Suppose that due to limited resources, we can only treat $100q\%$ of the population. We will assume that treatment is beneficial for at least $100q\%$ of the population i.e. $P(Y_1 - Y_0 > 0) > q$. Otherwise, if we know this in advance, the problem reduces to Context 2 described below. We desire to partition Ω into sets S and T such that $P(\omega \in T) = q$ so as to maximize the average outcome if all units in T were treated and all units in S were untreated. In other words, we wish to identify S and T to solve:

$$\arg\max_{S,T:S\cup T=\Omega,S\cap T=\emptyset,P(\omega\in T)=q}[qE(Y_1|\omega \in T) + (1-q)E(Y_0|\omega \in S)].$$

In fact, choosing S and T to maximize the average outcome if all units in T were treated and all units in S were untreated is equivalent to choosing S and T to maximize the treatment effect heterogeneity with $100q\%$ in one group, as stated in the following proposition.

Proposition 15.6.1. *The solution to*

$$\arg\max_{S,T:S\cup T=\Omega,S\cap T=\emptyset,P(\omega\in T)=q}[qE(Y_1|\omega \in T) + (1-q)E(Y_0|\omega \in S)]$$

is equivalent to the solution to

$$\arg\max_{S,T:S\cup T=\Omega,S\cap T=\emptyset,P(\omega\in T)=q}[E(Y_1 - Y_0|\omega \in T) - E(Y_1 - Y_0|\omega \in S)].$$

Proof. We have that

$$\begin{aligned}
& \arg\max_{S,T:S\cup T=\Omega,S\cap T=\emptyset,P(\omega\in T)=q}[E(Y_1 - Y_0|\omega \in T) \\
& \qquad -E(Y_1 - Y_0|\omega \in S)] \\
= \; & \arg\max_{S,T:S\cup T=\Omega,S\cap T=\emptyset,P(\omega\in T)=q}[E(Y_1|\omega \in T) - E(Y_1|\omega \in S) \\
& \qquad -E(Y_0|\omega \in T) + E(Y_0|\omega \in S) - \frac{1}{1-q}E(Y_1) + \frac{1}{q}E(Y_0) \\
= \; & \arg\max_{S,T:S\cup T=\Omega,S\cap T=\emptyset,P(\omega\in T)=q}[E(Y_1|\omega \in T) - E(Y_1|\omega \in S) \\
& \qquad -E(Y_0|\omega \in T) + E(Y_0|\omega \in S) - \frac{q}{1-q}E(Y_1|\omega \in T) \\
& \qquad -\frac{1-q}{1-q}E(Y_1|\omega \in S) + \frac{q}{q}E(Y_0|\omega \in T)
\end{aligned}$$

$$+\frac{(1-q)}{q}E(Y_0|\omega \in S)]$$

$$= \arg\max_{S,T:S\cup T=\Omega,S\cap T=\emptyset,P(\omega\in T)=q}[\frac{1-2q}{1-q}E(Y_1|\omega \in T)$$

$$+\frac{1-2q}{q}E(Y_0|\omega \in S)]$$

$$= \arg\max_{S,T:S\cup T=\Omega,S\cap T=\emptyset,P(\omega\in T)=q}[qE(Y_1|\omega \in T)$$

$$+(1-q)E(Y_0|\omega \in S)].$$

□

The solution to this maximization problem in fact takes a very simple form as stated in the next proposition.

Proposition 15.6.2. *The solution to*

$$\arg\max_{S,T:S\cup T=\Omega,S\cap T=\emptyset,P(\omega\in T)=q}[E(Y_1-Y_0|\omega \in T)-E(Y_1-Y_0|\omega \in S)]$$

almost surely takes the form, for some κ, *of* $T=\{\omega \in \Omega : Y_1(\omega)-Y_0(\omega) > \kappa\}$ *and* $S=\{\omega \in \Omega : Y_1(\omega)-Y_0(\omega) \leq \kappa\}$.

Proof. We prove the result by contradiction. Suppose S and T were not of this form. Then there must exist (possibly non-unique) disjoint sets $\Omega' \subseteq T$ and $\Omega^* \subseteq S$ of equal and positive probability such that $Y_1(\omega')-Y_0(\omega') < Y_1(\omega^*)-Y_0(\omega^*)$ for all $\omega' \in \Omega'$ and $\omega^* \in \Omega^*$. Let $T'=(T\cup\Omega^*)\backslash\Omega'$ and $S'=(S\cup\Omega')\backslash\Omega^*$. Then $E(Y_1-Y_0|\omega \in T')-E(Y_1-Y_0|\omega \in S') > E(Y_1-Y_0|\omega \in T)-E(Y_1-Y_0|\omega \in S)$ and thus S and T would not be the solution to $\arg\max_{S,T:S\cup T=\Omega,S\cap T=\emptyset,P(\omega\in T)=q}[E(Y_1-Y_0|\omega \in T)-E(Y_1-Y_0|\omega \in S)]$. □

If both counterfactual outcomes were known for all individuals, then κ could be obtained as the solution to $P(Y_1-Y_0>\kappa)=q$ and the average outcome for the population under the optimal treatment rule of giving treatment if $Y_1-Y_0>\kappa$ would be $qE(Y_1|Y_1-Y_0>\kappa)+(1-q)E(Y_0|Y_1-Y_0\leq\kappa)$. It is of course not possible to partition individuals in this way without complete knowledge of the counterfactual outcomes, which will in general not be available.

However, it is still possible to partition the covariate space to carry out a similar maximization. If we let Γ denote the support of C the task becomes

$$\arg\max_{S,T:S\cup T=\Gamma,S\cap T=\emptyset,P(C\in T)=q}[E(Y_1-Y_0|\omega \in T)-E(Y_1-Y_0|\omega \in S)].$$

By arguments similar to those presented above, the solution to this takes the form of $T=\{c \in \Gamma : E(Y|A=1,c)-E(Y|A=0,c) > k\}$ i.e. the treatment rule is then simply give treatment to those for whom $E(Y|A=1,c)-E(Y|A=0,c)>k$ with k given as the solution to

$$\int 1[E(Y_1-Y_0|C=c)>k]dP(c)=q.$$

In practice one must model $E(Y|A=1,C=c)-E(Y|A=0,C=c)$ and estimate k.

The average outcome under this treatment rule is then given by $q\int E(Y|A=1,c)dP(c|C\in T)+(1-q)\int E(Y|A=0,c)dP(c|C\notin T)$. Note that this average outcome will not, in general, be as high as the average outcome under the optimal decision rule if both counterfactual outcomes were themselves known for all individuals, in which case the average outcome would be given as above, $qE(Y_1|Y_1-Y_0>\kappa)+(1-q)E(Y_0|Y_1-Y_0\leq\kappa)$ where κ is defined as the solution to $P(Y_1-Y_0>\kappa)=q$. The extent to which the average outcome under the optimal treatment rule using the measured covariates C comes close to that which could be obtained under complete knowledge of the counterfactual outcomes will depend on the extent to which the covariates C are predictive of the outcome itself. Note that it is also thus of course the case that the average outcome under the optimal treatment rule using data on the measured covariates C will always be relative to C.

It may be of interest to compare the average outcome under this optimal treatment decision rule using the measured covariates C to the average outcome with no one treated, $E(Y|A=0)$, the outcome with $100q\%$ treated but selected randomly $qE(Y|A=1)+(1-q)E(Y|A=0)$, and the average outcome with everyone treated, $E(Y|A=1)$. It might also be of interest to compare the treatment effect for those treated under the optimal rule, $\int\{E(Y|A=1,c)-E(Y|A=0,c)\}dP(c|C\in T)$, to those left untreated by the rule $\int\{E(Y|A=1,c)-E(Y|A=0,c)\}dP(c|C\notin T)$, and also to the average treatment effect for the population $E(Y|A=1)-E(Y|A=0)$. Another relevant metric may be taken as the difference between the treatment effects comparing those who are assigned treatment by the rule versus those who are not:

$$\int\{E(Y|A=1,c)-E(Y|A=0,c)\}dP(c|C\in T)$$
$$-\int\{E(Y|A=1,c)-E(Y|A=0,c)\}dP(c|C\notin T).$$

This could be taken as a measure of effect heterogeneity introduced by the optimal treatment rule for the $100q\%$ to receive treatment. The analogous metric under treatment of a random $100q\%$ of the population selected for treatment would simply be 0.

Context 2: Unconstrained Treatment Subgroup Selection

Now suppose that resources are unconstrained and all could be treated who benefit from treatment. The optimal subgroup for treatment would then be

$$T=\{\omega:Y_1(\omega)-Y_0(\omega)>0\}.$$

Once again, we cannot determine this subgroup as, in general, we will not have information on both potential outcomes for all individuals. Instead, with covariate data on C, we would select the subgroup to treat as those with covariates C such that the expected value of the treatment effect conditional on C was positive. Thus we would treat those with covariate values that lie in the set

$$T=\{c\in\Gamma:E(Y|A=1,c)-E(Y|A=0,c)>0\}.$$

In practice with high dimensional C, the expectation $E(Y|a,c)$ would have to be modeled. If we were to follow this treatment rule, the average outcome under this rule would be

$$\int_{c\in T}E(Y|A=1,c)dP(c)+\int_{c\notin T}E(Y|A=0,c)dP(c).$$

Note that this average outcome will not, in general, be as high as the average outcome under the optimal decision rule if both counterfactual outcomes were themselves known in which case the average outcome would be $E(Y_1|Y_1-Y_0>0)P(Y_1-Y_0>0)+E(Y_0|Y_1-Y_0\leq 0)P(Y_1-Y_0\leq 0)$. The extent to which the average outcome under the optimal treatment rule using the measured covariates C comes close to that which could be obtained under complete knowledge of the counterfactual outcomes will depend on the extent to which the covariates C are predictive of the outcome itself. It is also thus of course the case that the average outcome under the optimal treatment rule using data on the measured covariates C will always be relative to C.

It may be of interest to compare this average outcome under the optimal treatment rule using the measured covariates C to the average outcome with no one treated, $E(Y|A=0)$, and to the average outcome with everyone treated, $E(Y|A=1)$. It might also be of interest to compare the treatment effect for those treated under the optimal rule $\int\{E(Y|A = 1,c) - E(Y|A=0,c)\}dP(c|C \in T)$, to those left untreated by the rule $\int\{E(Y|A=1,c) - E(Y|A = 0,c)\}dP(c|C \notin T)$, and also to the average treatment effect for the population $E(Y|A=1) - E(Y|A=0)$. Another relevant metric may be taken as the difference between the treatment effects comparing those who are assigned treatment by the rule versus those who are not:

$$\int\{E(Y|A=1,c) - E(Y|A=0,c)\}dP(c|C \in T)$$
$$-\int\{E(Y|A=1,c) - E(Y|A=0,c)\}dP(c|C \notin T).$$

This could be taken as a measure of effect heterogeneity.

Context 3: Unconstrained Treatment Subgroup Selection Under Costs or Side Effects

Another generalization of Setting 1 that might be considered is a setting in which there is a cost constraint. Typically this will require the investigator to only treat those with treatment effects greater than some threshold $\delta(c)$ that relies on the covariate value c. If all counterfactuals were known, we would use individual-level treatment effect $Y_1(\omega) - Y_0(\omega)$, and we will show that this can be replaced by $E(Y|A=1,c) - E(Y|A=0,c)$ in the realistic setting where only one counterfactual is observed for each individual.

To formalize our discussion, we wish to estimate the solution to

$$\text{Maximize} \int_{c\in T} E(Y|A=1,c)dP(c) + \int_{c\notin T} E(Y|A=0,c)dP(c)$$
$$\text{subject to} \int_{c\in T} \text{Cost}(c)dP(c) \leq \text{Cost Constraint},$$

where Cost$(\cdot)$ is pre-defined positive function giving the cost of treating someone in covariate strata and Cost Constraint is the pre-defined constraint. The results in this section easily generalize to the case where Cost(c) can equal zero, but we omit this case for simplicity. If $b = E[\text{Cost}(C)]$ is less than Cost Constraint then the constraint is not active and we revert to Context 2. Otherwise, the T maximizing the above objective takes the following form.

Proposition 15.6.3. *If b is finite and greater than* Cost Constraint*, then the T maximizing the objective function above takes the form, $\{\omega \in \Omega : E(Y|A=0,c) - E(Y|A=0,c) > k\,\text{Cost}(c)\}$, where k is the solution to*

$$\int 1\left[E(Y_1 - Y_0|C=c) > k\,\text{Cost}(c)\right]\text{Cost}(c)dP(c) = \text{Cost Constraint}\,.$$

Proof. Let P_c denote the probability measure with density $\frac{dP_c}{dP}(c) = \text{Cost}(c)/b$. Let $\tilde{Y} = bY/\text{Cost}(C)$, where we note that $\tilde{Y}$ is a deterministic function of Y conditional on $C=c$ so that $bE_P(Y|A=a,c)/\text{Cost}(c)$ is equal to $E_P(\tilde{Y}|A=a,c)$. We can write the mean outcome under the optimal rule as

$$\int_{c \in T} E(\tilde{Y}|A=1,c)dP_c(c) + \int_{c \notin T} E(\tilde{Y}|A=0,c)dP_c(c).$$

The cost constraint rewrites as $P_c(C \in T) \leq (\text{Cost Constraint})/b$. We are now in Context 1, so maximizing T takes the form $\{\omega \in \Omega : E(\tilde{Y}|A=0,c) - E(\tilde{Y}|A=0,c) > \tilde{k}\}$, where $\tilde{k}$ is the solution to

$$\int 1\left[E(\tilde{Y}|A=1,c) - E(\tilde{Y}|A=0,c) > \tilde{k}\right] dP_c(c) = (\text{Cost Constraint})/b$$

Multiplying both sides by b, using the definition of $\tilde{Y}$, and letting $k = \tilde{k}/b$ gives the result. □

It may be of interest to compare this average outcome under the optimal treatment rule to the average outcome with no one treated, $E(Y|A=0)$, and to the average outcome with everyone treated, $E(Y|A=1)$. It might also be of interest to compare the treatment effect for those treated under the optimal rule, $\int\{E(Y|A=1,c) - E(Y|A=0,c)\}dP(c|C \in T)$, to those left untreated by the rule $\int\{E(Y|A=1,c) - E(Y|A=0,c)\}dP(c|C \notin T)$, and also to the average treatment effect for the population $E(Y|A=1) - E(Y|A=0)$.

Context 4: Treatment Subgroup Selection to Maximize Treatment Effect Heterogeneity

In examining subgroup analyses reported in the literature one is sometimes under the impression that a central goal is to find a subgroup division that maximizes effect heterogeneity across the subgroups. While it is not clear that this goal is of principal policy importance, it can be carried out using a set of measured covariates C. The task could then be stated as finding a partition of individuals into sets T and S to maximize treatment effect heterogeneity when comparing the treatment effects among those in T versus S. The problem could thus formally be stated as

$$\arg\max_{S,T:S\cup T=\Omega,S\cap T=\emptyset}[E(Y_1 - Y_0|\omega \in T) - E(Y_1 - Y_0|\omega \in S)].$$

The solution to this maximization problem takes a relatively simple form as in the next Proposition.

Proposition 15.6.4. *The solution to*

$$\arg\max_{S,T:S\cup T=\Omega,S\cap T=\emptyset}[E(Y_1 - Y_0|\omega \in T) - E(Y_1 - Y_0|\omega \in S)]$$

takes the form, for some κ, *of* $T = \{\omega \in \Omega : Y_1(\omega) - Y_0(\omega) > \kappa\}$ *and* $S = \{\omega \in \Omega : Y_1(\omega) - Y_0(\omega) \leq \kappa\}$.

Proof. The proof is similar to that of Proposition 15.6.2 above. □

If we let $V = Y_1 - Y_0$ and let $p(v)$ denote the density of V. To determine κ, we wish to choose κ to maximize $E(Y_1 - Y_0|Y_1 - Y_0 > \kappa) - E(Y_1 - Y_0|Y_1 - Y_0 \leq \kappa)$ or equivalently,

$$\int_{\kappa}^{\infty} vp(v)dv \Big/ \int_{\kappa}^{\infty} p(v)dv - \int_{-\infty}^{\kappa} vp(v)dv \Big/ \int_{-\infty}^{\kappa} p(v)dv.$$

Differentiating with respect to κ we obtain:

$$\frac{\int_{\kappa}^{\infty} p(v)dv\Big[vp(v)\Big]_{v=\kappa}^{v=\infty} - \int_{\kappa}^{\infty} vp(v)dv\Big[p(v)\Big]_{v=\kappa}^{v=\infty}}{\Big[\int_{\kappa}^{\infty} p(v)dv\Big]^2}$$
$$-\frac{\int_{-\infty}^{\kappa} p(v)dv\Big[vp(v)\Big]_{v=-\infty}^{v=\kappa} - \int_{-\infty}^{\kappa} vp(v)dv\Big[p(v)\Big]_{v=-\infty}^{v=\kappa}}{\Big[\int_{-\infty}^{\kappa} p(v)dv\Big]^2}$$

Setting this equal to 0 and solving for κ gives

$$\begin{aligned}
&\Big[\int_{-\infty}^{\kappa} p(v)dv\Big]^2\Big\{\int_{\kappa}^{\infty} p(v)dv\Big[vp(v)\Big]_{v=\kappa}^{v=\infty} - \int_{\kappa}^{\infty} vp(v)dv\Big[p(v)\Big]_{v=\kappa}^{v=\infty}\Big\} \\
&\qquad -\Big[\int_{\kappa}^{\infty} p(v)dv\Big]^2\Big\{\int_{-\infty}^{\kappa} p(v)dv\Big[vp(v)\Big]_{v=-\infty}^{v=\kappa} \\
&\qquad -\int_{-\infty}^{\kappa} vp(v)dv\Big[p(v)\Big]_{v=-\infty}^{v=\kappa}\Big\} = 0 \\
&P(V \leq \kappa)^2 \quad \{-\kappa p(\kappa)P(V > \kappa) + p(\kappa)\int_{\kappa}^{\infty} vp(v)dv\} \\
&\qquad +P(V > \kappa)^2 \quad \{-\kappa p(\kappa)P(V \leq \kappa) + p(\kappa)\int_{-\infty}^{\kappa} vp(v)dv\} = 0 \\
&P(V \leq \kappa)^2 \quad \{-\kappa P(V > \kappa) + \int_{\kappa}^{\infty} vp(v)dv\} \\
&\qquad +P(V > \kappa)^2 \quad \{-\kappa P(V \leq \kappa) + \int_{-\infty}^{\kappa} vp(v)dv\} = 0.
\end{aligned}$$

The solution to the equation gives κ which could be obtained numerically.

The treatment rule that maximizes effect heterogeneity is then either $T = \{\omega \in \Omega : Y_1(\omega) - Y_0(\omega) \geq \kappa\}$ or $T = \{\omega \in \Omega : Y_1(\omega) - Y_0(\omega) > \kappa\}$. The maximum treatment effect heterogeneity that can thus be obtained comparing two subgroups that partition all individuals is thus $E(Y_1 - Y_0|Y_1 - Y_0 > \kappa) - E(Y_1 - Y_0|Y_1 - Y_0 \leq \kappa)$.

It is of course not possible to partition individuals in this manner without complete knowledge of the counterfactual outcomes. However, it is still possible to carry out a similar partitioning using measured covariates C. If we let Γ denote the support of C, the task becomes

$$\arg\max_{S,T \subseteq \Gamma: S \cup T = \Gamma, S \cap T = \emptyset}[E(Y_1 - Y_0|C \in T) - E(Y_1 - Y_0|C \in S)].$$

By arguments similar to those presented above, the sets S and T are then given by $T = \{c \in \Gamma : E(Y|A = 1, c) - E(Y|A = 0, c) > k\}$ and $S = \{c \in \Gamma : E(Y|A = 1, c) - E(Y|A = 0, c) \leq k\}$ for some k, and once again k could be solved for numerically.

The effect heterogeneity under this treatment rule for maximizing effect heterogeneity with measured covariates C is then given by:

$$\int \{E(Y|A=1,c) - E(Y|A=0,c)\}dP(c|C \in T)$$
$$-\int \{E(Y|A=1,c) - E(Y|A=0,c)\}dP(c|C \notin T).$$

Note that this measure of effect heterogeneity will not in general be as high as the maximum effect heterogeneity if both counterfactual outcomes for all individuals were known, which was given above as $E(Y_1 - Y_0|Y_1 - Y_0 \geq \kappa) - E(Y_1 - Y_0|Y_1 - Y_0 < \kappa)$. The extent to which the maximum effect heterogeneity under the treatment rule using the measured covariates C comes close to the maximum which can be obtained under complete knowledge of the counterfactual outcomes will depend on the extent to which the covariates C are predictive of the outcome itself. Note that it is also thus of course the case that the maximum effect heterogeneity under the treatment rule using data on the measured covariates C will always be relative to C. It might also be of interest to compare the treatment effect for those treated under the maximizing rule, $\int \{E(Y|A=1,c) - E(Y|A=0,c)\}dP(c|C \in T)$, to those left untreated by the rule $\int \{E(Y|A=1,c) - E(Y|A=0,c)\}dP(c|C \notin T)$, and also to the average treatment effect for the population $E(Y|A=1) - E(Y|A=0)$.

If using the treatment rule that maximizes effect heterogeneity, one can also estimate the average outcome under this rule as

$$\int_{c \in T} E(Y|A=1,c)dP(c) + \int_{c \notin T} E(Y|A=0,c)dP(c).$$

One could compare this to the average outcome with no one treated, $E(Y|A=0)$, and the average outcome with everyone treated, $E(Y|A=1)$. Note, however, this average outcome under the treatment rule that maximizes effect heterogeneity will in general be lower than the average outcome under the treatment rule that maximizes the average outcome itself as discussed in Context 2. It is thus not clear that this treatment rule that maximizes effect heterogeneity is of particular use in policy-making, unlike contexts 1, 2 and 3 above.

Further Comments on Observational Studies

The above approaches and results for randomized treatment A apply also to observational studies in which the covariates C suffice to control for confounding for the effect of A on Y but, when reference is made to the average outcome when no one is treated, $E(Y|A=0)$ must be replaced by $\int E(Y|A=0,c)dP(c)$; when reference is made to the average outcome when everyone is treated, $E(Y|A=1)$ must be replaced by $\int E(Y|A=1,c)dP(c)$; and when reference is made to the average treatment effect for the population $E(Y|A=1) - E(Y|A=0)$ must be replaced by $\int E(Y|A=1,c)dP(c) - \int E(Y|A=0,c)dP(c)$.

15.6.2 Statistical Estimation

Super-Learner for the Conditional Average Treatment Effect

The super-learner algorithm for this estimation problem is given below. For simplicity we use ten-fold cross-validation and assume that the sample size n is a multiple of ten. We suppose that the user has m candidate regression algorithms.

1. Define pseudo-observations $\tilde{Y}_1, \ldots, \tilde{Y}_n$.
2. For v in $\{1, \ldots, 10\}$:
   (a) For ℓ in $\{1, \ldots, m\}$:
      - Fit candidate algorithm ℓ on observations

$$\left((C_i, \tilde{Y}_i) : i \notin \left\{\frac{(v-1)n}{10} + 1, \ldots, \frac{vn}{10}\right\}\right)$$

      to generate the regression function estimate that takes as input c and outputs $\hat{E}_v^\ell[\tilde{Y}|c]$.

   (b) For i in $\left\{\frac{(v-1)n}{10} + 1, \ldots, \frac{vn}{10}\right\}$, define X_i^{CV} to be the m-length column vector $\left(\hat{E}_v^\ell[\tilde{Y}|c_i] : \ell = 1, \ldots, m\right)$.
3. Choose α_n be the convex m-length row vector minimizing $\frac{1}{n}\sum_{i=1}^n \left(\tilde{Y}_i - \alpha_n X_i^{\mathrm{CV}}\right)^2$.
4. For ℓ in $\{1, \ldots, m\}$:
   - Fit the candidates ℓ on all of the observations, yielding a function which takes as input c and outputs $\hat{E}^\ell[\tilde{Y}|c]$.
5. Return the function $\hat{b}$ defined by $\hat{b}(c) = \alpha_n X(c)$, where $X(c)$ is the column vector $\left(\hat{E}^\ell[\tilde{Y}|c] : \ell = 1, \ldots, m\right)$.

Estimator for Contexts 1 and 2

We now present a cross-validated targeted minimum loss-based estimator (CV-TMLE) for Contexts 1 and 2. We omit the derivation of this estimator from this work for brevity, and instead refer the reader to references given in the main text for the derivation of CV-TMLEs for nearly identical parameters as in Contexts 1 and 2. We assume that the outcome Y is bounded, and without loss of generality we assume that the lower bound is 0 and the upper bound is 1.

For simplicity, we use ten-fold cross-validation and assume that the sample size n is a multiple of ten. For each $v = 1, \ldots, 10$, we let T_v denote the observations (C_i, A_i, Y_i) with indices $i \notin \left\{\frac{(v-1)n}{10} + 1, \ldots, \frac{vn}{10}\right\}$, i.e. the observations included in the training sample for a given cross-validation split. We also let $v(i)$ denote the v such that $i \notin \left\{\frac{(v-1)n}{10} + 1, \ldots, \frac{vn}{10}\right\}$, i.e. the cross-validation index for which i is not in the training sample.

1. For v in $\{1, \ldots, 10\}$:
   (a) Obtain an estimate $\hat{E}_v[Y|\cdot]$ of the function mapping from (a, c) to $E[Y|a, c]$ using observations in T_v.
   (b) Obtain an estimate $\hat{b}_v$ of the CATE function using observations in T_v.
   Note: $\hat{b}_v(c)$ need not equal $\hat{E}[Y|A = 1, c] - \hat{E}[Y|A = 0, c]$.
2. Let $\delta_n = 0$ in Context 2, and in Context 1 let δ_n be the positive part of the smallest solution in δ to

$$\frac{1}{n}\sum_{i=1}^n 1(\hat{b}_{v(i)}(c) > \delta) \leq q.$$

3. Let ϵ_n be the slope estimate in an intercept-free logistic regression with outcome $(Y_i : i = 1, \ldots, n)$, covariate $\left(\frac{2A_i - 1}{P(A_i|C_i)} : i = 1, \ldots, n\right)$, offset $\left(\text{logit}\hat{E}_{v(i)}[Y|A_i, C_i] : i = 1, \ldots, n\right)$, and observation weights $\left(1\left\{\hat{b}_{v(i)}(C_i) > \delta_n\right\} : i = 1, \ldots, n\right)$.
   Note: The `glm` function in `R` will run a logistic regression on any outcome bounded in $[0, 1]$.
4. For each v in $\{1, \ldots, 10\}$ and any (a, c), let $\bar{Q}^*_v(a, c) = \text{logit}^{-1}\left[\text{logit}\left(\hat{E}_v[Y|a, c]\right) + \epsilon_n \frac{2a-1}{P(a|c)}\right]$ represent the fluctuated estimate of $E[Y|a, c]$.
5. Let $\hat{\psi} = \frac{1}{n}\sum_{i=1}^{n} 1(\hat{b}_{v(i)}(C_i) > \delta_n)\left[\bar{Q}^*_{v(i)}(1, C_i) - \bar{Q}^*_{v(i)}(0, C_i)\right]$.
6. Let $D_i = \frac{2A_i - 1}{P(A_i|C_i)}\left[Y_i - \bar{Q}^*_{v(i)}(A_i, C_i)\right] + \bar{Q}^*_{v(i)}(1, C_i) - \bar{Q}^*_{v(i)}(0, C_i) - \hat{\psi}$.
7. Let

$$\hat{\sigma}^2 = \frac{1}{n}\sum_{i=1}^{n}\left[1(\hat{b}_{v(i)}(C_i) > \delta_n)\left[D_i - \delta_n\right] + \delta_n q\right]^2,$$

   where we take $q = 1$ in Context 2.
8. Return the point estimate $\hat{\psi}$ and 95% confidence interval $\hat{\psi} \pm 1.96\frac{\hat{\sigma}}{\sqrt{n}}$.

15.6.3 Software Demonstration

In this section we present software for estimating the optimal treatment rule and for obtaining inference for the impact of implementing this rule in the population. This appendix uses functions that appear in version 0.31 of the `sg` package, which is available at `https://github.com/alexluedtke12/sg@v0.31`. The most recent version can be found at `https://github.com/alexluedtke12/sg`.

We first install the `sg` package from GitHub using the `devtools` package, and subsequently load the package.

```
library(devtools)
devtools::install_github("alexluedtke12/sg@v0.31")
library(sg)
```

The remainder of this demonstration is structured as follows. First, we show how to use the `sg` package to estimate the CATE function. Then, we show how to evaluate the impact of treating an optimal treatment rule, both in the presence and in the absence of a resource constraint.

Estimating the CATE Function

This demonstration will use the following simple simulated data set.

```
# set seed for random number generator
set.seed(1)
# function for simulating data
sim.data = function(nn){
# covariates
W = data.frame(W1=rnorm(nn),W2=rnorm(nn), W3=rnorm(nn))
# treatment indicator
A = rbinom(nn,1,1/2)
# binary outcome
Y = rbinom(nn,1,Qbar(A,W))
return(list(W=W,A=A,Y=Y))
}
# SuperLearner library
# Note: a restricted library is used in this example to reduce
#  runtime. In practice we recommend using a larger library.
#  Use command ``listWrappers()'' to see other prediction
#  algorithm wrappers.
SL.library = c('SL.mean','SL.glm','SL.gam')
# sample size
n = 1000
# E[Y|A,W]
Qbar = function(a,w){plogis(-1 - a*w$W1^2 + 2*a*w$W2)}
# data to use when running the methods
dat = sim.data(n)
W = dat$W
A = dat$A
Y = dat$Y
# data to use when evaluating true parameter values
n.mc = 2e4
dat = sim.data(n.mc)
W.mc = dat$W
A.mc = dat$A
Y.mc = dat$Y
# conditional average treatment effect function
cate.mc = Qbar(1,W.mc)-Qbar(0,W.mc)
```

We note that $A = 1$ and $A = 0$ can denote two different active treatments, or treatment and control.

The CATE function can be estimated using the `sg.SL` wrapper for the ensemble `SuperLearner` algorithm (van der Laan et al., 2007).

```
sl.out = sg.SL(W,A,Y,SL.library=SL.library,family=binomial())
# compare estimated CATE to true CATE in data set
plot(Qbar(1,W)-Qbar(0,W),sl.out$est,xlab="True CATE",ylab="Estimated CATE")
```

The output of the above plot is displayed in Figure 15.1.

The impact of different variables on the CATE function can be evaluated graphically. Here, we set `W2` and `W3` to their sample medians and plot the estimated CATE against `W1`.

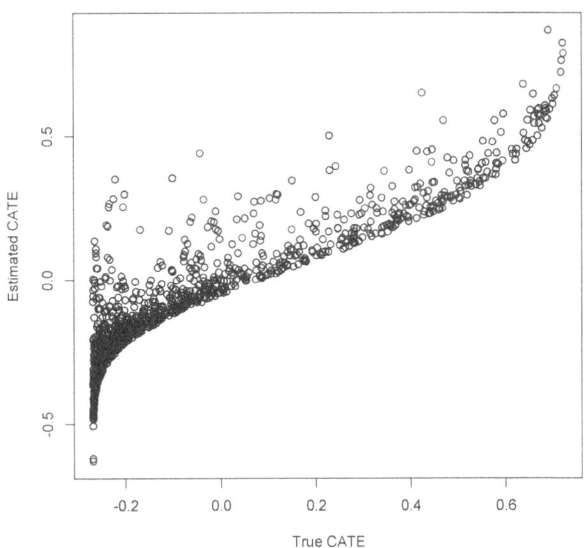

Figure 15.1 *Estimated versus true CATE in the software demonstration.*

```
# W1 values at which to evaluate the CATE
W1.vals = quantile(W$W1,seq(0.001,0.95,by=0.05))
# estimated CATE with W2 and W3 set to their medians
cate.W1 = predict(
sl.out$SL,
newdata=data.frame(
W1=W1.vals,
W2=median(W$W2),
W3=median(W$W3)))$pred
# plot estimated CATE against W2
plot(W1.vals,cate.W1,xlab="W1",ylab="CATE",type='l')
```

The output of the above plot is displayed in Figure 15.2.

Evaluating the Impact of Implementing the Optimal Treatment Rule

We now evaluate the impact of treating the optimal rule in the presence and the absence of resource constraints. Here we use the same simulated data set as was used to estimate the CATE function.

We start with a setting where at most 25% of the population can be treated. This function gives an additive contrast between the mean outcome under the estimated optimal treatment rule and the mean outcome under a stochastic baseline rule that treats all individuals in the population at random, regardless of the covariates. The probability of receiving (treatment $A = 0$, treatment $A = 1$) according to this stochastic baseline rule is dictated by the `baseline.probs` input argument. Larger values of `num.SL.rep` and `num.est.rep` reduce the stochasticity of output due to cross-validation splits but increases runtime.

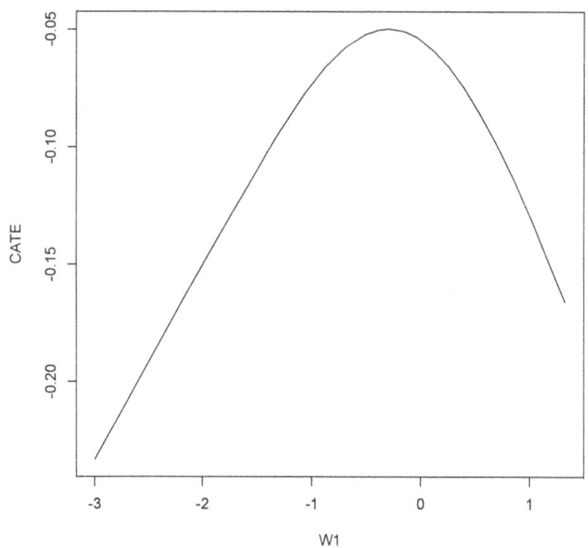

Figure 15.2 *CATE vs.* `W1` *in the software demonstration, where* `W2` *and* `W3` *are set to the sample medians.*

```
sg.cvtmle(W,A,Y,
baseline.probs=c(0.75,0.25), # baseline assigns A=1 with
# probability 25%
SL.library=SL.library,
family=binomial(),
kappa=0.25, # the optimal rule may treat at most
#25% of the population
num.SL.rep=2,
num.est.rep=2,
lib.ests=TRUE)
# R Console Output
# $est
# SuperLearner  SL.mean_All   SL.glm_All   SL.gam_All
#  0.107210896  0.008358105  0.098576837  0.107210896
#
# $ci
#                        lb         ub
# SuperLearner  0.083688690 0.13073310
# SL.mean_All  -0.004555034 0.02127124
# SL.glm_All    0.075308929 0.12184474
# SL.gam_All    0.083688690 0.13073310
#
# $est.mat
#               SuperLearner SL.mean_All SL.glm_All SL.gam_All
# Repetition 1     0.1048418 0.008381272 0.09828244  0.1048418
# Repetition 2     0.1095800 0.008334938 0.09887123  0.1095800
```

The output of `sg.cvtmle` is a three-argument list. The `est` argument displays the estimated impact of implementing the treatment strategy estimated by SuperLearner, and also the impact of implementing treatment rules estimated by the candidate algorithms included in the SuperLearner library. The `ci` argument contains the corresponding 95% level confidence intervals. The `est.mat` argument shows the separate estimates obtained during the `num.est.rep` repetitions of the estimation procedure. The final estimate is equal to the mean of these repetition-specific estimates.

The estimates presented above are close to the true improvement under the resource-constrained optimal rule, which can be evaluated in our simulation because we know the true data-generating distribution.

```
# truth
mean(
Qbar(1,W.mc)*((cate.mc>=max(quantile(cate.mc,1-0.25),0))-0.25) +
Qbar(0,W.mc)*((cate.mc<max(quantile(cate.mc,1-0.25),0))-0.75))
# R Console Output
# [1] 0.105269
```

Note that the `sg.cvtmle` function does not currently support individual-level treatment costs, i.e. it only allows estimating optimal treatment effects when the cost of assigning treatment is fixed across all individuals in the population. In these cases, when $A = 1$ is more expensive than $A = 0$ a cost constraint is equivalent to constraining the proportion of individuals in the population who can be treated.

Below we remove the resource constraint and contrast it against a baseline treating individuals with $A = 1$ with probability $1/2$.

```
sg.cvtmle(W,A,Y,
baseline.probs=c(0.50,0.50), # baseline assigns A=1 with
# probability 50%
SL.library=SL.library,
family=binomial(),
kappa=1, # no resource constraint
num.SL.rep=2,
num.est.rep=2,
lib.ests=TRUE)
# R Console Output
# $est
# SuperLearner  SL.mean_All   SL.glm_All   SL.gam_All
#   0.11078319   0.01672297   0.10478232   0.11078319
#
# $ci
#                        lb         ub
# SuperLearner  0.085855224 0.13571116
# SL.mean_All  -0.009112482 0.04255842
# SL.glm_All    0.079753790 0.12981086
# SL.gam_All    0.085855224 0.13571116
#
# $est.mat
#              SuperLearner SL.mean_All SL.glm_All SL.gam_All
# Repetition 1    0.1104028  0.01710950  0.1036115  0.1104028
# Repetition 2    0.1111636  0.01633644  0.1059532  0.1111636
```

To contrast against a baseline rule that treats everyone with $A = 0$, let `baseline.probs=c(1,0)`. To estimate the marginal mean outcome under the estimated optimal treatment rule without contrasting against a baseline treatment rule, let `baseline.probs=c(0,0)`.

The above estimate is close to the true improvement under the unconstrained optimal rule.

```
# truth
mean(Qbar(1,W.mc)*((cate.mc>=0)-0.50) + Qbar(0,W.mc)*((cate.mc<0)-0.50))
# R Console Output
# [1] 0.1162848
```

Chapter 16

Statistical Learning Methods for Estimating Optimal Individualized Treatment Rules from Observational Data

Qijia He, Ying-Qi Zhao

16.1 Introduction

Personalized medicine is an emerging practice that strives to improve the quality of healthcare by tailoring treatment to individual patient information. Individualized treatment rules (ITRs) formalize tailored treatment decisions a decision rule that maps patient information to a recommended treatment (Kosorok and Laber, 2019). An optimal ITR is the decision rule that leads to the best expected outcome overall, if followed by the whole population.

There is a wealth of literature on statistical methods for estimating an optimal ITR (Qian and Murphy, 2011; Zhang et al., 2012; Zhao et al., 2012; Zhang et al., 2012; Zhou et al., 2017; Zhao et al., 2019; Wu et al., 2020; Cui and Tchetgen Tchetgen, 2021). One approach is to express the optimal ITR as a function of the conditional mean of the outcome or contrast given treatment and covariates and then to estimate the ITR by first estimating these conditional expectations. Estimators of this form (e.g., Moodie et al., 2014; Qian and Murphy, 2011; Murphy, 2003; Robins, 2004; Moodie et al., 2007; Henderson et al., 2010; Shi et al., 2016) are often called indirect methods, as they indirectly specify the optimal ITRs based on a postulated mean model. A potential drawback associated with indirect estimators is the risk of misspecification of the requisite mean models. An alternative, is to optimize an estimator of the marginal mean outcome over a predefined set of ITRs. These methods are referred to as direct (Laber et al., 2014), value-search (Davidian et al., 2014), or policy learning (Athey et al., 2017) estimators. Direct methods may be less susceptible to misspecification. They have the additional benefit of allowing the researcher to specify a class of decision rules that satisfy logistic, interpretability, or other constraints.

Randomized controlled trials (RCTs) are the gold-standard for studying treatment effectiveness and learning causal relationships. However, RCTs are typically costly to run, require large sample sizes, and are conducted under strict enrollment criteria (Moodie et al., 2014; Song and Chung, 2010). Consequently, they may be limited in their generalization to a broader (e.g., real-world) patient population. In contrast, observational studies are often collected under less restrictive criteria and are therefore often larger and potentially more representative. There is a growing interest in estimating optimal ITRs from observational data, including electronic health records. However, these methods bear the risk of unmeasured confounding and selection bias (Liang et al., 2021).

To avoid unmeasured confounding of the treatment-outcome relationship, existing methods for estimating ITRs from observational data (Moodie et al., 2012) generally require a sufficiently rich set of covariates. Nevertheless, it is not always possible to rule out unmeasured confounding, particularly in observational studies and randomized trials with noncompliance as many important factors may be missing (Qiu et al., 2021). Recently, there

DOI: 10.1201/9781003216223-16

have been proposals to employ instrumental variable techniques (Cui and Tchetgen Tchetgen, 2021) or proximal causal inference (Qiu et al., 2021) to solve potential unmeasured confounding in the estimation of ITRs.

In this chapter, we present some approaches for estimating optimal ITRs from observational data. In Section 16.2, we review estimation for ITR estimation in observational studies under the no-unmeasured confounding assumption. We introduce two indirect methods, Q-learning and A-learning, as well as a direct method, outcome weighted learning. In section 16.3, we discuss estimation of ITRs under unmeasured confounding. The problem of optimal ITRs estimation under endogeneity can be addressed through the use of instrumental variables or the idea of proximal learning. A concluding discussion is provided in Section 16.4.

16.2 Individualized Treatment Rules Under No Unmeasured Confounding

16.2.1 Setup and Notation

We consider observational data in the single-stage setting. The complete data is composed of n independently identically distributed triples $(X_i, A_i, Y_i), i = 1, 2, \ldots, n$, where $X \in \mathscr{X}$ denotes covariates that are measured before the treatment decision is made, $A \in \mathscr{A} = \{0, 1\}$ denotes the binary treatment, and $Y \in \mathscr{Y} \subseteq \mathbb{R}$ denotes the observed outcome at the end of treatment. Without loss of generality, we assume that larger outcomes are more favorable. Note that X may contain confounding variables, i.e., variables which affect both treatment and outcome, which much be accounted for in estimating the treatment effect. (I.e., one cannot simply take the difference in means between the treatment and control groups.)

An individualized treatment rule (ITR), d, is a decision function that maps $\mathscr{X}$ to $\mathscr{A}$, so that under d a patient with $X = x$ will be assigned treatment $d(x)$. Let $\mathscr{D}$ be the set of all possible ITRs. We use the framework of potential outcomes (Rubin, 1974; Splawa-Neyman et al., 1990) to define the optimal ITR, denoted as d^*. Let $Y(a)$ be the potential outcome under treatment $a \in \{0, 1\}$, and define $Y(d) = \sum_{a \in \{0,1\}} Y(a) I\{a = d(X)\}$ to be the potential outcome under d. The value function, $V(d)$, is defined as the marginal mean outcome, $V(d) = E\{Y(d)\}$. The optimal ITR d^* is the ITR that maximizes $V(d)$ over all possible $d \in \mathscr{D}$, i.e., $V(d^*) \geq V(d), d \in \mathscr{D}$. To express the value in terms of the data-generating model and to derive the optimal ITRs from the observed data, we typically assume: (i) no unmeasured confounders, $\{Y(0), Y(1)\} \perp A|X$ (Rubin, 1974; Splawa-Neyman et al., 1990); (ii) consistency, $Y = Y(A)$; and (iii) positivity, there exists $\tau > 0$ so that $\tau < P(A = a|X)$ for each $a \in \mathscr{A}$ with probability one. These assumptions are satisfied in randomized clinical trials, but can be violated in observational studies. Hence, careful design and analysis techniques are required to develop ITRs from observational studies. In this section, we consider the situation where no unmeasured confounders assumption is satisfied. The next section considers estimation of ITRs when this assumption is violated.

16.2.2 Q-Learning

Q-learning is a two-step regression-based approach that has been used extensively in practice. We first describe a basic (vanilla) version of the algorithm with linear models that has been widely used, especially with data from randomized studies (Moodie et al., 2012). Define the so-called Q-function as $Q(x, a) = E(Y|X = x, A = a)$. It follows from the causal assumptions made in the preceding section that the value function can be expressed as $V(d) = EQ\{X, d(X)\}$. Thus, for any ITR d, it can be seen that $EQ\{X, d(X)\} \leq E\left[\max_{a \in \mathscr{A}} Q(X, a)\right]$, hence the optimal regime is given by $d^*(x) = \arg\max_{a \mathscr{A}} Q(x, a)$.

Given the preceding expression for the optimal ITR, a natural approach is to construct an estimator $\widehat{Q}_n$ of the Q-function and subsequently $\widehat{d_n}(x) = \arg\max_{a \in \mathscr{A}} \widehat{Q}_n(x, a)$ as the estimated optimal regime. To illustrate this idea, we assume the outcome is continuous and posit a linear model working model

$$Q(x, a; \xi) = x^T \beta + \left(x^T \psi\right) a, \tag{16.1}$$

where $\xi = (\beta^T, \psi^T)^T$. An intercept is assumed to be included in x. Under this model,

$$\max_{a \in \{0,1\}} Q(x, a; \xi) = x^T \beta + (x^T \psi) I(x^T \psi > 0),$$

and, if ξ^* is the true underlying parameter, then $d^*(x) = I\left(x^T \psi^* > 0\right)$. We can construct an estimator $\widehat{\xi}_n$ of ξ^* using least squares, so that

$$\widehat{\xi}_n = \arg\min_{\xi} \mathbb{E}_n \left\{Y - Q\left(X, A; \xi\right)\right\}^2,$$

where $\mathbb{E}_n$ denotes the empirical average. The optimal ITR can be estimated via $\widehat{d}_n(x) = I(x^T \hat{\psi}_n > 0)$.

The validity of applying Q-learning to observational data relies on the the assumption of no unmeasured confounding. Potential biases may arise from unmeasured confounding factors that affect the treatment assignment probabilities given the baseline covariates. This reflects a selection bias stemming from nonrandom treatment assignment. In such scenarioss, Q-learning could be implemented in combination with methodologies that adjust for confounding Robins (1999). Particularly, the Q-function could be estimated weighted linear regression using inverse probability of treatment weighting (IPTW) approach. IPTW balances the covariates by weighing subjects in the treatment group by $\pi(1|x)^{-1}$, and those in the control group by $\pi(0|x)^{-1}$. This creates a pseudo-sample in which treatment is independent of the variables that are included in the propensity score (Moodie et al., 2012). However, it should be noted that if the model for Q-function is correctly specified, weighting is ineffective since there is no bias to eliminate. When the model for Q-function is incorrectly specified, weighting may reduce bias if the propensity scores can be accurately estimated, albeit with an increase in variance Freedman and Berk (2008).

Recent developments have enhanced the robustness of Q-learning methodologies. Tian et al. (2014) developed an approach which models the treatment-covariate interaction effect directly within a regression framework, without the need to specify a main effect model or model the conditional mean function. A one-step "Direct Learning" approach using regression techniques and its extensions has been proposed with applications to multi-arm treatment settings (Qi and Liu, 2018; Qi et al., 2020). Ertefaie et al. (2021) proposed a robust Q-learning approach where the main effects in Q-function that do not influence the optimal decision rules are estimated using data-adaptive approaches, reducing the risk of estimation inconsistency.

16.2.3 A-Learning and G-Estimation

A-learning (Murphy, 2003; Robins, 2004; Blatt et al., 2004; Moodie et al., 2007) is an alternative method for estimating an optimal ITR that relies on modeling the contrast function, $C(x) = Q(x, 1) - Q(x, 0)$. To see why this is valuable. Consider again the working model $Q(x, a; \xi) = x^T \beta + \left(x^T \psi\right) a$. As mentioned previously, the optimal ITR $d^*(x)$, only depends on the sign of $x^T \psi^*$, which is equal to $I\{Q(x, 1; \xi^*) - Q(x, 0; \xi^*) > 0\} = I\{C(x; \psi^*) > 0\}$, where $C(x; \psi) = x^T \psi$. By focusing on the contrast function instead of the entire Q-function, A-learning is potentially more flexible and robust to modeling misspecification.

A-learning has appeared in multiple forms each with its own terminology (see Moodie et al., 2007; Tsiatis et al., 2019). When treatments are binary, $aC(x; \psi)$ corresponds to the so-called optimal-blip-to-zero function for g-estimation. Murphy (2003) refers

$C(x;\psi)[I\{C(x;\psi)>0\}-A]$ as the advantage or regret function. Intuitively, this expression represents the advantage brought by the optimal treatment, compared to the one actually received.

To implement A-learning, we first specify a model $C(x;\psi)$ for the contrast function, with ψ being an unknown parameter. We then impose a model $\pi(a|x;\gamma)$ for the propensity score, indexed by unknown parameter γ. All consistent and asymptotically normal estimators of ψ can be obtained via solving the equation given below (Robins, 2004; Zhang et al., 2013),

$$\sum_{i=1}^{n} \lambda(X_i)\left\{A_i-\pi(A_i|X_i;\gamma)\right\}\left\{Y_i-A_iC(X_i;\psi)-Q(X_i,0;\beta)\right\}=0, \tag{16.2}$$

where $\lambda(X_i)$ can be any function, the dimension of which is the same as ψ. Suppose the model $C(X_i;\psi)$ is correct, if $\text{var}(Y|X)$ is constant, then $\lambda(X_i)=\partial\{C(X;\psi)\}/\partial\psi$ provides the optimal choice for this function; if $\text{var}(Y|X)$ is not constant, Robins (2004) showed that the form of an optimal $\lambda(X_i)$ will be complex.

The propensity score $\pi(a|x;\gamma)$ and the main effect term $Q(x,0;\beta)$ are, of course, unknown and need to be estimated. We can model the propensity score using techniques such as logistic regression. If the outcome is continuous, we can model $Q(X,0;\beta)$ using linear regression. Semi-parametric and non-parametric methods can also be applied. If the contrast function is correctly specified, then as long as either propensity or main effect (not necessarily both) are correctly specified, the estimator $\widehat{\psi}_n$ generated by solving equation (16.2) will be consistent for ψ. The plug-in estimator $\widehat{d}_n(x)=I\{C(x;\widehat{\psi}_n)>0\}$ will also therefore be consistent. That only one of the two nuisance models needs to be correctly specified for consistency is the so-called double robustness property.

16.2.4 Value-Search Methods

Direct-search or value-search methods have gained popularity in recent years. This popularity is driven, at least in part, by the potential for increased robustness to model misspecification and the ability to explicitly pre-specify the class of ITRs which might be chosen to be clinically interpretable, parsimonious, or to satisfy cost or other constraints. Value-search methods estimate an optimal ITR by first constructing an estimator of the value function and then taking the maximizer over a pre-specified class of regimes as the estimator of the optimal regime (Zhang et al., 2012; Zhao et al., 2012).

Let $\widehat{Q}_n(x,a)$ denote an estimator of $Q(x,a)$, and $\widehat{\pi}_n(a|x)$ an estimator of the propensity score. The augmented inverse probability weighted estimator (AIPWE) of the value function is

$$\begin{aligned}\widehat{V}_n^{\text{AIPWE}}(d) \triangleq \mathbb{E}_n\Bigg[&\frac{YI\{A=d(X)\}}{\widehat{\pi}_n\{d(X)|X\}}\\ &-\frac{I\{A=d(X)\}-\widehat{\pi}_n\{d(X)|X\}}{\widehat{\pi}_n\{d(X)|X\}}\widehat{Q}_n\{X,d(X)\}\Bigg].\end{aligned} \tag{16.3}$$

It has been shown that $\widehat{V}_n^{\text{AIPWE}}(d)$ is doubly-robust in the sense that if either the propensity model or the model for the Q-function is correctly specified, but not necessarily both, then $\widehat{V}_n^{\text{AIPWE}}(d)$ is consistent for $V(d)$. The AIPWE can be viewed as an inverse probability weighted estimator (IPWE), plus an estimator of zero that is negatively correlated with the IPWE thereby reducing variance. If $\widehat{Q}_n\{X,d(X)\}\equiv 0$, then $\widehat{V}_n^{\text{AIPWE}}(d)$ reduces to the IPWE

$$\widehat{V}_n^{\text{IPWE}}(d)=\mathbb{E}_n\left[\frac{Y}{\widehat{\pi}_n(A|X)}I\{A=d(X)\}\right]. \tag{16.4}$$

Table 16.1 *Functional form of commonly used surrogates loss functions*

Loss Function	Expression
0-1 Loss	$I(t \geq 0) \cdot 0 + I(t < 0) \cdot 1$
Hinge Loss	$\max(1-t, 0)$
Exponential Loss	e^{-t}
Logistic Loss	$\log(1+e^{-t})$

We first review direct-search estimators based on the IPWE before proceeding to those based on the AIPWE.

Outcome weighted learning, proposed in Zhao et al. (2012), constructed the ITRs based on the IPWE as follows. Due to the discontinuous and nonconvex 0-1 indicator functions, it is computationally challenging to directly optimize $\widehat{V}^{\text{IPWE}}(d)$, especially over a large set of ITRs. A common method in classification literature is to minimize a surrogate objective, where the 0-1 loss function in the classification error is replaced by a convex surrogate loss function (Bartlett et al., 2006). This technique was employed by Zhao et al. (2012). Define $\mathcal{M}$ as the set of measurable functions $f : \mathbb{R}^p \to \mathbb{R}$. For any ITR d, we can write $I\{a = d(x)\} = I\{(2a-1)f(x) \geq 0\}$. Let $\mathcal{F} \subseteq \mathcal{M}$ be a Hilbert space equipped with norm $\|\cdot\|$. We can then minimize over $f \in \mathcal{F}$ the following surrogate objective function,

$$\mathbb{E}_n\left[\frac{Y}{\widehat{\pi}_n(A|X)}\phi\{(2A-1)f(X)\}\right] + \lambda_n\|f\|^2.$$

The penalty term is applied to prevent over-fitting, and $\lambda_n \geq 0$ is a tuning parameter controlling the amount of penalization. Popular choices of the surrogate loss functions include hinge loss and logistic loss. See Table 16.1 and Figure 16.1 for a list of common surrogate loss functions. However, the IPWE only takes into account outcomes from subjects who receive treatment consistent with d, and is therefore inefficient. Additionally, if the propensity model is incorrectly specified, the $\widehat{V}_n^{\text{IPWE}}(d)$ need not be consistent for $V(d)$, and the estimated ITR is subsequently need not be consistent for the optimal ITR. It is ideal to develop more efficient and robust methods for deriving ITRs from observational studies. Zhao et al. (2019) propose to estimate the optimal ITRs by maximizing a concave relaxation of $\widehat{V}_n^{\text{AIPWE}}(d)$, which is computationally and statistically efficient while maintaining the double robustness property.

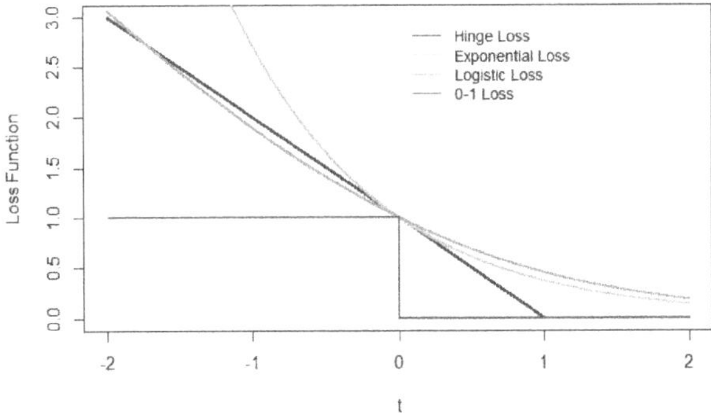

Figure 16.1 *Common convex surrogate loss functions*

Define

$$\widehat{W}_{a,n} = W_a(Y, X, A, \widehat{\pi}_n, \widehat{Q}_n) = \frac{YI\{A=a\}}{\widehat{\pi}_n(a|X)} - \frac{I\{A=a\} - \widehat{\pi}_n\{a|X\}}{\widehat{\pi}_n(a|X)} \widehat{Q}_n(X,a).$$

It can be shown that

$$\begin{aligned}\widehat{f}_n &= \arg\sup_{f \in \mathcal{F}} \widehat{V}^{\text{AIPWE}}(f) \\ &= \arg\inf_{f \in \mathcal{F}} \mathbb{E}_n \left[\left| \widehat{W}_{1,n} \right| I \left\{ \text{sign}\left(\widehat{W}_{1,n} \right) f(X) < 0 \right\} \right. \\ &\qquad \left. + \left| \widehat{W}_{n,0} \right| I \left\{ -\text{sign}\left(\widehat{W}_{0,n} \right) f(X) < 0 \right\} \right].\end{aligned}$$

Therefore, solving the optimal decision function is equivalent to minimizing a weighted 0-1 loss. In this case, the class labels are $(2a-1)\,\text{sign}\left(\widehat{W}_{a,n}\right)$ and the weights are $\left|\widehat{W}_{a,n}\right|$. By replacing the indicator function with a surrogate, the efficient augmentation and relaxation learning (EARL) estimator is defined as

$$\begin{aligned}\widetilde{f}_n^{\lambda_n} = \arg\inf_{f \in \mathcal{F}} \mathbb{E}_n & \left[\left| \widehat{W}_{1,n} \right| \phi \left\{ \text{sign}\left(\widehat{W}_{1,n} \right) f(X) \right\} \right. \\ & \left. + \left| \widehat{W}_{0,n} \right| \phi \left\{ -\text{sign}\left(\widehat{W}_{0,n} \right) f(X) \right\} \right] + \lambda_n \|f\|^2.\end{aligned} \tag{16.5}$$

That $\widehat{Q}_n$, $\widehat{\pi}_n$, and $\widetilde{f}_n^{\lambda_n}$ are all constructed from the same sample induces dependence which can complicate asymptotic arguments or require strong assumptions about the model classes for these estimators (see Chapter 9). To remove this dependency, one can employ sample splitting as follows. First, randomly partition the n samples into K subsets, $I_1, \ldots, I_K$, where K is a fixed integer. For each $k \in \{1, \ldots, K\}$, use I_k to construct estimators $\widehat{Q}_n^{(k)}$ and $\widehat{\pi}_n^{(k)}$. Use the remainder of the sample $I_{(-k)} = \{1, \ldots, K\} \backslash I_k$ to construct an estimator of the optimal ITR via (16.5) with $\widehat{Q}_n^{(k)}$ and $\widehat{\pi}_n^{(k)}$ plugged in. The final EARL estimator is constructed by aggregating over the K partitions. For a discussion of the asymptotic theory for this estimator, including the advantages of sample splitting, see Zhao et al. (2019).

There are other value-search methods. For example, Zhang et al. (2012) proposed to directly optimize $\widehat{V}_n^{\text{AIPWE}}(d)$ over a restricted class using a genetic algorithm. Zhou et al. (2017) proposed the residual weighted learning approach, which weights misclassification errors using residuals of outcome from regression fitting on covariates without considering treatment assignment. Tree-based methods are also proposed within the framework of value search approaches (Laber and Zhao, 2015; Cui et al., 2017; Kallus, 2018).

16.3 Individualized Treatment Rules Under Unmeasured Confounding

In order to mitigate confounding effects in observational studies, it is important to collect and adjust for as many relevant variables as possible. However, this still may not be sufficient to ensure the no unmeasured confounders assumption holds. An alternative approach, that does not require this assumption, is to use instrumental variables (IVs). An IV is a pre-treatment variable that is independent of all unmeasured confounding factors and has no direct causal effect on the outcome except through the treatment (Myers et al., 2011; Baiocchi et al., 2014; Cui and Tchetgen Tchetgen, 2021). Endogeneity occurs whenever an unobserved variable U is related to both explanatory variable A and response variable Y, but the U is not incorporated in the model, which means unmeasured confounding exists in the model. One can identify the unobserved correlation between the explanatory variable and the response variable by using an IV. We will denote an unmeasured confounder as U, and an observed binary pre-treatment IV as Z which we code to take values in $\{-1, 1\}$.

Cui and Tchetgen Tchetgen (2021) proposed a semiparametric instrumental variable method to estimate optimal ITRs with unmeasured confounding. It is necessary to make several assumptions in order to identify the optimal ITR under unmeasured confounding. Denote by $Y(z, a)$ the potential outcome when the IV is z and the treatment is a.
Assumption 1 (Latent unconfoundedness) $Y(z, a) \perp (Z, A) \mid X, U$ for each (z, a).
I.e., if U were known, then the confounding for Z and A on Y can be eliminated.
Assumption 2 (IV relevance) $Z \not\perp A \mid X$.
Assumption 3 (Exclusion restriction) $Y(z, a) = Y(a)$ for $z = \pm 1$, a=0, 1 almost surely.
Assumption 4 (IV independence) $Z \perp U \mid X$.
Assumptions 2 – 4 are general conditions for IVs. Assumption 2 states that Z and A are not independent given X. Assumption 3 claims that it is only through A that Z can have causal effect on Y. And assumption 4 says that Z and U are independent given X, which means the causal effect of Z on Y is not confounded given X.
In addition, we will make use of the following assumptions.
Assumption 5 (IV positivity) $0 < P(Z = 1 \mid X) < 1$ almost surely.
This assumption is required for nonparametric identification.
Assumption 6 (No unmeasured common effect modifier)

$$\operatorname{cov}\{\widetilde{\delta}(X, U), \widetilde{\gamma}(X, U) \mid X\} = 0$$

almost surely, where $\widetilde{\delta}(X, U) \equiv P(A = 1 \mid Z = 1, X, U) - P(A = 1 \mid Z = -1, X, U)$ and $\widetilde{\gamma}(X, U) \equiv E(Y(1) - Y(0) \mid X, U)$.
It indicates that there is no common effect modifier for the effect of treatment on the outcome and effect of IV on treatment.
Assumption 7 (Independent compliance type)

$$\delta(X) \equiv P(A = 1 \mid Z = 1, X) - P(A = 1 \mid Z = -1, X) = \widetilde{\delta}(H, U),$$

almost surely. This assumption would hold if U would be independent of the compliance type of a person (Wang and Tchetgen Tchetgen, 2018).

Under Assumptions 1–6 and the previously introduced positivity and consistency assumptions, Cui and Tchetgen Tchetgen (2021) proved that $\arg\max_{d \in \mathcal{D}} E\{Y(d)\}$ can be identified nonparametrically two different ways,

$$\arg\max_{d \in \mathcal{D}} E\{Y(d)\} = \arg\max_{d} E\left[\frac{Z(2A-1)YI\{A = d(X)\}}{\delta(X)P(Z \mid X)}\right], \text{and} \tag{16.6}$$

$$\arg\max_{d \in \mathcal{D}} E\{Y(d)\} = \arg\max_{d} E\left[\frac{YI\{Z = 2d(X) - 1\}}{\delta(X)P(Z \mid X)}\right]. \tag{16.7}$$

Equation (16.6) suggests that one may extend the prior identification of optimal treatment regimes to account for the confounding effect of an unmeasured factor by nonparametrically identifying optimal treatment regimes with valid IVs that satisfy Assumption 6. Equation (16.7) suggests that if Z and A are positively correlated, i.e., $\delta(X) > 0$, then the optimal ITR can potentially be identified even though treatment A is unobserved, by solving $\arg\max_d E\left[\widetilde{W}(X)YI\{Z = 2d(X) - 1\}P(Z \mid X)\right]$ given any possible weight $\widetilde{W}(X) > 0$. Moreover, if there is enough external information to estimate $\delta(X)$, then we can let $\widetilde{W}(X) = 1/\delta(X)$ to solve the optimization problem. This situation occurs if another data set consisting of $\{A, Z, X\}$ is available.

Two classification-based estimators are proposed by Cui and Tchetgen Tchetgen (2021). Equation (16.6) and (16.7) can be respectively expressed as

$$\arg\min_{d\in\mathcal{D}} E\left[W^{(1)} I\{A \neq d(X)\}\right], \tag{16.8}$$

$$\arg\min_{d\in\mathcal{D}} E\left[W^{(2)} I\{Z \neq 2d(X) - 1\}\right], \tag{16.9}$$

where $W^{(1)} = Z(2A-1)Y/\delta(X)P(Z \mid L)$, $W^{(2)} = Y/\delta(X)P(Z \mid X)$. Intuitively, either (16.8) or (16.9) can be interpreted as a classification problem aimed at sorting A (or Z) using X by minimizing the expectation of the weighted misclassification error. They adopted the same techniques as outcome-weighted learning (OWL), by replacing the indicator function with a surrogate loss function.

On the basis of the IV approach to weighted learning discussed above, Cui and Tchetgen Tchetgen (2021) developed a multiply robust classification-based estimator of optimal ITR to eliminate the restriction of treatment regimes. They proposed a statistic for the average treatment effect given X, which can be estimated by maximum likelihood estimation or machine learning methods. In addition, multiply robust estimators for both $E\left[W^{(1)} I\{A \neq d(X)\}\right]$ and $E\left[W^{(2)} I\{Z \neq 2d(X) - 1\}\right]$ were proposed for minimizing the weighted classification error (Cui and Tchetgen Tchetgen, 2021).

Weak IVs can pose problems, and the binary nature of the IV used in the method proposed by Cui and Tchetgen Tchetgen (2021) may limit its application (Qi et al., 2021). Recently, a new method for solving the optimal ITRs estimation problem under endogeneity has been developed (Qi et al., 2021), based on the idea of proximal causal inference (Miao et al., 2018; Tchetgen Tchetgen et al., 2020). Proximal causal inference allows causal effect identification based on the observed data through either treatment-inducing confounding proxies or outcome-inducing confounding proxies when the hypothesis that no unmeasured confounding is violated. Contrary to the IV approach discussed above, the proximal causal inference approach allows the use of flexible data types.

In this paper, Cui and Tchetgen Tchetgen (2021) presented a series of new identification results for several classes of value functions with regard to treatment-inducing or outcome-inducing confounding proxies when unmeasured confounding exists. They further proposed several effective methods for estimating restricted in-class optimal ITRs. By adopting Dikkala et al. (2020)'s min-max estimation method, the involved nuisance functions can be estimated nonparametrically. Thus, doubly robust methods for estimating an optimal ITR can be developed given a specific setting in which either a treatment-inducing or an outcome-inducing confounding bridge function is used to identify the causal effects. In practice, the sample splitting (cross fitting) technique is adopted to avoid dependence between the nuisance functions and the optimal ITR.

16.4 Conclusion

In this chapter, we have introduced several statistical learning methods for estimating an optimal ITR from observational data. Most existing methods for estimating optimal ITRs rely on the assumption of no unmeasured confounding. However, such an assumption is hard to guarantee in practice, especially in observational studies. IV-based approaches have been proposed to learn the optimal ITRs in the presence of potential unmeasured confounders. Further development to handle such situations is encouraged.

Chapter 17

Polygenic Risk Prediction for Precision Prevention

Jin Jin, Nilanjan Chatterjee

The rapidly developing modern genome-wide association studies (GWAS) have led to the discovery of tens of thousands of genetic susceptibility variants which together explain a substantial amount of variability in a large number of human traits and diseases (Visscher et al., 2017; Buniello et al., 2019). How to appropriately aggregate signals of a huge amount of genetic variants, specifically single nucleotide polymorphisms (SNPs), across the whole genome into a polygenic risk score (PRS) that can achieve considerable predictive power in the general population has become a key problem in genetic research (Chatterjee et al., 2016). With increasing predictive utility, PRSs been highlighted for their potential importance for predicting future risks of complex diseases and hence aiding development of risk-stratified strategies for prevention (Torkamani et al., 2018; Lambert et al., 2019; Sun et al., 2021). Real-world implementation of polygenic risk, prediction will require knowledge of how to choose the optimal method for constructing the PRS, and combine it with other critical socio-economic, lifestyle, and environmental risk factors to predict the absolute risk of an individual (Pal Choudhury et al., 2020). In addition, many important aspects that are often overlooked should be considered, such as population-specific genetic architectures potentially caused by differences in human demographic history (Eyre-Walker, 2010; Sanjak et al., 2017; O'Connor et al., 2019; Uricchio, 2020), and approaches to dealing with low ancestral diversity of the current genetic studies which could exacerbate potential health disparity issues (Kim et al., 2018; Duncan et al., 2019; Martin et al., 2019; Rosenberg et al., 2019; Lewis and Vassos, 2020; Lewis and Green, 2021).

This chapter aims to provide a comprehensive review of polygenic risk prediction, which will cover the basics of polygenic risk score (PRS), state-of-the-art methodologies for PRS development, polygenic risk prediction models that incorporate external genomic annotation and functional data, and recent focus on ancestry-specific polygenic risk prediction. We will also use case studies to illustrate the performance of different polygenic risk prediction models, and highlight important future challenges and opportunities in the end.

17.1 Definitions

17.1.1 Key Concepts

We will start with defining several key concepts in polygenic risk prediction.

SNP, which stands for single nucleotide polymorphism, refers to a genetic variant at a single base position in the DNA, and is the most common type of genetic variant among people. SNPs have been shown to be involved in the etiology of various human traits and diseases, and are predictive of the risk of many complex diseases and traits. A SNP usually consists of two alleles, and the SNPs that have two alleles observed in the population are called bi-allelic SNPs. The minor allele frequency (MAF) of a SNP is defined as the frequency of the rare (minor) allele in a given population. Humans have two alleles at each genetic

DOI: 10.1201/9781003216223-17

locus that were inherited separately from parents. The genotype of a SNP is represented as the corresponding pair of alleles - it is called homozygous if the two alleles are identical and heterozygous if the two alleles differ. A common way of SNP genotype encoding is to count the number of minor alleles in the genotype, which can be equal to 0, 1, or 2. This genotype encoding indicates measuring additive effect of the minor alleles.

A genome-wide association study (GWAS) is a research approach to identifying genetic variants that are statistically associated with the risk of a disease or a trait. Current PRS research has been mainly focusing on additive effects of generic variants as there has been little evidence of gene-gene interactions from current GWAS studies (Polderman et al., 2015; Aschard, 2016). GWAS have been identifying a large number of genetic loci associated with various human traits. A substantial proportion of these identified loci is identified to be associated with multiple traits. This is a phenomena known as "pleiotropy" (Zeng et al., 2018).

The heritability of a phenotype is defined as the proportion of the phenotype variation that is attributed to genetic variation, i.e., variance explained by the effect of genetic variants (SNPs), among individuals in a population. Instead of being determined by only a few susceptibility SNPs, many human phenotypes are found to be highly polygenic, i.e., there may be a large number of SNPs, each contributing to only a small amount of phenotypic heritability, but together they could explain a substantial proportion of the heritability in the general population. Recent development in GWAS and mixed-model techniques have made enhanced estimation of various components of heritability possible using genome-wide sets of variants (Yang et al., 2010; Bulik-Sullivan et al., 2015; Zheng et al., 2017; Yang et al., 2017; J Mayhew and Meyre, 2017; Zhu and Zhou, 2020). Heritability has also been shown to possibly vary with MAF, LD, and genotype certainty (Speed et al., 2017).

Another commonly seen terminology in the field is linkage disequilibrium (LD). LD is a phenomenon where genetic variations across two or more positions in DNA are not independently distributed. There are a variety of measures of LD in the genetics literature (Devlin and Risch, 1995; Fox et al., 2019; Hui and Burt, 2020), but for the purpose of this review LD between a pair of SNPs will be measured by the Pearson correlation coefficient (r^2) of their genotype values across individuals in the population.

Most of the PRS construction methods require an estimate of LD (and MAF) from external reference samples. One widely used reference database from is the 1000 Genomes project (Siva, 2008), which provides genotype data for approximately 2100 unrelated individuals in the U.S. that are of the five super-population origin, including 498 European (EUR), 659 African (AFR), 347 Hispanic/Latino (AMR), 503 East Asian (EAS), and 487 South Asian (SAS). Recently, an online tool called "TOP-LD" was also release which can be used to infer LD and MAF with high-coverage whole genome sequencing data from 15,578 individuals in the NHLBI Trans-Omics for Precision Medicine (TOPMed) program (Huang et al., 2022).

The total number of genetic variants that have been identified so far has reached to hundreds of millions (Taliun et al., 2021). However, research have shown that usually a few SNPs in each chromosome block, i.e., a set of nearby SNPs in a chromosome, are enough to uniquely identify the SNP patterns in the block (Gibbs et al., 2003; Berisa and Pickrell, 2016). HapMap 3, which is the third phase of the International HapMap project, published a list of approximately 1.2 million SNPs that are suggested to be sufficient for studying the entire genome for association with phenotypes among European-origin populations. This HapMap 3 SNP list has been widely used in genome-wide PRS construction, and has greatly helped the research on enhanced methods for PRS development. Furthermore, the Multi-Ethnic Global Array (MEGA) Consortium published a SNP list that has a better genotyping coverage of the ancestrally diverse populations.

17.1.2 Polygenic Risk Score (PRS)

Even though there are differences in different definitions of heritability based on the scale used (Witte et al., 2014), heritability essentially describes the degree of variation in the "true" polygenic risk for individuals in the underlying population (Chatterjee et al., 2016).

Polygenic risk score (PRS) is a weighted sum of the genetic variants an individual carries across different positions in their DNA. Specifically, under an additive model for genetic risk, PRS is typically defined as

$$PRS = \sum_{j=1}^{M} w_j G_j,$$

where M is the number of SNPs included in the score, w_j is the weight, i.e., estimated effect size, of SNP j, and $G_j = 0, 1$, or 2 is the number of effect alleles of SNP j in the individual. Conceptually, an individual's genetic risk of a specific trait refers to the underlying "true" score that captures the effect of all risk variants in the genome, and the variation of this true score in the population defines the heritability of the trait. In reality, however, we cannot construct this true score as our understanding of which genetic variants are causal and what are their true effect sizes are limited due to statistical uncertainty of inference from GWAS. But as the GWAS sample sizes increase, we expect to improve the predictive performance of the PRS towards the upper limit that is defined by heritability (Chatterjee et al., 2013; Dudbridge, 2013).

Due to limited access to individual-level genetic and phenotypic datasets, methodological research in statistical genetics has generally been focusing on utilizing GWAS summary-level association statistics, which were typically obtained from one-SNP-at-a-time regression analysis on the phenotype without accounting for LD (Park et al., 2010; Wen and Stephens, 2010; Yang et al., 2012; Pasaniuc and Price, 2017). As a result, methods for polygenic risk prediction have now been strongly encouraged to focus on GWAS summary-level association statistics only. To date, the majority of PRS were developed only based on common SNPs, i.e., SNPs with relatively high minor allele frequencies (MAFs), such as MAF$\geq$0.05 or MAF$\geq$0.01. Although methods have been proposed for handling summary-level association statistics of the rare variants (MAF$\leq$ 0.01), current GWAS sample sizes are still inadequate for obtaining stable effect size estimates with low uncertainty for the rare variants, and LD reference panels are still inadequate for rare variants as well.

17.2 State-of-the-Art Methods for PRS Construction

17.2.1 Overview

A common practice of PRS construction is through simple, methods, representative examples of which include constructing simple scores using only the top SNPs, SNPs that reach genome-wide significance ($p \leq 5 \times 10^{-8}$), and LD Pruning and Thresholding (P+T). These model-free methods construct PRS by directly utilizing the GWAS effect size estimates without accounting for LD structure, i.e., correlation structure between SNPs. Recently, a whole-genome Bayesian approach named LDpred (Vilhjálmsson et al., 2015) and its new version LDpred2 (Privé et al., 2020) have gained increasing popularity, and have shown enhanced predictive accuracy compared to simple score and P+T PRS in applications to a wide range of complex human traits/diseases. Unlike the simple score or P+T, LDpred re-weights the SNP effects by accounting for LD in the modeling process. Several other LD-based Bayesian methods have also been recently proposed, including SBLUP (Robinson et al., 2017), SBayesR (Lloyd-Jones et al., 2019), and PRS-CS (Ge et al., 2019). The main challenge in developing these LD-based methods is to reduce the extremely high computational burden of modeling high-dimensional LD structures in GWAS summary statistics. To avoid such computational burden, other methods such as EBPRS (Song et al., 2020) and

NPS (Chun et al., 2020) that do not directly model LD have also been proposed. Numerous PRS have been constructed based on these different methods and made available through open databases of polygenic scores such as PGS Catalog (Lambert et al., 2021) and Cancer PRSweb (Fritsche et al., 2020).

In this section, we give a brief overview of the representative summary-statistics methods for PRS construction and compare their performance via real-data examples. All algorithms for constructing PRS have two essential elements. The first is a "variable selection" procedure that determines which variants to include. The second is the estimation procedure for the association coefficients, i.e., effect sizes/weights, of the selected variants. Statistical imprecision in either of the two steps may cause dramatic loss in the predictive power of the PRS (see (Chatterjee et al., 2016), Box 2 for mathematical derivations). This is particularly tricky in genome-wide studies because the total heritability could be distributed over thousands, and in some cases tens of thousands, of common SNPs, each having extremely small effects. Under these highly polygenic architectures, selection of the true set of susceptibility SNPs for the model will be particularly challenging, and the rate of improvement in the precision of the model, as a function of GWAS sample size, is expected to be slow (see Figure 3 in Chatterjee et al., 2016).

17.2.2 Model-Free Methods

Simple Score Based on Top SNPs

A simple and straightforward approach to constructing PRS is to take the weighted sum of the number of effect alleles of a set of LD-clumped independent SNPs that reach the stringent genome-wide significance threshold, typically defined as $p \leq 5 \times 10^{-8}$ corresponding to multiple testing adjustment using Bonferroni criterion. Typically, in the "top" SNP approach, the selected SNPs are weighted by effect-size estimates (e.g., log-odds-ratio or linear regression coefficients) available from the GWAS summary data itself. A common method for generating independent SNPs from GWAS studies is called LD clumping, also known as informed LD pruning. It requires first sorting SNPs by p-values (from the smallest to the largest), then removing SNPs which are correlated at a given threshold level (r^2) or higher with other SNPs higher in the list. Sometimes, an additional criterion for removing SNPs based on genomic distance, e.g., SNPs within 500 kb of SNPs higher in the list, is added to ensure the clumped SNPs represent distinct genomic regions. Sorting the SNPs by p-value first is an important feature of LD clumping, as it preferentially keeps the SNPs with the strongest signals in a genomic region, and it often yields more accurate predictions than pruning random markers. LD clumping is crucial when working with GWAS summary-level data, as combining GWAS effect size estimates of the correlated SNPs as if they are independent will cause severe problems in PRS due to "double counting" association with correlated SNPs.

This simple top SNP PRS approach has been implemented in many studies due to its easy implementation, parsimony, and promising predictive accuracy on many complex traits/diseases (Wojcik et al., 2019; Thomas et al., 2020; Codd et al., 2021).

LD Pruning and Thresholding (P+T)

LD pruning and thresholding (P+T), also known as LD clumping and thresholding (C+T) or p-value-based clumping and thresholding (PC+T), constructs a polygenic score by applying two filtering steps based on LD and p-value. First, as in top SNP PRS, the variants are LD clumped so as to only keep variants with stronger signals and an absolute pairwise correlation weaker than a threshold, r^2. Then, instead of only selecting the genome-wide significant variants, it selects the remaining variants that have p-values smaller than a pre-defined threshold of significance, p_t. The score is then calculated by taking the weighted sum of the number of effect alleles of the selected variants, with weights set to the GWAS effect size estimates of the variants. Here, both r^2 and p_t are treated as tuning parameters: scores based on different settings of r^2 (e.g., 0.1, 0.2, 0.4, 0.6, and 0.8) and p_t (e.g., 5×10^{-8}, 5×10^{-6}, 5×10^{-4}, 5×10^{-2}, and 5×10^{-1}) are calculated for individuals in a validation dataset independent from the GWAS samples, then the set of "optimal" values for r^2 and p_t are selected with respect to predictive accuracy of the phenotype (e.g., explained variation, R^2, for continuous traits, and Area under the ROC curve, AUC, for dichotomous traits) on the validation dataset. P+T is by far the most commonly implemented simple method and has often been used as the benchmark for new method development (Vilhjálmsson et al., 2015; Márquez-Luna et al., 2017; Fritsche et al., 2020; Ni et al., 2021).

17.2.3 LD-Based Modeling Approaches

Summary Statistic Best Linear Unbiased Predictors (SBLUP)

The top SNP PRS and P+T PRS are constructed by taking a simple weighted sum of the effect of a small set of LD-clumped significant SNPs. The next set of methods we will introduce here estimate SNP effect sizes under a multivariate model accounting for LD and thus do not require the more ad-hoc LD clumping step described above.

SBLUP uses a random effects model to re-estimate SNP effects by converting the least-squares GWAS effect size estimates of the SNPs into approximate best linear unbiased predictors (BLUP) (Robinson et al., 2017). It is motivated by the fact that the resulting genetic predictor has maximized power among linear estimators with BLUP properties (Henderson, 1975).

Assume our goal is to predict some trait Y based on genotype $\{G_j, j = 1, \ldots, M\}$ where M denotes the number of SNPs considered. From a one-SNP-at-a-time regression analysis in GWAS, one obtains the least-squares estimate of the marginal effect size of each SNP j, $\widehat{\beta}_j$, which is the effect of SNP j on Y without adjusting for the effect of other SNPs, and its standard error estimate, $\widehat{\sigma}_j^2$, via one-SNP-at-a-time analysis using simple linear regression,

$$\boldsymbol{y} = \boldsymbol{g}_j \beta_j + \boldsymbol{\epsilon},$$

where $\boldsymbol{y}$ is the $N \times 1$ vector of the phenotype data, $\boldsymbol{g}_j$ is the $N \times 1$ vector of genotype data (coded as 0, 1 or 2) for SNP j that defines the number of effect alleles in the individuals, and $\boldsymbol{\epsilon}$ is the $N \times 1$ vector of residuals. The least-squares estimates $\widehat{\boldsymbol{\beta}} = (\widehat{\beta}_1, \ldots, \widehat{\beta}_M)^T$ can be written in the matrix form as $\text{diag}(\mathbf{G}^T\mathbf{G}) = \mathbf{G}^T\boldsymbol{y}$, where $\mathbf{G} = [\boldsymbol{g}_1, \ldots, \boldsymbol{g}_M]$.

The BLUP estimate of SNP effect size based on individual-level data is obtained by jointly modeling all SNPs in a random effects model,

$$\boldsymbol{y} = \mathbf{G}\boldsymbol{\beta}^{(J)} + \boldsymbol{e}, \tag{17.1}$$

where $\boldsymbol{\beta}^{(J)} = (\beta_1^{(J)}, \ldots, \beta_M^{(J)})^T$ denotes the vector of joint effect size of each SNP adjusting for the effects of other SNPs. Given a prior $\boldsymbol{\beta}^{(J)} \sim N(\mathbf{0}, h_g^2\mathbf{I}_M)$ and $\boldsymbol{e} \sim N(\mathbf{0}, \sigma_e^2\mathbf{I}_N)$, where h_g^2 denotes the prior per-SNP heritability, the BLUP estimate becomes $\widehat{\beta}^{(J)} = \left(\mathbf{G}^T\mathbf{G} + \sigma_e^2/h_g^2\mathbf{I}_M\right)^T \mathbf{G}^T\boldsymbol{y}$. When the individual-level data $\mathbf{G}$ and $\boldsymbol{y}$ are unavailable, SBLUP approximates $\mathbf{G}^T\mathbf{G}$ by the quantity from a reference cohort which is assumed to have similar LD and allele frequency, $\mathbf{B} = (N/N_0)\mathbf{G}_0^T\mathbf{G}_0$, with N_0 being the sample size of the reference sample. SBLUP additionally uses the approximation $\mathbf{G}^T\boldsymbol{y} \approx \text{diag}\,(\mathbf{B})\,\widehat{\boldsymbol{\beta}}$. SBLUP is therefore calculated as $\boldsymbol{\beta}_{\text{SBLUP}}^{(J)} = \left(\mathbf{B} + \sigma_e^2/h_g^2\mathbf{I}_M\right)^T \text{diag}\,(\mathbf{B})\,\widehat{\boldsymbol{\beta}}$.

LDpred and LDpred2

Similar to SBLUP, the LDpred method infers joint SNP effect sizes by a shrinkage estimator that combines GWAS summary statistics with a prior to the effect sizes while leveraging LD information from an external reference panel (Vilhjálmsson et al., 2015). Different from SBLUP which assumes the same normal prior for the effect size of all SNPs, LDpred assumes a spike-and-slab prior in the form,

$$\beta_j^{(J)} \overset{i.i.d.}{\sim} \begin{cases} N(0, h_g^2) & \text{with probability } p_t, \\ 0 & \text{with probability } (1 - p_t), \end{cases}$$

meaning that only a small proportion (p_t) of the SNPs are assumed to have non-zero causal effects that follow a common normal prior, $N(0, h_g^2)$, while all other SNPs are assumed to have no contribution to the phenotypic variation. Here p_t is treated as a tuning parameter that will be estimated via parameter tuning on a validation dataset, and the a priori per-SNP heritability, h_g^2, is estimated via constrained LD score regression (LDSC) (Bulik-Sullivan et al., 2015). When we fix p_t at 1, i.e., assuming an "infinitesimal" prior, the model is called "LDpred-inf", and the posterior mean effects can be derived analytically with a closed-form approximation. To reduce computational burden, LDpred assumes that distant variants are unlinked, in which case the posterior mean effect sizes within a small region l under an infinitesimal model can be well approximated by

$$E\left(\boldsymbol{\beta}_l^{(J)} | \widehat{\boldsymbol{\beta}}_l, \mathbf{D}\right) \approx \left(\frac{M}{Nh_g^2}\mathbf{I} + \mathbf{D}_l\right)^{-1} \widehat{\boldsymbol{\beta}}_l,$$

where $\mathbf{D}_l$ denotes the regional LD matrix within the LD region l, and $\widehat{\boldsymbol{\beta}}_l$ denotes the vector of GWAS effect size estimates of the SNPs within the region. This approximation assumes that both the heritability explained by the region and the LD with SNPs outside of the region are negligible. Note that under these assumptions, the resulting effect size estimates approximate the standard genomic BLUP estimates (Yang et al., 2010), i.e., LDpred-inf is a natural extension of the SBLUP. The LD radius, i.e., the number of SNPs adjusted for on each side of a given SNP, is recommended to be set to approximately $M/3000$ (i.e., a 2 MB LD window on average) to balance the predictive accuracy and computational efficiency of the algorithm.

Under a non-infinitesimal Gaussian mixture prior, it is hard to derive an analytical expression for the posterior mean effect sizes, and thus LDpred adopts an approximate MCMC Gibbs sampler which obtains effect size estimation from the posterior distribution instead of posterior mean. To ensure convergence, Ldpred shrinks the posterior probability of being causal by a fixed factor, $c = \min\left(1, \widehat{h}_g^2 / \left(\tilde{h}_g^2\right)_{(i)}\right)$ at each iteration step i, where $\widehat{h}_g^2$ is the estimated heritability based on constrained LDSC, and $\left(\tilde{h}_g^2\right)_{(i)}$ is the estimated genome-wide heritability at each iteration. LDpred further uses Rao-Blackwellization to speed up the convergence. The LDpred software is available at `https://bitbucket.org/bjarni_vilhjalmsson/ldpred`.

Recently, a new version of LDpred algorithm called LDpred2 was published (Privé et al., 2020), which, according to the follow-up applications, shows similar or higher predictive accuracy than the original LDpred algorithm. LDpred2 comes with two major extensions of LDpred: (1) a hyperparameter-free version called "LDpred2-auto", which estimates p_t (the proportion of causal SNPs) and h_g^2 (prior per-SNP heritability) within the model instead of treating p_t as a tuning parameter and estimating h_g^2 using constrained LDSC; (2) an option for generating sparse effect size estimates, where the effect size estimates for the SNPs whose posterior probabilities of being causal are below the prior probability p_t are set to 0.

LDpred2 also suggests that the LD window size (the total number of SNPs divided by 3000, which corresponds to a 2 Mb LD window on average) recommended by the original LDpred algorithm is not large enough and adopts a larger window size of 3 cM when computing the correlation between variants. Finally, LDpred2 also comes with an option "LDpred2-grid", which, similar to the original LDpred algorithm, treats p_t, h_g^2 and the indicator of "sparse" option as tuning parameters and estimates them using a validation dataset. LDpred2 can be implemented using the "bigsnpr" R package (Privé et al., 2018).

Regarding the choice of an appropriate set of candidate SNPs for PRS construction, it is recommended that HapMap3 variants (Consortium et al., 2010) with a minor allele frequency (MAF) greater than 0.01 can be used. When constructing the LD reference panel, it is recommended that at least 300 unrelated samples are included, whose ancestry should match that of the discovery sample, such as the commonly used unrelated samples from the 1000 Genomes project (Siva, 2008).

LDpred and LDpred2 (Privé et al., 2020) have been applied to a wide range of human traits/diseases such as BMI, height (Khera et al., 2019), coronary heart diseases (Dikilitas et al., 2020; Mosley et al., 2020), type-2 diabetes, breast cancer (Khera et al., 2018; Mars et al., 2020), kidney function biomarkers (Yu et al., 2021), tobacco and alcohol use (Liu et al., 2019), and psychiatric disorders (Ni et al., 2021).

SBayesR

SBayesR was proposed under a similar Bayesian framework as LDpred, but with a slightly different prior distribution for SNP effect sizes and a different estimation procedure (Lloyd-Jones et al., 2019). Instead of assuming the effects of causal SNPs follow a common normal prior, SBayesR considers a mixture of normals. Specifically, it assumes the following prior distribution,

$$\beta_j^{(J)} \overset{i.i.d.}{\sim} \begin{cases} N(0, \gamma_2 h^2) & \text{with probability } \pi_1, \\ \vdots & \\ N(0, \gamma_C h^2) & \text{with probability } \pi_C, \\ 0 & \text{with probability } \left(1 - \sum_{c=1}^{C} \pi_c\right), \end{cases}$$

where C denotes the pre-specified number of components in the normal mixture, γ_cs are pre-specified scaling parameters that constrain how the common variance h^2 scales in each normal distribution. The model further assumes an inverse χ^2 prior distribution for h^2 and a $Dirichlet(\mathbf{1})$ prior distribution for $(\pi_1, \ldots, \pi_C)^T$, and estimates these model parameters along with the posterior mean effects of variants via a Gibbs sampling algorithm, where a right-hand side updating scheme is adopted along with the use of sparse matrix operations on the reference LD correlation matrix to maximize the computational efficiency. SBayesR does not require parameter tuning. SBayesR can be implemented using the GCTB software, which is available at `http://cnsgenomics.com/software/gctb/`.

PRS-CS

Under a Bayesian framework similar to the ones for LDpred and SBayesR, PRS-CS assumes a continuous shringkage prior for the SNP effect sizes,

$$\beta_j^{(J)} \sim N\left(0, \frac{\sigma^2}{N}\phi\psi_j\right), \ \psi_j \sim g,$$

where the variance of $\beta_j^{(J)}$ scales with the residual variance and GWAS sample size N, ϕ is a global scaling parameter shared across variants that controls the degree of sparseness of the model, ψ_j is a local, SNP-specific parameter, and g is an absolutely continuous mixing density function as opposed to a finite mixture of densities. This type of prior is known as a global-local scale mixture of normals.

Appropriate choices of the continuous mixing density g can produce various shapes of the prior distribution on $\beta_j^{(J)}$ that have a sizable amount of mass near 0 to impose strong shrinkage on noise, while at the same time have heavy tails to avoid over-shrinkage of the non-zero effects. To reduce the computational burden in simultaneous, genome-wide update of the effect sizes, PRS-CS uses a genome partition (Berisa and Pickrell, 2016), which divides the genome into 1703 largely independent genomic regions. In this case, posterior SNP effect sizes can be estimated via block updates within each LD block, i.e., chromosome region where bases are likely to be coinherited and thus the SNPs are correlated, assuming no LD between blocks. PRS-CS comes with two algorithms, where the standard algorithm treats ϕ as tuning parameters, and the alternative algorithm, "PRS-CS-auto", estimates all model parameters automatically without parameter tuning. A Python-based command line tool "PRS-CS" is available at `https://github.com/getian107/PRScs`.

Lassosum

Besides Bayesian hierarchical models, another LD-based method called lassosum was proposed under a penalized regression framework which also constructs PRS based on GWAS summary statistics and an external LD reference panel (Mak et al., 2017). Under the joint linear regression model (17.1), the classical LASSO (Tibshirani, 1996) obtains estimates of $\widehat{\beta}^{(J)}$ by minimizing the objective function

$$f(\boldsymbol{\beta}^{(J)}) = \boldsymbol{y}^T\boldsymbol{y} + \boldsymbol{\beta}^{(J)^T}\mathbf{R}\boldsymbol{\beta}^{(J)} - 2\boldsymbol{\beta}^{(J)^T}\boldsymbol{r} + 2\lambda\|\boldsymbol{\beta}^{(J)}\|_1^1,$$

where $\|\cdot\|_1^1$ denotes the $\mathcal{L}_1$ norm, $\mathbf{R} = \mathbf{G}^T\mathbf{G}$, under the assumption of standardized genotype ($\mathbf{G}$) and phenotype ($\boldsymbol{y}$) data, is equal to the LD correlation matrix, and $\boldsymbol{r} = \mathbf{G}^T\boldsymbol{y}$ represents the correlation between genotype and phenotype.

When only the GWAS summary statistics are available, we can approximate $\mathbf{R} = \mathbf{G}^T\mathbf{G}$ by its estimate based on an external LD reference data, $\mathbf{R}_0 = \mathbf{G}_r^T\mathbf{G}_r$, and approximate $\boldsymbol{r} = \mathbf{G}^T\boldsymbol{y}$ using GWAS summary statistics. This leads to an objective function

$$f(\boldsymbol{\beta}^{(J)}) = \boldsymbol{y}^T\boldsymbol{y} + \boldsymbol{\beta}^{(J)^T}\mathbf{R}_0\boldsymbol{\beta}^{(J)} - 2\boldsymbol{\beta}^{(J)^T}\boldsymbol{r} + 2\lambda\|\boldsymbol{\beta}^{(J)}\|_1^1. \tag{17.2}$$

Since the reference genotype $\mathbf{G}_r^T$ used to estimate $\mathbf{R}_0$ is different from the genotype $\mathbf{G}^T$ used to calculate $\boldsymbol{r}$, (17.2) will no longer be a LASSO problem, and the solutions to minimizing (17.2) is possibly unstable and non-unique. lassosum then proposes to regularize (17.2) by replacing $\mathbf{R}_0$ by $\mathbf{R_s} = (\mathbf{1} - \mathbf{s})\mathbf{R_0} + \mathbf{sI}$, which gives an objective function

$$f(\boldsymbol{\beta}^{(J)}) = \boldsymbol{y}^T\boldsymbol{y} + (1-s)\boldsymbol{\beta}^{(J)^T}\mathbf{R}_s\boldsymbol{\beta}^{(J)} + s\boldsymbol{\beta}^{(J)^T}\boldsymbol{\beta}^{(J)} - 2\boldsymbol{\beta}^{(J)^T}\boldsymbol{r} + 2\lambda\|\boldsymbol{\beta}^{(J)}\|_1^1.$$

Here, λ and s can either be treated as tuning parameters and selected based on a validation dataset, or be estimated along with other unknown parameters ("lassosum-auto"). An R package "lassosum" is available on Github at `https://github.com/tshmak/lassosum`.

DBSLMM

Yang and Zhou (2020) proposed a Deterministic Bayesian Sparse Linear Mixed Model (DB-SLMM), which assumes that all SNPs are causal, i.e., having non-zero effects on the phenotype, but partitions SNPs into a large-effect group and a small-effect group. In other words, its assumption of prior effect size distribution is a hybrid of the sparse assumption (e.g., in LDpred) and the polygenic assumption (e.g., in SBLUP). Different from most of the other summary statistics Bayesian methods that require computationally intensive MCMC algorithms for parameter estimation, DBSLMM first utilizes a simple deterministic search algorithm to effectively select SNPs with potentially large effects, then obtain the effect size estimates for all SNPs through an analytic solution.

DBSLMM rewrites model 17.1 in the form

$$\boldsymbol{y} = \mathbf{G}_l\boldsymbol{\beta}^{(J)}{}_l + \mathbf{G}_s\boldsymbol{\beta}^{(J)}{}_s + \boldsymbol{e}, \tag{17.3}$$

where $\mathbf{G}_l$ and $\mathbf{G}_s$ respectively denote the $N \times M_l$ genotype matrix for the M_l likely large-effect SNPs and the $N \times M_s$ genotype matrix for the remaining $M_s = M - M_l$ likely small-effect SNPs, $\boldsymbol{\beta}^{(J)}{}_l$ and $\boldsymbol{\beta}^{(J)}{}_s$ are the corresponding joint effect sizes. The M_l large-effect SNPs can be selected by simple methods such as P + T. A normal mixture effect size assumption on $\boldsymbol{\beta}^{(J)}$ is first induced, which, under model17.3, is then converted to two normal priors: $\beta^{(J)}_{l,j} \sim N(0, h_l^2)$ and $\beta^{(J)}_{s,j} \sim N(0, h_s^2)$, where h_l^2 and h_s^2 are prior per-SNP heritability controlled by some hyperparameters. DBSLMM further assumes that under a large GWAS sample size N, the information contained in the GWAS summary statistics overwhelms the information provided by the prior, and therefore sets h_l^2 to infinity and treats $\boldsymbol{\beta}^{(J)}{}_l$ as fixed effects. In this way, the posterior estimates of $\boldsymbol{\beta}^{(J)}{}_l$ and $\boldsymbol{\beta}^{(J)}{}_s$ can be computed analytically with a closed-form solution (see Supplemental Methods in Yang and Zhou, 2020).

DBSLMM additionally uses a block-diagonal matrix approximation to the LD matrix as in PRS-CS, and a fast preconditioned conjugate gradient algorithm for solving linear systems. With these tricks, DBSLMM is able to construct genome-wide PRS based on biobank-scale data with tens of millions of SNPs in a computationally efficient fashion Yang and Zhou, 2020. The "DBSLMM" software is available at `https://github.com/biostat0903/DBSLMM`.

In general, the computationally intensive LD-based methods including LDpred, SBayesR and PRS-CS, including too many SNP, such as SNPs in strong LD, may not further improve the performance of the LD-based Bayesian methods, including SNPs with extremely low MAF could even lower the predictive accuracy due to additional noises included. A reasonable SNP selection criterion is required to achieve a desirable performance of these methods. For example, one can select the common SNPs, i.e., SNPs that have MAF greater than 0.05 or 0.01, from approximately 2.6 million biallelic SNPs in the combination of HapMap 3 SNP list and the Multi-Ethnic Genotyping Array (MEGA) SNP list, where the latter was developed to equitably capture the global genetic variation of ancestrally distinct populations (Bien et al., 2016).

17.2.4 Advanced Methods that do not Incorporate External LD Information

A major obstacle in PRS construction is the computational burden since it requires identifying causal SNPs from millions or tens of millions of correlated variants and estimating their joint effect sizes based on extremely high-dimensional marginal effect size estimates. We have introduced methods that have shown improved prediction accuracy compared to top SNP PRS and P+T PRS. These methods model LD by borrowing information from external LD reference panels and are thus computationally intensive. Recently, several other methods were proposed that avoid directly modeling LD to improve computational efficiency. One example is the EB-PRS method that leverages information of effect sizes across all variants without accounting for LD or parameter tuning (Song et al., 2020). It assumes a spike-and-slab type of prior on effect sizes similar to that in SBayesR, where the slab is a K-component mixture normal. It constructs an "optimal" polygenic risk score under an independent-SNP assumption by minimizing the overall Bayes risk.

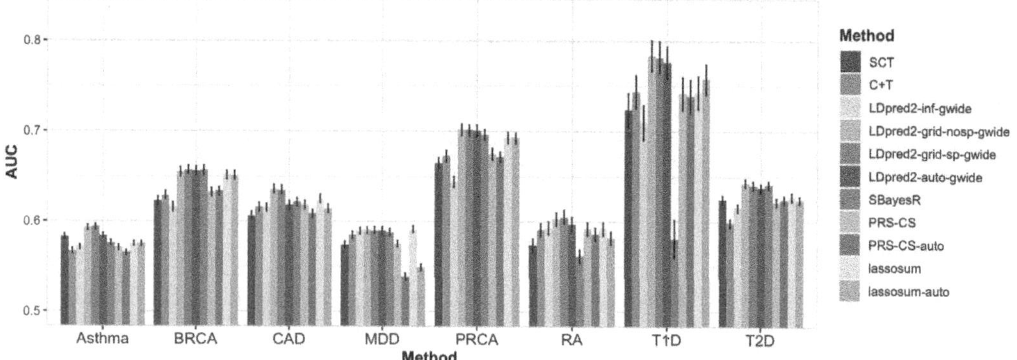

Figure 17.1 *Comparison of AUC across different PRS methods on eight complex diseases using publicly available summary data of European ancestry (Privé et al., 2020). The "grid" and "auto" models are compared for LDpred2, lassosum and PRS-CS. The bars present estimated AUC on a testing sample of European ancestry from UK Biobank (mean and 95% CI from 10,000 bootstrap samples).*

Another method uses a partitioning-based, non-parametric shrinkage (NPS) method which does not require explicitly modeling any underlying genetic architecture (Chun et al., 2020). NPS accounts for correlation structures in GWAS summary statistics arising due to LD, specifically, the correlations in true genetic effects and in sampling errors, by applying eigenvalue decomposition of LD matrix instead of using high-dimensional sampling techniques.

17.2.5 Data Examples

We now illustrate the relative performance of various summary statistics PRS methods via published applications on several different traits/diseases. Privé et al. (2020) presented a comparison of methods on predicting the polygenic risk of eight common diseases including asthma, breast cancer (BRCA), coronary artery disease (CAD), depressive disorder (MDD), prostate cancer (PRCA), Type 1 or 2 diabetes (T1D and T2D), and rheumatoid arthritis (RA). Figure 17.1 shows the area under the ROC curve (AUC) of the PRS constructed by stacked P+T (SCT), P+T (i.e., C+T), LDpred2-inf, LDpred2-grid without the "sparse" option, LDpred2-auto, SBayesR, lassosum, and lassosum-auto. A summary of the GWAS summary statistics used and the estimated tuning parameters can be found in (Privé et al., 2020). We can observe that LDpred2-grid and LDpred2-auto which assume a spike-and-slab prior have more or less similar performance that is stable and consistently similar to or better than that of the other methods considered. PRS-CS, which assumes a more flexible and complex prior effect size distribution than LDpred2, consistently performs worse than LDpred2 and lassosum instead of showing significant improvements; SBayesR performs similarly as LDpred2 on T2D and similarly as lassosum on most of the other diseases except for RA and T1D, where it has the lowest AUC among all methods. In general, the majority of the LD-based Bayesian methods (LDpred2, PRS-CS and SBayesR) and penalized regression-based method (lassosum) outperform the simple methods without accounting for LD (C+T and SCT). We can further observe that for the LD-based methods including LDpred2, PRS-CS and lassosum, the "grid" models usually perform better than their "auto" counterparts, i.e., the models that directly estimate parameters from the data without parameter tuning.

In a recent application to schizophrenia (SCZ) and MDD, ten PRS methods were applied, which include the previously introduced P+T (i.e., PC+T or C+T), SBLUP, LDpred2-inf, LDpred2, lassosum, PRS-CS, PRS-CS-auto, SBayesR. Two other methods were also considered: LDpred-funct, which incorporates external functional annotations (see Marquez-Luna et al. (2021) and Section 17.3 for details), and MegaPRS, a software that implements a suite of methods and selects the method and the "optimal" model via parameter tuning on a validation dataset utilizing the BLD-LDAK model (see (Speed and Balding, 2019) and Section 17.3 for details). The methods were compared on a pooled dataset of 37 European ancestry cohorts that include approximately 31,000 cases and 41,000 controls (Ni et al., 2021). Model performance was reported on one of the 30 cohorts in the target sample, after parameter tuning using a separate cohort based on GWAS summary statistics obtained from a meta-analysis of the remaining 35 cohorts. P+T is outperformed by the other nine methods, especially MegaPRS, LDPred2 and SBayesR which are estimated to explain up to 9.2% variance in liability for SCZ, with an increase of 44% compared to that of P+T (see Figure 1A in Ni et al. (2021)). Similar results can be observed for MDD.

Pain et al. (2021) compared the performance of various PRS methods on two target populations: (1) UK Biobank (UKB) (Buniello et al., 2019), and the Twins Early Development Study (TEDS) (Rimfeld et al., 2019). The analysis involved 8 binary phenotypes including depression, T2D, CAD, Inflammatory Bowel Disease (IBD), RA, Multiple Sclerosis (MultiScler), BRCA, and PRCA, and three continuous phenotypes including intelligence, height and body mass index (BMI). Details of the GWAS summary statistics and target samples are summarized in Table 1 in Pain et al. (2021). The following methods were considered: P + T, lassosum, PRS-CS, SBLUP, SBayesR, LDpred (LDpred1), LDpred2, DBSLMM, and a "all" model, which combines scores from all methods in an elastic net model. The methods were implemented in four possible ways: (1) "10FCVal", which is a single PRS based on the optimal parameter estimated using 10-fold cross-validation, (2) "Multi-PRS", which is an elastic net model combining PRS under a range of model parameters, where the elastic net shrinkage parameters are derived using 10-fold cross-validation, (3) "PseudoVal", which is a single PRS based on the predicted optimal parameter estimated using pseudo-validation, i.e., a single optimal parameter is estimated based on the GWAS summary statistics alone, and therefore do not require parameter tuning, and (4) "Inf", which is a single PRS based on the infinitesimal model that does not require parameter tuning.

In general, "MultiPRS" outperforms their "10FCVal" counterpart (i.e., single polygenic score based on the optimal parameter as identified using 10-fold cross-validation) which outperfoms its "PseudoVal" counterpart (i.e., single polygenic score based on the predicted optimal parameter as identified using pseudovalidation, no tuning sample required), if there is any (Figure 17.2). Among the Bayesian hierarchical models that account for LD, "10FCVal" and "MultiPRS" PRS constructed by LDpred2 and PRS-CS outperform those constructed by P+T, LDpred1, and SBayesR. lassosum performs similarly as LDpred2. The "all" model that further combines the PRS from all methods in an elastic net model performs better than or at least similarly as the single best method.

From the three examples above, we can see that even though many novel methods have been claimed to possibly outperform other methods in terms of predictive accuracy, it is safe to say that there is no uniformly optimal PRS method that shows the highest predictive accuracy on all phenotypes. In general, the LD-based methods including LDpred, LDpred2, SBayesR and PRS-CS show more or less similar predictive accuracies that are higher than those of the simple scores and P+T. In real-world applications, a reasonable strategy is to apply all applicable PRS methods and select the "optimal" ones according to their performance on an independent validation dataset, instead of always sticking to one single method.

17.3 Incorporation of External Genomic Information

There has been extensive evidence that GWAS signals tend to be enriched for functional variants (Hu et al., 2017; Broekema et al., 2020; Weissbrod et al., 2020). Continuously

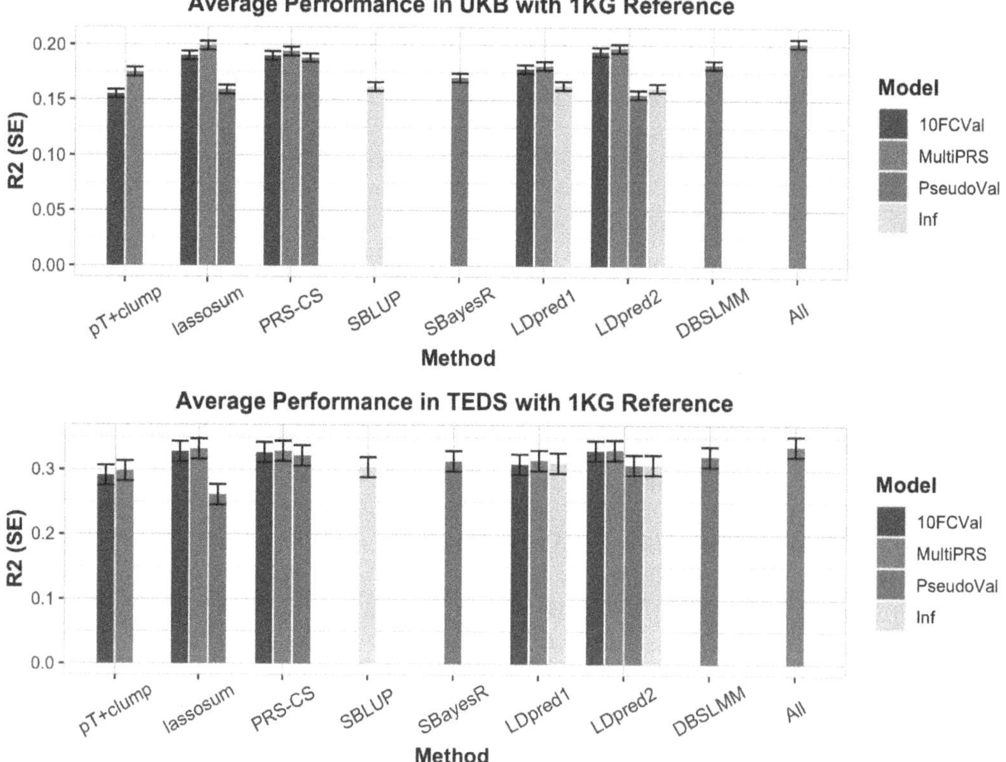

Figure 17.2 *Comparison of the various PRS methods on UKB and TEDS target samples with 1KG reference. Average cross-validated correlation between predicted and observed values across 11 phenotypes is displayed. "10FCVal": a single PRS based on the optimal parameter estimated using 10-fold cross-validation. "Multi-PRS": an elastic net model containing PRS based on a range of parameters, with shrinkage parameters estimated using 10-fold cross-validation. "PseudoVal": a single PRS based on the predicted optimal parameter estimated using pseudo-validation that do not require parameter tuning. "Inf": a single PRS based on the infinitesimal model that do not require parameter tuning.*

refined high-throughput sequencing technologies and annotation algorithms are generating various types of tissue-, cell type-, and ancestry-specific annotations of genetic variants across the whole genome (Kim-Hellmuth et al., 2020; van der Wijst et al., 2020; Liu et al., 2016; Gay et al., 2020; Lu et al., 2017). These advancements in data resources have made the incorporation of various types of external annotations more easily, which could better prioritize SNPs and lead to major enhancement of the predictive power of PRS. There are three main types of annotations: (1) pleiotropic annotation, (2) population genetic annotations such as MAF, LD patterns, and annotations based on specific genomic elements (e.g., conserved genomic regions), and (3) functional annotations based on various type of QTL-type studies and laboratory experiments to determine functional characteristics of different regions of the genome.

The external genomic information can be incorporated to inform "priors" for the effect-size distribution using mixed models, Bayesian hierarchical models, and penalized regression methods. Typically, the association parameters (or log odds ratio association parameters for binary traits) are assumed to have a symmetric distribution with zero mean and variance specified by some variance component parameters that are determined by a function of prior information including the functional annotations. These prior distributions induce "shrinkage" of the estimated association coefficients of the SNPs towards or away from the null to provide more efficient effect size estimates in terms of bias and variance.

More and more recent studies have demonstrated that utilizing well-informed priors, including information on both pleiotropic and functional annotations can accelerate the discovery of susceptibility loci. Information from pleiotropic analysis, functional annotation, and expression and methylation-quantitative traits loci can all be incorporated into a structured manner to form differential priors for the association parameters of different SNPs. The benefit of incorporating functional annotations in improving the predictive power of PRS models have been extensively investigated and shown by many recently proposed methods such as the variable thresholding approach in (Shi et al., 2016), PleioPred (Hu et al., 2017), LDpred-funct (Marquez-Luna et al., 2021), MegaPRS (Speed and Balding, 2019), and PolyFun-Pred (Weissbrod et al., 2021).

17.4 Recent Focus on Ancestry-Specific Risk Predictions

Over the last several years, there have been more and more extensive discussions on important health disparity issues in genomic studies (Gurdasani et al., 2019), including the lower power of the European-based PRS models on the general population of mixed ancestry background (Gurdasani et al., 2019). Reducing health disparities is a key value for public health, but evidence suggests that clinical use of the current PRS which are constructed mainly for the European population could exacerbate race-based health disparities due to differences in predictive power across ancestry groups (Kim et al., 2018; Duncan et al., 2019; Martin et al., 2019; Rosenberg et al., 2019; Lewis and Vassos, 2020; Lewis and Green, 2021). The debate focuses on the crucial issue that, while having shown great potential in risk prediction for individuals of European ancestry, the utility of PRS in clinical practice encounters obstacles due to the typically low genetic heritability explained for the various non-European populations that have substantially lower sample sizes compared to the European population in the current genomic databases (Curtis, 2018).

Given the extremely low accessibility of non-European datasets, the majority of the studies have been applying PRS constructed for European population to other populations, most of which suffer from considerable decrease in predictive accuracy (Yu et al., 2021; Liu et al., 2021; Vassos et al., 2017). This low transferability of European PRS to other populations may be due to several reasons. First, alleles have different effect sizes in different populations, which is possible due to the differences in interactions with the environment (Novembre and Barton, 2018). Second, differences in LD pattern across populations means that causal variants may be linked with other variants differently in different populations, leading to differences in joint effect sizes (Martin et al., 2017; Wojcik et al., 2019). Third, the estimated predictive accuracy of the PRS in European populations may be inflated for the other populations because of population stratification, meaning that populations can be distinguished by observing genotypes (Berg et al., 2019; Sohail et al., 2019). Lastly, each population may have its own genetic architecture formed by different evolutionary paths across populations. It is therefore reasonable to assume that one population's demographic history influences the number of causal variants and their allele frequencies, which in turn results in the part of phenotypic variance contributed by the population-specific causal variants. The number of such variants can be large, in which case the European-based PRS will fail to capture a considerable amount of heritability explained by these variants.

As improving the applicability of PRS in diverse populations has become a primary focus of genetic research, methods for constructing enhanced PRS for the minority populations have started to emerge, which seek to appropriately combine GWAS data of the target populations with that of the European population or/and various types of functional annotations. The resultant population-specific PRS can not only be used to enhance disease risk prediction/prevention for the under-represented minor populations, but also be applied in other applications, such as phenome-wide association studies (PheWAS) (Bush et al., 2016) and Mendelian Randomization (MR) studies Lawlor et al. (2008); Sanderson et al. (2022) that further identify novel population-specific causal links among complex human traits and diseases.

A simple method for constructing enhanced non-European PRS is to combine the discovery summary statistics of the target population with those of European and all other available populations by a meta-analysis on ancestry-specific GWAS. Another similar method called "weighted PRS" was proposed in 2017 (Márquez-Luna et al., 2017), which, instead of combining GWAS summary statistics, seeks an "optimal" weighted combination of the ancestry-specific PRS constructed separately on GWAS of each ancestry group. In the case of LDpred PRS, suppose we have constructed the ancestry-specific LDpred PRS for three ancestry groups, PRS_{EUR}, PRS_{AFR}, and PRS_{AMR}. The weighted LDpred PRS, $\text{PRS}_{\text{w-LDpred}}$, is then constructed as follows,

$$\text{PRS}_{\text{w-LDpred}} = \alpha_1 \text{PRS}_{\text{EUR}} + \alpha_2 \text{PRS}_{\text{AFR}} + \alpha_3 \text{PRS}_{\text{AMR}},$$

where the weights α_is are estimated by fitting a regression model on a validation dataset. Weighted PRS has been implemented using P+T in many applications and has shown substantially improved predictive power on non-European populations compared to single-ancestry PRS methods (Bogdan et al., 2018; Li et al., 2018; Martin et al., 2019; Chen et al., 2020).

Recently, a multi-ancestry version of PRS-CS called "PRS-CSx" was proposed to borrow information across ancestry groups by jointly modeling ancestry-specific GWAS summary statistics (Ruan et al., 2022). Briefly, PRS-CSx assumes the following prior to the ancestry-specific effect sizes $\beta_{j,k}^{(J)}$,

$$\beta_{j,k}^{(J)} \sim N\left(0, \frac{\sigma_k^2}{N_k}\psi_j\right), \ \psi_j \sim \text{Gamma}(a, \delta_j), \ \delta_j \sim \text{Gamma}(b, \phi),$$

where ϕ is a global shrinkage parameter shared by all SNPs that controls the overall sparseness of the genetic architecture, and ψ_j is a local, SNP-specific shrinkage parameter. By assigning a Gamma-Gamma hierarchical prior on ψ_j, the marginal prior density of $\beta_{j,k}^{(J)}$ has a considerably large amount of mass near 0 to ensure a strong shrinkage on small noises, and heavy tails that help avoid over-shrinkage of true effects. We can see that when a SNP is available in multiple populations, the continuous shrinkage prior is coupled across populations, enabling information sharing between summary statistics while allowing for the estimation of ancestry-specific effect sizes to retain model flexibility. After the Bayesian modeling step, PRS-CSx conducts an additional step of linearly combining the PRS based on the posterior effect size estimates for EUR and target population. The weights for the linear combination are estimated based on the tuning dataset.

Several other multi-ancestry methods were proposed. For example, there is another recent method called "XPASS" which, similar to the first step of PRS-CSx, seeks to borrow information across populations using a similar Bayesian modeling framework but under an infinitesimal model (Cai et al., 2021). (Zhang et al., 2022) proposed a computationally efficient, model-free method called "CT-SLEB", which first conducts P + T for selecting SNPs to be included in the target population PRS, then uses an Empirical Bayesian approach to estimate SNP effect sizes, and finally implements a Super Learning (SL) model to combine multiple PRS generated under different SNP selection thresholds.

Recent studies have shown the multi-ancestry methods borrowing information across populations can lead to improved PRS performance for each distinct population, and in particular for the non-European minority populations, for various human traits and diseases

(Wu et al., 2021; Ho et al., 2022; Ruan et al., 2022; Cai et al., 2021; Zhang et al., 2022; Ge et al., 2022). There are also studies which indicate that the several current multi-ancestry PRS methods, such as PRS-CSx, do not provide further improvement to single-ancestry PRS or the simple meta-analyzed PRS (Privé et al., 2022; Tsuo et al., 2022; Barr et al., 2022; Nurnberger Jr et al., 2021). This suggests that further research should be conducted on developing more enhanced multi-ancestry methods.

17.5 Future Directions

Although polygenic risk prediction has been thoroughly investigated for over a decade and much advancement has been made in terms of developing algorithms for building PRS from genome-wide datasets, many obstacles remain. For example, as data from less common and rare variants emerges from future studies, there might be opportunities to incorporate them to further improve performance of PRS. However, studies of heritability indicate that uncommon and rare variants, which individually can point to important biology, may not explain significant heritability (Weiner et al., 2022).

One key question is how to improve performance of PRS in multi-ancestry population. To date, there is still a lack of large-scale GWAS for populations of non-European origin. Such imbalance in data sources is a major obstacle in achieving significant improvement in the predictive performance of PRS in the general, ancestrally diverse population. Further research is also required for understanding the diversity in genetic architecture across ancestry groups, so as to further improve ancestry-specific polygenic risk prediction. Besides multi-ancestry polygenic risk prediction, there are also special challenges in dealing with admixed populations, where individuals cannot be categorized into distinct ancestry groups as their genomes are mixtures of several different populations (Duncan et al., 2019). This is a unique challenge that has not been addressed by current multi-ancestry methods. Fortunately, grants and consortia/centers for polygenic risk prediction in diverse populations have been rapidly emerging in recent years, such as NHGRI's eMERGE consortium (Gottesman et al., 2013), Population Architecture Using Genomics and Epidemiology (PAGE) Consortium, PRS Diversity Consortium, NIA's Alzheimer's Disease Genetics Consortium, All of Us research program, and Center for Admixed Populations and Health Equity (CAPE) (Ojo, 2018). Such resources will help facilitate the development and application of PRS for individuals of diverse ancestries and alleviate health disparity issues.

With continuously improved predictive accuracy, PRS has received a growing interest in its practical utility for predicting the risk of common diseases responsive to early therapeutic interventions (Nguyen and Eisman, 2020). The PRS only describes a genetic component of an individual's risk of a disease relative to others with a different genetic profile. Research on the etiology of human diseases have identified many other risk factors and show extensive evidence of complex interactions of genetic and environmental risk factors in disease progression. Thus, the clinical utility of PRS depends on many other factors including the absolute risk of the disease that describes the probability of the occurring of the disease within a specific future time frame, information on other important factors such as family history, rare high-penetrant genetic variants not captured in PRS, socio-economic and environmental factors, and the types of interventions available to individuals to mitigate their risk (Chatterjee et al., 2016; Pal Choudhury et al., 2020).

Classical statistical methods often assume that data on the outcome and all risk factors are available from a single study with an adequately large sample size. In the future, however, complex model development incorporating a wide variety of risk factors will require combining information across disparate data sources (Kundu et al., 2019; Jin et al., 2021). Further absolute risk models can be calibrated to population risk using various types of disease registries and surveillance datasets (Pal Choudhury et al., 2020; Jin et al., 2021).

Future research is needed to develop more advanced data integration tools for building models in high-dimensional settings using disparate data sources.

In summary, with increasing sample sizes for genome-wide association studies and implementation of advanced methods, PRS is showing promises for their predictive utility across a variety of complex diseases and traits. However, clinical applications of PRS need improved methods for increasing transportability of PRS to non-European populations and flexible tools for integrating PRS with other types of risk-factors to estimate individualized absolute risks of diseases.

Chapter 18

Post-Selection Inference for Individualized Treatment Rules with Nonparametric Confounding Control

Jeremiah Jones, Ashkan Ertefaie, Robert L. Strawderman

18.1 Introduction

It can be difficult to construct desirable individualized treatment rules (ITRs) in the presence of a large number of potential tailoring variables. Often, it is important to encourage sparsity in the estimated rule through some form of variable selection. The statistical community has long recognized that the advantages of sparsity are introduced at the cost of complicating classical statistical inference. Classical inference frameworks fail to accommodate selection because of bias that is introduced by only performing inference on those variable coefficients which are estimated to be further away from zero than others (Leeb and Pötscher, 2005, 2008; Berk et al., 2013). Several authors have proposed techniques that address this issue. For a recent review of this body of work, see Kuchibhotla et al. (2020), who motivate the study of post-selection inference as a response to the replicability crisis in the sciences. The importance of this issue to scientific replication is detailed in Benjamini (2020).

Typical formulations cast the problem of estimating ITRs as one in which a "best" rule is targeted among a class of decision rules. This "best" rule is estimated either directly, as in direct-policy methods, or through outcome modeling algorithms such as one-stage Q-learning (Zhao et al., 2015; Schulte et al., 2014; Zhao et al., 2012). One strength of ITR methods is that the concepts of reward or utility can be used to balance patient outcomes with other considerations, such as side effects. Although tradeoffs may be evaluated with respect to individual patients, other factors may be relevant when comparing decision rules. For example, some rules may differ in the cost or difficulty to implement in practice.

Sparsity may be one factor to weigh when comparing multiple ITRs. For example, when comparing two decision rules with very similar performance in terms of patient utility, the rule which uses fewer tailoring variables might be preferred. This is because the comparatively sparse rule may reduce the cost of individualized treatment by eliminating variables that are costly to measure and only slightly improve expected patient utility (Flores et al., 2013). Additionally, the future performance of the sparse rule may be improved relative to the non-sparse rule by increased precision and elimination of spurious or weak predictors (Lu et al., 2013). When the in-sample estimates of patient utility are relatively similar between these two rules, these other considerations might lead an analyst to prefer the sparse rule.

An additional complication for outcome-modeling methods such as Q-learning is the role of confounding in the outcome model. The form of the decision rules in Q-learning do not depend on the full outcome model, but on the so-called "blip" (Robins, 2004; Robins et al., 2008) or "contrast" function (Zhang et al., 2012; Schulte et al., 2014). However, as we discuss in Section 18.2, misspecifications in the confounding model may impact the targets of the

DOI: 10.1201/9781003216223-18

Q-learning model. This complicates the variable selection problem by allowing the possibility that decision rules are constructed on the basis of confounding. To address this, we provide a method for controlling confounding in a way that eliminates explicit dependence on the confounding model. This approach was explored in partial linear models by Robinson (1988) and expanded to general Q-learning problems by Ertefaie et al. (2021). We further establish that the targets of this method are given as the coefficients from the best weighted linear approximation to the true contrast function.

In Section 18.3, some additional discussion of the variable selection problem as it applies to ITR estimation is given. The model selection problem is formally described, adapting the ideas explored in previous work on selection (e.g., Berk et al., 2013; Kuchibhotla et al., 2020) to the ITR estimation problem. The effect of model selection on both the set of decision rules and the targeted rules are established. We also present the Lasso problem corresponding to the methods presented in Section 18.2. The Lasso solution paths for the proposed estimator are shown to approximate those of the Oracle Lasso estimator with high probability.

In Section 18.4, we introduce two methods for valid inference for linear regression parameters after model selection. The Polyhedral method has been explored in various contexts (Lee et al., 2016; Tibshirani et al., 2018; Tian and Taylor, 2017) as a method to provide inference after model selection by a so-called "affine selection procedure" such as the Lasso with a fixed tuning parameter. In contrast, the UPoSI method (Kuchibhotla et al., 2020) has been developed to provide inference for any variable selection technique. For both of these methods, results are presented to justify the use of the proposed method of Section 18.2.3 within each of these frameworks. In the case of the Polyhedral method, these results are based on the work of Zhao et al. (2017); we present a novel application of the results of Kuchibhotla et al. (2020).

We illustrate these ideas through simulation studies and examine the ability of different methods to provide statistically valid inference for the targeted rule parameter. Comparisons are drawn between the coverage properties guaranteed by each method. The performance of each method in terms of confidence interval length is also explored. We conclude with some general discussion of the particular issues that competing post-selection inference frameworks offer, as well as challenges in moving to multi-stage decision-making problems.

Since we focus on ITR estimation in one stage, subscripts will not be used to indicate stage as elsewhere. Throughout this chapter, we will often use $\|W\|_q$ to represent the ℓ_q norm of the vector W and $W^{\otimes 2}$ to represent the outer product of the vector W. For a matrix A, we may denote the maximal element as $\|A\|_\infty$, and the (ℓ_2, ℓ_2) operator norm as $\|A\|_{2,2}$, otherwise known as the spectral norm or maximal singular value of the matrix A. Other norms $\|\cdot\|$ will be defined as necessary.

18.2 One-Stage Q-Learning Algorithm with Nonparametric Confounding Control

18.2.1 Decision Rule Estimation via One-Stage Q-Learning

In our ITR setting, we suppose that we observe n i.i.d. trajectories of $O_i \equiv (X_i^\top, A_i, Y_i)$ for $i = 1, \dots, n$ from an unknown distribution P_0. The tailoring variables $X_i \in \mathcal{X} \subseteq \mathbb{R}^p$ are assumed to be pre-treatment covariates, $A_i \in \{0, 1\}$ represents a binary treatment with propensity $\mu_A(x) = \mathbb{E}(A_1 | X_1 = x)$, and Y_i represents the continuous outcome $i = 1, \dots, n$.

Let $Y_i^*(a)$ denote the potential outcome of Y_i if the treatment is set to $A_i = a$. We make the commonly used assumptions for studying causal effects: stable unit treatment value assumption, no unmeasured confounders and positivity assumption (Rubin, 1978; Robins, 1986, 1989). Let $d(\cdot) \in \mathcal{D}$ be a decision rule that maps the observed covariates to a treatment where $\mathcal{D}$ is the set of all such rules. Assuming that higher outcomes are more desirable, we are interested in rules that maximize expected outcomes under that rule. We call the function $V : \mathcal{D} \mapsto \mathbb{R}$ defined as $V(d) := \mathbb{E}\{Y_1^*(d)\}$ the value function. A value-optimal decision rule is one that, if implemented, leads to an optimized expected outcome–i.e., $d^{opt} \in \arg\max_{d \in \mathcal{D}} V(d)$.

In general, an optimal decision rule d^{opt} satisfies

$$\begin{aligned} d^{opt}(x) &\in \arg\max_{a\in\{0,1\}} \mathbb{E}\left\{Y_1^*(a)|X_1 = x\right\} \\ &= \arg\max_{a\in\{0,1\}} \mathbb{E}\left\{Y_1^*(0) + a\big(Y_1^*(1) - Y_1^*(0)\big)\big|X_1 = x\right\} \\ &= \arg\max_{a\in\{0,1\}} \left\{\eta^*(x) + a\Delta^*(x)\right\}. \end{aligned}$$

This final expression decomposes the expected potential outcomes into a "treatment-free outcome model," $\eta^*(x)$, and a "contrast" or "blip" function, $\Delta^*(x)$ (Robins, 2004; Robins et al., 2008; Zhang et al., 2012; Schulte et al., 2014). The maximization only depends on

$$\Delta^*(x) = \mathbb{E}\left\{Y_1(1) - Y_1(0)|X_1 = x\right\},$$

and, consequently, $d^*(x) = \mathbb{1}\left\{\Delta^*(x) > 0\right\}$ maximizes $V(d)$.

The binary treatments considered here allow the expression of a saturated model for the observed outcome:

$$Y_i = \eta(X_i) + A_i\Delta(X_i) + \epsilon_{0i}, \tag{18.1}$$

where $\mathbb{E}(\epsilon_{01}|X_1, A_1) = 0$. The function $Q(x, a) = \mathbb{E}(Y_1|X_1 = x, A_1 = a)$ is decomposed by the functions $\eta(x) = Q(x, 0)$ and $\Delta(x) = Q(x, 1) - Q(x, 0)$. The previous causal assumptions imply that $\Delta(x) \equiv \Delta^*(x)$ and $\eta(x) \equiv \eta^*(x)$, so that optimization of expected potential outcomes is accomplished through study of $\Delta(x)$.

In the absence of additional information other than baseline tailoring variables, this contrast function would be the basis for making value-optimal treatment decisions for future patients. The usual approach to Q-learning imposes models on both the η and Δ functions. For example, linear parametric models are commonly used as a class of functions for the treatment-free outcome model. However, the validity this approach relies heavily on the accuracy of the η model. For example, if models $\eta(x;\gamma)$ and $\Delta(x;\theta)$ are imposed, then we may write the no-longer saturated version of (18.1) as

$$Y_i = \eta(X_i;\gamma) + A_i\Delta(X_i;\theta) + \epsilon_{1i}. \tag{18.2}$$

The formulation (18.2) gives rise to some complications. To see this, consider the residuals in this scheme, ϵ_{1i}, which are defined by

$$\epsilon_{1i} \equiv \epsilon_{1i}(\gamma, \theta) = \epsilon_{0i} + \{\eta(X_i) - \eta(X_i;\gamma)\} + A_i\{\Delta(X_i) - \Delta(X_i;\theta)\}.$$

Minimizing the expected squared-error loss is a common technique for identifying these parameters. Least-squares estimators from this model can be shown to target parameters which minimize the risk function

$$\begin{aligned} \mathbb{E}\Big[&\{\eta(X_1) - \eta(X_1;\gamma)\}^2 + \{\Delta(X_1) - \Delta(X_1;\theta)\}^2 \\ &+ 2A_1\{\eta(X_1) - \eta(X_1;\gamma)\}\{\Delta(X_1) - \Delta(X_1;\theta)\}\Big]. \end{aligned} \tag{18.3}$$

From the last line of this representation, we can see that the minimizer in θ is affected by misspecifications in the $\eta(\cdot)$ model. Only when $\eta(x)$ is contained in the span of parametric models $\eta(x;\gamma)$ could the contrast model become unaffected by the treatment-free outcome model. It would be preferable if the latter did not affect interpretations of θ, since it is irrelevant to the ITR estimation problem.

18.2.2 A Nonparametric Confounding Control Method

Progress can be made by re-expressing the model (18.1). By taking the conditional expectation of each side with respect to X_i, we obtain

$$\mu_Y(X_i) = \eta(X_i) + \mu_A(X_i)\Delta(X_i).$$

Subtracting this last expression from both sides of the equality in (18.1), we obtain equivalent the model

$$Y_i - \mu_Y(X_i) = \{A_i - \mu_A(X_i)\}\,\Delta(X_i) + \epsilon_{0i}. \tag{18.4}$$

In contrast to (18.2), this model exhibits a number of features. First, the explicit dependence upon the treatment-free outcome model $\eta(X_i)$ is eliminated by introducing the conditional expectations μ_A and μ_Y. Second, the residual ϵ_{i0} is the same as that of the saturated model (18.1), since no assumptions have yet been placed on the data-generating distribution. Further, the mean functions μ_A, μ_Y are relatively easy to estimate and are disentangled from the contrast model. If μ_Y and μ_A were known exactly, an analyst could impose a blip model, yielding

$$Y_i - \mu_Y(X_i) = \{A_i - \mu_A(X_i)\}\,\Delta(X_i;\theta) + \epsilon_{2i}, \tag{18.5}$$

where

$$\epsilon_{2i} \equiv \epsilon_{2i}(\theta) = \epsilon_{0i} + \{A_i - \mu_A(X_i)\}\,\{\Delta(X_i) - \Delta(X_i;\theta)\}. \tag{18.6}$$

At first glance, it doesn't appear that this model offers any improvement upon the previous working model (18.2). A fundamental difference between the two models, however, is the centering of $A_i - \mu_A(X_i)$, which has profound implications for the error variable. Specifically, this term has mean zero when conditioned upon X_i, and both the true function $\Delta(X_i)$ and working model $\Delta(X_i;\theta)$ are considered fixed on this conditioning variable. Examining the form of $\epsilon_{2i}(\theta)$, we see that it satisfies $\mathbb{E}\left(\epsilon_{2i}|X_i\right) = 0$ for any fixed θ. Notably, this implies the residuals have mean zero even when the contrast model is misspecified.

Using a class of linear working models $\Delta(X_1;\theta) = X_1^\top\theta$ along with squared-error loss, it is apparent that (18.5) falls into a class of linear-least squares regression problems with "response" $Y_i - \mu_Y(X_i)$ and "predictors" given by the vector $\{A_i - \mu_A(X_i)\}\,X_i$. In such problems, relevant fundamental quantities are the "Gram matrix" constructed from the predictors and the vector of inner products between predictors and response. Anticipating these needs, we define several of these quantities here for use throughout the remainder of the chapter. In the expressions below, we recall the definition of $W^{\otimes 2} = WW^\top$ for any vector W:

$$\begin{aligned}
H_0 =& \mathbb{E}\left[\{A_1 - \mu_A(X_1)\}^2 X_1^{\otimes 2}\right] \\
H_n =& n^{-1}\sum_{i=1}^{n} \{A_i - \mu_A(X_i)\}^2 X_i^{\otimes 2} \\
G_0 =& \mathbb{E}\left[\{A_1 - \mu_A(X_1)\}^2 \Delta(X_1)X_1\right] \\
G_n =& n^{-1}\sum_{i=1}^{n} X_i\{A_i - \mu_A(X_i)\}^2 \Delta(X_i) \\
\tilde{G}_n =& n^{-1}\sum_{i=1}^{n} X_i\{A_i - \mu_A(X_i)\}\{Y_i - \mu_Y(X_i)\}.
\end{aligned}$$

In these definitions, H_n and H_0 represent the Gram matrix and its expectation, respectively. The column vector $\tilde{G}_n$ represents the vector of inner products, $G_n = \mathbb{E}(\tilde{G}_n|X_1, A_1, \ldots, X_n, A_n)$, and $G_0 = \mathbb{E}(G_n)$.

The risk under squared-error loss of any θ takes the form

$$R(\theta) = \mathbb{E}\left(\left[Y_1 - \mu_Y(X_1) - \{A_1 - \mu_A(X_1)\} X_1^\top \theta\right]^2\right)$$
$$= \mathbb{E}\left(\left[\{A_1 - \mu_A(X_1)\}\{\Delta(X_1) - X_1^\top \theta\}\right]^2 + \epsilon_{01}^2\right).$$

The second line follows by making the substitution (18.4), grouping terms, and using the property $\mathbb{E}(\epsilon_{01}|X_1, A_1) = 0$. Since the second term in the final line does not depend on θ, we see that the minimizer of $R(\theta)$ equivalently minimizes the weighted risk function

$$R^*(\theta) = \mathbb{E}\left[\{A_1 - \mu_A(X_1)\}^2 \{\Delta(X_1) - X_1^\top \theta\}^2\right]. \tag{18.7}$$

Compared to (18.3), (18.7) does not depend on the treatment-free outcome model, which implies that the minimizer in θ is free of this model. The first-order condition for a minimizer θ^*_{0,M^F}, where the subscript M^F indicates use of the all p predictors in X_1, generally requires

$$0 = G_0 - H_0 \theta^*_{0,M^F}, \tag{18.8}$$

which results in the closed form solution

$$\theta^*_{0,M^F} = H_0^{-1} G_0, \tag{18.9}$$

provided that H_0 is positive definite. If we instead conditioned the expectation in (18.7) on the design elements $X_1, A_1, \ldots, X_n, A_n$, a similar argument would lead to a minimizer

$$\theta^*_{n,M^F} = H_n^{-1} G_n, \tag{18.10}$$

provided that H_n is positive definite.

18.2.3 Least-Squares Estimation

When μ_A and μ_Y are known exactly, the empirical risk under least-squares loss is given by

$$\tilde{R}_n(\theta) = \frac{1}{n} \sum_{i=1}^{n} \left[Y_i - \mu_Y(X_i) - \{A_i - \mu_A(X_i)\} X_i^\top \theta\right]^2 \tag{18.11}$$

which is equivalent to the linear least-squares regression of the transformed outcomes $Y_i - \mu_Y(X_i)$ on the transformed design variables $\{A_i - \mu_A(X_i)\} X_i$. Hence, the minimizer of (18.11) is given by

$$\tilde{\theta}_{n,M^F} = H_n^{-1} \tilde{G}_n.$$

The previous development gives an intuition for this transformed regression procedure in the unlikely case that both μ_A and μ_Y are known exactly. When the observed treatment is assigned with known randomization probability, it may be reasonable that the function $\mu_A(\cdot)$ is known exactly. Even in this case, the same cannot usually be said of $\mu_Y(\cdot)$. Because these functions are not of direct interest to the estimation problem, we may consider them to be infinite-dimensional nuisance parameters which generally must be estimated based on the data.

Previous work has proposed estimating these nuisance parameters using flexible machine learning techniques in a cross-fitting framework (Zhao et al., 2017; Ertefaie et al., 2021). Cross-fitting has been considered previously as a way to ensure these observation-specific errors are uncorrelated with each observation's contribution to the estimator (Klaassen, 1987; Zheng and van der Laan, 2011; Chernozhukov et al., 2018). The setup is similar to that used for K-fold cross-validation. Consider a fixed number $K > 0$ of folds used to randomly partition the data indices $\{1,\dots,n\}$ into K roughly-equally sized partitions $\boldsymbol{I}_1,\dots \boldsymbol{I}_K$. Let $\boldsymbol{I}_k^c$ represent the complement of the kth partition $\boldsymbol{I}_k$ with $\boldsymbol{I}_k^c = \cup_{j\neq k}\boldsymbol{I}_j$. For any collection of indices $\boldsymbol{I} \subseteq \{1,\dots,n\}$, let $\boldsymbol{D_I} = (X_i, A_i, Y_i)_{i\in \boldsymbol{I}}$ represent the corresponding data from the full sample. Cross-fitted estimators predict the values $\mu_A(X_i)$, $\mu_Y(X_i)$ for those observations $i \in \boldsymbol{I}_k$ by training the learners on the observations in $\boldsymbol{I}_k^c$. We will represent these predictions by $\hat{\mu}_A(X_i;\boldsymbol{D}_{\boldsymbol{I}_k^c})$, $\hat{\mu}_Y(X_i;\boldsymbol{D}_{\boldsymbol{I}_k^c})$. Many statistical software packages that implement machine learning methods utilize cross-validation as a matter of course. In practice, using these packages to obtain the cross-fitted predictions can require very little time or effort.

The cross-fitted least-squares estimator is constructed analogously to $\tilde{\theta}_{n,M^F}$ by replacing the true means with the cross-fitted predictions. Beginning with the least-squares objective function, the cross-fitted empirical risk is given by

$$\hat{R}_n(\theta) = \frac{1}{n}\sum_{k=1}^{K}\sum_{i\in\boldsymbol{I}_k}\left[Y_i - \hat{\mu}_Y(X_i;\boldsymbol{D}_{\boldsymbol{I}_k^c}) - \left\{A_i - \hat{\mu}_A(X_i;\boldsymbol{D}_{\boldsymbol{I}_k^c})\right\}X_i^\top\theta\right]^2. \tag{18.12}$$

The minimizer of $\hat{R}_n(\theta)$ equals

$$\hat{\theta}_{n,M^F} = \hat{H}_n^{-1}\hat{G}_n,$$

provided that $\hat{H}_n$ is positive definite, where

$$\begin{aligned}
\hat{H}_n =& n^{-1}\sum_{k=1}^{K}\sum_{i\in\boldsymbol{I}_k}\left[\left\{A_i - \hat{\mu}_A(X_i;\boldsymbol{D}_{\boldsymbol{I}_k^c})\right\}^2 X_i^{\otimes 2}\right]\\
\hat{G}_n =& n^{-1}\sum_{k=1}^{K}\sum_{i\in\boldsymbol{I}_k} X_i\left\{A_i - \hat{\mu}_A(X_i;\boldsymbol{D}_{\boldsymbol{I}_k^c})\right\}\left\{Y_i - \hat{\mu}_Y(X_i;\boldsymbol{D}_{\boldsymbol{I}_k^c})\right\}.
\end{aligned}$$

Throughout the remainder, we make use of Assumptions 2-5 presented in Section 18.7.1. In addition to regularity conditions on the unknown distribution P_0 and conditions on the positive definiteness of H_n and $\hat{H}_n$, these assumptions specify certain rates of approximation of the estimated mean functions. These rates allow nonparametric estimators under certain conditions; see Remark 8 for a discussion.

The Proposition below establishes that the estimator using cross-fitting approximates the Oracle estimator with known μ_A and μ_Y. With high probability, the error from cross-fitting is much smaller than the sampling variability of the oracle estimator.

Proposition 18.2.1. *Suppose Assumptions 2-5 in Section 18.7.1 hold. Then*

$$\|\hat{\theta}_{n,M^F} - \tilde{\theta}_{n,M^F}\|_\infty = o_p(n^{-1/2}).$$

Proof. This will follow as a result of Proposition 18.3.1. □

18.2.4 Decision Rule Targets under M^F

In Section 18.2.1, the goal of ITR estimation was presented as identifying a decision rule maximizing $V(d)$ over the space of all rules $\mathcal{D}$. It was shown that $d^*(x) = \mathbb{1}\{\Delta^*(x) > 0\}$ maximizes $V(d)$ over $d \in \mathcal{D}$. Machine learning algorithms to estimate the optimal rules from large classes which cannot be described by a finite-dimensional parameter have been proposed (Zhao et al., 2012; Zhang et al., 2012; van der Laan and Luedtke, 2015). However, we focus on finite-dimensional subspaces of $\mathcal{D}$ for four reasons: (1) these finite-dimensional models lead to more interpretable and understandable decision rules; (2) effect modifier selection may be performed via existing regularization methods; (3) the targeted finite-dimensional parameters have a valid causal interpretation in terms of the conditional average treatment effect; and (4) the class of parametric rules, while not containing d^*, may nonetheless result in rules with competitive value while providing parametric rates of convergence and better finite-sample efficiency.

Mimicking the construction of d^*, we could identify any linear parametric model $\Delta(x;\theta) = x^\top\theta$ with a parametric decision rule $d_\theta(x) = \mathbb{1}(x^\top\theta > 0)$. In this way, we may also view a decision rule as a function-valued map $\theta \mapsto d_\theta$. Since X_1 is p-dimensional, the space of all such rules is the image of the set of $\theta \in \mathbb{R}^p$ under the mapping d_θ. We will write this space as

$$\mathcal{D}_{M^F} = \left\{d_\theta : \theta \in \mathbb{R}^p\right\} \subset \mathcal{D},$$

where the subscript M^F is used to indicate that this space corresponds to the full model with dimension p.

The notion of which decision rule is targeted by Q-learning-based estimators such as those in Section 18.2.3 is complicated by both the heuristic construction of the decision rules as well as the sources of randomness. Here, we consider three different parameters as relevant targets. The first parameter is the target of the ITR estimation problem over the restricted space, $\theta^{opt}_{M^F} \in \arg\max_{\theta\in\mathbb{R}^p} V(\theta)$, where we consider the value function $V(\theta) \equiv V(d_\theta)$ as a map directly from the parameter θ to a measure of performance. It is possible that $\theta^{opt}_{M^F}$ is non-unique. Another target considers the outcome variables $Y_1, \ldots, Y_n$ to be random, but the other components of $O_1, \ldots, O_n$ to be fixed. This leads to the target vector $\theta^*_{n,M^F} = H_n^{-1}G_n$. The final vector considers all forms of randomness in the observed data, $\theta^*_{0,M^F} = H_0^{-1}G_0$.

The three parameters have slightly different interpretations. The first parameter, $\theta^{opt}_{M^F}$, corresponds to an optimal rule in the class $\mathcal{D}_{M^F}$. The second parameter, θ^*_{n,M^F}, corresponds to the unbiased target of the method described in Section 18.2.3 in populations with the same realizations of H_n and G_n. The final parameter, θ^*_{0,M^F}, corresponds to the unbiased target of this method across the entire distribution of $O_1, \ldots, O_n$. It is not necessarily the case that any of these three parameters are equivalent, except in the case where θ^*_{0,M^F} completely parametrizes the true blip function. In this restrictive case, all three parameters are equivalent.

As such, $\hat{\theta}_{n,M^F} = \hat{H}_n^{-1}\hat{G}_n$ cannot in general be expected to converge in probability to $\theta^{opt}_{M^F}$. The other two parameters may be considered targets of this estimator in the sense that the ℓ_∞-distance between either of θ^*_{n,M^F} or θ^*_{0,M^F} and $\hat{\theta}_{n,M^F}$ tends to zero as $n \to \infty$, as expected from Proposition 18.2.1 and Chebyshev's inequality. Because these targets are well-defined, related to interpretable projections of the underlying blip function, and may relate to useful decision rules, these parameters are relevant to ITR estimation even if not necessarily value-optimal. The vector $\hat{\theta}_{n,M^F}$ provides an interpretable measure of the importance of each variable in this targeted rule, subject to sampling variation. Classical inference methods such as confidence intervals and tests provide a quantitative measure of replicability for these results.

18.3 Variable Selection in this ITR Estimation Framework

18.3.1 Defining the Set of Models

Throughout this section, we will make frequent use of the following matrices and column vectors. These quantities have been previously defined; we reprint them here to simplify their comparison. The expressions given for H_n, G_n and $\tilde{G}_n$ are equivalent to those given earlier since the double sum over all folds and all indices within each fold just reduce to the sum over all subjects; the expressions for $H_0, \hat{H}_n, G_0$,and $\hat{G}_n$ are identical to those given earlier:

$$
\begin{aligned}
H_0 =& \mathbb{E}\left[\{A_1 - \mu_A(X_1)\}^2 X_1^{\otimes 2}\right] \\
H_n =& n^{-1}\sum_{k=1}^{K}\sum_{i\in \boldsymbol{I}_k} \{A_i - \mu_A(X_i)\}^2 X_i^{\otimes 2} \\
\hat{H}_n =& n^{-1}\sum_{k=1}^{K}\sum_{i\in \boldsymbol{I}_k} \{A_i - \hat{\mu}_A(X_i; \boldsymbol{D}_{\boldsymbol{I}_k^c})\}^2 X_i^{\otimes 2} \\
G_0 =& \mathbb{E}\left[\{A_1 - \mu_A(X_1)\}^2 \Delta(X_1)X_1\right] \\
G_n =& n^{-1}\sum_{k=1}^{K}\sum_{i\in \boldsymbol{I}_k} X_i \{A_i - \mu_A(X_i)\}^2 \Delta(X_i) \\
\tilde{G}_n =& n^{-1}\sum_{k=1}^{K}\sum_{i\in \boldsymbol{I}_k} X_i \{A_i - \mu_A(X_i)\}\{Y_i - \mu_Y(X_i)\} \\
\hat{G}_n =& n^{-1}\sum_{k=1}^{K}\sum_{i\in \boldsymbol{I}_k} X_i \{A_i - \hat{\mu}_A(X_i; \boldsymbol{D}_{\boldsymbol{I}_k^c})\}\{Y_i - \hat{\mu}_Y(X_i; \boldsymbol{D}_{\boldsymbol{I}_k^c})\}.
\end{aligned}
$$

The development in Section 18.2 assumed the full information in X_1 would be used in decision rule creation. Next we define the model selection event as it acts upon the decision rules. The observed data defines a maximal amount of information which can be used, or a "full model" represented through the entire vector X_1. Sub-models are created by subsetting this full vector. We may identify this subsetting operation with the indices of X_1 used to create the sub-vector. That is, the "full model" may be identified with the object $M^F := \{1, \ldots, p\}$ and sub-models of M^F can be identified as any $M \subseteq M^F$. The maximal set of all possible sub-models is given by the power set $\mathcal{M} := \{M : M \subseteq M^F\}$.

We will often use the notation of $M \in \mathcal{M}$ to refer to an arbitrary (fixed) sub-model. That is, M represents a particular specification of the elements of X_1 that will be used to assess effect modification and thereby tailor future treatment. Based on the description of $\mathcal{M}$, we may think of any *apriori*-specified model $M \in \mathcal{M}$ as representing the set of indices j corresponding to the covariates X_{1j} to be included in said model; that is, the jth element of X_1, X_{1j}, is included as part of the model M if and only if $j \in M$. We adopt the notation of Kuchibhotla et al. (2020) of $X_1(M)$ representing a sub-matrix or sub-vector of X_1 corresponding to the model indices M. For example, when X_1 is a column vector of dimension 5 and $M = \{1, 2\}$, then $X_1(M)$ represents the 2-dimensional sub-vector of X_1 constructed from the first two elements of X_1. Similarly, $H_n(M)$ represents the $|M| \times |M|$ sub-matrix of the $p \times p$ matrix H_n with entries corresponding to the rows and columns indexed by M.

18.3.2 The ITR Estimation Problem for Sub-Models

Restricting the set of variables used for tailoring induces several changes to the problems described in 18.2.4. The restriction impacts the working model for $\Delta(\cdot)$, the class of decision rules, and the three target parameters listed for the full-model case. Because of the link between the linear working models $\Delta(x; \theta) = x^\top\theta$ and the resulting decision rules $\mathbb{1}(x^\top\theta > 0)$, analysts may decide not to include all of the information in the covariates X_1 in the working model in order to limit which variables are used for tailoring. By choosing a sub-model prior to data analysis, the analyst creates a specific working model of the form $x(M)^\top\theta_M$, where $\theta_M \in \mathbb{R}^{|M|}$. This corresponds to only including the covariates related to M

in the regression model. Such a choice induces a decision rule $d_{M,\theta_M}(x) = \mathbb{1}\{x(M)^\top \theta_M > 0\}$, which analogously to Section 18.2.4, may be viewed as a function-valued map $(M, \theta_M) \mapsto d_{M,\theta_M}$ for any $M \in \mathcal{M}$ and $\theta_M \in \mathbb{R}^{|M|}$. The set of all decision rules under this restriction is defined for any $M \in \mathcal{M}$ as the image of $\theta_M \in \mathbb{R}^{|M|}$ under this mapping, which in set notation can be written

$$\mathcal{D}_M = \left\{ d_{M,\theta_M} : \theta_M \in \mathbb{R}^{|M|} \right\}. \tag{18.13}$$

Analogues of the full-model target parameters may also be defined for any particular sub-model. For any $M \in \mathcal{M}$, a corresponding optimal decision rule maximizes the value function as $d_M^{opt} \in \arg\max_{d \in \mathcal{D}_M} V(d)$. Equivalently, the parameter of this rule satisfies $\theta_M^{opt} \in \arg\max_{\theta_M \in \mathbb{R}^{|M|}} V(d_{M,\theta_M})$. As in Section 18.2.4, the estimator of Section 18.2.3 obeying the sub-model restriction does not in general target such a rule. Using straightforward generalizations of the arguments in that section, the oracle and cross-fitted estimators for the sub-model are respectively

$$\tilde{\theta}_{n,M} = H_n(M)^{-1} \tilde{G}_n(M) \tag{18.14}$$
$$\hat{\theta}_{n,M} = \hat{H}_n(M)^{-1} \hat{G}_n(M). \tag{18.15}$$

The targets of these estimators can be shown to be represented by

$$\theta_{n,M}^* = H_n(M)^{-1} G_n(M) \tag{18.16}$$
$$\theta_{0,M}^* = H_0(M)^{-1} G_0(M). \tag{18.17}$$

When a particular sub-model M is specified prior to data analysis, standard inference techniques for M-estimators apply. It is important to emphasize here that, when considering models M' and M such that $M \subset M'$, the target coefficients (18.16) and (18.17) under M will generally differ from those under M' for the variables included in both models except under restrictive conditions on the data-generating process.

We now describe some considerations for restricting the rule space. Recall that in general, $\theta_{0,M^F}^* \in \mathbb{R}^p$ is not equal to $\theta_{M^F}^{opt}$. Since $V(d_{M^F,\theta_{0,M^F}^*}) \leq V(d_{M^F,\theta_{M^F}^{opt}})$, there may exist some $M' \in \mathcal{M}$ yielding $V(d_{M',\theta_{0,M'}^*}) \geq V(d_{M^F,\theta_{0,M^F}^*})$. Even if this isn't the case, it is possible that $V(d_{M',\theta_{0,M'}^*}) \approx V(d_{M^F,\theta_{0,M^F}^*})$, with the relative sparsity of M' compared to M^F leading one to prefer the sparse decision rule. Based on these possibilities, certain sub-models may be very relevant to the ITR estimation problem, while others may not be so useful–e.g. those models that lead to value functions which are substantially lower than $V(d_{M^F,\theta_{0,M^F}^*})$.

Because the analyst may not be able to anticipate which sub-models are inferior to M^F in terms of value function, making use of the data to adapt to the underlying distribution may be desirable. Random model selection is formally described as a random variable $\hat{M}$ that (i) depends at least in part on the observed data $O_1, \ldots, O_n$ and (ii) takes its values in the space $\mathcal{M}$. In this interpretation, we may view each $M \in \mathcal{M}$ as a potential realization of the random variable $\hat{M}$. Thus, model selection acts to select the "relevant" sub-space $\mathcal{D}_{\hat{M}}$ and targets $\theta_{0,\hat{M}}^*$ or $\theta_{n,\hat{M}}^*$. However, unlike the case where the choice of model is not influenced by sampling variation in the observed data, inference is complicated by the data-dependent choice of model. For example, consider the definitions of the targets (18.16)-(18.17) evaluated at $M = \hat{M}$. These targets have dimension of $\mathbb{R}^{|\hat{M}|}$ depending on the selected model. One impact on the inferential problem is that the number of tests or intervals to be constructed for each element of the target vector depends on the data. Techniques accounting for this complication are presented in Section 18.4.

18.3.3 Lasso Penalization for Selection

There are many possible approaches to variable selection in regression problems. The Lasso (Tibshirani, 1996) is a popular penalized-regression technique that employs the ℓ_1 penalty. The geometric structure of the ℓ_1 penalty encourages sparsity, and thereby performs variable selection while allowing one to simultaneously produce a corresponding coefficient estimate. Indeed, the popularity of the Lasso stems in part from the fact that it can be viewed as an estimation procedure, a model selection procedure, or both.

In the current context of ITR estimation, we defined the Oracle risk function $\tilde{R}_n(\theta)$; see (18.12). Through the use of cross-fitting, we also defined the related risk function $\hat{R}_n(\theta)$ in (18.11). When penalization is desired, a natural estimator is then derived by regularizing these risks. The ℓ_1-penalized, or Lasso-type, estimators derived from these risks are defined for any $\lambda \geq 0$ as

$$\hat{\theta}_n^\lambda = \arg\min_{\theta \in \mathbb{R}^p} \left\{ \hat{R}_n(\theta) + \lambda \|\theta\|_1 \right\} \tag{18.18}$$

$$\tilde{\theta}_n^\lambda = \arg\min_{\theta \in \mathbb{R}^p} \left\{ \tilde{R}_n(\theta) + \lambda \|\theta\|_1 \right\}. \tag{18.19}$$

Like the original Lasso, and for a given $\lambda \geq 0$, the nonzero coefficient estimates in the Lasso-type estimator $\hat{\theta}_n^\lambda$ can be used to define a selected model $\hat{M}$; similarly, the nonzero coefficient estimates in the Lasso-type estimator $\tilde{\theta}_n^\lambda$ can be used to define a selected model $\tilde{M}$. The Proposition below establishes that the impact of cross-fitted estimation is of order smaller than $n^{-1/2}$.

Proposition 18.3.1. *Suppose Assumptions 2-5 in Section 18.7.1 hold. Then*

$$\sup_{0 \leq \lambda < \infty} \|\hat{\theta}_n^\lambda - \tilde{\theta}_n^\lambda\|_\infty = o_p(n^{-1/2}).$$

Viewed from the perspective of model selection, the previous Proposition establishes that the models $\hat{M}$ and $\tilde{M}$ respectively generated by $\hat{\theta}_n^\lambda$ and $\tilde{\theta}_n^\lambda$ agree with high probability asymptotically for those $\tilde{\theta}_n^\lambda$ components outside of any $n^{-1/2}$-neighborhood of zero.

The variable selection consistency of the Lasso was demonstrated contemporaneously by a few authors: a necessary condition was presented in Zou (2006), and necessary and "almost" sufficient conditions were detailed in Zhao and Yu (2006); with modification, similar results can be established for models derived from $\hat{\theta}_n^\lambda$ and/or $\tilde{\theta}_n^\lambda$. Moreover, previous work has established the asymptotic behavior of estimators like $\hat{\theta}_n^\lambda$ (e.g., Knight and Fu, 2000). However, statistical inference procedures based on this asymptotic distribution are known to have potentially serious deficiencies (e.g., Leeb and Pötscher, 2005, 2008). More recently, new procedures for inference have been proposed that focus on least squares estimators, equivalently the sub-model estimators described in Section 18.3.2, that are derived under the selected model $\hat{M}$ (e.g., Lee et al., 2016; Tian and Taylor, 2017; Tibshirani et al., 2018; Kuchibhotla et al., 2020). In Section 18.4, this latter inferential perspective is developed in greater detail for the ITR estimation problem; as such, the Lasso-type coefficient vector $\hat{\theta}_n^\lambda$ will not be of direct interest outside of its role in generating a data-dependent model $\hat{M}$.

18.4 Post-Selection Inference for ITR Estimation

18.4.1 Description of the Problem

When $\hat{M}$ is selected on the basis of the data, standard inference procedures which do not take into account this dependence may fail. At the same time, the data-driven model $\hat{M}$ may allow the sparse working model to adapt better to the underlying blip function, which may lead to better rules in terms of value or sparsity, as discussed in 18.3.2. Data-dependent models then may be very relevant to the ITR estimation problem. Accounting for sampling variation represents a challenge in this setting, as randomness in the data affects both the variation of $\hat{\theta}_{n,\hat{M}}$ around its target, the model $\hat{M}$, and consequently the underlying dimension of the parameter for inference. Usual statistical inference techniques might target components of the full-model parameter θ^*_{0,M^F} under sparsity assumptions. Post-selection estimators in general do not seem to target these types of parameters when these sparsity assumptions fail (Leeb and Pötscher, 2008). Rather, such methods target the importance measures $\theta^*_{0,\hat{M}}$ or $\theta^*_{n,\hat{M}}$, which may be viewed as the targets of estimation by future researchers that able to treat the model $\hat{M}$ as being chosen in advance. Due to the relevance of these randomly-selected targets to the ITR estimation problem, performing inference in the form of confidence intervals or hypothesis tests for these chosen parameters is desirable. However, the fact that the parameters and their relevant dimensions are randomly selected based on the data requires generalizations of classical fixed-parameter inference frameworks.

In this section, we will consider two methods for performing post-selection inference. The UPoSI method is *universally valid* across all possible model selectors $\hat{M}$ taking values in $\mathcal{M}$ (Kuchibhotla et al., 2020). The polyhedral method arises from studying the exact distribution of a particular class of model selectors, which includes the Lasso for non-random tuning parameters (Lee et al., 2016). The UPoSI method has the benefit of admitting variants which explicitly handle either of the target parameters $\theta^*_{0,\hat{M}}$ or $\theta^*_{n,\hat{M}}$, while the polyhedral method only handles $\theta^*_{n,\hat{M}}$. Some high-level arguments based on one-step estimator updates (Taylor and Tibshirani, 2018, Sec. 3.4) suggest that the polyhedral method may be modified to accommodate $\theta^*_{0,\hat{M}}$. However, due to computational considerations and the lack of established results, we will compare the UPoSI and polyhedral methods for targeting $\theta^*_{n,\hat{M}}$.

We are specifically interested in using the ℓ_1-penalized estimator (18.18) presented in Section 18.3.3 as a model selection mechanism $\hat{M}$. As indicated earlier, the selected model corresponds to the indices of the non-zero elements of $\hat{\theta}^{\lambda}_n$. This model $\hat{M}$ will then be used to perform inference for $\theta^*_{n,\hat{M}}$. We will consider the λ tuning parameter as non-random in order to accommodate the Polyhedral method, although no such assumption is needed for the UPoSI derivation. Throughout this section, we take the asymptotic perspective of $p < \infty$ fixed and not growing with n. While it is possible that many of the following results hold under relaxations of this assumption, such possibilities serve to complicate the presentation. This assumption will be highlighted at certain relevant opportunities, even though this is included in Assumption 4.

18.4.2 Polyhedral Method

The Lasso is often used as a model selection procedure due to the sparsity induced from its solutions. The Lasso model selection procedure identifies the covariates having non-zero coefficients in the Lasso solution. The zero coefficients are then considered "removed" from the model. The polyhedral method for post-selection inference was derived for the Lasso selection procedure by Lee et al. (2016). It provides a non-asymptotic procedure for controlling the False Coverage Rate (FCR) of confidence intervals under a certain data-generating process. This procedure was shown to hold in an asymptotic sense under certain relaxations of the distributional assumptions in Tian and Taylor (2017).

We provide a derivation of the main features of the polyhedral approach in the transformed saturated model (18.4). We may write this model in vector form as

$$\tilde{\boldsymbol{Y}}_n = \tilde{\boldsymbol{\Delta}}_n + \boldsymbol{\epsilon}_n \tag{18.20}$$

where $\tilde{\boldsymbol{Y}}_n = (Y_1 - \mu_Y(X_1), \ldots, Y_n - \mu_Y(X_n))^\top$, $\boldsymbol{\epsilon}_n = (\epsilon_{01}, \ldots, \epsilon_{0n})^\top$, and the ith element of the n-dimensional vector $\tilde{\boldsymbol{\Delta}}_n$ is given by $\{A_i - \mu_A(X_i)\}\,\Delta(X_i)$. Suppose momentarily that

$\boldsymbol{\epsilon}_n$ is generated from a multivariate Gaussian distribution with mean zero and covariance matrix $\Sigma \equiv \Sigma(A, X)$. Under the independence assumption, Σ is diagonal with elements $\text{diag}(\Sigma) = (\sigma_1^2, \ldots, \sigma_n^2)$. The general method follows by examining the Karush-Kuhn-Tucker (KKT) conditions of the Lasso solution (18.19) and re-writing them in the form of an affine inequality

$$\begin{pmatrix} \tilde{A}_0(M,s) \\ \tilde{A}_1(M,s) \end{pmatrix} \tilde{\boldsymbol{Y}}_n \leq \begin{pmatrix} \tilde{b}_0(M,s) \\ \tilde{b}_1(M,s) \end{pmatrix}.$$

The variable s may be interpreted as the signs of the non-zero Lasso coefficients. The matrices $\tilde{A}_0, \tilde{b}_0$ are related to the "inactive" constraints of the Lasso solution–i.e. constraints upon the unselected covariates–while $\tilde{A}_1, \tilde{b}_1$ are related to the "active" constraints on the selected variables. In the display above, we make explicit the dependence of $\tilde{A}_0, \tilde{b}_0, \tilde{A}_1$, and $\tilde{b}_1$ upon the possible selected models $M \in \mathcal{M}$ and $s \in \{-1,1\}^{|M|}$. Notably, these components also depend on the tuning parameter λ and "transformed design matrix" resulting from the linear working models considered here. This matrix is given by $\tilde{\boldsymbol{X}}_n = \tilde{\boldsymbol{W}}_n(X_1 \ \cdots \ X_n)^\top$ where $\tilde{\boldsymbol{W}}_n$ is the diagonal matrix with i^{th} diagonal entry given by $A_i - \mu_A(X_i)$. In other words, we have $H_n = n^{-1}\tilde{\boldsymbol{X}}_n^\top \tilde{\boldsymbol{X}}_n$ and $\tilde{G}_n = n^{-1}\tilde{\boldsymbol{X}}_n^\top \tilde{\boldsymbol{Y}}_n$. It will be convenient to write the previous display in the form $\tilde{A}\tilde{\boldsymbol{Y}}_n \leq \tilde{b}$.

Recall that $\tilde{\theta}_n^\lambda$ represents the Lasso solution to (18.19) for a nonrandom tuning parameter λ and $\tilde{M}$ represents the indices of the nonzero coefficients. Let $\tilde{s}$ represent the signs of the nonzero coefficients. Because a model selection event $\{\tilde{M} = M, \tilde{s} = s\} \equiv \{A(M,s)\boldsymbol{Y}_n \leq b(M,s)\}$, the Lasso selector is termed an "affine selection procedure". Such affine selectors have the property that the distribution of any linear combination of the outcome may be described over the affine region. Define the truncated Gaussian pivot as

$$F\left(x; \omega, c^2, L, U\right) = \frac{\Phi((x-\omega)/c) - \Phi((L-\omega)/c)}{\Phi((U-\omega)/c) - \Phi((L-\omega)/c)},$$

for any real-valued ω, L, U and any $c > 0$. For any fixed vector $v \in \mathbb{R}^n$, Lee et al. (2016) established the result

$$F\left(v^\top \tilde{\boldsymbol{Y}}_n; v^\top \tilde{\boldsymbol{\Delta}}_n, v^\top \Sigma v, L(M,s), U(M,s)\right) |\{\tilde{M} = M, \tilde{s} = s\} \sim \mathcal{U}[0,1] \tag{18.21}$$

where $\mathcal{U}[0,1]$ represents the uniform distribution on the interval $[0,1]$.

In the case where $\boldsymbol{\epsilon}_n$ is Gaussian, the distributional result (18.21) holds exactly. When the errors are not Gaussian, the distribution may be shown to be approximate in the sense that the pivot converges to this limiting distribution under some regularity conditions (see Tian and Taylor (2017) and Tibshirani et al. (2018)). This pivotal statistic may be used as the basis for inferential procedures such as confidence intervals and hypothesis tests–in the former setting as an exact procedure, and in the latter as an asymptotic one.

Since the Polyhedral method focuses on targets which are linear combinations of the conditional mean vector $\tilde{\boldsymbol{\Delta}}_n$, we consider targets of the form $\theta_{n,M}^*$ in this chapter. To put the components of this target into the relevant form $v^\top \tilde{\boldsymbol{\Delta}}_n$, we must identify the appropriate vector v. Let e_k be a conformable vector of zero with an entry of 1 in the kth position. Define the vectors $v_{M,j}$ and $\hat{v}_{M,j}$ for $j = 1, \ldots, |M|, M \in \mathcal{M}$ with respective i^{th} elements given by

$$e_i^\top v_{M,j} = \{A_i - \mu_A(X_i)\} e_j^\top H_n(M)^{-1} X_i \tag{18.22}$$

$$e_i^\top \hat{v}_{M,j} = \{A_i - \hat{\mu}_A(X_i)\} e_j^\top \hat{H}_n(M)^{-1} X_i \tag{18.23}$$

so that $e_j^\top \tilde{\theta}_{n,M} = v_{M,j}^\top \tilde{\boldsymbol{Y}}_n$, $e_j^\top \hat{\theta}_{n,M} = v_{M,j}^\top \hat{\boldsymbol{Y}}_n$, and $e_j^\top \theta_{n,M}^* = v_{M,j}^\top \tilde{\boldsymbol{\Delta}}_n$. Here, $\hat{\boldsymbol{Y}}_n$ is defined similarly to $\tilde{\boldsymbol{Y}}_n$ except using the cross-fitted estimates for the μ_Y function. The remaining components that must be handled in the pivot (18.21) are the variance $v^\top \Sigma v$ and the truncation limits $L(M,s), U(M,s)$. The general form of the truncation limits are presented in Lee et al. (2016). To simplify the presentation, we restrict the diagonal matrix Σ to have constant diagonal elements: $\sigma^2 \equiv \sigma_1^2 = \cdots = \sigma_n^2$. Then the choice of v given in (18.22) corresponds to $v_{M,j}^\top \Sigma v_{M,j} = \sigma^2 e_j^\top H_n(M)^{-1} e_j$, and that of (18.23) corresponds to $\hat{v}_{M,j}^\top \Sigma \hat{v}_{M,j} = \sigma^2 e_j^\top \hat{H}_n(M)^{-1} e_j$. This simplification allows the expression of the pivot, for $j = 1, \ldots, |M|$, as

$$F\Big(e_j^\top \tilde{\theta}_{n,M}\ ;\ e_j^\top \theta_{n,M}^*,\ \sigma^2 e_j^\top H_n(M)^{-1} e_j,\ L_j(M,s),\ U_j(M,s)\Big) \tag{18.24}$$

and also simplifies the form of the truncation limits (Zhao et al., 2017), which may be written as

$$\begin{aligned} L_j(M,s) =& e_j^\top \tilde{\theta}_{n,M} + \max_{k=1,\ldots,|M|: s_k z_{jk}(M)<0} c_{jk}(M,s) \\ U_j(M,s) =& e_j^\top \tilde{\theta}_{n,M} + \min_{k=1,\ldots,|M|: s_k z_{jk}(M)>0} c_{jk}(M,s) \\ c_{jk}(M,s) =& \frac{e_k^\top H_n(M)^{-1}\{\tilde{G}_n(M) - 2\lambda s\}}{z_{jk}} \\ z_{jk}(M) =& -e_k^\top H_n(M)^{-1} e_j. \end{aligned} \tag{18.25}$$

Because the condition (18.21) holds exactly, the simplified pivot (18.24) may be used to construct confidence intervals after selection by the Lasso solution (18.19). The constructed confidence intervals satisfy an exact conditional coverage condition, as reported in Lee et al. (2016). However, this development uses the unknown μ_A and μ_Y throughout the pivot. Define $\hat{L}_j(M,s)$ and $\hat{U}_j(M,s)$ as in (18.25), except with $\tilde{\theta}_{n,M}$, H_n, and $\tilde{G}_n$ replaced by the estimated values $\hat{\theta}_{n,M}$, $\hat{H}_n$, and $\hat{G}_n$, respectively. Further, let $\hat{M}$ and $\hat{s}$ be defined similarly to $\tilde{M}$ and $\tilde{s}$, respectively, using the cross-fitted penalized estimator $\hat{\theta}_n^\lambda$. In the following Theorem, cross-fitting is shown to have a negligible impact in an asymptotic sense.

Theorem 18.4.1. *(Zhao et al., 2017, Thm. 2) Suppose Assumptions 2-9 in Section 18.7.1 hold and the noise variables* $\epsilon_{01}, \ldots, \epsilon_{0n}$ *in* (18.4) *are i.i.d.* $\mathrm{N}(0,\sigma^2)$. *Then for any* $M \in \mathcal{M}$ *and* $s \in \{-1,1\}^{|M|}$ *such that* $P(\hat{M} = M, \hat{s} = s) > 0$, *the pivot*

$$F\Big(e_j^\top \hat{\theta}_{n,M}\ ;\ e_j^\top \theta_{n,M}^*,\ \sigma^2 e_j^\top \hat{H}_n(M)^{-1} e_j,\ \hat{L}_j(M,s),\ \hat{U}_j(M,s)\Big) \tag{18.26}$$

converges in distribution to that of $\mathcal{U}[0,1]$ *conditional on* $\hat{M} = M, \hat{s} = s$.

Through the probability integral transform, this result implies that confidence intervals $C_{n,\hat{M},j}, j = 1, \ldots, |\hat{M}|$ satisfy the asymptotic conditional coverage criterion

$$\liminf_{n\to\infty} P\Big(e_j^\top \theta_{n,\hat{M}}^* \in C_{n,\hat{M},j} \Big| \hat{M} = M, \hat{s} = s\Big) \geq 1 - \alpha, \tag{18.27}$$

which in turn implies the asymptotic FCR condition

$$\liminf_{n\to\infty} \mathbb{E}\left[|\hat{M}|^{-1} \sum_{j=1}^{|\hat{M}|} \mathbb{1}\{e_j^\top \theta_{n,\hat{M}}^* \notin C_{n,\hat{M},j}\} \middle| |\hat{M}| > 0 \right] \leq \alpha. \tag{18.28}$$

See Lee et al. (2016) for additional information on these criteria. In particular, (18.27) implies a marginal condition which involves a similar guarantee without the condition within the probability statement.

Theorem 18.4.1 requires the errors to have an identical Gaussian distribution. Relaxations of Gaussianity have been explored in several papers, under various assumptions (Tian and Taylor, 2017; Tibshirani et al., 2018). Exact results for Gaussian errors with heterogeneous variance are handled in Lee et al. (2016), although the inactive constraints A_0, b_0 are no longer trivially satisfied. Additionally, the theoretical results require estimation of the heterogeneous variance matrix Σ. Notice that the ith diagonal element of Σ represents the variance component $\mathbb{E}(\epsilon_{0i}^2|X_i, A_i)$, where ϵ_{0i} represents the error from the saturated model (18.4). The dimensionality and difficulty of learning the unknown function $\Delta(X)$ represents a challenge in estimation of Σ. On the other hand, Tibshirani et al. (2018) has noticed sufficient performance of tests based on the Truncated Gaussian statistics even under the false assumption of homogeneous variance. General results on robustness of the pivot to heterogeneity are unknown to these authors.

Some drawbacks to the Polyhedral method have been recently explored in the literature. The Polyhedral method has been shown to create confidence intervals with infinite expected length under many situations (Kivaranovic and Leeb, 2020). The issue occurs due to the truncation of the Gaussian distribution: specifically, there is no restriction on the pivot $F(x;\omega,c^2,L,U)$ that $L \le \omega \le U$. In other words, the pre-truncation Gaussian mean ω may fall outside of the truncation limits. Confidence intervals for the true mean based on the pivot may then extend beyond the truncation limits when searching for plausible values of ω. In terms of (18.25), confidence intervals may have infinite length with positive probability whenever $e_j^\top \tilde{\theta}_{n,M}$ is very close to L_j or U_j, as one must search beyond the truncation limits to find values of $e_j^\top \theta_{n,M}^*$ consistent with the data, in the sense that the pivot (18.26) evaluated at some candidate value of $e_j^\top \theta_{n,M}^*$ is at least $\alpha/2$.

Another issue with this approach is the development of exact finite-sample results for fixed tuning parameter λ. It is common to use the data to select a value for this tuning parameter, e.g. using cross-validation. However, the finite-sample results do not allow this parameter to depend on the data. It is possible that asymptotic arguments for cross-validation (e.g., van der Vaart et al., 2006) could be used to infer asymptotic convergence results that could justify the use of these random values. However, such results have not yet been established in the literature.

18.4.3 UPoSI

18.4.3.1 Deriving the UPoSI Regions

The UPoSI method provides an alternative framework in which post-selection inference is conducted. The post-selection inference problem is formulated as providing coverage guarantees for confidence regions that are constructed for parameters, like those defined in (18.16)-(18.17), after a random model selection event takes place. Unlike the Polyhedral method, the UPoSI framework is agnostic to the specific random model selection mechanism. While we may continue to think of the model $\hat{M}$ as being determined by the Lasso as defined in Section 18.3.3, this is not required in the construction of the UPoSI confidence region.

The UPoSI regions are derived by examining the post-selection inference problem through the lens of simultaneous inference. The post-selection inference problem is defined for general parameters and confidence region construction methods. For any parameter vector $\bar{\theta}_{n,\hat{M}}$, where the parameter is selected based on the random model, the goal is to construct a confidence region $\bar{\mathcal{R}}_{n,\hat{M}}$ containing this selected parameter at the desired confidence level. Such a region satisfies the Full-Vector False-Coverage Probability (FVFCP) criterion:

$$P\left(\bar{\theta}_{n,\hat{M}} \notin \bar{\mathcal{R}}_{n,\hat{M}}\right) \le \alpha. \qquad (18.29)$$

The following Theorem, proved in Kuchibhotla et al. (2020), establishes the equivalence between this criterion and simultaneous inference.

Theorem 18.4.2. *(Kuchibhotla et al., 2020, Thm. 3.1) Let $\bar{\mathcal{R}}_{n,M}$ be a confidence region for a parameter $\bar{\theta}_{n,M}$. Let $\hat{M}$ be a data-dependent model taking values almost surely in $\mathcal{M}$. Then (18.29) is equivalent to*

$$P\Big(\bigcap_{M\in\mathcal{M}}\Big\{\bar{\theta}_{n,M}\in\bar{\mathcal{R}}_{n,M}\Big\}\Big)\geq 1-\alpha. \tag{18.30}$$

In the remainder, we will derive the form of the UPoSI confidence regions in the context of our ITR estimation framework. The idea is to examine the normal equations for any sub-model M, along with the system resulting from taking expectations. Using the previously-established notation regarding sub-matrices and sub-vectors, we may write the sets of first-order equations as

$$\hat{H}_n(M)\hat{\theta}_{n,M} = \hat{G}_n(M) \qquad\qquad H_0(M)\theta^*_{0,M} = G_0(M).$$

By subtracting the rightmost system from the leftmost one, it is shown in Theorem 4.1 of Kuchibhotla et al. (2020) that

$$\begin{aligned}\|\hat{H}_n(M)\{\hat{\theta}_{n,M}-\theta^*_{0,M}\}\|_\infty \leq&\|\hat{G}_n-G_0\|_\infty+\|\hat{H}_n-H_0\|_\infty\|\theta^*_{0,M}\|_1\\ =&D_n^G+D_n^H\|\theta^*_{0,M}\|_1.\end{aligned} \tag{18.31}$$

The final line results from defining $D_n^G=\|\hat{G}_n-G_0\|_\infty$ and $D_n^H=\|\hat{H}_n-H_0\|_\infty$. Since this is an almost-sure inequality resulting from the normal equations, we might interpret the random variables D_n^G and D_n^H as almost-surely bounding the scaled distance of $\hat{\theta}_{n,M}$ from its target. This interpretation leads to two UPoSI confidence regions, the first with a finite-sample guarantee and the second with an asymptotic one:

$$\hat{\mathcal{R}}^*_{n,M} := \Big\{\theta\in\mathbb{R}^{|M|}:\|\hat{H}_n(M)\{\hat{\theta}_{n,M}-\theta\}\|_\infty\leq C_n^G(\alpha)+C_n^H(\alpha)\|\theta\|_1\Big\} \tag{18.32}$$

$$\hat{\mathcal{R}}^{\dagger *}_{n,M} := \Big\{\theta\in\mathbb{R}^{|M|}:\|\hat{H}_n(M)\{\hat{\theta}_{n,M}-\theta\}\|_\infty\leq C_n^G(\alpha)+C_n^H(\alpha)\|\hat{\theta}_{n,M}\|_1\Big\}. \tag{18.33}$$

Here, the critical values $C_n^G(\alpha)$ and $C_n^H(\alpha)$ are bivariate quantiles of D_n^G and D_n^H, which for any α satisfy

$$P(D_n^G\leq C_n^G(\alpha),\ D_n^H\leq C_n^H(\alpha))\geq 1-\alpha. \tag{18.34}$$

The first region (18.32) is an exact $(1-\alpha)\%$ post-selection region in the sense of (18.30) because it is created by pivoting the exact bound (18.31) in the unknown parameter $\theta^*_{0,M}$ and replacing the random variables D_n^G and D_n^H by their respective quantiles. The second region (18.33) is an asymptotically valid region because the second term in the last line of (18.31) has the unknown parameter replaced by its consistent estimate.

In this development, we arrived at the regions above for the fixed target $\theta^*_{0,M}$ by manipulating the normal equations associated with both $\hat{\theta}_{n,M}$ and $\theta^*_{0,M}$. Notably, we might instead replace the equations associated with the latter by

$$H_n(M)\theta^*_{n,M} = G_n(M),$$

from which we would bound

$$\begin{aligned}\|\hat{H}_n(M)\{\hat{\theta}_{n,M}-\theta^*_{n,M}\}\|_\infty \leq&\|\hat{G}_n-G_n\|_\infty+\|\hat{H}_n-H_n\|_\infty\|\theta^*_{n,M}\|_1\\ =&D_n^{G_n}+D_n^{H_n}\|\theta^*_{n,M}\|_1.\end{aligned}$$

Under Assumptions 2-5 in Section 18.7.1, the first term of the final line is $O_p(n^{-1/2})$ and the second term is $o_p(n^{-1/2})$, so that a simplification of the UPoSI regions is given as

$$\hat{\mathcal{R}}_{n,M} := \Big\{\theta\in\mathbb{R}^{|M|}:\|\hat{H}_n(M)\{\hat{\theta}_{n,M}-\theta\}\|_\infty\leq C_n^{G_n}(\alpha)\Big\}. \tag{18.35}$$

The definition of $C_n^{G_n}(\alpha)$ is also simplified as

$$C_n^{G_n}(\alpha) = \inf_{c>0} P(D_n^{G_n} \le c) \ge 1-\alpha,$$

a standard univariate $1-\alpha$ quantile.

This region asymptotically satisfies both (18.30) and (18.29), in the sense that the probability statements hold for all large enough n by setting $\bar{\mathcal{R}}_{n,M} \equiv \hat{\mathcal{R}}_{n,M}$ and $\bar{\theta}_{n,M} \equiv \theta^*_{n,M}$.

Theorem 18.4.3. *Suppose Assumptions 2-5 in Section 18.7.1 hold with $p<\infty$ fixed in n. Then the confidence region* (18.35) *satisfies*

$$\liminf_{n\to\infty} P\left(\cap_{M\in\mathcal{M}}\{\theta^*_{n,M} \in \hat{\mathcal{R}}_{n,M}\}\right) \ge 1-\alpha, \tag{18.36}$$

and asymptotically controls the Full-Vector False Coverage Probability

$$\limsup_{n\to\infty} P\left(\theta^*_{n,\hat{M}} \notin \hat{\mathcal{R}}_{n,\hat{M}}\right) \le \alpha. \tag{18.37}$$

Due to our focus on the target parameter $\theta^*_{n,\hat{M}}$, we will continue to examine the region (18.35) as "the UPoSI region" throughout the remainder. Generalizations of the remaining arguments could be used to target $\theta^*_{0,\hat{M}}$ through the regions (18.32) and (18.33). General properties for these regions without nuisance parameter estimation are detailed in Kuchibhotla et al. (2020).

18.4.3.2 Implied Confidence Intervals

The confidence region (18.35) has a more complicated geometry than desired when the goal is to build intervals for each coordinate of the parameter vector. The smallest hyperrectangle enclosing the region is useful since the coordinate-wise projections of this hyperrectangle correspond to commonly used confidence intervals. An analytic solution is available for the UPoSI region (18.35) by straightforward generalizations of the arguments in Kuchibhotla et al. (2020). The bounds of the rectangle in the jth coordinate of $\theta^*_{n,M}$ is given by

$$e_j^\top \hat{\theta}_{n,M} \pm \|e_j^\top(\hat{H}_n(M))^{-1}\|_1 C_n^{G_n}(\alpha), \ \forall j \in M \tag{18.38}$$

where e_j represents a conformable column vector with 1 in the jth position and 0 elsewhere. This analytic formula can be used directly in the construction of confidence intervals for each coordinate of the $\theta^*_{n,M}$ vector. This representation also demonstrates that these confidence intervals are symmetric about the point estimates $e_j^\top \hat{\theta}_{n,M}$. The critical value $C_n^{G_n}(\alpha)$ need only be estimated to create these intervals.

Because these regions are based on $\hat{\mathcal{R}}_{n,M}$, we may specify the interval $\hat{\mathcal{R}}_{n,M,j} = \{u \in \mathbb{R} : |u - e_j^\top \hat{\theta}_{n,M}| \le \|e_j^\top(\hat{H}_n(M))^{-1}\|_1 C_n^{G_n}(\alpha)\}$. Then the coverage condition (18.36) may be stated for these intervals as

$$\liminf_{n\to\infty} P\left(\cap_{M\in\mathcal{M}} \cap_{j\in M} \{e_j^\top \hat{\theta}_{n,M} \in \hat{R}_{n,M,j}\}\right) \ge 1-\alpha,$$

which would be implied by Theorem 18.4.3 along with the observation that the hyperrectangle $\prod_{j\in M} \hat{\mathcal{R}}_{n,M,j}$ contains the region $\hat{\mathcal{R}}_{n,M}$.

18.4.3.3 The Multiplier Bootstrap and its Algorithm

From the expression (18.38), it may be apparent that the overall size of the confidence region is controlled by the critical value $C_n^{G_n}(\alpha)$. The previous development has not yet provided a method for choosing appropriate values of these two components. One approach could be to make a parametric assumption on the distributions of X_1 and Y_1. However, this approach would tie inference to a particular set of assumed distributions, as well as an assumed dependence structure.

Kuchibhotla et al. (2020) instead consider a multiplier bootstrap approach to estimate the quantiles of the appropriate distributions. The multiplier bootstrap framework makes comparatively fewer assumptions and is robust to various dependence structures. This approach can further be justified using high-dimensional central limit theorems, allowing one to use such methods in higher-dimensional problems.

Recall that the distribution of $\sqrt{n}D_n^{G_n} = \sqrt{n}\|\hat{G}_n - G_n\|_\infty$ must be approximated to construct the region (18.35). We proceed by defining, for each $i \in \boldsymbol{I}_k, k = 1, \ldots, K$,

$$\begin{aligned}\tilde{W}_i :=& X_i \{A_i - \mu_A(X_i)\} \{Y_i - \mu_Y(X_i)\} \\ \hat{W}_{i(k)} :=& X_i \{A_i - \hat{\mu}_A(X_i; \boldsymbol{D}_{\boldsymbol{I}_k^c})\} \{Y_i - \hat{\mu}_Y(X_i; \boldsymbol{D}_{\boldsymbol{I}_k^c})\}\end{aligned}$$

so that $\tilde{G}_n = n^{-1}\sum_{i=1}^n \tilde{W}_i$ and $\hat{G}_n = n^{-1}\sum_{k=1}^K \sum_{i\in\boldsymbol{I}_k} \hat{W}_{i(k)}$. We examine two quantities, corresponding to known and estimated mean functions, respectively:

$$\begin{aligned}\tilde{S}_n^* :=& n^{-1/2} \sum_{i=1}^n Z_i \left(\tilde{W}_i - \tilde{G}_n\right) \\ \hat{S}_n^* :=& n^{-1/2} \sum_{k=1}^K \sum_{i\in\boldsymbol{I}_k} Z_i \left(\hat{W}_{i(k)} - \hat{G}_n\right)\end{aligned} \tag{18.39}$$

where $Z_1, \ldots, Z_n$ are a set of independent standard normal random variables that do not depend on the data. One may expect to be able to approximate the distribution of $\sqrt{n}D_n^{G_n}$ by $\|\tilde{S}_n^*\|_\infty$. In our framework, we expect $\sqrt{n}D_n^{G_n} = O_p(1)$, so that this is the appropriate scale for distributional approximation. Since $C_n^{G_n}(\alpha)$ was defined as an upper $1-\alpha$ quantile of $D_n^{G_n}$, we define $\tilde{C}_n^{G_n}(\alpha)$ on a similar scale via the expression

$$\tilde{C}_n^{G_n}(\alpha) = \inf_{c>0} P^*\left(n^{-1/2}\|\tilde{S}_n^*\|_\infty \leq c \middle| O_1, \ldots, O_n\right) \geq 1 - \alpha,$$

where $P^*(\cdot|O_1, \ldots, O_n)$ represents probability according to the multiplier bootstrap distribution conditioned upon the observed data. Similarly, we may define the marginal version $P^*(\cdot)$ which does not condition on the observed data. The quantity $\tilde{C}_n^{G_n}(\alpha)$ depends on unknown nuisance parameters. Instead, cross-fitting may be used in $\hat{C}_n^{G_n}(\alpha)$, defined similarly by

$$\hat{C}_n^{G_n}(\alpha) = \inf_{c>0} P^*\left(n^{-1/2}\|\hat{S}_n^*\|_\infty \leq c \middle| O_1, \ldots, O_n\right) \geq 1 - \alpha. \tag{18.40}$$

The following conjecture establishes that the bootstrap distribution of $\|\tilde{S}_n^*\|_\infty$ can be used to uniformly approximate the distribution of $\sqrt{n}D_n^{G_n}$. Because the critical values $C_n^{G_n}(\alpha)$ are based on quantiles of this distribution, this implies that the quantiles of the approximated distribution are close as well. The impact of cross-fitting is also shown to be asymptotically negligible.

Conjecture 5. *Under Assumptions 2-5 in Section 18.7.1,*

$$\sup_{c\geq 0}\left|P^*\left(\|\tilde{S}_n^*\|_\infty \leq c \middle| O_1, \ldots, O_n\right) - P\left(\sqrt{n}D_n^{G_n} \leq c\right)\right| \to 0$$

$$\sup_{c\geq 0}\left|P^*\left(\|\hat{S}_n^*\|_\infty \leq c\right) - P^*\left(\|\tilde{S}_n^*\|_\infty \leq c\right)\right| \to 0.$$

In practice, the bootstrap distribution of $\|\tilde{S}_n^*\|_\infty$ may be approximated by that of $\|\hat{S}_n^*\|_\infty$ using Monte-Carlo methods. This can be implemented drawing B independent realizations of the vector $Z = (Z_1, \ldots, Z_n)$, where B is chosen to be suitably large. The construction (18.39) would lead to B realizations of $\hat{S}_n^*$ which are independent, conditional upon $O_1, \ldots, O_n$. Then an approximation of $\hat{C}_n^{G_n}(\alpha)$ would replace P^* in (18.40) by the empirical distribution of the Monte-Carlo realizations of $\|\hat{S}_n^*\|_\infty$.

18.5 Simulations

We compared UPoSI and the Polyhedral method through several simulations on the basis of confidence interval length and coverage properties. Data were generated on the basis of the saturated model (18.1) by varying the functional form of the treatment-free outcome model $\eta(X)$, the conditional average treatment effect function $\Delta(X)$, and the propensity $\mu_A(X)$. The baseline tailoring and confounding variables $X \in \mathbb{R}^{5+q}$ for $q = 5$ were generated independently as uniform random variables on $(-1, 1)$, and the residuals ϵ_0 were independently and identically generated from the standard normal distribution.

Different functional forms were specified for $\eta(X)$, $\Delta(X)$, or as the component of the propensity $\mu_A(X) = \text{expit}\{.2f(X)\}$ where the constant .2 was chosen to ensure the positivity assumption while providing a sufficient confounding effect and $f(X)$ represents one of the functions in the display below. These forms were chosen to represent different complexities of association: no association, linear, slightly nonlinear, and extremely nonlinear association. In the case of $\eta(X)$, departures from linearity are not relevant to decision rule construction, but may nonetheless impact estimation and inference if a linear model is assumed to hold. On the other hand, the form of the $\Delta(X)$ function directly impacts the sub-model parameter (18.17) indexing the targeted decision rule. The functions used are presented below.

$$\begin{aligned} f_{zero}(X) &= 0 && \text{Z} \\ f_{lin}(X) &= 3X_1 - X_2 - X_3 - X_4 + X_5 && \text{L} \\ f_{quad}(X) &= 2X_1 - 2X_2 - X_3 - X_4 + X_5^2 && \text{Q} \\ f_{fgs}(X) &= 2\sin(\pi X_1 X_2) + 2(X_2 - 0.5)^2 && \text{N} \end{aligned}$$

We use the letters printed alongside each function to abbreviate the simulation settings in order of specification of $\mu_A(\cdot)$, $\eta(\cdot)$ and $\Delta(\cdot)$. For example, ZLQ refers to the setting in which treatment was randomized with $\mu_A(X) \equiv 1/2$, $\eta(\cdot)$ was specified as the linear model $f_{lin}(\cdot)$, and $\Delta(\cdot)$ was specified as the quadratic model $f_{quad}(\cdot)$.

The Robinson's transformation model (18.5) was used for all methods. Five-fold cross-fitting was used with a machine learning ensemble to fit the unknown mean functions. The ensemble was fit by the `SuperLearner` R package and included a library of base learners including linear or logistic regression, Multivariate Adaptive Regression Splines provided by the `earth` R package, Generalized Additive Models from the `mgcv` package, and the marginal mean. The model was selected using the Lasso with tuning parameter chosen by adapting the choice of Negahban et al. (2012), later used in Lee et al. (2016). Specifically, λ was chosen as $\lambda = \mathbb{E}\left(\|\tilde{G}_n - G_n\|_\infty | X_1, A_1, \ldots, X_n, A_n\right)$. Since the exact value of λ was unknown, it was approximated by 500 Monte-Carlo simulations.

Performance of the UPoSI and Polyhedral methods are compared with the naive method which ignores selection when constructing confidence intervals using standard Gaussian likelihood-based inference. To examine the role of cross-fitting, we also performed the Lasso-based selection along with these three inference techniques on the oracle model with known μ_A and μ_Y. The inference techniques are compared in Tables 18.1 and 18.2 on the basis of median confidence interval length, FCR as used in (18.28), and the FVFCP as presented in

Table 18.1 *Simulation Results for the UPoSI, Polyhedral (SI), and Naive methods. The oracle model ("True") results are presented. Comparisons are based on Median Confidence Interval Length (Med. CI. Len.), False Coverage Rate (FCR), and Full-vector False Coverage Probability (FVFCP).*

			Med. CI. Len.			FCR			FVFCP		
$\hat{\mu}$	Setting	n	UPoSI	SI	Naive	UPoSI	SI	Naive	UPoSI	SI	Naive
True	ZLL	500	1.91	0.96	0.88	0	0.06	0.05	0.00	0.23	0.21
		1000	1.27	0.64	0.62	0	0.06	0.07	0.00	0.25	0.30
		2000	0.86	0.44	0.44	0	0.06	0.07	0.01	0.26	0.29
	ZLF	500	1.73	1.20	1.05	0	0.03	0.08	0.00	0.04	0.11
		1000	1.19	0.83	0.74	0	0.03	0.08	0.00	0.04	0.11
		2000	0.84	0.57	0.52	0	0.02	0.07	0.00	0.03	0.10
	ZQQ	500	1.73	0.91	0.85	0	0.06	0.06	0.00	0.20	0.21
		1000	1.17	0.61	0.60	0	0.05	0.06	0.00	0.19	0.23
		2000	0.79	0.43	0.42	0	0.06	0.07	0.01	0.20	0.24
	ZFF	500	1.73	1.20	1.05	0	0.03	0.08	0.00	0.04	0.11
		1000	1.19	0.83	0.74	0	0.03	0.08	0.00	0.04	0.11
		2000	0.84	0.57	0.52	0	0.02	0.07	0.00	0.03	0.10
	LLL	500	1.95	1.04	0.93	0	0.06	0.05	0.00	0.26	0.24
		1000	1.30	0.67	0.65	0	0.05	0.06	0.00	0.22	0.27
		2000	0.88	0.47	0.46	0	0.05	0.06	0.00	0.22	0.27
	LLF	500	1.81	1.20	1.05	0	0.02	0.06	0.00	0.02	0.09
		1000	1.24	0.79	0.74	0	0.02	0.06	0.00	0.03	0.08
		2000	0.87	0.55	0.53	0	0.03	0.07	0.00	0.03	0.11
	LQQ	500	1.75	1.00	0.91	0	0.05	0.06	0.00	0.19	0.21
		1000	1.17	0.66	0.64	0	0.05	0.06	0.00	0.19	0.22
		2000	0.80	0.46	0.45	0	0.05	0.06	0.01	0.17	0.23
	LFF	500	1.81	1.20	1.05	0	0.02	0.06	0.00	0.02	0.09
		1000	1.24	0.79	0.74	0	0.02	0.06	0.00	0.03	0.08
		2000	0.87	0.55	0.53	0	0.03	0.07	0.00	0.03	0.11
	QQL	500	1.92	1.04	0.93	0	0.07	0.05	0.00	0.27	0.22
		1000	1.28	0.67	0.66	0	0.06	0.07	0.00	0.26	0.31
		2000	0.87	0.47	0.46	0	0.05	0.06	0.01	0.24	0.28

(18.29) and (18.37). Based on the results in the table, we can identify several trends. First, the UPoSI method is very conservative for the FCR criterion, with FCR of 0 across all sample sizes and simulation settings. The UPoSI method also tends to be conservative for the Full-Vector False Coverage Probability that it is set up to target. This is likely due to the hyper-rectangle containing the UPoSI region being larger than the UPoSI region itself. The median lengths of the UPoSI confidence intervals also tend to be larger than the other two methods. On the other hand, the UPoSI intervals covered the full parameter vector at the nominal rate even with cross-fitting, as seen in Table 18.2.

Compared to the UPoSI intervals, the Polyhedral intervals (SI) tend to be smaller on median. The Full-Vector False Coverage Probability criterion controlled by UPoSI is not controlled well by the SI intervals, as these only provide coordinate-wise inference guarantees. On the other hand, the FCR criterion tends to be controlled at or close to the nominal 0.05 level. This occurs even in the more nonlinear scenarios. Under cross-fitting, the FCR

Table 18.2 *Simulation Results for the UPoSI, Polyhedral (SI), and Naive methods. The SuperLearner-estimated functions with cross-fitting ("SL") results are presented. Comparisons are based on Median Confidence Interval Length (Med. CI. Len.), False Coverage Rate (FCR), and Full-vector False Coverage Probability (FVFCP).*

			Med. CI. Len.			FCR			FVFCP		
$\hat{\mu}$	Setting	n	UPoSI	SI	Naive	UPoSI	SI	Naive	UPoSI	SI	Naive
True	ZLL	500	1.91	0.96	0.88	0	0.06	0.05	0.00	0.23	0.21
		1000	1.27	0.64	0.62	0	0.06	0.07	0.00	0.25	0.30
		2000	0.86	0.44	0.44	0	0.06	0.07	0.01	0.26	0.29
	ZLF	500	1.73	1.20	1.05	0	0.03	0.08	0.00	0.04	0.11
		1000	1.19	0.83	0.74	0	0.03	0.08	0.00	0.04	0.11
		2000	0.84	0.57	0.52	0	0.02	0.07	0.00	0.03	0.10
	ZQQ	500	1.73	0.91	0.85	0	0.06	0.06	0.00	0.20	0.21
		1000	1.17	0.61	0.60	0	0.05	0.06	0.00	0.19	0.23
		2000	0.79	0.43	0.42	0	0.06	0.07	0.01	0.20	0.24
	ZFF	500	1.73	1.20	1.05	0	0.03	0.08	0.00	0.04	0.11
		1000	1.19	0.83	0.74	0	0.03	0.08	0.00	0.04	0.11
		2000	0.84	0.57	0.52	0	0.02	0.07	0.00	0.03	0.10
	LLL	500	1.95	1.04	0.93	0	0.06	0.05	0.00	0.26	0.24
		1000	1.30	0.67	0.65	0	0.05	0.06	0.00	0.22	0.27
		2000	0.88	0.47	0.46	0	0.05	0.06	0.00	0.22	0.27
	LLF	500	1.81	1.20	1.05	0	0.02	0.06	0.00	0.02	0.09
		1000	1.24	0.79	0.74	0	0.02	0.06	0.00	0.03	0.08
		2000	0.87	0.55	0.53	0	0.03	0.07	0.00	0.03	0.11
	LQQ	500	1.75	1.00	0.91	0	0.05	0.06	0.00	0.19	0.21
		1000	1.17	0.66	0.64	0	0.05	0.06	0.00	0.19	0.22
		2000	0.80	0.46	0.45	0	0.05	0.06	0.01	0.17	0.23
	LFF	500	1.81	1.20	1.05	0	0.02	0.06	0.00	0.02	0.09
		1000	1.24	0.79	0.74	0	0.02	0.06	0.00	0.03	0.08
		2000	0.87	0.55	0.53	0	0.03	0.07	0.00	0.03	0.11
	QQL	500	1.92	1.04	0.93	0	0.07	0.05	0.00	0.27	0.22
		1000	1.28	0.67	0.66	0	0.06	0.07	0.00	0.26	0.31
		2000	0.87	0.47	0.46	0	0.05	0.06	0.01	0.24	0.28

remains close to the nominal 0.05 level. On the other hand, the Naive intervals do not control either coverage criterion at the nominal level. After selection, the naive intervals failed to cover their targets at a rate of up to 8%.

While the median confidence interval length is smaller for UPoSI compared to SI, other features of confidence interval length are also of interest. To get a closer look at the confidence interval lengths, the results from Setting ZQQ with $n = 1000$ and cross-fitting are presented in Figure 18.1A. In this plot, the SI intervals tend to have much more variable lengths. In Setting ZQQ, the true $\Delta(X)$ model is linear in variables 1-4 and quadratic in variable 5. For the linear variables, the SI intervals tend to be close in length to those of the Naive intervals. For the other variables, the SI intervals tend to be larger. The UPoSI intervals don't seem to suffer from the extreme lengths of the Polyhedral method. In Figure 18.1B, the coverage rates for each variable are presented under the same simulation setting.

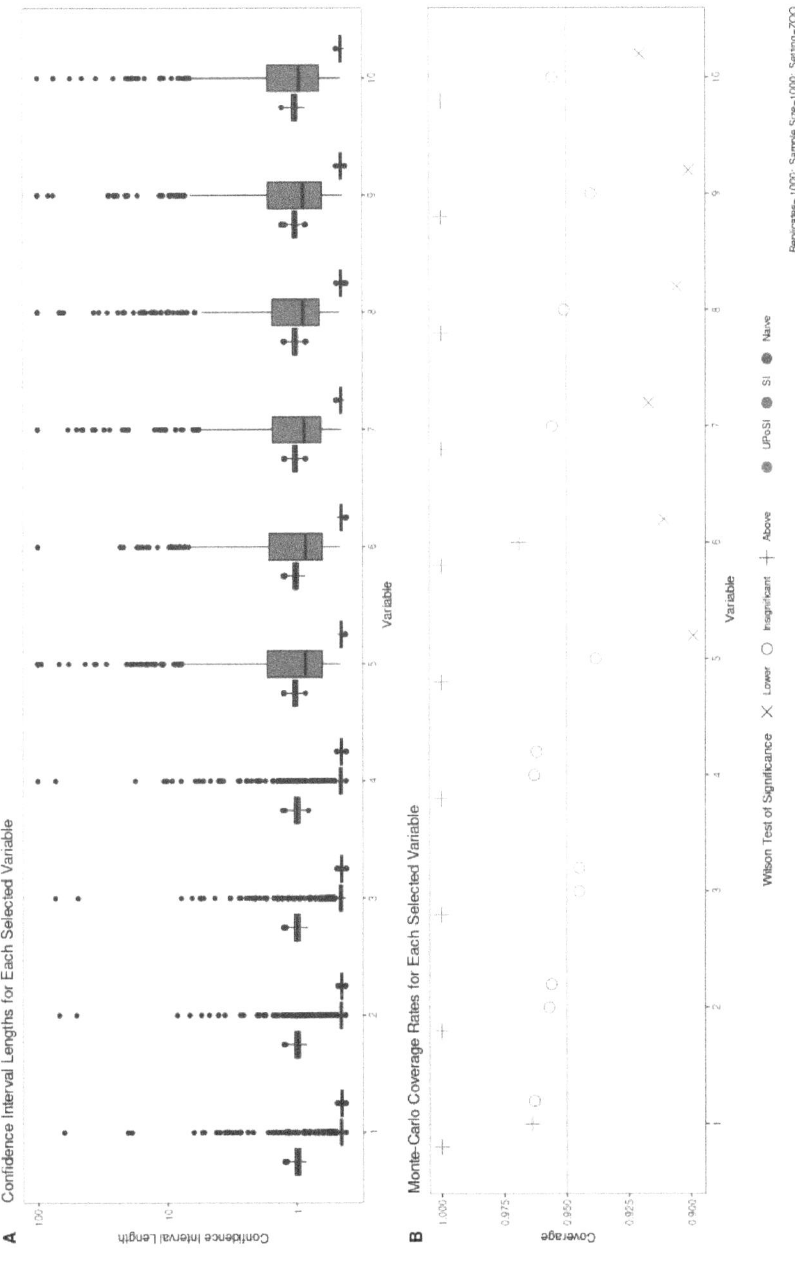

Figure 18.1 ***A***: *A boxplot of confidence interval lengths for each inference method. Variables 1-5 are involved in the true model, while variables 6-10 are noise.* ***B***: *Coverage rates for the intervals for each variable after selection.*

From this we see that the UPoSI intervals tend to be conservative in terms of coverage, while the SI intervals tend to cover at the nominal level. The Naive intervals suffer from poor coverage when one of the noise variables is selected by the Lasso. Since this translates to erroneously concluding that the unimportant variables have nonzero parameter values, this behavior is highly undesirable.

18.6 Conclusion

Several competing methods for performing inference on model coefficients after a selection event have been proposed in the statistical literature. These typically focus on the coefficients of association in some postulated model. We have shown how Robinson's Transformation can be used to eliminate, or at least mitigate, the effects of estimating an infinite dimensional nuisance parameter that is not relevant to the ITR estimation problem. We have additionally proposed natural extensions of the UPoSI and Polyhedral methods to facilitate inference after model selection in the resulting transformed model. The general properties of these inference methods are seen to be maintained even when estimating unknown conditional mean functions via cross-fitting, under some performance assumptions.

The UPoSI and Polyhedral methods themselves have very different characteristics. The Polyhedral method is based on a specific model selection strategy: that of the Lasso. It also depends on the tuning parameter λ_n being fixed in advance. The UPoSI method does not depend on any specific model selection technique, and hence does not depend on this restriction on how the tuning parameter is selected. It additionally admits any selection method, including alternative penalization methods with favorable properties compared to the Lasso (e.g. Fan and Li, 2001; Zou, 2006; Zhang, 2010). Other intriguing cases handled by the UPoSI framework are those informal methods which involve human judgement and intervention to select the model (c.f., Sec. 1.2 in Kuchibhotla et al., 2020). While the UPoSI intervals tend to be larger in median than those from the Polyhedral method, the Polyhedral intervals may suffer from drastically large–even infinite–confidence interval lengths. The UPoSI intervals tend to be more resistant to these extreme values.

We presented these methods in the case of a one-stage individualized treatment rule. When moving to a multi-stage setting, the Robinson's transformation approach may be extended (Ertefaie et al., 2021). One complication in developing this theory is that a model is selected in each stage, and the model fitting that takes place in the earlier stage depends implicitly on this random model. Another concerns the pseudo-outcomes constructed in earlier stages, which cannot be assumed to have Gaussian errors or homogeneous variance. Future work will examine the conditions under which these methods generalize to this setting.

18.7 Technical Details

18.7.1 Assumptions

Use the notation established in Section 18.2. Define the norm $\|f\|_{2kP_0}$ for $k = 1, \ldots, K$ as

$$\|f\|_{2kP_0} = \left\{\mathbb{E}_{P_0}\left[f(O_{n+1}; \boldsymbol{D}_{\boldsymbol{I}_k^c})^2\right]\right\}^{1/2},$$

which depends on the "training" data $\boldsymbol{D}_{\boldsymbol{I}_k^c}$. Also let $n_k = |\boldsymbol{I}_k|$ and $\bar{n}_k = n - n_k$ for $k = 1, \ldots, K$.

We make the following assumptions, which are essentially those of Ertefaie et al. (2021).

Assumption 2. $O_1, \ldots, O_n$ are i.i.d. realizations of an underlying distribution P_0. Further, the causal assumptions of Sec. 18.2 hold:

1. $Y_1 = Y_1^*(A_1)$
2. $Y_1^*(a) \perp\!\!\!\perp A_1|X_1,\ a \in \{0,1\}$
3. $\delta < \mu_A(X_1) < 1-\delta$ almost-surely for some $\delta > 0$.

Assumption 3. $|\Delta(X_1)| < C$ and $\|X_1\|_\infty < C$ almost-surely for some $0 < C < \infty$. Furthermore, $\mathbb{E}(\epsilon_{01}^2|X_1, A_1) < C$ almost-surely.

Assumption 4. H_n and $\hat{H}_n$ are positive-definite for all $n \geq n_0$ and some $n_0 > 0$. Further assume that $p < \infty$ is fixed in n and $\lambda_{min}(H_n)$, the minimum eigenvalue of H_n, satisfies $1/\lambda_{min}(H_n) = O_p(1)$.

Assumption 5. The cross-fitting setup described in Section 18.2.3 is used for some fixed $K > 1$. The estimated nuisance parameters satisfy the following rates for $k = 1, \ldots, K$.

$$\begin{aligned}\|\hat{\mu}_Y - \mu_Y\|_{2kP_0} =& o_p(1)\\ \|\hat{\mu}_A - \mu_A\|_{2kP_0} =& o_p(\bar{n}_k^{-1/4})\\ \|\hat{\mu}_A - \mu_A\|_{2kP_0}\|\hat{\mu}_Y - \mu_Y\|_{2kP_0} =& o_p(\bar{n}_k^{-1/2})\end{aligned}$$

Remark 8. In the cross-fitting setup described previously, $\bar{n}_k/n \to (K-1)/K$, so that $O_p(\bar{n}_k^r) = O_p(n^r)$ for any $r \in \mathbb{R}$. The first rate merely requires that the outcome model converges in root-mean-squared error (RMSE), while the second rate requires that the treatment model converges in RMSE faster than $n^{-1/4}$. The final rate requires a balance between the accuracy of the treatment and outcome models, so that the product of the rates converges faster than $n^{-1/2}$. This may occur, e.g. if the first rate is refined to achieve $n^{-1/4}$ convergence. Importantly, these rates are slower than the parametric rates of convergence of $n^{-1/2}$, although they may be achieved by several nonparametric techniques under varied assumptions (Xiaohong Chen and White, 1999; Chen, 2007; Biau, 2012).

Remark 9. The results of Zhao et al. (2017), which will be referenced in Section 18.4.2, use a slightly different norm. For example, instead of $\|\hat{\mu}_Y - \mu_Y\|_{2kP_0} = o_p(1)$, that work requires

$$\left\{\frac{1}{n}\sum_{k=1}^{K}\sum_{i\in\boldsymbol{I}_k}\left(\hat{\mu}_Y(X_i;\boldsymbol{D}_{\boldsymbol{I}_k^c}) - \mu_Y(X_i)\right)^2\right\}^{1/2} = o_p(1).$$

In Ertefaie et al. (2021), Assumptions 2-5 are shown to have a similar effect on estimation error. In Section 18.4.2, we will continue to assume the previous assumptions hold.

The following assumptions are made for Theorem 18.4.1.

Assumption 6. (Size of the selected model) For some constant m, $P(|\hat{M}| \leq m) \to 1$.

Remark 10. In the context of 4, this is trivially satisfied. However, the presentation of Zhao et al. (2017) does not require p fixed with n, and so replaces the fixed p assumption included in 4 with this restriction on the model size.

Assumption 7. (Sparse eigenvalue assumption) For all $M \in \mathcal{M}$ such that $|M| \leq m$, the smallest eigenvalue of $\mathbb{E}[X_1(M)^{\otimes 2}]$ is greater than or equal to $1/C$.

Assumption 8. (Truncation threshold) Using $\hat{L}_j(M,s)$ and $\hat{U}_j(M,s)$ as defined in Sec. 18.4.2, the truncation lengths satisfy

$$P\left(\frac{\hat{U}_j(\hat{M},\hat{s}) - \hat{L}_j(\hat{M},\hat{s})}{\sigma\|\hat{v}_{\hat{M},j}\|_2} \geq 1/C\right) \to 1$$

for $j = 1, \ldots, |\hat{M}|$.

Assumption 9. (Lasso solution) Let e_k represent a conformable column vector of zeroes with a 1 in the kth position. There exists $C > 0$ such that

$$P\left(|e_k^\top \hat{\theta}_n^{\lambda_n}| \geq 1/(C\sqrt{n}),\ \forall k \in \hat{M}\right) \to 1.$$

Remark 11. Assumption 9 in the setup of Proposition 18.3.1 implies that $P(\hat{M} = \tilde{M}, \hat{s} = \tilde{s}) \to 1$ as $n \to \infty$, where $\tilde{M}, \tilde{s}$ are the nonzero elements and signs, respectively, of $\tilde{\theta}_n^{\lambda_n}$ defined in (18.19).

18.7.2 Proofs

Proof of Proposition 18.3.1. First, notice the minimand represented in (18.18) is equivalent to

$$\hat{R}_n^*(\theta; \lambda_n) = \theta^\top \hat{H}_n \theta - 2\theta^\top \hat{G}_n + \lambda_n \|\theta\|_1,$$

and similarly that of (18.19) is equivalent to

$$\tilde{R}_n^*(\theta; \lambda_n) = \theta^\top H_n \theta - 2\theta^\top \tilde{G}_n + \lambda_n \|\theta\|_1.$$

Note that $\tilde{R}_n^*(0; \lambda_n) = 0$ for all $\lambda_n \geq 0$, $n \geq 0$. First, we draw attention to the fact that $\tilde{\theta}_n \equiv \tilde{\theta}_n^0$ is $O_p(n^{-1/2})$ under our assumptions. Next, note that at each n, $\|\tilde{\theta}_n^\lambda\|_1$ is non-increasing in λ. Therefore, we have $\|\tilde{\theta}_n^\lambda\|_1 \leq \|\tilde{\theta}_n^0\|_1 = O_p(n^{-1/2})$, where the bound in probability is uniform in $\lambda \geq 0$.

Taking the transformation $\theta = \tilde{\theta}_n^{\lambda_n} + n^{-1/2}u$, let the following functions be defined:

$$\begin{aligned}
\hat{F}_n(u; \lambda_n) =& n[\hat{R}_n^*(\tilde{\theta}_n^{\lambda_n} + n^{-1/2}u; \lambda_n) - \hat{R}_n^*(\tilde{\theta}_n^{\lambda_n}; \lambda_n)] \\
\tilde{F}_n(u; \lambda_n) =& n[\tilde{R}_n^*(\tilde{\theta}_n^{\lambda_n} + n^{-1/2}u; \lambda_n) - \tilde{R}_n^*(\tilde{\theta}_n^{\lambda_n}; \lambda_n)] \\
N_n(u; \lambda_n) =& n\lambda_n(\|\tilde{\theta}_n^{\lambda_n} + n^{-1/2}u\|_1 - \|\tilde{\theta}_n^{\lambda_n}\|_1).
\end{aligned}$$

Then we may write

$$\begin{aligned}
\hat{F}_n(u; \lambda_n) &= 2n^{1/2}\tilde{\theta}_n^{\lambda_n \top} \hat{H}_n u + u^\top \hat{H}_n u - 2n^{1/2}\tilde{\theta}_n^{\lambda_n \top} \hat{G}_n + N_n(u; \lambda_n) \\
\tilde{F}_n(u; \lambda_n) &= 2n^{1/2}\tilde{\theta}_n^{\lambda_n \top} H_n u + u^\top H_n u - 2n^{1/2}\tilde{\theta}_n^{\lambda_n \top} \tilde{G}_n + N_n(u; \lambda_n).
\end{aligned}$$

Notice that under Assumption 4, there exists $n_0 > 0$ such that both $\hat{F}_n(u)$ and $F_n(u)$ are convex in the argument $u \in \mathbb{R}^p$ with unique minima, for every $n \geq n_0$. In the top line expression for $\hat{F}_n(u)$, add and subtract H_n wherever $\hat{H}_n$ appears, and do similarly with $\tilde{G}_n$ for $\hat{G}_n$. This yields

$$\begin{aligned}
\hat{F}_n(u; \lambda_n) - \tilde{F}_n(u; \lambda_n) = 2n^{1/2}\tilde{\theta}_n^{\lambda_n \top}(\hat{H}_n - H_n)u + u^\top(\hat{H}_n - H_n)u \\
- 2n^{1/2}\tilde{\theta}_n^{\lambda_n \top}(\hat{G}_n - \tilde{G}_n).
\end{aligned}$$

Finally, the proof of Lemma 5 in the Supplement of Ertefaie et al. (2021) establishes $\|\hat{H}_n - H_n\|_\infty = o_p(n^{-1/2})$, and similarly the proof of Theorem 1 in the same reference establishes that $\|\hat{G}_n - \tilde{G}_n\|_\infty = o_p(n^{-1/2})$. Thus we have that $\hat{F}_n(u; \lambda_n) = \tilde{F}_n(u; \lambda_n) + o_p(1)$, with the $o_p(1)$ remainder holding pointwise in u. To see that this implies uniform convergence in probability both over compacts of u and over λ_n, use the inequalities $|u^\top W v| \leq \|u\|_1 \|v\|_1 \|W\|_\infty$ for vectors u and v and matrix W:

$$\begin{aligned}
|\hat{F}_n(u; \lambda_n) - \tilde{F}_n(u; \lambda_n)| \leq 2\|n^{1/2}\tilde{\theta}_n^{\lambda_n}\|_1 \|\hat{H}_n - H_n\|_\infty \|u\|_1 \\
+ \|u\|_1^2 \|\hat{H}_n - H_n\|_\infty + 2\|n^{1/2}\tilde{\theta}_n^{\lambda_n}\|_1 \|\hat{G}_n - \tilde{G}_n\|_\infty.
\end{aligned}$$

Now take the supremum over an ℓ_1 compact, and use the previous rates:

$$\sup_{\|u\|_1 \leq K} |\hat{F}_n(u; \lambda_n) - \tilde{F}_n(u; \lambda_n)| \leq K o_p(n^{-1/2}) + K^2 o_p(n^{-1/2}) + O_p(n^{-1/2})$$

which does not depend on the sequence λ_n. This shows

$$\sup_{0\le\lambda<\infty}\sup_{\|u\|_1\le K}|\hat{F}_n(u;\lambda)-\tilde{F}_n(u;\lambda)|\to 0 \text{ in probability.} \tag{18.41}$$

Finally, we connect this to the minimizers $\hat{\theta}_n^{\lambda_n}$ and $\tilde{\theta}_n^{\lambda_n}$. Based on the change of variables, $\tilde{F}_n(u;\lambda_n)$ is uniquely minimized at $u=0$ and $\hat{F}_n(u;\lambda_n)$ is uniquely minimized at $\hat{u}_n^{\lambda_n}=\sqrt{n}(\hat{\theta}_n^{\lambda_n}-\tilde{\theta}_n^{\lambda_n})$, where we may write $\hat{u}_n$ to suppress the dependence on the sequence of λ_n. The desired result $\sup_{0\le\lambda<\infty}\|\hat{u}_n^{\lambda}\|_\infty=\sup_{0\le\lambda<\infty}\|\sqrt{n}(\hat{\theta}_n^{\lambda}-\tilde{\theta}_n^{\lambda})\|_\infty=o_p(1)$ follows by straightforward generalizations of standard arguments for convex functions (Davis et al., 1992, Lem. 2.2). To see this, first let $\delta>0$ and define $B_\delta:=\{v:\|v\|_1\le\delta\}$. Due to (18.41), we can argue along subsequences n_j of n for which the in-probability convergence above is strengthened:

$$\sup_{0\le\lambda<\infty}\sup_{u\in B_\delta}|\hat{F}_{n_j}(u;\lambda)-\tilde{F}_{n_j}(u;\lambda)|\to 0 \text{ almost-surely.} \tag{18.42}$$

Suppose that $\|\hat{u}_{n_j}^{\lambda_{n_j}}\|_1>\delta$ occurs infinitely often along such a subsequence. By (18.42) and the minimization of $\tilde{F}_{n_j}(u;\lambda_{n_j})$ uniquely at 0, we have

$$\hat{F}_{n_j}(v;\lambda_{n_j})>\hat{F}_{n_j}(0;\lambda_{n_j})\ge\hat{F}_{n_j}(\hat{u}_{n_j};\lambda_{n_j}),$$

almost surely for infinitely many n_j, any $v\in B_\delta$, and any sequence of λ_{n_j} satisfying $0\le\lambda_{n_j}<\infty$ at each n_j. This contradicts the convexity of $\hat{F}_n(u;\lambda_n)$ by choosing v to lie on the line segment between the origin and $\hat{u}_n$. Hence, we must have $\|\hat{u}_{n_j}^{\lambda_{n_j}}\|_1>\delta$ for only finitely many n_j.

Note that $\hat{F}_n(u;\lambda)$ is made up of terms which are $O_p(1)$ for each bounded u and the $N_n(u;\lambda)$ term. For each n, as λ increases, the latter term dominates and $\hat{F}_n(u;\lambda)$ is minimized near $u=0$. Then we may find a sequence of constants L_{n_j} such that $\sup_{\lambda>L_{n_j}}\|\hat{u}_{n_j}^{\lambda}\|_1<\delta$. Therefore, to establish that $\sup_{0\le\lambda<\infty}\|\hat{u}_n^{\lambda}\|_1>\delta$ occurs only finitely often, we may restrict the supremum at each n_j to the set $0\le\lambda\le L_{n_j}<\infty$. Since this is a compact set, we may choose $\lambda_{n_j}=\arg\max_{0\le\lambda\le L_{n_j}}\|\hat{u}_{n_j}^{\lambda}\|_1$ which implies, due to the continuity of $F_n(u;\lambda)$,

$$\|\hat{u}_{n_j}^{\lambda_{n_j}}\|_1=\sup_{0\le\lambda\le L_{n_j}}\|\hat{u}_{n_j}^{\lambda}\|_1.$$

The preceding arguments imply that this choice of λ_{n_j} satisfies $\|\hat{u}_n^{\lambda_{n_j}}\|_1>\delta$ only finitely often. Since L_{n_j} was chosen to bound the supremum on the set of large λ, we have established

$$\sup_{0\le\lambda\le\infty}\|\hat{u}_{n_j}^{\lambda}\|_1>\delta$$

occurs only finitely often along any subsequence n_j satisfying (18.42). Going back to the original sequence, this implies $\sup_{0\le\lambda<\infty}\|\hat{u}_n^{\lambda}\|_1=o_p(1)$.

□

The following Lemma is used in the proof of Theorem 18.4.3.

Lemma 18.7.1. *Suppose Assumptions 2-4 hold. Let $p<\infty$ be fixed with n. Then*

$$\max_{M\in\mathcal{M}}\|\theta_{n,M}^*\|_1=O_p(1).$$

Proof. Use the relationship between ℓ_q norms to bound

$$\|\theta_{n,M}^*\|_1\le\sqrt{|M|}\|\theta_{n,M}^*\|_2$$

$$=\sqrt{|M|}\|H_n(M)^{-1}G_n(M)\|_2.$$

Now use the definition of the $\|\cdot\|_{2,2}$ operator norm as the maximum singular value of a matrix to upper-bound this final quantity by

$$\sqrt{|M|}\lambda_{max}\left(H_n(M)^{-1}\right)\|G_n(M)\|_2 = \sqrt{|M|}\left\{\lambda_{min}\left(H_n(M)\right)\right\}^{-1}\|G_n(M)\|_2.$$

By the Cauchy Interlace Theorem, $\lambda_{min}(H_n(M)) \geq \lambda_{min}(H_n)$ for all $M \in \mathcal{M}$. By Assumption 4, $\lambda_{min}(H_n)^{-1} = O_p(1)$. From here, we take the max over $M \in \mathcal{M}$ to find

$$\max_{M\in\mathcal{M}} \|\theta^*_{n,M}\|_1 \leq \sqrt{p}O_p(1)\|G_n\|_2,$$

where the trivial inequality $\|G_n(M)\|_2 \leq \|G_n\|_2$ for any sub-vector indexed by $M \in \mathcal{M}$ is used in this final line. Since $p < \infty$ is considered fixed, $\|G_0\|_2 = O(1)$ by Assumptions 2-3, and $\|G_n - G_0\|_2 = O_p(n^{-1/2})$ by the CLT, we have established the result. □

Proof of Theorem 18.4.3. As in the proof of Theorem 4.1 in Kuchibhotla et al. (2020), we start with the probability statement

$$\liminf_{n\to\infty} P\left(\cap_{M\in\mathcal{M}}\left\{\|\hat{H}_n(M)\{\hat{\theta}_{n,M} - \theta^*_{n,M}\}\|_\infty \leq D_n^{G_n} + D_n^{H_n}\|\theta^*_{n,M}\|_1\right\}\right) = 1.$$

With $p < \infty$ fixed, $|\mathcal{M}| < \infty$ is fixed in n. Hence with probability one,

$$\begin{aligned}\max_{M\in\mathcal{M}} \|\hat{H}_n(M)\sqrt{n}\{\hat{\theta}_{n,M} - \theta^*_{n,M}\}\|_\infty &\leq \sqrt{n}D_n^{G_n} + \sqrt{n}D_n^{H_n}\max_{M\in\mathcal{M}}\|\theta^*_{n,M}\|_1 \\ &= \sqrt{n}D_n^{G_n} + o_p(1).\end{aligned}$$

Due to Lemma 18.7.1, this final line would follow if $D_n^{H_n} = o_p(n^{-1/2})$. Since $D_n^{H_n} = \|\hat{H}_n - H_n\|_\infty$, this property is established in the proof of Lemma 5 in the Supplement of Ertefaie et al. (2021). Hence,

$$\liminf_{n\to\infty} P\left(\cap_{M\in\mathcal{M}}\left\{\|\hat{H}_n(M)\{\hat{\theta}_{n,M} - \theta^*_{n,M}\}\|_\infty \leq D_n^{G_n}\right\}\right) = 1,$$

which yields the asymptotic coverage criterion.

The Full-Vector False Coverage probability statement follows directly from Theorem 18.4.2. □

Bibliography

107th Congress (2002). Rare diseases act of 2002. *Public Law* pages 107–280.

Aas, K., Czado, C., and Brechmann, E. (2012). Truncated regular vines in high dimensions with application to financial data. *Canadian Journal of Statistics* **40,** 68–85.

Aas, K., Czado, C., Frigessi, A., and Bakken, H. (2009). Pair-copula constructions of multiple dependence. *Insurance, Mathematics and Economics* **44,** 182–198.

Abadi, M., Agarwal, A., Barham, P., Brevdo, E., Chen, Z., Citro, C., Corrado, G. S., Davis, A., Dean, J., Devin, M., et al. (2016). Tensorflow: Large-scale machine learning on heterogeneous distributed systems. *arXiv preprint arXiv:1603.04467.*

Abadie, A. (2005). Semiparametric difference-in-differences estimators. *The Review of Economic Studies* **72,** 1–19.

Abadie, A., Chingos, M. M., and West, M. R. (2018). Endogenous stratification in randomized experiments. *Review of Economics and Statistics* **100,** 567–580.

Abadie, A., Diamond, A., and Hainmueller, J. (2010). Synthetic control methods for comparative case studies: Estimating the effect of california's tobacco control program. *Journal of the American Statistical Association* **105,** 493–505.

Abbas, R., Rossoni, C., Jaki, T., Paoletti, X., and Mozgunov, P. (2020). A comparison of phase I dose-finding designs in clinical trials with monotonicity assumption violation. *Clinical Trials* **17,** 522–534.

Abbasi-Yadkori, Y., Pál, D., and Szepesvári, C. (2011). Improved algorithms for linear stochastic bandits. *Advances in Neural Information Processing Systems* **24,** 2312–2320.

Abbasi-Yadkori, Y., Pal, D., and Szepesvari, C. (2012). Online-to-confidence-set conversions and application to sparse stochastic bandits. In *Artificial Intelligence and Statistics*, pages 1–9. PMLR.

Acemoglu, D. and Angrist, J. D. (2001). Consequences of employment protection? The case of the Americans with Disabilities Act. *Journal of Political Economy* **109,** 915–957.

Adcock, C. (1988). A Bayesian approach to calculating sample sizes. *Journal of the Royal Statistical Society: Series D (The Statistician)* **37,** 433–439.

Agrawal, S. and Devanur, N. (2016). Linear contextual bandits with knapsacks. *Advances in Neural Information Processing Systems* **29,** 3450–3458.

Agrawal, S. and Devanur, N. R. (2014). Bandits with concave rewards and convex knapsacks. In *Proceedings of the fifteenth ACM conference on Economics and computation*, pages 989–1006.

Agrawal, S. and Goyal, N. (2012). Analysis of thompson sampling for the multi-armed bandit problem. In *Conference on learning theory*, pages 39.1–39.26. JMLR Workshop and Conference Proceedings.

Agrawal, S. and Goyal, N. (2013a). Further optimal regret bounds for thompson sampling. In *Artificial intelligence and statistics*, pages 99–107. PMLR.

Agrawal, S. and Goyal, N. (2013b). Thompson sampling for contextual bandits with linear payoffs. In *International Conference on Machine Learning*, pages 127–135. PMLR.

Aguilera, A., Figueroa, C. A., Hernandez-Ramos, R., Sarkar, U., Cemballi, A., Gomez-Pathak, L., Miramontes, J., Yom-Tov, E., Chakraborty, B., Yan, X., et al. (2020). mhealth app using machine learning to increase physical activity in diabetes and depression: clinical trial protocol for the diamante study. *BMJ open* **10,** e034723.

Albert, J. H. and Chib, S. (1993). Bayesian analysis of binary and polychotomous response data. *Journal of the American Statistical Association* **88,** 669–679.

Ameko, M. K., Beltzer, M. L., Cai, L., Boukhechba, M., Teachman, B. A., and Barnes, L. E. (2020). Offline contextual multi-armed bandits for mobile health interventions: A case study on emotion regulation. In *Fourteenth ACM Conference on Recommender Systems*, pages 249–258.

An, G., Mi, Q., Dutta-Moscato, J., and Vodovotz, Y. (2009). Agent-based models in translational systems biology. *Wiley Interdisciplinary Reviews: Systems Biology and Medicine* **1(2),** 159–171.

Andrews, D. W. (1994). Empirical process methods in econometrics. *Handbook of Econometrics* **4,** 2247–2294.

Andrews, S., Ellis, D. A., Shaw, H., and Piwek, L. (2015). Beyond self-report: tools to compare estimated and real-world smartphone use. *PLoS One* **10,** e0139004.

Angrist, J. D. and Kugler, A. D. (2008). Rural windfall or a new resource curse? Coca, income, and civil conflict in colombia. *The Review of Economics and Statistics* **90,** 191–215.

Angrist, J. D. and Pischke, J.-S. (2008). *Mostly Harmless Econometrics: An Empiricist's Companion.* Princeton University Press.

Antognini, A. B. and Zagoraiou, M. (2012). Multi-objective optimal designs in comparative clinical trials with covariates: the reinforced doubly adaptive biased coin design. *The Annals of Statistics* **40,** 1315–1345.

Anzia, S. F. and Berry, C. R. (2011). The Jackie (and Jill) Robinson effect: Why do congresswomen outperform congressmen? *American Journal of Political Science* **55,** 478–493.

Arjas, E. and Saarela, O. (2010). Optimal dynamic regimes: Presenting a case for predictive inference. *The International Journal of Biostatistics* **6(2),** Article 10.

Arjovsky, M., Chintala, S., and Bottou, L. (2017). Wasserstein generative adversarial networks. In *International conference on machine learning*, pages 214–223. PMLR.

Arkhangelsky, D. (2018). Dealing with a technological bias: The difference-in-difference approach. Technical report, CEMFI.

Arkhangelsky, D., Athey, S., Hirshberg, D. A., Imbens, G. W., and Wager, S. (2019). Synthetic difference in differences. Technical report, National Bureau of Economic Research.

Armitage, P. (1960). *Sequential Medical Trials.* Blackwell Scientific Publications.

Aschard, H. (2016). A perspective on interaction effects in genetic association studies. *Genetic Epidemiology* **40,** 678–688.

Ashford, J. and Sowden, R. (1970). Multi-variate probit analysis. *Biometrics* **26(3),** 535–546.

Assmann, S. F., Pocock, S. J., Enos, L. E., and Kasten, L. E. (2000). Subgroup analysis and other (mis) uses of baseline data in clinical trials. *The Lancet* **355,** 1064–1069.

Athey, S., Bayati, M., Doudchenko, N., Imbens, G., and Khosravi, K. (2018). Matrix completion methods for causal panel data models. Technical report, National Bureau of Economic Research.

Athey, S. and Imbens, G. (2016). Recursive partitioning for heterogeneous causal effects. *Proceedings of the National Academy of Sciences* **113,** 7353–7360.

Athey, S. and Imbens, G. W. (2006). Identification and inference in nonlinear difference-in-differences models. *Econometrica* **74,** 431–497.

Athey, S., Tibshirani, J., Wager, S., et al. (2019). Generalized random forests. *The Annals of Statistics* **47,** 1148–1178.

Athey, S. and Wager, S. (2019). Estimating treatment effects with causal forests: An application. *Observational Studies* **5,** 37–51.

Athey, S., Wager, S., et al. (2017). Efficient policy learning. Technical report.

Atkinson, A., Biswas, A., and Pronzato, L. (2011). Covariate-balanced response-adaptive designs for clinical trials with continuous responses that target allocation probabilities. Technical report, Technical Report NI11042-DAE, Isaac Newton Institute for Mathematical Sciences.

Atkinson, A. C. and Biswas, A. (2019). *Randomised response-adaptive designs in clinical trials*. Chapman and Hall/CRC.

Audibert, J.-Y., Bubeck, S., et al. (2009). Minimax policies for adversarial and stochastic bandits. In *COLT*, volume 7, pages 1–122.

Auer, P. (2002). Using confidence bounds for exploitation-exploration trade-offs. *Journal of Machine Learning Research* **3,** 397–422.

Auer, P., Cesa-Bianchi, N., Freund, Y., and Schapire, R. E. (2002). The nonstochastic multiarmed bandit problem. *SIAM Journal on Computing* **32,** 48–77.

Auer, P., Gajane, P., and Ortner, R. (2019). Adaptively tracking the best bandit arm with an unknown number of distribution changes. In *Conference on Learning Theory*, pages 138–158. PMLR.

Auer, P. and Ortner, R. (2010). Ucb revisited: Improved regret bounds for the stochastic multi-armed bandit problem. *Periodica Mathematica Hungarica* **61,** 55–65.

Azriel, D. (2014). Optimal sequential designs in phase I studies. *Computational Statistics & Data Analysis* **71,** 288–297.

Azriel, D., Mandel, M., and Rinott, Y. (2011). The treatment versus experimentation dilemma in dose finding studies. *Journal of Statistical Planning and Inference* **141,** 2759–2768.

Babb, J., Rogatko, A., and Zacks, S. (1998). Cancer phase I clinical trials: efficient dose escalation with overdose control. *Statistics in Medicine* **17,** 1103–1120.

Babb, J. S. and Rogatko, A. (2001). Patient specific dosing in a cancer phase I clinical trial. *Statistics in Medicine* **20,** 2079–2090.

Badanidiyuru, A., Kleinberg, R., and Slivkins, A. (2018). Bandits with knapsacks. *Journal of the ACM (JACM)* **65,** 1–55.

Baiocchi, M., Cheng, J., and Small, D. S. (2014). Instrumental variable methods for causal inference. *Statistics in Medicine* **33,** 2297–2340.

Baird, L. (1995). Residual algorithms: Reinforcement learning with function approximation. In *Machine Learning Proceedings 1995*, pages 30–37. Elsevier.

Baldi Antognini, A. and Zagoraiou, M. (2011). The covariate-adaptive biased coin design for balancing clinical trials in the presence of prognostic factors. *Biometrika* **98,** 519–535.

Ballarini, N. M., Burnett, T., Jaki, T., Jennison, C., König, F., and Posch, M. (2021). Optimizing subgroup selection in two-stage adaptive enrichment and umbrella designs. *Statistics in Medicine* **40,** 2939–2956.

Bang, H. and Robins, J. M. (2005). Doubly robust estimation in missing data and causal inference models. *Biometrics* **61,** 962–973.

Bang, H. and Robins, J. M. (2008). Correction to "Doubly Robust Estimation in Missing Data and Causal Inference Models," by H. Bang and J. M. Robins; 61, 962–972, December 2005. *Biometrics* **64,** 650–650.

Bareinboim, E., Forney, A., and Pearl, J. (2015). Bandits with unobserved confounders: A causal approach. *Advances in Neural Information Processing Systems* **28,** 1342–1350.

Barker, A., Sigman, C., Kelloff, G., Hylton, N., Berry, D., and Esserman, L. (2009). I-SPY 2: an adaptive breast cancer trial design in the setting of neoadjuvant chemotherapy. *Clinical Pharmacology & Therapeutics* **86,** 97–100.

Barnett, H. Y., Villar, S. S., Geys, H., and Jaki, T. (2023). A novel statistical test for treatment differences in clinical trials using a response-adaptive forward-looking gittins index rule. *Biometrics* **79(1)**, 86–97.

Barocas, S., Hardt, M., and Narayanan, A. (2021). *Fairness and Machine Learning.* fairmlbook.org. `http://www.fairmlbook.org`.

Barr, P. B., Driver, M. N., Kuo, S. I.-C., Stephenson, M., Aliev, F., Linnér, R. K., Marks, J., Anokhin, A. P., Bucholz, K., Chan, G., Edenberg, H. J., Edwards, A. C., Francis, M. W., Hancock, D. B., Harden, K. P., Kamarajan, C., Kaprio, J., Kinreich, S., Kramer, J., Kuperman, S., Latvala, A., Meyers, J. L., Palmer, A. A., Plawecki, M. H., Porjesz, B., Rose, R. J., Schuckit, M. A., Salvatore, J. E., and Dick, D. M. (2022). Clinical, environmental, and genetic risk factors for substance use disorders: Characterizing combined effects across multiple cohorts. *medRxiv* doi: https://doi.org/10.1101/2022.01.27.22269750.

Bartlett, P. L., Jordan, M. I., and McAuliffe, J. D. (2006). Convexity, classification, and risk bounds. *Journal of the American Statistical Association* **101,** 138–156.

Bartroff, J. and Lai, T. L. (2010). Approximate dynamic programming and its applications to the design of phase I cancer trials. *Statistical Science* **25,** 245–257.

Bastani, H. and Bayati, M. (2020). Online decision making with high-dimensional covariates. *Operations Research* **68,** 276–294.

Bauer, P., Bretz, F., Dragalin, V., König, F., and Wassmer, G. (2016). Twenty-five years of confirmatory adaptive designs: opportunities and pitfalls. *Statistics in Medicine* **35,** 325–347.

Bauer, P. and Kieser, M. (1999). Combining different phases in the development of medical treatments within a single trial. *Statistics in Medicine* **18,** 1833–1848.

Bauer, P. and Köhne, K. (1994). Evaluation of experiments with adaptive interim analyses. *Biometrics* **50,** 1029–1041.

Bedford, T. and Cooke, R. (2001). Probability density decomposition for conditionally dependent random variables modeled by vines. *Annals of Mathematics and Artificial Intelligence* **32,** 245–268.

Bedford, T. and Cooke, R. (2002). Vines: A new graphical model for dependent random variables. *Annals of Statistics* **30,** 1031–1068.

Bekele, B. N. and Thall, P. F. (2004). Dose-finding based on multiple toxicities in a soft tissue sarcoma trial. *Journal of the American Statistical Association* **99,** 26–35.

Bellman, R. (1952). On the theory of dynamic programming. *Proceedings of the National Academy of Sciences* **38,** 716–719.

Bellman, R. (1957). *Dynamic programming.* Princeton University Press.

Belloni, A., Chernozhukov, V., and Wang, L. (2011). Square-root lasso: pivotal recovery of sparse signals via conic programming. *Biometrika* **98,** 791–806.

Ben-Michael, E., Feller, A., and Rothstein, J. (2021). The augmented synthetic control method. *Journal of the American Statistical Association* **116,** 1789–1803.

Benjamini, Y. (2020). Selective inference: The silent killer of replicability. *Harvard Data Science Review,* **2(4)**. https://doi.org/10.1162/99608f92.fc62b261

Berg, J. J., Harpak, A., Sinnott-Armstrong, N., Joergensen, A. M., Mostafavi, H., Field, Y., Boyle, E. A., Zhang, X., Racimo, F., Pritchard, J. K., et al. (2019). Reduced signal for polygenic adaptation of height in UK biobank. *Elife* **8,** e39725.

Berger, J. O. (1985). *Statistical Decision Theory and Bayesian Analysis.* Springer Science & Business Media.

Berger, J. O., Wang, X., and Shen, L. (2014). A Bayesian approach to subgroup identification. *Journal of Biopharmaceutical Statistics* **24,** 110–129.

Berisa, T. and Pickrell, J. K. (2016). Approximately independent linkage disequilibrium blocks in human populations. *Bioinformatics* **32,** 283.

Berk, R., Brown, L., Buja, A., Zhang, K., and Zhao, L. (2013). Valid post-selection inference. *The Annals of Statistics* **41,** 802–837.

Berkson, J. (1950). Are there two regressions? *Journal of the American Statistical Association* **45(250),** 164.

Berry, D. A. (2006). Bayesian clinical trials. *Nature Reviews Drug Discovery* **5,** 27–36.

Berry, D. A. (2010). Adaptive clinical trials: The promise and the caution. *Journal of Clinical Oncology* **29,** 606–609.

Berry, D. A. and Fristedt, B. (1985). Bandit problems: sequential allocation of experiments (monographs on statistics and applied probability). *London: Chapman and Hall* **5,** 7–7.

Berry, S. M., Broglio, K. R., Groshen, S., and Berry, D. A. (2013). Bayesian hierarchical modeling of patient subpopulations: efficient designs of phase II oncology clinical trials. *Clinical Trials* **10,** 720–734.

Berry, S. M., Carlin, B. P., Lee, J. J., and Muller, P. (2010). *Bayesian adaptive methods for clinical trials.* CRC Press, Raton, FL.

Bertrand, M., Duflo, E., and Mullainathan, S. (2004). How much should we trust differences-in-differences estimates? *The Quarterly Journal of Economics* **119,** 249–275.

Bertsekas, D. (2012). *Dynamic programming and optimal control: Volume I,* volume 1. Athena scientific.

Besbes, O., Gur, Y., and Zeevi, A. (2014). Stochastic multi-armed-bandit problem with non-stationary rewards. *Advances in Neural Information Processing Systems* **27,** 199–207.

Bian, Z., Moodie, E. E. M., Shortreed, S. M., and Bhatnagar, S. (2021). Variable selection in regression-based estimation of dynamic treatment regimes. *arXiv preprint arXiv:2101.07359.*

Biau, G. (2012). Analysis of a random forests model. *The Journal of Machine Learning Research* **13,** 1063–1095. Publisher: JMLR. org.

Bibaut, A., Dimakopoulou, M., Kallus, N., Chambaz, A., and van der Laan, M. (2021). Post-contextual-bandit inference. *Advances in Neural Information Processing Systems* **34,** NIPS'21: Proceedings of the 35th International Conference on Neural Information Processing Systems December 2021 Article No.: 2187, Pages 28548–28559.

Bickel, P. J., Klaassen, C. A., Bickel, P. J., Ritov, Y., Klaassen, J., Wellner, J. A., and Ritov, Y. (1993). *Efficient and adaptive estimation for semiparametric models*, volume 4. Springer.

Bickel, P. J. and Ritov, Y. (1988). Estimating integrated squared density derivatives: sharp best order of convergence estimates. *Sankhyā* pages 381–393.

Bien, S. A., Wojcik, G. L., Zubair, N., Gignoux, C. R., Martin, A. R., Kocarnik, J. M., Martin, L. W., Buyske, S., Haessler, J., Walker, R. W., et al. (2016). Strategies for enriching variant coverage in candidate disease loci on a multiethnic genotyping array. *PLoS One* **11,** e0167758.

Bilge, U. and Saka, O. (2006). Agent based simulations in healthcare. *Stud Health Technol Inform* **124,** 699–704.

Birgé, L. and Massart, P. (1995). Estimation of integral functionals of a density. *The Annals of Statistics* **23,** 11–29.

Bland, J. M. and Bland, D. (1994). Statistics notes: One and two sided tests of significance. *British Medical Journal* **309,** 248.

Blatt, D., Murphy, S. A., and Zhu, J. (2004). A-learning for approximate planning. *Ann Arbor* **1001,** 48109–48122.

Blundell, R., Dias, M. C., Meghir, C., and van Reenen, J. (2004). Evaluating the employment impact of a mandatory job search program. *Journal of the European Economic Association* **2,** 569–606.

Bogdan, R., Baranger, D. A., and Agrawal, A. (2018). Polygenic risk scores in clinical psychology: bridging genomic risk to individual differences. *Annual Review of Clinical Psychology* **14,** 119–157.

Bohmer, M., Hecht, B., Schoning, J., Kruger, A., and Bauer, G. (2011). Falling asleep with angry birds, facebook and kindle - a large scale study on mobile application usage. In *MobileHCI*, pages 47–56.

Bornkamp, B., Pinheiro, J., Bretz, F., et al. (2009). Mcpmod: An R package for the design and analysis of dose-finding studies. *Journal of Statistical Software* **29,** 1–23.

Bradic, J., Chernozhukov, V., Newey, W. K., and Zhu, Y. (2019). Minimax semiparametric learning with approximate sparsity. *arXiv preprint arXiv:1912.12213.*

Bradic, J., Wager, S., and Zhu, Y. (2019). Sparsity double robust inference of average treatment effects. *arXiv preprint arXiv:1905.00744.*

Brannath, W., Koenig, F., and Bauer, P. (2007). Multiplicity and flexibility in clinical trials. *Pharmaceutical Statistics: The Journal of Applied Statistics in the Pharmaceutical Industry* **6,** 205–216.

Brannath, W., König, F., and Bauer, P. (2006). Estimation in flexible two stage designs. *Statistics in Medicine* **25,** 3366–3381.

Brannath, W., Posch, M., and Bauer, P. (2002). Recursive combination tests. *Journal of the American Statistical Association* **97,** 236–244.

Brannath, W., Zuber, E., Branson, M., Bretz, F., Gallo, P., Posch, M., and Racine-Poon, A. (2009). Confirmatory adaptive designs with Bayesian decision tools for a targeted therapy in oncology. *Statistics in Medicine* **28,** 1445–1463.

Bratton, D. (2014). NSTAGEBIN: Stata module to perform sample size calculation for multi-arm multi-stage randomised controlled trials with binary outcomes. Statistical Software Components, Boston College Department of Economics.

Braun, T. M., Kang, S., and Taylor, J. M. (2016). A phase I/II trial design when response is unobserved in subjects with dose-limiting toxicity. *Statistical Methods in Medical Research* **25,** 659–673.

Braun, T. M., Thall, P. F., Nguyen, H., and De Lima, M. (2007). Simultaneously optimizing dose and schedule of a new cytotoxic agent. *Clinical Trials* **4,** 113–124.

Braun, T. M., Yuan, Z., and Thall, P. F. (2005). Determining a maximum-tolerated schedule of a cytotoxic agent. *Biometrics* **61,** 335–343.

Breslow, N. E. and Clayton, D. G. (1993). Approximate inference in generalized linear mixed models. *Journal of the American Statistical Association* **88,** 9–25.

Bretz, F., Koenig, F., Brannath, W., Glimm, E., and Posch, M. (2009). Adaptive designs for confirmatory clinical trials. *Statistics in Medicine* **28,** 1181–1217.

Bretz, F., Pinheiro, J. C., and Branson, M. (2005). Combining multiple comparisons and modeling techniques in dose-response studies. *Biometrics* **61,** 738–748.

Bretz, F., Schmidli, H., König, F., Racine, A., and Maurer, W. (2006). Confirmatory seamless phase II/III clinical trials with hypotheses selection at interim: general concepts. *Biometrical Journal* **48,** 623–634.

Brindley, P. and Dunn, W. (2009). Simulation for clinical research trials: a theoretical outline. *Journal of Critical Care* **24,** 164–167.

Brodeur, A., Clark, A. E., Fleche, S., and Powdthavee, N. (2021). Covid-19, lockdowns and well-being: Evidence from google trends. *Journal of Public Economics* **193,** 104346.

Broekema, R., Bakker, O., and Jonkers, I. (2020). A practical view of fine-mapping and gene prioritization in the post-genome-wide association era. *Open Biology* **10,** 190221.

Bubeck, S., Munos, R., and Stoltz, G. (2009). Pure exploration in multi-armed bandits problems. In *International conference on Algorithmic learning theory*, pages 23–37. Springer.

Bui, N. Q. and Kummar, S. (2018). Evolution of early phase clinical trials in oncology. *Journal of Molecular Medicine* **96,** 31–38.

Bulik-Sullivan, B. K., Loh, P.-R., Finucane, H. K., Ripke, S., Yang, J., Patterson, N., Daly, M. J., Price, A. L., and Neale, B. M. (2015). LD score regression distinguishes confounding from polygenicity in genome-wide association studies. *Nature Genetics* **47,** 291–295.

Buniello, A., MacArthur, J. A. L., Cerezo, M., Harris, L. W., Hayhurst, J., Malangone, C., McMahon, A., Morales, J., Mountjoy, E., Sollis, E., et al. (2019). The NHGRI-EBI GWAS catalog of published genome-wide association studies, targeted arrays and summary statistics 2019. *Nucleic Acids Research* **47,** D1005–D1012.

Buonaccorsi, J. (2010). *Measurement Error: Models, Methods, and Applications.* Chapman and Hall; Boca Raton, FL.

Burnett, T. (2017). *Bayesian Decision Making in Adaptive Clinical Trials.* Phd thesis, University of Bath.

Burnett, T. and Jennison, C. (2021). Adaptive enrichment trials: What are the benefits? *Statistics in Medicine* **40,** 690–711.

Burnett, T., König, F., and Jaki, T. (2020). Adding experimental treatment arms to multi-arm multi-stage platform trials in progress. *arXiv preprint arXiv:2007.04951.*

Burnett, T., Mozgunov, P., Pallmann, P., Villar, S. S., Wheeler, G. M., and Jaki, T. (2020). Adding flexibility to clinical trial designs: an example-based guide to the practical use of adaptive designs. *BMC Medicine* **18,** 1–21.

Bursaux, E. (1996). La mesure de la charge virale en VIH-1 permet d'affiner le pronostic de la maladie. volume 12. Médecine/Sciences. [Cited 2018 April 18].

Bush, W. S., Oetjens, M. T., and Crawford, D. C. (2016). Unravelling the human genome–phenome relationship using phenome-wide association studies. *Nature Reviews Genetics* **17,** 129–145.

Cai, M., Xiao, J., Zhang, S., Wan, X., Zhao, H., Chen, G., and Yang, C. (2021). A unified framework for cross-population trait prediction by leveraging the genetic correlation of polygenic traits. *The American Journal of Human Genetics* **108,** 632–655.

Cai, T., Tian, L., Wong, P. H., and Wei, L. (2011). Analysis of randomized comparative clinical trial data for personalized treatment selections. *Biostatistics* **12,** 270–282.

Cain, L. E., Robins, J. M., Lanoy, E., Logan, R., Costagliola, D., and Hernán, M. A. (2010). When to start treatment? A systematic approach to the comparison of dynamic regimes using observational data. *The International Journal of Biostatistics* **6,** 18.

Caisse Nationale d'Assurance Maladie (2009). Technical report 2009. Technical report. [Cited 2015 August 10].

Candes, E. and Tao, T. (2007). The Dantzig selector: Statistical estimation when p is much larger than n. *The Annals of Statistics* **35,** 2313–2351.

Cao, Y., Wen, Z., Kveton, B., and Xie, Y. (2019). Nearly optimal adaptive procedure with change detection for piecewise-stationary bandit. In *The 22nd International Conference on Artificial Intelligence and Statistics*, pages 418–427. PMLR.

Card, D. and Krueger, A. B. (1994). Minimum wages and employment: A case study of the fast-food industry in New Jersey and Pennsylvania. *American Economic Review* **84,** 772–793.

Carpenter, S. M., Menictas, M., Nahum-Shani, I., Wetter, D. W., and Murphy, S. A. (2020). Developments in mobile health just-in-time adaptive interventions for addiction science. *Current Addiction Reports* **7,** 280–290.

Carpentier, A., Vernade, C., and Abbasi-Yadkori, Y. (2020). The elliptical potential lemma revisited. *arXiv preprint arXiv:2010.10182.*

Carroll, R., Ruppert, D., Stefanski, L., and Crainiceanu, C. (2006). *Measurement Error in Nonlinear Models: A Modern Perspective.* Chapman and Hall; Boca Raton, FL.

Carroll, R. J. and Stefanski, L. A. (1990). Approximate quasi-likelihood estimation in models with surrogate predictors. *Journal of the American Statistical Association* **85(411),** 652–663.

Casella, G. and Berger, R. L. (2001). *Statistical Inference.* Duxbury Press.

Cesa-Bianchi, N., Gentile, C., and Zappella, G. (2013). A gang of bandits. In *Proceedings of the 26th International Conference on Neural Information Processing Systems-Volume 1*, pages 737–745.

Cesa-Bianchi, N. and Lugosi, G. (2012). Combinatorial bandits. *Journal of Computer and System Sciences* **78,** 1404–1422.

Chakraborty, B. and Moodie, E. E. M. (2013). *Statistical Methods for Dynamic Treatment Regimes.* New York: Springer-Verlag.

Chakraborty, B. and Murphy, S. A. (2014). Dynamic treatment regimes. *Annual Review of Statistics and Its Application* **1,** 447–464.

Chamberlain, G. (2000). Econometric applications of maxmin expected utility. *Journal of Applied Econometrics* **15,** 625–644.

Chamberlain, G. and Imbens, G. W. (2003). Nonparametric applications of Bayesian inference. *Journal of Business & Economic Statistics* **21,** 12–18.

Chang, N.-C. (2020). Double/debiased machine learning for difference-in-differences models. *The Econometrics Journal* **23,** 177–191.

Chao, Y.-C., Braun, T. M., Tamura, R. N., and Kidwell, K. M. (2020). A Bayesian group sequential small n sequential multiple-assignment randomized trial. *Journal of the Royal Statistical Society: Series C (Applied Statistics)* **69,** 663–680.

Chapelle, O. and Li, L. (2011). An empirical evaluation of thompson sampling. *Advances in Neural Information Processing Systems* **24,** NIPS'11: Proceedings of the 24th International Conference on Neural Information Processing Systems December 2011 Pages 2249–2257.

Chapple, A. G. and Thall, P. F. (2018). Subgroup-specific dose finding in phase I clinical trials based on time to toxicity allowing adaptive subgroup combination. *Pharmaceutical Statistics* **17,** 734–749.

Chapple, A. G. and Thall, P. F. (2019). A hybrid phase I-II/III clinical trial design allowing dose re-optimization in phase III. *Biometrics* **75,** 371–381.

Charles, D., Chickering, M., and Simard, P. (2013). Counterfactual reasoning and learning systems: The example of computational advertising. *Journal of Machine Learning Research* **14,** 3207–3260.

Chatterjee, N., Shi, J., and García-Closas, M. (2016). Developing and evaluating polygenic risk prediction models for stratified disease prevention. *Nature Reviews Genetics* **17,** 392.

Chatterjee, N., Wheeler, B., Sampson, J., Hartge, P., Chanock, S. J., and Park, J.-H. (2013). Projecting the performance of risk prediction based on polygenic analyses of genome-wide association studies. *Nature Genetics* **45,** 400–405.

Chatterjee, S. and Bose, A. (2005). Generalized bootstrap for estimating equations. *Annals of Statistics* **33,** 414–436.

Chen, M.-H., Raffield, L. M., Mousas, A., Sakaue, S., Huffman, J. E., Moscati, A., Trivedi, B., Jiang, T., Akbari, P., Vuckovic, D., et al. (2020). Trans-ethnic and ancestry-specific blood-cell genetics in 746,667 individuals from 5 global populations. *Cell* **182,** 1198–1213.

Chen, X. (2007). Chapter 76 Large Sample Sieve Estimation of Semi-Nonparametric Models. In Heckman, J. J. and Leamer, E. E., editors, *Handbook of Econometrics,* **6,** 5549–5632. Elsevier.

Chen, Y., Cuellar, A., Luo, H., Modi, J., Nemlekar, H., and Nikolaidis, S. (2020). The fair contextual multi-armed bandit. In *Proceedings of the 19th International Conference on Autonomous Agents and MultiAgent Systems,* pages 1810–1812.

Chen, Y., Lee, C.-W., Luo, H., and Wei, C.-Y. (2019). A new algorithm for non-stationary contextual bandits: Efficient, optimal and parameter-free. In *Conference on Learning Theory,* pages 696–726. PMLR.

Chernoff, H. (1959). Sequential design of experiments. *The Annals of Mathematical Statistics* **30,** 755–770.

Chernozhukov, V., Chetverikov, D., Demirer, M., Duflo, E., Hansen, C., Newey, W., and Robins, J. M. (2018). Double/debiased machine learning for treatment and structural parameters. *The Econometrics Journal* **21,** C1–C68.

Chernozhukov, V., Escanciano, J. C., Ichimura, H., Newey, W. K., and Robins, J. M. (2016). Locally robust semiparametric estimation. *arXiv preprint arXiv:1608.00033.*

Cheung, K. and Duan, N. (2014). Design of implementation studies for quality improvement programs: an effectiveness–cost-effectiveness framework. *American Journal of Public Health* **104,** e23–e30.

Cheung, K., Ling, W., Karr, C. J., Weingardt, K., Schueller, S. M., and Mohr, D. C. (2018). Evaluation of a recommender app for apps for the treatment of depression and anxiety: An analysis of longitudinal user engagement. *Journal of the American Medical Informatics Association* **25,** 955–962.

Cheung, Y. K. (2011). *Dose Finding by the Continual Reassessment Method.* CRC Press.

Cheung, Y. K., Chakraborty, B., and Davidson, K. W. (2015). Sequential multiple assignment randomized trial (SMART) with adaptive randomization for quality improvement in depression treatment program. *Biometrics* **71,** 450–459.

Cheung, Y. K. and Chappell, R. (2000). Sequential designs for phase I clinical trials with late-onset toxicities. *Biometrics* **56,** 1177–1182.

Chevret, S. (2006). *Statistical methods for dose-finding experiments*, volume 24. Wiley.

Chevret, S. (2012). Bayesian adaptive clinical trials: A dream for statisticians only? *Statistics in Medicine* **31,** 1002–1013.

Chib, S. and Greenberg, E. (1998). Analysis of multivariate probit models. *Biometrika* **85,** 347–361.

Chipman, H. A., George, E. I., and McCulloch, R. E. (2010). BART: Bayesian additive regression trees. *The Annals of Applied Statistics* **4,** 266–298.

Cho, H., Wang, P., and Qu, A. (2017). Personalize treatment for longitudinal data using unspecified random-effects model. *Statistica Sinica* pages 187–206.

Chow, S.-C., Chang, M., and Pong, A. (2005). Statistical consideration of adaptive methods in clinical development. *Journal of Biopharmaceutical Statistics* **15,** 575–591.

Chow, S.-C. and Chang, Y.-W. (2019). Statistical considerations for rare diseases drug development. *Journal of Biopharmaceutical Statistics* **29,** 874–886.

Chow, S.-C., Corey, R., and Lin, M. (2012). On the independence of data monitoring committee in adaptive design clinical trials. *Journal of Biopharmaceutical Statistics* **22,** 853–867.

Christian, B. (2020). *The Alignment Problem: Machine Learning and Human Values.* W. W. Norton.

Christmann, C. A., Hoffmann, A., and Bleser, G. (2009). Adherence in internet interventions for anxiety and depression. *Journal of Medical Internet Research* **11,** e13.

Chu, W., Li, L., Reyzin, L., and Schapire, R. (2011). Contextual bandits with linear payoff functions. In *Proceedings of the Fourteenth International Conference on Artificial Intelligence and Statistics*, pages 208–214. JMLR Workshop and Conference Proceedings.

Chu, Y. and Yuan, Y. (2018). A Bayesian basket trial design using a calibrated Bayesian hierarchical model. *Clinical Trials* **15,** 149–158.

Chun, S., Imakaev, M., Hui, D., Patsopoulos, N. A., Neale, B. M., Kathiresan, S., Stitziel, N. O., and Sunyaev, S. R. (2020). Non-parametric polygenic risk prediction via partitioned GWAS summary statistics. *The American Journal of Human Genetics* **107,** 46–59.

Clayton, M. K. (1989). Covariate models for bernoulli bandits. *Sequential Analysis* **8,** 405–426.

Cochran, W. (1968). Errors of measurement in statistics. *Technometrics* **10(4),** 637–666.

Codd, V., Denniff, M., Swinfield, C., Warner, S. C., Papakonstantinou, M., Sheth, S., Nanus, D. E., Budgeon, C. A., Musicha, C., Bountziouka, V., et al. (2021). A major population resource of 474,074 participants in UK biobank to investigate determinants and biomedical consequences of leukocyte telomere length. *medRxiv.*

Cohn, D. L. (2013). *Measure theory.* Springer.

Collins, F. S. and Varmus, H. (2015). A new initiative on precision medicine. *New England Journal of Medicine* **372,** 793–795.

Collins, L. M., Murphy, S. A., and Bierman, K. L. (2004). A conceptual framework for adaptive preventive interventions. *Prevention Science* **5,** 185–196.

Committee for Medicinal Products for Human Use (2007). Reflection paper on methodological issues in confirmatory clinical trials planned with an adaptive design. *London: EMEA.* https://www.ema.europa.eu/en/documents/scientific-guideline/reflection-paper-methodological-issues-confirmatory-clinical-trials-planned-adaptive-design_en.pdf.

Conaway, M. R. and Petroni, G. R. (2019). The impact of early-phase trial design in the drug development process. *Clinical Cancer Research* **25,** 819–827.

Consortium, I. H., et al. (2010). Integrating common and rare genetic variation in diverse human populations. *Nature* **467,** 52.

Cook, S. and Bies, R. (2016). Disease progression modeling: Key concepts and recent developments. *Current Pharmacology Reports* **2,** 221–230.

Cotterill, A. and Jaki, T. (2018). Dose-escalation strategies which use subgroup information. *Pharmaceutical Statistics* **17,** 414–436.

Crump, R. K., Hotz, V. J., Imbens, G. W., and Mitnik, O. A. (2009). Dealing with limited overlap in estimation of average treatment effects. *Biometrika* **96,** 187–199.

Cuadros, D., Abu-Raddad, L., Awad, S., and Garcia-Ramos, G. (2014). Use of agent-based simulations to design and interpret HIV clinical trials. *Computers in Biology and Medicine* **50,** 1–8.

Cuffe, R. L., Lawrence, D., Stone, A., and Vandemeulebroecke, M. (2014). When is a seamless study desirable? case studies from different pharmaceutical sponsors. *Pharmaceutical Statistics* **13,** 229–237.

Cui, Y. and Tchetgen Tchetgen, E. (2021). A semiparametric instrumental variable approach to optimal treatment regimes under endogeneity. *Journal of the American Statistical Association* **116,** 162–173.

Cui, Y., Zhu, R., and Kosorok, M. (2017). Tree based weighted learning for estimating individualized treatment rules with censored data. *Electronic Journal of Statistics* **11,** 3927.

Curtis, D. (2018). Polygenic risk score for schizophrenia is more strongly associated with ancestry than with schizophrenia. *Psychiatric Genetics* **28,** 85–89.

Cybenko, G. (1989). Approximation by superpositions of a sigmoidal function. *Mathematics of Control, Signals and Systems* **2,** 303–314.

Dani, V., Hayes, T. P., and Kakade, S. M. (2008). Stochastic linear optimization under bandit feedback.

Davidian, M., Tsiatis, A., and Laber, E. (2014). Value search estimators. *Dynamic Treatment Regimes* pages 1–40.

Davis, R. A., Knight, K., and Liu, J. (1992). M-estimation for autoregressions with infinite variance. *Stochastic Processes and their Applications* **40,** 145–180.

Dawson, R. and Lavori, P. W. (2012). Efficient design and inference for multistage randomized trials of individualized treatment policies. *Biostatistics* **13,** 142–152.

De Luna, X., Waernbaum, I., and Richardson, T. S. (2011). Covariate selection for the nonparametric estimation of an average treatment effect. *Biometrika* **98,** 861–875.

Deliu, N., Williams, J. J., and Villar, S. S. (2021). Efficient inference without trading-off regret in bandits: An allocation probability test for thompson sampling. *arXiv preprint arXiv:2111.00137.*

Demeulemeester, R., Savy, N., Mounié, M., Molinier, L., Delpierre, C., Dellamonica, P., Allavena, C., Pugliesse, P., Cuzin, L., Saint-Pierre, P., and Costa, N. (2021). Economic impact of generic antiretrovirals in france for HIV patients' care: a simulation between 2019 and 2023. *Value In Health* Submitted.

Depp, C. A., Ceglowski, J., Wang, V. C., Yaghouti, F., Mausbach, B. T., Thompson, W. K., and Granholm, E. L. (2015). Augmenting psychoeducation with a mobile intervention for bipolar disorder: A randomized controlled trial. *Journal of Affective Disorders* **174,** 23–30.

Deshmukh, A. A., Dogan, U., and Scott, C. (2017). Multi-task learning for contextual bandits. *arXiv preprint arXiv:1705.08618.*

Devlin, B. and Risch, N. (1995). A comparison of linkage disequilibrium measures for fine-scale mapping. *Genomics* **29,** 311–322.

Diaz, F. J., Rivera, T. E., Josiassen, R. C., and Leon, J. d. (2007). Individualizing drug dosage by using a random intercept linear model. *Statistics in Medicine* **26,** 2052–2073.

Díaz, I. (2020). Machine learning in the estimation of causal effects: targeted minimum loss-based estimation and double/debiased machine learning. *Biostatistics* **21,** 353–358.

Díaz, I. and van der Laan, M. J. (2012). Population intervention causal effects based on stochastic interventions. *Biometrics* **68,** 541–549.

Díaz, I. and van der Laan, M. J. (2013). Targeted data adaptive estimation of the causal dose-response curve. *Journal of Causal Inference* **1,** 171–192.

Diggle, P. J., Heagerty, P. J., Liang, K.-Y., and Zeger, S. (2002). *Analysis of longitudinal data.* Oxford University Press.

Dikilitas, O., Schaid, D. J., Kosel, M. L., Carroll, R. J., Chute, C. G., Denny, J. A., Fedotov, A., Feng, Q., Hakonarson, H., Jarvik, G. P., et al. (2020). Predictive utility of polygenic risk scores for coronary heart disease in three major racial and ethnic groups. *The American Journal of Human Genetics* **106,** 707–716.

Dikkala, N., Lewis, G., Mackey, L., and Syrgkanis, V. (2020). Minimax estimation of conditional moment models. *arXiv preprint arXiv:2006.07201.*

Dimairo, M., Boote, J., Julious, S. A., Nicholl, J. P., and Todd, S. (2015). Missing steps in a staircase: a qualitative study of the perspectives of key stakeholders on the use of adaptive designs in confirmatory trials. *Trials* **16,** 430.

Dimairo, M., Julious, S. A., Todd, S., Nicholl, J. P., and Boote, J. (2015). Cross-sector surveys assessing perceptions of key stakeholders towards barriers, concerns and facilitators to the appropriate use of adaptive designs in confirmatory trials. *Trials* **16,** 585.

Dimairo, M., Pallmann, P., Jaki, T., Wheeler, G., Bradburn, M., Flight, L., Cooper, C., and Marsh, J. A practical adaptive & novel designs and analysis (PANDA) toolkit. Accessed: 26/04/2020.

Dimairo, M., Pallmann, P., Wason, J., Todd, S., Jaki, T., Julious, S. A., Mander, A. P., Weir, C. J., Koenig, F., Walton, M. K., et al. (2020). The Adaptive designs CONSORT Extension (ACE) statement: a checklist with explanation and elaboration guideline for reporting randomised trials that use an adaptive design. *British Medical Journal* **369,** BMJ 2020;369:m115.

Dimick, J. B. and Ryan, A. M. (2014). Methods for evaluating changes in health care policy: the difference-in-differences approach. *Journal of the American Medical Association* **312,** 2401–2402.

Ding, P. and Li, F. (2019). A bracketing relationship between difference-in-differences and lagged-dependent-variable adjustment. *Political Analysis* **27,** 605–615.

Ding, W., Qin, T., Zhang, X.-D., and Liu, T.-Y. (2013). Multi-armed bandit with budget constraint and variable costs. In *Proceedings of the AAAI Conference on Artificial Intelligence*, volume 27.

Dissmann, J., Brechmann, E. C., Czado, C., and Kurowicka, D. (2013). Selecting and estimating regular vine copulae and application to financial returns. *Computational Statistics & Data Analysis* **59,** 52–69.

Dragalin, V. (2006). Adaptive designs: terminology and classification. *Drug Information Journal* **40,** 425–435.

Dudbridge, F. (2013). Power and predictive accuracy of polygenic risk scores. *PLoS Genetics* **9,** e1003348.

Dudík, M., Erhan, D., Langford, J., and Li, L. (2014). Doubly robust policy evaluation and optimization. *Statistical Science* **29,** 485–511.

Dudík, M., Langford, J., and Li, L. (2011). Doubly robust policy evaluation and learning. *arXiv preprint arXiv:1103.4601.*

Dumville, J., Hahn, S., Miles, J., and Torgerson, D. (2006). The use of unequal randomisation ratios in clinical trials: a review. *Contemporary Clinical Trials* **27,** 1–12.

Duncan, L., Shen, H., Gelaye, B., Meijsen, J., Ressler, K., Feldman, M., Peterson, R., and Domingue, B. (2019). Analysis of polygenic risk score usage and performance in diverse human populations. *Nature Communications* **10,** 1–9.

Dunnett, C. W. (1955). A multiple comparison procedure for comparing several treatments with a control. *Journal of the American Statistical Association* **50,** 1096–1121.

Dunnett, C. W. and Tamhane, A. C. (1991). Step-down multiple tests for comparing treatments with a control in unbalanced one-way layouts. *Statistics in Medicine* **10,** 939–947.

Dunnett, C. W. and Tamhane, A. C. (1998). Some new multiple-test procedures for dose finding. *Journal of Biopharmaceutical Statistics* **8,** 353–366.

Efron, B. (1992). Bootstrap methods: Another look at the jackknife. In *Breakthroughs in Statistics*, pages 569–593. Springer.

Ernst, D., Geurts, P., and Wehenkel, L. (2005). Tree-based batch mode reinforcement learning. *Journal of Machine Learning Research* **6,** 503–556.

Ertefaie, A., McKay, J. R., Oslin, D., and Strawderman, R. L. (2021). Robust q-learning. *Journal of the American Statistical Association* **116,** 368–381.

Ertefaie, A. and Strawderman, R. L. (2018). Constructing dynamic treatment regimes over indefinite time horizons. *Biometrika* **105,** 963–977.

Even-Dar, E., Mannor, S., Mansour, Y., and Mahadevan, S. (2006). Action elimination and stopping conditions for the multi-armed bandit and reinforcement learning problems. *Journal of Machine Learning Research* **7,** 1079–1105.

Eyre-Walker, A. (2010). Evolution in health and medicine sackler colloquium: Genetic architecture of a complex trait and its implications for fitness and genome-wide association studies. *Proceedings of the National Academy of Sciences of the United States of America* **107,** 1752–1756.

Fan, A., Lu, W., and Song, R. (2016). Sequential advantage selection for optimal treatment regime. *The Annals of Applied Statistics* **10,** 32–53.

Fan, J. and Li, R. (2001). Variable selection via nonconcave penalized likelihood and its oracle properties. *Journal of the American Statistical Association* **96,** 1348–1360.

Fang, F., Hochstedler, K. A., Tamura, R. N., Braun, T. M., and Kidwell, K. M. (2021). Bayesian methods to compare dose levels with placebo in a small n, sequential, multiple assignment, randomized trial. *Statistics in Medicine* **40,** 963–977.

Farrell, M. H. (2015). Robust inference on average treatment effects with possibly more covariates than observations. *Journal of Econometrics* **189,** 1–23.

Farrell, M. H., Liang, T., and Misra, S. (2021). Deep neural networks for estimation and inference. *Econometrica* **89,** 181–213.

Fernholz, L. T. (1983). *Von Mises calculus for statistical functionals*, volume 19. Springer Science & Business Media.

Ferrari, P., Friedenreich, C., and Matthews, C. E. (2007). The role of measurement error in estimating levels of physical activity. *American Journal of Epidemiology* **166(7),** 832–840.

Finn, C., Abbeel, P., and Levine, S. (2017). Model-agnostic meta-learning for fast adaptation of deep networks. In *Proceedings of the 34th International Conference on Machine Learning-Volume 70*, pages 1126–1135. JMLR. org.

Firth, J., Torous, J., Nicholas, J., Carney, R., Pratap, A., Rosenbaum, S., and Sarris, J. (2017). The efficacy of smartphone-based mental health interventions for depressive symptoms: a meta-analysis of randomized controlled trials. *World Psychiatry* **16,** 287–298.

Fisher, A. and Kennedy, E. H. (2021). Visually communicating and teaching intuition for influence functions. *The American Statistician* **75,** 162–172.

Fisher, H. M., Winger, J. G., Miller, S. N., Wright, A. N., Plumb Vilardaga, J. C., Majestic, C., Kelleher, S. A., and Somers, T. J. (2021). Relationship between social support, physical symptoms, and depression in women with breast cancer and pain. *Supportive Care in Cancer* **29,** 5513–5521.

Fisher, L. D. (1991). The use of one-sided tests in drug trials: an FDA advisory committee member's perspective. *Journal of Biopharmaceutical Statistics* **1,** 151–156.

Flores, M., Glusman, G., Brogaard, K., Price, N. D., and Hood, L. (2013). P4 medicine: how systems medicine will transform the healthcare sector and society. *Personalized Medicine* **10,** 565–576.

Food and Administration. (2015). Rare diseases: Common issues in drug development. Guidance for industry (draft).

Forman, E. M., Kerrigan, S. G., Butryn, M. L., Juarascio, A. S., Manasse, S. M., Ontañón, S., Dallal, D. H., Crochiere, R. J., and Moskow, D. (2019). Can the artificial intelligence technique of reinforcement learning use continuously-monitored digital data to optimize treatment for weight loss? *Journal of behavioral medicine* **42,** 276–290.

Foster, D. J. and Syrgkanis, V. (2019). Orthogonal statistical learning. *arXiv preprint arXiv:1901.09036.*

Fox, E. A., Wright, A. E., Fumagalli, M., and Vieira, F. G. (2019). ngsld: evaluating linkage disequilibrium using genotype likelihoods. *Bioinformatics* **35,** 3855–3856.

Fox, K., Poole-Wilson, P., Clayton, T. C., Henderson, R., Shaw, T., Wheatley, D., Knight, R., and Pocock, S. (2005). 5-year outcome of an interventional strategy in non-ST-elevation acute coronary syndrome: the British Heart Foundation RITA 3 randomised trial. *The Lancet* **366,** 914–920.

Freedman, D. A. and Berk, R. A. (2008). Weighting regressions by propensity scores. *Evaluation review* **32,** 392–409.

Friedman, L. M., Furberg, C., DeMets, D. L., Reboussin, D. M., Granger, C. B., et al. (2010). *Fundamentals of clinical trials*, volume 4. Springer, New York.

Fritsche, L. G., Patil, S., Beesley, L. J., VandeHaar, P., Salvatore, M., Ma, Y., Peng, R. B., Taliun, D., Zhou, X., and Mukherjee, B. (2020). Cancer PRSweb: an online repository with polygenic risk scores for major cancer traits and their evaluation in two independent biobanks. *The American Journal of Human Genetics* **107,** 815–836.

Fu, W. J. (2003). Penalized estimating equations. *Biometrics* **59,** 126–132.

Gail, M. and Simon, R. (1985). Testing for qualitative interactions between treatment effects and patient subsets. *Biometrics* **41(2)**, 361–372.

Garcelon, E., Ghavamzadeh, M., Lazaric, A., and Pirotta, M. (2020a). Conservative exploration in reinforcement learning. In *International Conference on Artificial Intelligence and Statistics*, pages 1431–1441. PMLR.

Garcelon, E., Ghavamzadeh, M., Lazaric, A., and Pirotta, M. (2020b). Improved algorithms for conservative exploration in bandits. In *Proceedings of the AAAI Conference on Artificial Intelligence*, volume 34, pages 3962–3969.

Garès, V., Dimeglio, C., Guernec, G., Fantin, R., Lepage, B., Kosorok, M., and Savy, N. (2020). On the use of optimal transportation theory to recode variables and application to database merging. *The International Journal of Biostatistics*, **16(1)**, 20180106. https://doi.org/10.1515/ijb-2018-0106.

Garivier, A. and Moulines, E. (2011). On upper-confidence bound policies for switching bandit problems. In *International Conference on Algorithmic Learning Theory*, pages 174–188. Springer.

Garnelo, M., Rosenbaum, D., Maddison, C., Ramalho, T., Saxton, D., Shanahan, M., Teh, Y. W., Rezende, D., and Eslami, S. A. (2018). Conditional neural processes. In *International Conference on Machine Learning*, pages 1704–1713. PMLR.

Gasparini, M. and Eisele, J. (2000). A curve-free method for phase I clinical trials. *Biometrics* **56,** 609–615.

Gauthier, J., Thall, P., and Yuan, Y. (2019). Bayesian phase 1/2 trial designs and cellular immunotherapies: a practical primer. *Cell Gene Ther. Insights* **5,** 1483–1494.

Gay, N. R., Gloudemans, M., Antonio, M. L., Abell, N. S., Balliu, B., Park, Y., Martin, A. R., Musharoff, S., Rao, A. S., Aguet, F., et al. (2020). Impact of admixture and ancestry on eQTL analysis and GWAS colocalization in GTEx. *Genome Biology* **21,** 1–20.

Ge, T., Chen, C.-Y., Ni, Y., Feng, Y.-C. A., and Smoller, J. W. (2019). Polygenic prediction via Bayesian regression and continuous shrinkage priors. *Nature Communications* **10,** 1–10.

Ge, T., Irvin, M. R., Patki, A., Srinivasasainagendra, V., Lin, Y.-F., Tiwari, H. K., Armstrong, N. D., Benoit, B., Chen, C.-Y., Choi, K. W., et al. (2022). Development and validation of a trans-ancestry polygenic risk score for type 2 diabetes in diverse populations. *Genome Medicine* **14,** 1–16.

Gentile, C., Li, S., and Zappella, G. (2014). Online clustering of bandits. In *International Conference on Machine Learning*, pages 757–765. PMLR.

Gerchinovitz, S. (2011). Sparsity regret bounds for individual sequences in online linear regression. In *Proceedings of the 24th Annual Conference on Learning Theory*, pages 377–396. JMLR Workshop and Conference Proceedings.

Gertler, P., Martinez, S., Premand, P., Rawlings, L. B., and Vermeersch, C. M. J. (2011). Impact evaluation in practice, Chapter 6. *World Bank Training Series: Washington DC.*

Gibbs, R. A., Belmont, J. W., Hardenbol, P., Willis, T. D., Yu, F., Yang, H., Ch'ang, L.-Y., Huang, W., Liu, B., Shen, Y., et al. (2003). The international HapMap project. Nature 426, 89–796.

Gillen, S., Jung, C., Kearns, M., and Roth, A. (2018). Online learning with an unknown fairness metric. *arXiv preprint arXiv:1802.06936.*

Gleser, L. J. (1990). Improvements of the naive approach to estimation in nonlinear errors-in-variables regression models. *Contemporary Mathematics* **112,** 99–114.

Glynn, P. W. (1987). Likelilood ratio gradient estimation: an overview. In *Proceedings of the 19th conference on Winter simulation*, pages 366–375.

Godambe, V. P. (1991). *Estimating Functions.* Oxford science publications. Clarendon Press.

Goldenshluger, A. and Zeevi, A. (2011). A note on performance limitations in bandit problems with side information. *IEEE transactions on information theory* **57,** 1707–1713.

Goldenshluger, A. and Zeevi, A. (2013). A linear response bandit problem. *Stochastic Systems* **3,** 230–261.

Goodfellow, I. J., Shlens, J., and Szegedy, C. (2014). Explaining and harnessing adversarial examples. *arXiv preprint https://doi.org/10.48550/arXiv.1412.6572.*

Goodman-Bacon, A. and Marcus, J. (2020). Using difference-in-differences to identify causal effects of COVID-19 policies. Survey Research Methods, 14, 153–158.

Götte, H., Donica, M., and Mordenti, G. (2015). Improving probabilities of correct interim decision in population enrichment designs. *Journal of Biopharmaceutical Statistics* **25,** 1020–1038.

Gottesman, O., Kuivaniemi, H., Tromp, G., Faucett, W. A., Li, R., Manolio, T. A., Sanderson, S. C., Kannry, J., Zinberg, R., Basford, M. A., et al. (2013). The electronic medical records and genomics (eMERGE) network: past, present, and future. *Genetics in Medicine* **15,** 761–771.

Graham, D. J., McCoy, E. J., and Stephens, D. A. (2016). Approximate Bayesian inference for doubly robust estimation. *Bayesian Analysis* **11,** 47–69.

Graham, E., Jaki, T., and Harbron, C. (2019). A comparison of stochastic programming methods for portfolio level decision-making. *Journal of Biopharmaceutical Statistics* **13,** 1–25.

Grayling, M. J. (2019). DESMA: Stata module to design and simulate (adaptive) multi-arm clinical trials. Statistical Software Components, Boston College Department of Economics.

Green, D. P. and Kern, H. L. (2012). Modeling heterogeneous treatment effects in survey experiments with Bayesian additive regression trees. *Public Opinion Quarterly* **76,** 491–511.

Greenland, S. (2008). Invited commentary: Variable selection versus shrinkage in the control of multiple confounders. *American Journal of Epidemiology* **167,** 523–529.

Griggs, R. C., Batshaw, M., Dunkle, M., Gopal-Srivastava, R., Kaye, E., Krischer, J., Nguyen, T., Paulus, K., Merkel, P. A., et al. (2009). Clinical research for rare disease: opportunities, challenges, and solutions. *Molecular Genetics and Metabolism* **96,** 20–26.

Grimes, D. A. and Schulz, K. F. (2002). An overview of clinical research: the lay of the land. *The Lancet* **359,** 57–61.

Grimm, V., Berger, U., Bastiansen, F., Eliassen, S., Ginot, V., Giske, J., Goss-Custard, J., Grand, T., Heinz, S. K., Huse, G., Huth, A., Jepsen, J. U., Jorgensen, C., Mooij, W. M., Müller, B., Pe'er, G., Piou, C., Railsback, S. F., Robbins, A. M., Robbins, M. M., Rossmanith, E., Rüger, N., Strand, E., Souissi, S., Stillman, R. A., Vabo, R., Visser, U., and DeAngelis, D. L. (2006). A standard protocol for describing individual-based and agent-based models. *Ecological Modelling* **198,** 115–126.

Gruber, L. and Czado, C. (2015). Sequential Bayesian model selection of regular vine copulas. *Bayesian Analysis* **10,** 937–963.

Guan, Q., Reich, B. J., Laber, E. B., and Bandyopadhyay, D. (2020). Bayesian nonparametric policy search with application to periodontal recall intervals. *Journal of the American Statistical Association* **115,** 1066–1078.

Gunter, L., Zhu, J., and Murphy, S. (2011). Variable selection for qualitative interactions. *Statistical Methodology* **8,** 42–55.

Guo, B. and Yuan, Y. (2017). Bayesian phase I/II biomarker-based dose finding for precision medicine with molecularly targeted agents. *Journal of the American Statistical Association* **112,** 508–520.

Gupta, A., Koren, T., and Talwar, K. (2019). Better algorithms for stochastic bandits with adversarial corruptions. In *Conference on Learning Theory*, pages 1562–1578. PMLR.

Gupta, S., Faughnan, M. E., Tomlinson, G. A., and Bayoumi, A. M. (2011). A framework for applying unfamiliar trial designs in studies of rare diseases. *Journal of Clinical Epidemiology* **64,** 1085–1094.

Gurdasani, D., Barroso, I., Zeggini, E., and Sandhu, M. S. (2019). Genomics of disease risk in globally diverse populations. *Nature Reviews Genetics* **20,** 520–535.

Gustafson, P. (2004). *Measurement Error and Misclassification in Statistics and Epidemiology: Impacts and Bayesian Adjustments.* Chapman and Hall; Boca Raton, FL.

Györfi, L., Kohler, M., Krzykaz, A., and Walk, H. (2002). *A Distribution-Free Theory of Nonparametric Regression.* Springer.

Haapala, I., Barengo, N., Biggs, S., L, S., and Manninen, P. (2009). Weight loss by mobile phone: a 1-year effectiveness study. *Public Health Nutr.* **12,** 2382–2391.

Hadad, V., Hirshberg, D. A., Zhan, R., Wager, S., and Athey, S. (2021). Confidence intervals for policy evaluation in adaptive experiments. *Proceedings of the National Academy of Sciences* **118,** e2014602118.

Hahn, P. R., Murray, J. S., and Carvalho, C. M. (2020). Bayesian regression tree models for causal inference: Regularization, confounding, and heterogeneous effects (with discussion). *Bayesian Analysis* **15,** 965–1056.

Haines, L. M. and Clark, A. E. (2014). The construction of optimal designs for dose-escalation studies. *Statistics and Computing* **24,** 101–109.

Haines, L. M., Perevozskaya, I., and Rosenberger, W. F. (2003). Bayesian optimal designs for phase I clinical trials. *Biometrics* **59,** 591–600.

Hall, P. and Heyde, C. C. (2014). *Martingale limit theory and its application.* Academic press.

Haneuse, S. and Rotnitzky, A. (2013). Estimation of the effect of interventions that modify the received treatment. *Statistics in Medicine* **32,** 5260–5277.

Hansen, B. B. (2008). The prognostic analogue of the propensity score. *Biometrika* **95,** 481–488.

Hao, B., Lattimore, T., and Wang, M. (2020). High-dimensional sparse linear bandits. *arXiv preprint arXiv:2011.04020.*

Harrington, J. A., Wheeler, G. M., Sweeting, M. J., Mander, A. P., and Jodrell, D. I. (2013). Adaptive designs for dual-agent phase I dose-escalation studies. *Nature Reviews Clinical Oncology* **10,** 277–288.

Hartford, J., Graham, D. R., Leyton-Brown, K., and Ravanbakhsh, S. (2018). Deep models of interactions across sets. *arXiv preprint arXiv:1803.02879.*

Hartman, H., Tamura, R. N., Schipper, M. J., and Kidwell, K. M. (2021). Design and analysis considerations for utilizing a mapping function in a small sample, sequential, multiple assignment, randomized trials with continuous outcomes. *Statistics in Medicine* **40,** 312–326.

Hartung, J. (1999). A note on combining dependent tests of significance. *Biometrical Journal* **41,** 849–855.

Hasminskii, R. Z. and Ibragimov, I. A. (1978). On the nonparametric estimation of functionals. *Proceedings of the 2nd Prague Symposium on Asymptotic Statistics* pages 41–51.

Haussler, D. and Warmuth, M. (2018). The probably approximately correct (PAC) and other learning models. *The Mathematics of Generalization* pages 17–36.

Haute Autorité de Santé (2012). Guide du parcours de soins-maladie rénale chronique de l'adulte. Technical report.

Hayward, R. A., Kent, D. M., Vijan, S., and Hofer, T. P. (2006). Multivariable risk prediction can greatly enhance the statistical power of clinical trial subgroup analysis. *BMC Medical Research Methodology* **6,** 1–11.

Heckman, J. J., Ichimura, H., and Todd, P. (1998). Matching as an econometric evaluation estimator. *The Review of Economic Studies* **65,** 261–294.

Henderson, C. R. (1975). Best linear unbiased estimation and prediction under a selection model. *Biometrics* pages 423–447.

Henderson, R., Ansell, P., and Alshibani, D. (2010). Regret-regression for optimal dynamic treatment regimes. *Biometrics* **66,** 1192–1201.

Henmi, M. and Eguchi, S. (2004). A paradox concerning nuisance parameters and projected estimating functions. *Biometrika* **91,** 929–941.

Hernández-Neuta, I., Neumann, F., Brightmeyer, J., Ba Tis, T., Madaboosi, N., Wei, Q., Ozcan, A., and Nilsson, M. (2019). Smartphone-based clinical diagnostics: towards democratization of evidence-based health care. *Journal of Internal Medicine* **285,** 19–39.

Hernán, M. A. and Robins, J. M. (2020). *Causal Inference: What If.* Chapman & Hall/CRC, Boca Raton.

Heron, K. E. and Smyth, J. M. (2010). Ecological momentary interventions: incorporating mobile technology into psychosocial and health behaviour treatments. *British Journal of Health Psychology* **15,** 1–39.

Heusel, M., Ramsauer, H., Unterthiner, T., Nessler, B., and Hochreiter, S. (2017). GANs trained by a two time-scale update rule converge to a local Nash equilibrium. In *Advances in neural information processing systems*, pages 6626–6637.

Heyde, C. C. (1997). *Quasi-likelihood and its application: a general approach to optimal parameter estimation.* Springer.

Hill, A., Hill, T., Jose, S., and Pozniak, A. (2014). Predicted savings to the UK National Health Service from switching to generic antiretrovirals, 2014-2018. *Journal of the International AIDS Society* **17,** 19497.

Hill, J. L. (2011). Bayesian nonparametric modeling for causal inference. *Journal of Computational and Graphical Statistics* **20,** 217–240.

Hines, O., Dukes, O., Diaz-Ordaz, K., and Vansteelandt, S. (2022). Demystifying statistical learning based on efficient influence functions. *The American Statistician* **76,** 292–304.

Hirano, K. and Porter, J. R. (2012). Impossibility results for nondifferentiable functionals. *Econometrica* **80,** 1769–1790.

Hirshberg, D. A. and Wager, S. (2021). Augmented minimax linear estimation. *The Annals of Statistics* **49,** 3206–3227.

Ho, W.-K., Tai, M.-C., Dennis, J., Shu, X., Li, J., Ho, P. J., Millwood, I. Y., Lin, K., Jee, Y.-H., Lee, S.-H., et al. (2022). Polygenic risk scores for prediction of breast cancer risk in Asian populations. *Genetics in Medicine* **24,** 586–600.

Hochreiter, S., Younger, A. S., and Conwell, P. R. (2001). Learning to learn using gradient descent. In *International Conference on Artificial Neural Networks*, pages 87–94. Springer.

Hoeper, M. M., Barst, R. J., Bourge, R. C., Feldman, J., Frost, A. E., Galié, N., Gómez-Sánchez, M. A., Grimminger, F., Grünig, E., Hassoun, P. M., et al. (2013). Imatinib mesylate as add-on therapy for pulmonary arterial hypertension: results of the randomized IMPRES study. *Circulation* **127,** 1128–1138.

Holford, N., Kimko, H., Monteleone, J., and Peck, C. (2000). Simulation of clinical trials. *Annual Review of Pharmacology and Toxicology* **40,** 209–234.

Holford, N., Ma, S., and Ploeger, B. (2010). Clinical trial simulation: a review. *Clin. Pharmacol. Ther.* **88,** 166–182.

Hommel, G. (2001). Adaptive modifications of hypotheses after an interim analysis. *Biometrical Journal* **43,** 581–589.

Hornik, K. (1991). Approximation capabilities of multilayer feedforward networks. *Neural Networks* **4,** 251–257.

Hosmer, D. W. and Lemeshow, S. (1992). Confidence interval estimation of interaction. *Epidemiology* pages 452–456.

Hu, F. and Rosenberger, W. F. (2003). Optimality, variability, power: evaluating response-adaptive randomization procedures for treatment comparisons. *Journal of the American Statistical Association* **98,** 671–678.

Hu, X., Qian, M., Cheng, B., and Cheung, Y.-Y. (2021). Personalized policy learning using longitudinal mobile health data. *Journal of the American Statistical Association* **116,** 410–420.

Hu, Y., Lu, Q., Liu, W., Zhang, Y., Li, M., and Zhao, H. (2017). Joint modeling of genetically correlated diseases and functional annotations increases accuracy of polygenic risk prediction. *PLoS Genetics* **13,** e1006836.

Hua, W., Mei, H., Zohar, S., Giral, M., and Xu, Y. (2022). Personalized dynamic treatment regimes in continuous time: a Bayesian approach for optimizing clinical decisions with timing. *Bayesian Analysis* **17,** 849–878.

Huang, J., Ma, S., and Zhang, C.-H. (2008). Adaptive lasso for sparse high-dimensional regression models. *Statistica Sinica* pages 1603–1618.

Huang, L., Rosen, J. D., Sun, Q., Chen, J., Wheeler, M. M., Zhou, Y., Min, Y.-I., Kooperberg, C., Conomos, M. P., Stilp, A. M., et al. (2022). TOP-LD: A tool to explore linkage disequilibrium with topmed whole-genome sequence data. *The American Journal of Human Genetics* **109,** 1175–1181.

Huang, W., Labille, K., Wu, X., Lee, D., and Heffernan, N. (2020). Achieving user-side fairness in contextual bandits. *arXiv preprint arXiv:2010.12102.*

Hui, T.-Y. J. and Burt, A. (2020). Estimating linkage disequilibrium from genotypes under Hardy-Weinberg equilibrium. *BMC Genetics* **21,** 1–11.

Hunt, G. and Stein, C. (1946). Most stringent tests of statistical hypotheses. *Unpublished Manuscript.*

Hwang, S. (2015). Some characterizations of non-ergodic estimating functions for stochastic processes. *Journal of the Korean Statistical Society* **44,** 661–667.

Hwang, S. and Basawa, I. (2011). Godambe estimating functions and asymptotic optimal inference. *Statistics & Probability Letters* **81,** 1121–1127.

Hwang, S. and Basawa, I. (2014). Martingale estimating functions for stochastic processes: A review toward a unifying tool. *Contemporary Developments in Statistical Theory: A Festschrift for Hira Lal Koul* pages 9–28.

Hyman, D. M., Puzanov, I., Subbiah, V., Faris, J. E., Chau, I., Blay, J.-Y., Wolf, J., Raje, N. S., Diamond, E. L., Hollebecque, A., et al. (2015). Vemurafenib in multiple nonmelanoma cancers with BRAF v600 mutations. *New England Journal of Medicine* **373,** 726–736.

Ichimura, H. and Newey, W. K. (2022). The influence function of semiparametric estimators. *Quantitative Economics* **13,** 29–61.

Imai, K., Keele, L., and Yamamoto, T. (2010). Identification, inference and sensitivity analysis for causal mediation effects. *Statistical Science* **25,** 51–71.

Imai, K. and Ratkovic, M. (2013). Estimating treatment effect heterogeneity in randomized program evaluation. *The Annals of Applied Statistics* **7,** 443–470.

Imbens, G. W. and Rubin, D. B. (2015). *Causal Inference in Statistics, Social, and Biomedical Sciences.* Cambridge University Press.

Immorlica, N., Sankararaman, K. A., Schapire, R., and Slivkins, A. (2019). Adversarial bandits with knapsacks. In *2019 IEEE 60th Annual Symposium on Foundations of Computer Science (FOCS)*, pages 202–219. IEEE.

J Mayhew, A. and Meyre, D. (2017). Assessing the heritability of complex traits in humans: methodological challenges and opportunities. *Current Genomics* **18,** 332–340.

Jaki, T. (2013). Uptake of novel statistical methods for early-phase clinical studies in the UK public sector. *Clinical Trials* **10,** 344–346.

Jaki, T. (2015). Multi-arm clinical trials with treatment selection: what can be gained and at what price? *Clinical Investigation* **5,** 393–399.

Jaki, T., Clive, S., and Weir, C. J. (2013). Principles of dose finding studies in cancer: a comparison of trial designs. *Cancer Chemotherapy and Pharmacology* **71,** 1107–1114.

Jaki, T., Pallmann, P., and Magirr, D. (2019). The R package MAMS for designing multi-arm multi-stage clinical trials. *Journal of Statistical Software* **88,**.

Javanmard, A. and Montanari, A. (2014). Confidence intervals and hypothesis testing for high-dimensional regression. *The Journal of Machine Learning Research* **15,** 2869–2909.

Jeng, X. J., Lu, W., and Peng, H. (2018). High-dimensional inference for personalized treatment decision. *Electronic Journal of Statistics* **12,** 2074–2089.

Jennison, C. and Turnbull, B. W. (1999). *Group sequential methods with applications to clinical trials*. Chapman and Hall/CRC, Raton, FL.

Jennison, C. and Turnbull, B. W. (2006). Confirmatory seamless phase II/III clinical trials with hypotheses selection at interim: opportunities and limitations. *Biometrical Journal* **48,** 650–655.

Jiang, N. and Li, L. (2016). Doubly robust off-policy value evaluation for reinforcement learning. In *International Conference on Machine Learning*, pages 652–661. PMLR.

Jin, J., Agarwala, N., Kundu, P., Harvey, B., Zhang, Y., Wallace, E., and Chatterjee, N. (2021). Individual and community-level risk for COVID-19 mortality in the United States. *Nature Medicine* **27,** 264–269.

Jin, T., Xu, P., Shi, J., Xiao, X., and Gu, Q. (2020). MOTS: Minimax optimal Thompson sampling. *arXiv preprint arXiv:2003.01803*.

Jin, Y., Yang, Z., and Wang, Z. (2021). Is pessimism provably efficient for offline RL? In *International Conference on Machine Learning*, pages 5084–5096. PMLR.

Joe, H. (1994). Multivariate extreme-value distributions with applications to environmental data. *Canadian Journal of Statistics* **22,** 47–64.

Joe, H. (1996). Families of m-variate distributions with given margins and m (m-1)/2 bivariate dependence parameters. *Lecture Notes-Monograph Series* pages 120–141.

Johnson, M. (1987). *Multivariate Statistical Simulation*. John Wiley, New York, NY.

Jones, R. L., Ravi, V., Brohl, A.S., Chawla, S.P., Ganjoo, K. Italiano, A., Attia, S., Burgess, M., Thornton, K., Cranmer, L., Liu, L., Theuer, C., Maki, R. (2019). Results of the TAPPAS trial: An adaptive enrichment phase III trial of TRC105 and pazopanib (P) versus pazopanib alone in patients with advanced angiosarcoma (AS). *Annals of Oncology*, **30 (Supplement 5)**, 683–709.

Joseph, M., Kearns, M., Morgenstern, J., and Roth, A. (2016). Fairness in learning: Classic and contextual bandits. *arXiv preprint arXiv:1605.07139*.

Kallus, N. (2018). Balanced policy evaluation and learning. *Advances in Neural Information Processing Systems* **31,** https://proceedings.neurips.cc/paper_files/paper/2018/file/66167 58da438b02b8d360ad83a5b3d77-Paper.pdf.

Kandasamy, K., Krishnamurthy, A., Poczos, B., Wasserman, L., and Robins, J. M. (2015). Nonparametric von mises estimators for entropies, divergences and mutual informations. *Advances in Neural Information Processing Systems* **28,** https://proceedings.neurips.cc/paper_files/paper/2015/file/06138bc5af6023646ede0e1f7c1eac75-Paper.pdf.

Kang, D., S Coffey, C., J Smith, B., Yuan, Y., Shi, Q., and Yin, J. (2021). Hierarchical Bayesian clustering design of multiple biomarker subgroups (HCOMBS). *Statistics in Medicine* **40,** 2893–2921.

Kapoor, S., Patel, K. K., and Kar, P. (2019). Corruption-tolerant bandit learning. *Machine Learning* **108,** 687–715.

Kaptein, M. (2019). A practical approach to sample size calculation for fixed populations. *Contemporary Clinical Trials Communications* **14,** 100339.

Karyotaki, E., Riper, H., Twisk, J., Hoogendoorn, A., Kleiboer, A., Mira, A., Mackinnon, A., Meyer, B., Botella, C., Littlewood, E., et al. (2017). Efficacy of self-guided internet-based cognitive behavioral therapy in the treatment of depressive symptoms: a meta-analysis of individual participant data. *JAMA Psychiatry* **74,** 351–359.

Kaufmann, E., Korda, N., and Munos, R. (2012). Thompson sampling: An asymptotically optimal finite-time analysis. In *International conference on algorithmic learning theory*, pages 199–213. Springer.

Kazerouni, A., Ghavamzadeh, M., Abbasi-Yadkori, Y., and Van Roy, B. (2016). Conservative contextual linear bandits. *arXiv preprint arXiv:1611.06426.*

Keele, L. and Minozzi, W. (2013). How much is Minnesota like Wisconsin? assumptions and counterfactuals in causal inference with observational data. *Political Analysis* **21,** 193–216.

Kempthorne, P. J. (1987). Numerical specification of discrete least favorable prior distributions. *SIAM Journal on Scientific and Statistical Computing* **8,** 171–184.

Kennedy, E. H. (2016). Semiparametric theory and empirical processes in causal inference. *In: Statistical Causal Inferences and Their Applications in Public Health Research* pages 141–167.

Kennedy, E. H. (2018). Semiparametric theory. *Wiley StatsRef: Statistics Reference Online.* doi:10.1002/9781118445112.stat08083 (arxiv:1709.06418).

Kennedy, E. H. (2019). Nonparametric causal effects based on incremental propensity score interventions. *Journal of the American Statistical Association* **114,** 645–656.

Kennedy, E. H. (2020). Towards optimal doubly robust estimation of heterogeneous causal effects. *arXiv preprint arXiv:2004.14497v5.*

Kennedy, E. H., Balakrishnan, S., and G'Sell, M. (2020). Sharp instruments for classifying compliers and generalizing causal effects. *The Annals of Statistics* **48,** 2008–2030.

Kennedy, E. H., Balakrishnan, S., and Wasserman, L. (2021). Semiparametric counterfactual density estimation. *arXiv preprint arXiv:2102.12034.*

Kennedy, E. H., Balakrishnan, S., and Wasserman, L. (2022). Minimax rates for heterogeneous causal effect estimation. *arXiv preprint arXiv:2203.00837.*

Kennedy, E. H., Ma, Z., McHugh, M. D., and Small, D. S. (2017). Nonparametric methods for doubly robust estimation of continuous treatment effects. *Journal of the Royal Statistical Society: Series B (Statistical Methodology)* **79,** 1229–1245.

Kent, D. M. and Hayward, R. A. (2007). Limitations of applying summary results of clinical trials to individual patients: the need for risk stratification. *Journal of the American Medical Association* **298,** 1209–1212.

Kent, D. M., Hayward, R. A., Griffith, J. L., Vijan, S., Beshansky, J. R., Califf, R. M., and Selker, H. P. (2002). An independently derived and validated predictive model for selecting patients with myocardial infarction who are likely to benefit from tissue plasminogen activator compared with streptokinase. *The American Journal of Medicine* **113,** 104–111.

Keogh, R. H., Shaw, P. A., Gustafson, P., Carroll, R. J., Deffner, V., Dodd, K. W., Küchenhoff, H., Tooze, J. A., Wallace, M. P. amd Kipnis, V., and Freedman, L. S. (2020). STRATOS guidance document on measurement error and misclassification of variables in observational epidemiology: Part 1 - basic theory, validation studies and simple methods of adjustment. *Statistics in Medicine* **39(16),** 2197–2231.

Khera, A. V., Chaffin, M., Aragam, K. G., Haas, M. E., Roselli, C., Choi, S. H., Natarajan, P., Lander, E. S., Lubitz, S. A., Ellinor, P. T., et al. (2018). Genome-wide polygenic scores for common diseases identify individuals with risk equivalent to monogenic mutations. *Nature Genetics* **50,** 1219–1224.

Khera, A. V., Chaffin, M., Wade, K. H., Zahid, S., Brancale, J., Xia, R., Distefano, M., Senol-Cosar, O., Haas, M. E., Bick, A., et al. (2019). Polygenic prediction of weight and obesity trajectories from birth to adulthood. *Cell* **177,** 587–596.

Kidwell, K. M., Seewald, N. J., Tran, Q., Kasari, C., and Almirall, D. (2018). Design and analysis considerations for comparing dynamic treatment regimens with binary outcomes from sequential multiple assignment randomized trials. *Journal of Applied Statistics* **45,** 1628–1651.

Kim, E. S., Herbst, R. S., Wistuba, I. I., Lee, J. J., Blumenschein, G. R., Tsao, A., Stewart, D. J., Hicks, M. E., Erasmus, J., Gupta, S., et al. (2011). The BATTLE trial: personalizing therapy for lung cancer. *Cancer Discovery* **1,** 44–53.

Kim, K., Kim, J., and Kennedy, E. H. (2018). Causal effects based on distributional distances. *arXiv preprint arXiv: 1806.02935.*

Kim, M. S., Patel, K. P., Teng, A. K., Berens, A. J., and Lachance, J. (2018). Genetic disease risks can be misestimated across global populations. *Genome Biology* **19,** 1–14.

Kim, W., Kim, G.-s., and Paik, M. C. (2021). Doubly robust Thompson sampling for linear payoffs. *arXiv preprint arXiv:2102.01229.*

Kim-Hellmuth, S., Aguet, F., Oliva, M., Muñoz-Aguirre, M., Kasela, S., Wucher, V., Castel, S. E., Hamel, A. R., Viñuela, A., Roberts, A. L., et al. (2020). Cell type–specific genetic regulation of gene expression across human tissues. *Science* **369(6509),** doi: 10.1126/science.aaz8528.

Kivaranovic, D. and Leeb, H. (2020). On the length of post-model-selection confidence intervals conditional on polyhedral constraints. *Journal of the American Statistical Association* pages 1–13. Publisher: Taylor & Francis.

Klaassen, C. A. J. (1987). Consistent estimation of the influence function of locally asymptotically linear estimators. *The Annals of Statistics* **15,** 1548–1562.

Klasnja, P., Hekler, E. B., Shiffman, S., Boruvka, A., Almirall, D., Tewari, A., and Murphy, S. A. (2015). Microrandomized trials: An experimental design for developing just-in-time adaptive interventions. *Health Psychology* **34,** 1220.

Knight, K. and Fu, W. (2000). Asymptotics for lasso-type estimators. *The Annals of Statistics* **28,** 1356–1378.

Knottnerus, J. A. and Bouter, L. M. (2001). The ethics of sample size:: Two-sided testing and one-sided thinking. *Journal of Clinical Epidemiology* **54,** 109–110.

Kocsis, L. and Szepesvári, C. (2006). Discounted UCB. In *2nd PASCAL Challenges Workshop*, volume 2.

Koenig, F., Brannath, W., Bretz, F., and Posch, M. (2008). Adaptive Dunnett tests for treatment selection. *Statistics in Medicine* **27,** 1612–1625.

Konstantinidou, M. K., Karaglani, M., Panagopoulou, M., Fiska, A., and Chatzaki, E. (2017). Are the origins of precision medicine found in the Corpus Hippocraticum? *Molecular Diagnosis & Therapy* **21,** 601–606.

Korn, E. L. and Freidlin, B. (2011). Outcome-adaptive randomization: is it useful? *Journal of Clinical Oncology* **29,** 771.

Kosorok, M. R. (2008). *Introduction to empirical processes and semiparametric inference.* Springer.

Kosorok, M. R. and Laber, E. B. (2019). Precision medicine. *Annual Review of Statistics and its Application* **6,** 263–286.

Kosorok, M. R. and Moodie, E. E. M. (2015). *Adaptive Treatment Strategies in Practice.* SIAM.

Kravitz R. L., Duan N., eds, and the DEcIDE Methods Center N-of-1 Guidance Panel (Duan N, Eslick I, Gabler NB, Kaplan HC, Kravitz RL, Larson EB, Pace WD, Schmid CH, Sim I, Vohra S). Design and Implementation of N-of-1 Trials: A User's Guide.

AHRQ Publication No. 13(14)-EHC122-EF. Rockville, MD: Agency for Healthcare Research and Quality; January 2014.

Kuchibhotla, A. K., Brown, L. D., Buja, A., Cai, J., George, E. I., and Zhao, L. H. (2020). Valid post-selection inference in model-free linear regression. *The Annals of Statistics* **48,** 2953–2981.

Kundu, P., Tang, R., and Chatterjee, N. (2019). Generalized meta-analysis for multiple regression models across studies with disparate covariate information. *Biometrika* **106,** 567–585.

Künzel, S. R., Sekhon, J. S., Bickel, P. J., and Yu, B. (2019). Metalearners for estimating heterogeneous treatment effects using machine learning. *Proceedings of the National Academy of Sciences* **116,** 4156–4165.

Kunzmann, K., Grayling, M. J., Lee, K. M., Robertson, D. S., Rufibach, K., and Wason, J. M. (2021). A review of Bayesian perspectives on sample size derivation for confirmatory trials. *The American Statistician* **75,** 1–9.

Kurowicka, D. (2011). Optimal truncation of vines. In Kurowicka, D. and Joe, H., editors, *Dependence Modeling: Vine Copula Handbook.* World Scientific Publishing Co.

Kurowicka, D. and Cooke, R. (2006). *Uncertainty analysis with high dimensional dependence modelling.* John Wiley & Sons.

Kusner, M. J., Loftus, J. R., Russell, C., and Silva, R. (2017). Counterfactual fairness. *arXiv preprint arXiv:1703.06856.*

Laber, E. and Zhao, Y. (2015). Tree-based methods for individualized treatment regimes. *Biometrika* **102,** 501–514.

Laber, E. B., Linn, K. A., and Stefanski, L. A. (2014). Interactive model building for Q-learning. *Biometrika* **101,** 831–847.

Laber, E. B., Lizotte, D. J., Qian, M., Pelham, W. E., and Murphy, S. A. (2014). Dynamic treatment regimes: Technical challenges and applications. *Electronic Journal of Statistics* **8,** 1225.

Laber, E. B. and Staicu, A.-M. (2018). Functional feature construction for individualized treatment regimes. *Journal of the American Statistical Association* **113,** 1219–1227.

Lagakos, S. W. et al. (2006). The challenge of subgroup analyses-reporting without distorting. *New England Journal of Medicine* **354,** 1667.

Lai, T. L. and Robbins, H. (1985). Asymptotically efficient adaptive allocation rules. *Advances in Applied Mathematics* **6,** 4–22.

Lai, T. L. and Wei, C. Z. (1982). Least squares estimates in stochastic regression models with applications to identification and control of dynamic systems. *The Annals of Statistics* **10,** 154–166.

Laird, N. M. and Ware, J. H. (1982). Random-effects models for longitudinal data. *Biometrics* pages 963–974.

Lambert, S. A., Abraham, G., and Inouye, M. (2019). Towards clinical utility of polygenic risk scores. *Human Molecular Genetics* **28,** R133–R142.

Lambert, S. A., Gil, L., Jupp, S., Ritchie, S. C., Xu, Y., Buniello, A., McMahon, A., Abraham, G., Chapman, M., Parkinson, H., et al. (2021). The polygenic score catalog as an open database for reproducibility and systematic evaluation. *Nature Genetics* **53,** 420–425.

Lambert, S. D., Grover, S., Laizner, A. M., McCusker, J., Belzile, E., Moodie, E. E. M., Kayser, J. W., Lowensteyn, I., Vallis, M., Walker, M., Da Costa, D., Pilote, L., Ibberson, C., Sabetty, J., and de Raad, M. (2022). Adaptive web-based stress management programs among adults with a cardiovascular disease (CVD): A pilot Sequential Multiple Assignment Randomized Trial (SMART). *Patient Education and Counseling* **105(6),** 1587–1597.

Langford, J. and Zhang, T. (2007). Epoch-greedy algorithm for multi-armed bandits with side information. *Advances in Neural Information Processing Systems (NIPS 2007)* **20,** 1.

Lattimore, F., Lattimore, T., and Reid, M. D. (2016). Causal bandits: Learning good interventions via causal inference. *arXiv preprint arXiv:1606.03203.*

Lattimore, T. (2015). Optimally confident UCB: Improved regret for finite-armed bandits. *arXiv preprint arXiv:1507.07880.*

Lattimore, T. (2018). Refining the confidence level for optimistic bandit strategies. *The Journal of Machine Learning Research* **19,** 765–796.

Lattimore, T. and Szepesvári, C. (2020). *Bandit algorithms.* Cambridge University Press.

Lavori, P. and Dawson, R. (2004). Dynamic treatment regimes: Practical design considerations. *Clinical Trials (London, England)* **1,** 9–20.

Lavori, P. W. and Dawson, R. (2000). A design for testing clinical strategies: biased adaptive within-subject randomization. *Journal of the Royal Statistical Society: Series A (Statistics in Society)* **163,** 29–38.

Lawlor, D. A., Harbord, R. M., Sterne, J. A., Timpson, N., and Davey Smith, G. (2008). Mendelian randomization: using genes as instruments for making causal inferences in epidemiology. *Statistics in Medicine* **27,** 1133–1163.

Le Tourneau, C., Lee, J. J., and Siu, L. L. (2009). Dose escalation methods in phase I cancer clinical trials. *JNCI: Journal of the National Cancer Institute* **101,** 708–720.

Lechner, M. (2011). The estimation of causal effects by difference-in-difference methods. *Foundations and Trends in Econometrics* **4,** 165–224.

Lee, J., Thall, P. F., Ji, Y., and Müller, P. (2015). Bayesian dose-finding in two treatment cycles based on the joint utility of efficacy and toxicity. *Journal of the American Statistical Association* **110,** 711–722.

Lee, J., Thall, P. F., Ji, Y., and Müller, P. (2016). A decision-theoretic phase I–II design for ordinal outcomes in two cycles. *Biostatistics* **17,** 304–319.

Lee, J., Thall, P. F., and Rezvani, K. (2019). Optimizing natural killer cell doses for heterogeneous cancer patients on the basis of multiple event times. *Journal of the Royal Statistical Society. Series C, Applied Statistics* **68,** 461.

Lee, J. D., Sun, D. L., Sun, Y., Taylor, J. E., et al. (2016). Exact post-selection inference, with application to the lasso. *Annals of Statistics* **44,** 907–927.

Lee, K. M., Brown, L. C., Jaki, T., Stallard, N., and Wason, J. (2021). Statistical consideration when adding new arms to ongoing clinical trials: the potentials and the caveats. *Trials* **22,** 1–10.

Lee, S. and Bareinboim, E. (2018). Structural causal bandits: where to intervene? *Advances in Neural Information Processing Systems 31* **31.**

Lee, S. and Bareinboim, E. (2019). Structural causal bandits with non-manipulable variables. In *Proceedings of the AAAI Conference on Artificial Intelligence*, **33,** 4164–4172.

Lee, S. M. and Cheung, Y. K. (2009). Model calibration in the continual reassessment method. *Clinical Trials* **6,** 227–238.

Leeb, H. and Pötscher, B. M. (2005). Model Selection and Inference: Facts and Fiction. *Econometric Theory* **21,** 21–59.

Leeb, H. and Pötscher, B. M. (2008). Sparse estimators and the oracle property, or the return of Hodges' estimator. *Journal of Econometrics* **142,** 201–211.

Leete, O. and Laber, E. (2022). Model-assisted v-learning. Technical report, Duke University.

Lehmacher, W. and Wassmer, G. (1999). Adaptive sample size calculations in group sequential trials. *Biometrics* **55,** 1286–1290.

Lei, H., Nahum-Shani, I., Lynch, K., Oslin, D., and Murphy, S. (2012). A" smart" design for building individualized treatment sequences. *Annual Review of Clinical Psychology* **8,** 21–48.

Lei, H., Tewari, A., and Murphy, S. (2017). An actor-critic contextual bandit algorithm for personalized interventions using mobile devices. arXiv preprint arXiv:1706.09090.

Lewis, A. C. and Green, R. C. (2021). Polygenic risk scores in the clinic: new perspectives needed on familiar ethical issues. *Genome Medicine* **13,** 1–10.

Lewis, C. M. and Vassos, E. (2020). Polygenic risk scores: from research tools to clinical instruments. *Genome Medicine* **12,** 1–11.

Li, F. and Li, F. (2019). Double-robust estimation in difference-in-differences with an application to traffic safety evaluation. *arXiv preprint arXiv:1901.02152.*

Li, F., Morgan, K. L., and Zaslavsky, A. M. (2018). Balancing covariates via propensity score weighting. *Journal of the American Statistical Association* **113,** 390–400.

Li, J. and Chan, I. S. (2006). Detecting qualitative interactions in clinical trials: an extension of range test. *Journal of Biopharmaceutical Statistics* **16,** 831–841.

Li, J., Zhang, X., Li, A., Liu, S., Qin, W., Yu, C., Liu, Y., Liu, B., and Jiang, T. (2018). Polygenic risk for Alzheimer's disease influences precuneal volume in two independent general populations. *Neurobiology of Aging* **64,** 116–122.

Li, L., Chu, W., Langford, J., and Schapire, R. E. (2010). A contextual-bandit approach to personalized news article recommendation. In *Proceedings of the 19th international conference on World wide web*, pages 661–670.

Li, L., Chu, W., Langford, J., and Wang, X. (2011). Unbiased offline evaluation of contextual-bandit-based news article recommendation algorithms. In *Proceedings of the fourth ACM international conference on Web search and data mining*, pages 297–306.

Li, L., Munos, R., and Szepesvári, C. (2015). Toward minimax off-policy value estimation. In *Artificial Intelligence and Statistics*, pages 608–616. PMLR.

Li, L., Tchetgen, E. T., van der Vaart, A., and Robins, J. M. (2011). Higher order inference on a treatment effect under low regularity conditions. *Statistics & Probability Letters* **81,** 821–828.

Li, R. and Chambless, L. (2007). Test for additive interaction in proportional hazards models. *Annals of Epidemiology* **17,** 227–236.

Li, S., Karatzoglou, A., and Gentile, C. (2016). Collaborative filtering bandits. In *Proceedings of the 39th International ACM SIGIR conference on Research and Development in Information Retrieval*, pages 539–548.

Li, Y., Bekele, B. N., Ji, Y., and Cook, J. D. (2008). Dose–schedule finding in phase I/II clinical trials using a Bayesian isotonic transformation. *Statistics in Medicine* **27,** 4895–4913.

Li, Z., Laber, E., and Meyer, N. (2022). Thompson sampling for pursuit-evasion problems. In *2022 International Conference on Electrical, Computer, Communications and Mechatronics Engineering (ICECCME)*, pages 1–8. IEEE.

Liang, M., Choi, Y.-G., Ning, Y., Smith, M. A., and Zhao, Y.-Q. (2021). Estimation and inference on high-dimensional individualized treatment rule in observational data using split-and-pooled de-correlated score. *arXiv preprint arXiv:2007.04445.*

Liao, P., Greenewald, K., Klasnja, P., and Murphy, S. (2020). Personalized heartsteps: A reinforcement learning algorithm for optimizing physical activity. *Proceedings of the ACM on Interactive, Mobile, Wearable and Ubiquitous Technologies* **4,** 1–22.

Lieberman, J. A., Stroup, T. S., McEvoy, J. P., Swartz, M. S., Rosenheck, R. A., Perkins, D. O., Keefe, R. S. E., Davis, S., Davis, C. E., Lebowitz, B. D., and Severe, J. (2005). Effectiveness of antipsychotic drugs in patients with chronic schozophrenia. *New England Journal of Medicine* **353,** 1209–1223.

Lillie, E., Patay, B., Diamant, J., Issell, B., Topol, E., and Schork, N. (2011). The n-of-1 clinical trial: the ultimate strategy for individualizing medicine. *Personalized Medicine* **8,** 161–173.

Lin, J. and Bunn, V. (2017). Comparison of multi-arm multi-stage design and adaptive randomization in platform clinical trials. *Contemporary Clinical Trials* **54,** 48–59.

Lin, R., Thall, P. F., and Yuan, Y. (2020). An adaptive trial design to optimize dose-schedule regimes with delayed outcomes. *Biometrics* **76,** 304–315.

Lin, R., Thall, P. F., and Yuan, Y. (2021). A phase I–II basket trial design to optimize dose-schedule regimes based on delayed outcomes. *Bayesian Analysis* **16,** 179–202.

Lin, T., Jin, C., and Jordan, M. I. (2019). On gradient descent ascent for nonconvex-concave minimax problems. *arXiv preprint arXiv:1906.00331v6.*

Little, R. J., D'Agostino, R., Cohen, M. L., Dickersin, K., Emerson, S. S., Farrar, J. T., Frangakis, C., Hogan, J. W., Molenberghs, G., Murphy, S. A., et al. (2012). The prevention and treatment of missing data in clinical trials. *New England Journal of Medicine* **367,** 1355–1360.

Liu, C., Zeinomar, N., Chung, W. K., Kiryluk, K., Ghravi, A. G., Hripcsak, G., Crew, K. D., Shang, N., Khan, A., Fasel, D., et al. (2021). Generalizability of polygenic risk scores for breast cancer in the multiethnic emerge study. *medRxiv* doi:10.1001/jamanetworkopen.2021.19084.

Liu, C.-T., Raghavan, S., Maruthur, N., Kabagambe, E. K., Hong, J., Ng, M. C., Hivert, M.-F., Lu, Y., An, P., Bentley, A. R., et al. (2016). Trans-ethnic meta-analysis and functional annotation illuminates the genetic architecture of fasting glucose and insulin. *The American Journal of Human Genetics* **99,** 56–75.

Liu, M., Jiang, Y., Wedow, R., Li, Y., Brazel, D. M., Chen, F., Datta, G., Davila-Velderrain, J., McGuire, D., Tian, C., et al. (2019). Association studies of up to 1.2 million individuals yield new insights into the genetic etiology of tobacco and alcohol use. *Nature Genetics* **51,** 237–244.

Liu, Q., Proschan, M. A., and Pledger, G. W. (2002). A unified theory of two-stage adaptive designs. *Journal of the American Statistical Association* **97,** 1034–1041.

Liu, S., See, K. C., Ngiam, K. Y., Celi, L. A., Sun, X., and Feng, M. (2020). Reinforcement learning for clinical decision support in critical care: comprehensive review. *Journal of Medical Internet Research* **22,** e18477.

Liu, S. and Yuan, Y. (2015). Bayesian optimal interval designs for phase I clinical trials. *Journal of the Royal Statistical Society: Series C (Applied Statistics)* **64,** 507–523.

Liu, Y., Radanovic, G., Dimitrakakis, C., Mandal, D., and Parkes, D. C. (2017). Calibrated fairness in bandits. *arXiv preprint arXiv:1707.01875.*

Lloyd-Jones, L. R., Zeng, J., Sidorenko, J., Yengo, L., Moser, G., Kemper, K. E., Wang, H., Zheng, Z., Magi, R., Esko, T., et al. (2019). Improved polygenic prediction by Bayesian multiple regression on summary statistics. *Nature Communications* **10,** 1–11.

London, A. J. (2018). Learning health systems, clinical equipoise and the ethics of response adaptive randomisation. *Journal of Medical Ethics* **44,** 409–415.

Lot, F., Cazein, F., and Ndeikoundam, D. (2019). VIH et autres IST: activité de dépistage et de diagnostic en France. Technical report, Santé Publique France. Journée de la Société Française de Lutte contre le Sida. [Cited 2018 April 18].

Lovibond, S. H. and Lovibond, P. F. (1996). *Manual for the depression anxiety stress scales.* Psychology Foundation of Australia.

Lu, A., Frazier, P. I., and Kislev, O. (2018). Surge pricing moves Uber's driver-partners. In *Proceedings of the 2018 ACM Conference on Economics and Computation*, page 3. ACM.

Lu, C., Nie, X., and Wager, S. (2019). Robust nonparametric difference-in-differences estimation. *arXiv preprint arXiv:1905.11622v1.*

Lu, N. T., Crespi, C. M., Liu, N. M., Vu, J. Q., Ahmadieh, Y., Wu, S., Lin, S., McClune, A., Durazo, F., Saab, S., et al. (2016). A phase I dose escalation study demonstrates quercetin safety and explores potential for bioflavonoid antivirals in patients with chronic hepatitis c. *Phytotherapy Research* **30,** 160–168.

Lu, Q., Powles, R. L., Abdallah, S., Ou, D., Wang, Q., Hu, Y., Lu, Y., Liu, W., Li, B., Mukherjee, S., et al. (2017). Systematic tissue-specific functional annotation of the human genome highlights immune-related DNA elements for late-onset Alzheimer's disease. *PLoS Genetics* **13,** e1006933.

Lu, W., Zhang, H. H., and Zeng, D. (2013). Variable selection for optimal treatment decision. *Statistical Methods in Medical Research* **22,** 493–504.

Lu, Y., Meisami, A., and Tewari, A. (2021a). Causal bandits with unknown graph structure. *arXiv preprint arXiv:2106.02988.*

Lu, Y., Meisami, A., and Tewari, A. (2021b). Low-rank generalized linear bandit problems. In *International Conference on Artificial Intelligence and Statistics*, pages 460–468. PMLR.

Lu, Y., Meisami, A., Tewari, A., and Yan, W. (2020). Regret analysis of bandit problems with causal background knowledge. In *Conference on Uncertainty in Artificial Intelligence*, pages 141–150. PMLR.

Luckett, D. J., Laber, E. B., Kahkoska, A. R., Maahs, D. M., Mayer-Davis, E., and Kosorok, M. R. (2020). Estimating dynamic treatment regimes in mobile health using v-learning. *Journal of the American Statistical Association* **115(530),** 692–706.

Luedtke, A., Carone, M., Simon, N. R., and Sofrygin, O. (2020). Learning to learn from data: using deep adversarial learning to construct optimal statistical procedures. *Science Advances* (in Press; available online late Feb or Mar 2020).

Luedtke, A., Chung, I., and Sofrygin, O. (2021). Adversarial Monte Carlo meta-learning of optimal prediction procedures. *Journal of Machine Learning Research* **22,** 1–67.

Luedtke, A. R., Diaz, I., and van der Laan, M. J. (2015). The statistics of sensitivity analyses. *UC Berkeley Division of Biostatistics Working Paper Series* Paper 341.

Luedtke, A. R. and van der Laan, M. J. (2016c). Optimal dynamic treatments in resource-limited settings. *The International Journal of Biostatistics* **12,** 283–303.

Luedtke, A. R. and van der Laan, M. J. (2016a). Statistical inference for the mean outcome under a possibly non-unique optimal treatment strategy. *The Annals of Statistics* **44,** 713–742.

Luedtke, A. R. and van der Laan, M. J. (2016b). Super-learning of an optimal dynamic treatment rule. *The International Journal of Biostatistics* **12,** 305–332.

Lunceford, J. K., Davidian, M., and Tsiatis, A. A. (2002). Estimation of survival distributions of treatment policies in two-stage randomization designs in clinical trials. *Biometrics* **58,** 48–57.

Lyden, P., Pryor, K. E., Coffey, C. S., Cudkowicz, M., Conwit, R., Jadhav, A., Sawyer Jr, R. N., Claassen, J., Adeoye, O., Song, S., et al. (2019). Randomized, controlled, dose escalation trial of a protease-activated receptor-1 agonist in acute ischemic stroke: Final results of the rhapsody trial: A multi-center, phase 2 trial using a continual reassessment method to determine the safety and tolerability of 3k3a-apc, a recombinant variant of human activated protein c, in combination with tissue plasminogen activator, mechanical thrombectomy or both in moderate to severe acute ischemic stroke. *Annals of Neurology* **85,** 125.

Lykouris, T., Mirrokni, V., and Paes Leme, R. (2018). Stochastic bandits robust to adversarial corruptions. In *Proceedings of the 50th Annual ACM SIGACT Symposium on Theory of Computing*, pages 114–122.

Ma, C., Zhu, B., Jiao, J., and Wainwright, M. J. (2021). Minimax off-policy evaluation for multi-armed bandits. *arXiv preprint arXiv:2101.07781.*

Ma, T., Cai, H., Qi, Z., Shi, C., and Laber, E. B. (2023). Sequential knockoffs for variable selection in reinforcement learning. *arXiv preprint arXiv:2303.14281.*

Maei, H., Szepesvári, C., Bhatnagar, S., and Sutton, R. (2010). Toward off-policy learning control with function approximation. In *Proceedings of the 27th International Conference on Machine Learning*, 719–726.

Magirr, D., Jaki, T., Posch, M., and Klinglmueller, F. (2013). Simultaneous confidence intervals that are compatible with closed testing in adaptive designs. *Biometrika* **100,** 985–996.

Magirr, D., Jaki, T., and Whitehead, J. (2012). A generalized dunnett test for multi-arm multi-stage clinical studies with treatment selection. *Biometrika* **99,** 494–501.

Maglio, P. and Mabry, P. (2011). Agent-based models and systems science approaches to public health. *American Journal of Preventive Medicine* **40,** 392–394.

Magnusson, B. P. and Turnbull, B. W. (2013). Group sequential enrichment design incorporating subgroup selection. *Statistics in Medicine* **32,** 2695–2714.

Mak, T. S. H., Porsch, R. M., Choi, S. W., Zhou, X., and Sham, P. C. (2017). Polygenic scores via penalized regression on summary statistics. *Genetic Epidemiology* **41,** 469–480.

Mander, A. P. and Sweeting, M. J. (2015). A product of independent beta probabilities dose escalation design for dual-agent phase I trials. *Statistics in Medicine* **34,** 1261–1276.

Mandrekar, S. J., Cui, Y., and Sargent, D. J. (2007). An adaptive phase I design for identifying a biologically optimal dose for dual agent drug combinations. *Statistics in Medicine* **26,** 2317–2330.

Manolis, E., Brogren, J., Cole, S., Hay, J., Nordmark, A., Karlsson, K., Lentz, F., Benda, N., Wangorsch, G., Pons, G., Zhao, W., Gigante, V., Serone, F., Standing, J.,

Dokoumetzidis, A., Vakkilainen, J., van den Heuvel, M., Mangas S, V., Taminiau, J., Kerwash, E., Khan, D., Musuamba, F., and Skottheim Rusten, I. (2017). Commentary on the MID3 Good Practices Paper. *CPT Pharmacometrics Syst Pharmacol* **6,** 416–417.

Manschot, C., Laber, E., and Davidian, M. (2023). Interim monitoring of sequential multiple assignment randomized trials using partial information. *Biometrics* **79,** 2881–2894.

Marcus, R., Peritz, E., and Gabriel, K. R. (1976). On closed testing procedures with special reference to ordered analysis of variance. *Biometrika* **63,** 655–660.

Maron, H., Fetaya, E., Segol, N., and Lipman, Y. (2019). On the universality of invariant networks. *arXiv preprint arXiv:1901.09342.*

Marquez-Luna, C., Gazal, S., Loh, P.-R., Kim, S. S., Furlotte, N., Auton, A., Price, A. L., 23andMe Research Team, et al. (2021). Ldpred-funct: incorporating functional priors improves polygenic prediction accuracy in UK biobank and 23andMe data sets. Nature Communications volume 12, Article number: 6052

Márquez-Luna, C., Loh, P.-R., Consortium, S. A. T., Consortium, S. T., and Price, A. L. (2017). Multiethnic polygenic risk scores improve risk prediction in diverse populations. *Genetic Epidemiology* **41,** 811–823.

Mars, N., Widén, E., Kerminen, S., Meretoja, T., Pirinen, M., della Briotta Parolo, P., Palta, P., Palotie, A., Kaprio, J., Joensuu, H., et al. (2020). The role of polygenic risk and susceptibility genes in breast cancer over the course of life. *Nature Communications* **11,** 1–9.

Marschner, I. C. (2021). A general framework for the analysis of adaptive experiments. *Statistical Science* **36,** 465–492.

Marshall, S., Burghaus, R., Cosson, V., Cheung, S., Chenel, M., DellaPasqua, O., Frey, N., Hamren, B., Harnisch, L., Ivanow, F., Kerbusch, T., Lippert, J., Milligan, P., Rohou, S., Staab, A., Steimer, J., Torne, C., and Visser, S. (2016). Good Practices in Model-Informed Drug Discovery and Development: Practice, Application, and Documentation. *CPT Pharmacometrics Syst Pharmacol* **5,** 93–122.

Martin, A. R., Daly, M. J., Robinson, E. B., Hyman, S. E., and Neale, B. M. (2019). Predicting polygenic risk of psychiatric disorders. *Biological Psychiatry* **86,** 97–109.

Martin, A. R., Gignoux, C. R., Walters, R. K., Wojcik, G. L., Neale, B. M., Gravel, S., Daly, M. J., Bustamante, C. D., and Kenny, E. E. (2017). Human demographic history impacts genetic risk prediction across diverse populations. *The American Journal of Human Genetics* **100,** 635–649.

Martin, A. R., Kanai, M., Kamatani, Y., Okada, Y., Neale, B. M., and Daly, M. J. (2019). Clinical use of current polygenic risk scores may exacerbate health disparities. *Nature Genetics* **51,** 584–591.

Mary, J., Preux, P., and Nicol, O. (2014). Improving offline evaluation of contextual bandit algorithms via bootstrapping techniques. In *International Conference on Machine Learning*, pages 172–180. PMLR.

Maurer, A., Pontil, M., and Romera-Paredes, B. (2016). The benefit of multitask representation learning. *Journal of Machine Learning Research* **17,** 1–32.

Mehta, C., Liu, L., and Theuer, C. (2019). An adaptive population enrichment phase III trial of TRC105 and pazopanib versus pazopanib alone in patients with advanced angiosarcoma (TAPPAS trial). *Annals of Oncology* **30,** 103–108.

Mehta, C. R. and Pocock, S. J. (2011). Adaptive increase in sample size when interim results are promising: A practical guide with examples. *Statistics in Medicine* **30,** 3267–3284.

Metelkina, A. and Pronzato, L. (2017). Information-regret compromise in covariate-adaptive treatment allocation. *The Annals of Statistics* **45,** 2046–2073.

Meurer, W. J., Lewis, R. J., and Berry, D. A. (2012). Adaptive clinical trials: a partial remedy for the therapeutic misconception? *Journal of the American Medical Association* **307,** 2377–2378.

Meyer, B. D. (1995). Natural and quasi-experiments in economics. *Journal of Business & Economic Statistics* **13,** 151–161.

Miao, W., Shi, X., and Tchetgen, E. T. (2018). A confounding bridge approach for double negative control inference on causal effects. *arXiv preprint arXiv:1808.04945.*

Micheletti, R. G., Pagnoux, C., Tamura, R. N., Grayson, P. C., McAlear, C. A., Borchin, R., Krischer, J. P., and Merkel, P. A. (2020). Protocol for a randomized multicenter study for isolated skin vasculitis (ARAMIS) comparing the efficacy of three drugs: azathioprine, colchicine, and dapsone. *Trials* **21,** 1–9.

Mijoule, G., Savy, N., and Savy, S. (2012). Models for patients recruitment in clinical trials and sensitivity analysis. *Statistics in Medicine* **31,** 1655–1674.

Minois, N., Savy, S., Lauwers-Cances, V., Andrieu, S., and Savy, N. (2017). How to deal with the Poisson-gamma model to forecast patients' recruitment in clinical trials when there are pauses in recruitment dynamic? *Contemporary Clinical Trials Communications* **5,** 144–152.

Mishchenko, K., Kovalev, D., Shulgin, E., Richtárik, P., and Malitsky, Y. (2020). Revisiting stochastic extragradient. In *International Conference on Artificial Intelligence and Statistics*, pages 4573–4582. PMLR.

Mohr, D., Schueller, S., Riley, W., Brown, C., Cuijpers, P., Duan, N., Kwasny, M., Stiles-Shields, C., and Cheung, K. (2015). Trials of intervention principles: Evaluation methods for evolving behavioral intervention technologies. *Journal of Medical Internet Research* **17,** e166.

Mohr, D. C., Cheung, K., Schueller, S. M., Brown, C. H., and Duan, N. (2013). Continuous evaluation of evolving behavioral intervention technologies. *American Journal of Preventive Medicine* **45,** 517–523.

Mohr, D. C., Tomasino, K. N., Lattie, E. G., Palac, H. L., Kwasny, M. J., Weingardt, K., Karr, C. J., Kaiser, S. M., Rossom, R. C., Bardsley, L. R., et al. (2017). Intellicare: an eclectic, skills-based app suite for the treatment of depression and anxiety. *Journal of Medical Internet Research* **19(1),** e10. doi: 10.2196/jmir.6645.

Moodie, E. E. M., Chakraborty, B., and Kramer, M. S. (2012). Q-learning for estimating optimal dynamic treatment rules from observational data. *Canadian Journal of Statistics* **40,** 629–645.

Moodie, E. E. M., Dean, N., and Sun, Y. R. (2014). Q-learning: Flexible learning about useful utilities. *Statistics in Biosciences* **6,** 223–243.

Moodie, E. E. M., Richardson, T. S., and Stephens, D. A. (2007). Demystifying optimal dynamic treatment regimes. *Biometrics* **63,** 447–455.

Moodie, E. E. M. and Richardson, T. S. (2010). Estimating optimal dynamic regimes: Correcting bias under the null. *Scandinavian Journal of Statistics* **37,** 126–146.

Moore, J. H., Gilbert, J. C., Tsai, C.-T., Chiang, F.-T., Holden, T., Barney, N., and White, B. C. (2006). A flexible computational framework for detecting, characterizing, and interpreting statistical patterns of epistasis in genetic studies of human disease susceptibility. *Journal of Theoretical Biology* **241,** 252–261.

Morita, S., Thall, P. F., and Müller, P. (2010). Evaluating the impact of prior assumptions in Bayesian biostatistics. *Statistics in Biosciences* **2,** 1–17.

Mosley, J. D., Gupta, D. K., Tan, J., Yao, J., Wells, Q. S., Shaffer, C. M., Kundu, S., Robinson-Cohen, C., Psaty, B. M., Rich, S. S., et al. (2020). Predictive accuracy of a polygenic risk score compared with a clinical risk score for incident coronary heart disease. *Journal of the American Medical Association* **323,** 627–635.

Mozgunov, P. and Jaki, T. (2019). An information theoretic phase I-II design for molecularly targeted agents that does not require an assumption of monotonicity. *Journal of the Royal Statistical Society: Series C (Applied Statistics)* **68,** 347–367.

Murphy, S. A. (2003). Optimal dynamic treatment regimes. *Journal of the Royal Statistical Society: Series B (Statistical Methodology)* **65,** 331–355.

Murphy, S. A. (2005a). An experimental design for the development of adaptive treatment strategies. *Statistics in Medicine* **24,** 1455–1481.

Murphy, S. A. (2005b). A generalization error for q-learning. *Journal of Machine Learning Research* **6,** 1073–1097.

Murray, R. P., Connett, J. E., Lauger, G. G., and Voelker, H. T. (1993). Error in smoking measures: effects of intervention on relations of cotinine and carbon monoxide to self-reported smoking. The Lung Health Study Research Group. *American Journal of Public Health* **83(9),** 1251–1257.

Murray, T. A., Yuan, Y., and Thall, P. F. (2018). A Bayesian machine learning approach for optimizing dynamic treatment regimes. *Journal of the American Statistical Association* **113,** 1255–1267.

Mustanski, B., Saber, R., Macapagal, K., Matson, M., Laber, E., Rodrgiuez-Diaz, C., Moran, K. O., Carrion, A., Moskowitz, D. A., and Newcomb, M. E. (2022). Effectiveness of the smart sex ed program among 13–18 year old English and Spanish speaking adolescent men who have sex with men. *AIDS and Behavior* pages 1–12.

Myers, J. A., Rassen, J. A., Gagne, J. J., Huybrechts, K. F., Schneeweiss, S., Rothman, K. J., Joffe, M. M., and Glynn, R. J. (2011). Effects of adjusting for instrumental variables on bias and precision of effect estimates. *American Journal of Epidemiology* **174,** 1213–1222.

Nagler, T. and Vatter, T. (2019). *rvinecopulib: High Performance Algorithms for Vine Copula Modeling.* R package version 0.5.1.1.0.

Nahum-Shani, I., Qian, M., Almirall, D., Pelham, W. E., Gnagy, B., Fabiano, G. A., Waxmonsky, J. G., Yu, J., and Murphy, S. A. (2012). Experimental design and primary data analysis methods for comparing adaptive interventions. *Psychological Methods* **17,** 457.

Nair, V., Patil, V., and Sinha, G. (2021). Budgeted and non-budgeted causal bandits. In *International Conference on Artificial Intelligence and Statistics*, pages 2017–2025. PMLR.

Nash, S. G. (2000). A survey of truncated-Newton methods. *Journal of Computational and Applied Mathematics* **124,** 45–59.

National Research Council, Division on Earth and Life Studies, Board on Life Sciences, Committee on A Framework for Developing a New Taxonomy of Disease (2011). Toward precision medicine: building a knowledge network for biomedical research and a new taxonomy of disease.

Negahban, S. N., Ravikumar, P., Wainwright, M. J., and Yu, B. (2012). A unified framework for high-dimensional analysis of M-estimators with decomposable regularizers. *Statistical Science* **27,** 538–557.

Nelsen, R. (2007). *An introduction to copulas.* Springer Science & Business Media.

Nelson, W. (1966). Minimax solution of statistical decision problems by iteration. *The Annals of Mathematical Statistics* pages 1643–1657.

Nemirovski, A., Juditsky, A., Lan, G., and Shapiro, A. (2009). Robust stochastic approximation approach to stochastic programming. *SIAM Journal on Optimization* **19,** 1574–1609.

Neu, G. (2015). Explore no more: Improved high-probability regret bounds for non-stochastic bandits. *arXiv preprint arXiv:1506.03271.*

Neuenschwander, B., Wandel, S., Roychoudhury, S., and Bailey, S. (2016). Robust exchangeability designs for early phase clinical trials with multiple strata. *Pharmaceutical Statistics* **15,** 123–134.

Newey, W. K. (1994). The asymptotic variance of semiparametric estimators. *Econometrica: Journal of the Econometric Society* **62,** 1349–1382.

Nguyen, T. V. and Eisman, J. A. (2020). Post-GWAS polygenic risk score: Utility and challenges. *JBMR Plus* **4,** e10411.

Ni, G., Zeng, J., Revez, J. A., Wang, Y., Zheng, Z., Ge, T., Restuadi, R., Kiewa, J., Nyholt, D. R., Coleman, J. R., and Smoller, J. W. (2021). A comparison of ten polygenic score methods for psychiatric disorders applied across multiple cohorts. *Biological Psychiatry* **90(9)**, 611–620.

Nie, X. and Wager, S. (2021). Quasi-oracle estimation of heterogeneous treatment effects. *Biometrika* **108,** 299–319.

NIH (2014). National cancer institute. NCI dictionary of cancer terms. Accessed: 26/04/2020. https://www.cancer.gov/ publications/dictionaries/cancer-terms/def/mtd.

NIHR. Adopting an adaptive approach to help HIV patients on antiretroviral therapy (cART). Accessed: 28/01/2020. https://www.nihr.ac.uk/documents/case-studies/adopting-an-adaptive-approach-to-help-hiv-patients-on-antiretroviral-therapy-cart/22259.

Niss, L. and Tewari, A. (2020). What you see may not be what you get: UCB bandit algorithms robust to ε-contamination. In *Conference on Uncertainty in Artificial Intelligence*, pages 450–459. PMLR.

Norwood, P., Davidian, M., and Laber, E. (2022). Adapative randomization methods for sequential multiple assignment randomized trials (SMARTs) via Thompson sampling. arxiv https://doi.org/10.48550/arXiv.2401.03268.

Noubiap, R. F. and Seidel, W. (2001). An algorithm for calculating γ-minimax decision rules under generalized moment conditions. *The Annals of Statistics* **29,** 1094–1116.

Novembre, J. and Barton, N. H. (2018). Tread lightly interpreting polygenic tests of selection. *Genetics* **208,** 1351–1355.

Nshimyumukiza, L., Durand, A., Gagnon, M., Douville, X., Morin, S., Lindsay, C., Duplantie, J., Gagne, C., Jean, S., Giguere, Y., Dodin, S., Rousseau, F., and Reinharz, D. (2013). An economic evaluation: Simulation of the cost-effectiveness and cost-utility of universal prevention strategies against osteoporosis-related fractures. *J. Bone Miner. Res.* **28,** 383–394.

Nurnberger Jr, J. I., Wang, Y., Zang, Y., Lai, D., Wetherill, L., Edenberg, H. J., Aliev, F., Plawecki, M. H., Chorlian, D., Chan, G., et al. (2021). High polygenic risk scores are associated with early age of onset of alcohol use disorder in adolescents and young adults at risk. *Biological Psychiatry Global Open Science.*

Nuventra, E. (2018). Lessons from FDA's grand rounds: "how simulation can transform regulatory pathways". Nuventra, Blog.

Obenauer, M. L. and von der Nienburg, B. (1915). Effect of minimum-wage determinations in Oregon. *Bulletin of the United States Bureau of Labor Statistics* **1,** 5–8.

Obermeyer, Z., Powers, B., Vogeli, C., and Mullainathan, S. (2019). Dissecting racial bias in an algorithm used to manage the health of populations. *Science* **366,** 447–453.

O'Connor, L. J., Schoech, A. P., Hormozdiari, F., Gazal, S., Patterson, N., and Price, A. L. (2019). Extreme polygenicity of complex traits is explained by negative selection. *The American Journal of Human Genetics* **105,** 456–476.

Oganisian, A. and Roy, J. A. (2021). A practical introduction to Bayesian estimation of causal effects: Parametric and nonparametric approaches. *Statistics in Medicine* **40,** 518–551.

Ogburn, E. L., Rotnitzky, A., and Robins, J. M. (2015). Doubly robust estimation of the local average treatment effect curve. *Journal of the Royal Statistical Society: Series B (Statistical Methodology)* **77,** 373–396.

Ogburn, E. L., Sofrygin, O., Diaz, I., and van der Laan, M. J. (2017). Causal inference for social network data. *arXiv preprint arXiv:1705.08527*.

Oh, E. J., Qian, M., and Cheung, Y. K. (2022). Generalization error bounds of dynamic treatment regimes in penalized regression-based learning. *The Annals of Statistics* **50,** 2047–2071.

Ojo, A. (2018). The NIH All of Us Research Program (AoU RP). *Innovation in Aging* **2,** 768.

Ondra, T., Jobjörnsson, S., Beckman, R. A., Burman, C.-F., König, F., Stallard, N., and Posch, M. (2019). Optimized adaptive enrichment designs. *Statistical Methods in Medical Research* **28,** 2096–2111.

O'Quigley, J., Hughes, M. D., and Fenton, T. (2001). Dose-finding designs for HIV studies. *Biometrics* **57,** 1018–1029.

O'Quigley, J., Pepe, M., and Fisher, L. (1990). Continual reassessment method: a practical design for phase 1 clinical trials in cancer. *Biometrics* pages 33–48.

O'Quigley, J. and Shen, L. Z. (1996). Continual reassessment method: a likelihood approach. *Biometrics* **52,** 673–684.

Orellana, L., Rotnitzky, A., and Robins, J. M. (2010). Dynamic regime marginal structural mean models for estimation of optimal dynamic treatment regimes, part I: Main content. *The International Journal of Biostatistics* **6,**.

Pain, O., Glanville, K. P., Hagenaars, S. P., Selzam, S., Fürtjes, A. E., Gaspar, H. A., Coleman, J. R., Rimfeld, K., Breen, G., Plomin, R., et al. (2021). Evaluation of polygenic prediction methodology within a reference-standardized framework. *PLoS Genetics* **17,** e1009021.

Pal Choudhury, P., Maas, P., Wilcox, A., Wheeler, W., Brook, M., Check, D., Garcia-Closas, M., and Chatterjee, N. (2020). iCARE: An R package to build, validate and apply absolute risk models. *PLoS One* **15,** e0228198.

Pallmann, P., Bedding, A. W., Choodari-Oskooei, B., Dimairo, M., Flight, L., Hampson, L. V., Holmes, J., Mander, A. P., Sydes, M. R., Villar, S. S., et al. (2018). Adaptive designs in clinical trials: why use them, and how to run and report them. *BMC Medicine* **16,** 29.

Pan, G. and Wolfe, D. A. (1997). Test for qualitative interaction of clinical significance. *Statistics in Medicine* **16,** 1645–1652.

Panagiotelis, A., Czado, C., and Joe, H. (2012). Pair copula constructions for multivariate discrete data. *Journal of the American Statistical Association* **107,** 1063–1072.

Pane, J. F., Griffin, B. A., McCaffrey, D. F., and Karam, R. (2014). Effectiveness of cognitive tutor algebra I at scale. *Educational Evaluation and Policy Analysis* **36,** 127–144.

Paoletti, X., Ezzalfani, M., and Le Tourneau, C. (2015). Statistical controversies in clinical research: requiem for the 3+3 design for phase I trials. *Annals of Oncology* **26,** 1808–1812.

Paredes, P., Gilad-Bachrach, R., Czerwinski, M., Roseway, A., Rowan, K., and Hernandez, J. (2014). Poptherapy: Coping with stress through pop-culture. In *Proceedings of the 8th International Conference on Pervasive Computing Technologies for Healthcare*, pages 109–117.

Park, J.-H., Wacholder, S., Gail, M. H., Peters, U., Jacobs, K. B., Chanock, S. J., and Chatterjee, N. (2010). Estimation of effect size distribution from genome-wide association studies and implications for future discoveries. *Nature Genetics* **42,** 570–575.

Park, J. J., Siden, E., Zoratti, M. J., Dron, L., Harari, O., Singer, J., Lester, R. T., Thorlund, K., and Mills, E. J. (2019). Systematic review of basket trials, umbrella trials, and platform trials: a landscape analysis of master protocols. *Trials* **20,** 1–10.

Parmar, M. K., Barthel, F. M.-S., Sydes, M., Langley, R., Kaplan, R., Eisenhauer, E., Brady, M., James, N., Bookman, M. A., Swart, A.-M., et al. (2008). Speeding up the evaluation of new agents in cancer. *Journal of the National Cancer Institute* **100,** 1204–1214.

Pasaniuc, B. and Price, A. L. (2017). Dissecting the genetics of complex traits using summary association statistics. *Nature Reviews Genetics* **18,** 117–127.

Paszke, A., Gross, S., Massa, F., Lerer, A., Bradbury, J., Chanan, G., Killeen, T., Lin, Z., Gimelshein, N., and Antiga, L. (2019). Pytorch: An imperative style, high-performance deep learning library. In *Advances in Neural Information Processing Systems*, pages 8024–8035.

Patil, V., Ghalme, G., Nair, V., and Narahari, Y. (2020). Achieving fairness in the stochastic multi-armed bandit problem. In *Proceedings of the AAAI Conference on Artificial Intelligence*, volume 34, pages 5379–5386.

Paulus, J. K. and Kent, D. M. (2020). Predictably unequal: understanding and addressing concerns that algorithmic clinical prediction may increase health disparities. *NPJ digital medicine* **3,** 1–8.

Pearl, J. (2009). *Causality: Models, Reasoning, and Inference.* Cambridge University Press.

Peck, L. R. (2003). Subgroup analysis in social experiments: Measuring program impacts based on post-treatment choice. *American Journal of Evaluation* **24,** 157–187.

Pepe, M. S. and Anderson, G. L. (1994). A cautionary note on inference for marginal regression models with longitudinal data and general correlated response data. *Communications in Statistics-Simulation and Computation* **23,** 939–951.

Petersen, A. (2018). *flam: Fits Piecewise Constant Models with Data-Adaptive Knots.* R package version 3.2.

Petersen, A., Witten, D., and Simon, N. (2016). Fused lasso additive model. *Journal of Computational and Graphical Statistics* **25,** 1005–1025.

Petersen, M. L. and van der Laan, M. J. (2014). Causal models and learning from data: integrating causal modeling and statistical estimation. *Epidemiology* **25,** 418.

Pfanzagl, J. (1982). *Contributions to a general asymptotic statistical theory,* volume 13. Springer.

Piantadosi, S. and Gail, M. (1993). A comparison of the power of two tests for qualitative interactions. *Statistics in Medicine* **12,** 1239–1248.

Piette, J. D., Farris, K. B., Newman, S., An, L., Sussman, J., and Singh, S. (2015). The potential impact of intelligent systems for mobile health self-management support: Monte Carlo simulations of text message support for medication adherence. *Annals of Behavioral Medicine* **49,** 84–94.

Piette, J. D., Krein, S. L., Striplin, D., Marinec, N., Kerns, R. D., Farris, K. B., Singh, S., An, L., and Heapy, A. A. (2016). Patient-centered pain care using artificial intelligence and mobile health tools: protocol for a randomized study funded by the US Department of Veterans Affairs Health Services Research and Development Program. *JMIR Research Protocols* **5,** e53.

Pinheiro, J., Bornkamp, B., Glimm, E., and Bretz, F. (2014). Model-based dose finding under model uncertainty using general parametric models. *Statistics in Medicine* **33,** 1646–1661.

Pocock, S. J. (1977). Group sequential methods in the design and analysis of clinical trials. *Biometrika* **64,** 191–199.

Pocock, S. J., Assmann, S. E., Enos, L. E., and Kasten, L. E. (2002). Subgroup analysis, covariate adjustment and baseline comparisons in clinical trial reporting: current practiceand problems. *Statistics in Medicine* **21,** 2917–2930.

Pocock, S. J. and Lubsen, J. (2008). More on subgroup analyses in clinical trials. *The New England Journal of Medicine* **358,** 2076.

Polderman, T. J., Benyamin, B., De Leeuw, C. A., Sullivan, P. F., Van Bochoven, A., Visscher, P. M., and Posthuma, D. (2015). Meta-analysis of the heritability of human traits based on fifty years of twin studies. *Nature Genetics* **47,** 702–709.

Pombo-Romero, J., Varela, L., and Ricoy, C. (2013). Diffusion of innovations in social interaction systems. An agent-based model for the introduction of new drugs in markets. *European Journal of Health Economics* **14,** 443–455.

Posch, M. and Bauer, P. (1999). Adaptive two stage designs and the conditional error function. *Biometrical Journal* **41,** 689–696.

Posch, M., Koenig, F., Branson, M., Brannath, W., Dunger-Baldauf, C., and Bauer, P. (2005). Testing and estimation in flexible group sequential designs with adaptive treatment selection. *Statistics in Medicine* **24,** 3697–3714.

Prakasa Rao, B. L. S. (1987). *Asymptotic theory of statistical inference.* John Wiley & Sons, Inc.

Privé, F., Arbel, J., and Vilhjálmsson, B. J. (2020). LDpred2: better, faster, stronger. *Bioinformatics* **36,** 5424–5431.

Privé, F., Aschard, H., Carmi, S., Folkersen, L., Hoggart, C., O'Reilly, P. F., and Vilhjálmsson, B. J. (2022). Portability of 245 polygenic scores when derived from the UK biobank and applied to 9 ancestry groups from the same cohort. *The American Journal of Human Genetics* **109,** 12–23.

Privé, F., Aschard, H., Ziyatdinov, A., and Blum, M. G. (2018). Efficient analysis of large-scale genome-wide data with two R packages: bigstatsr and bigsnpr. *Bioinformatics* **34,** 2781–2787.

Proschan, M. and Evans, S. (2020). The temptation of response-adaptive randomization. *Clinical Infectious Diseases* **31,** 3002–3004.

Proschan, M. A. and Hunsberger, S. A. (1995). Designed extension of studies based on conditional power. *Biometrics* **51,** 1315–1324.

Pugliese, P., Cuzin, L., and Enel, P. (2003). Nadis 2000: développement d'un dossier médical informatisé pour les patients infectés par VIH, VHB et VHC. *Presse Medicale* **32,** 299–303.

Pushpakom, S., Kolamunnage-Dona, R., Taylor, C., Foster, T., Spowart, C., García-Fiñana, M., Kemp, G. J., Jaki, T., Khoo, S., Williamson, P., Pirmohamed, M., and for the TAILoR Study Group (2020). TAILoR (TelmisArtan and InsuLin Resistance in Human Immunodeficiency Virus [HIV]): An Adaptive-design, dose-ranging phase IIb randomized trial of telmisartan for the teduction of insulin resistance in HIV-positive individuals on combination antiretroviral therapy. *Clinical Infectious Diseases* **6,** 2062–2072.

Pushpakom, S. P., Taylor, C., Kolamunnage-Dona, R., Spowart, C., Vora, J., García-Fiñana, M., Kemp, G. J., Whitehead, J., Jaki, T., Khoo, S., et al. (2015). Telmisartan and insulin resistance in HIV (TAILoR): protocol for a dose-ranging phase II randomised open-labelled trial of telmisartan as a strategy for the reduction of insulin resistance in HIV-positive individuals on combination antiretroviral therapy. *BMJ Open* **5,**.

Puterman, M. L. (2014). *Markov decision processes: discrete stochastic dynamic programming.* John Wiley & Sons.

Qi, Z., Liu, D., Fu, H., and Liu, Y. (2020). Multi-armed angle-based direct learning for estimating optimal individualized treatment rules with various outcomes. *Journal of the American Statistical Association* **115,** 678–691.

Qi, Z. and Liu, Y. (2018). D-learning to estimate optimal individual treatment rules. *Electronic Journal of Statistics* **12,** 3601–3638.

Qi, Z., Miao, R., and Zhang, X. (2021). Proximal learning for individualized treatment regimes under unmeasured confounding. *arXiv preprint arXiv:2105.01187.*

Qian, M. and Murphy, S. A. (2011). Performance guarantees for individualized treatment rules. *The Annals of Statistics* **39,** 1180.

Qian, T., Klasnja, P., and Murphy, S. A. (2020). Linear mixed models under endogeneity: modeling sequential treatment effects with application to a mobile health study. *Statistical Science* **35,** 375–390.

Qiu, H., Carone, M., Sadikova, E., Petukhova, M., Kessler, R. C., and Luedtke, A. (2021). Optimal individualized decision rules using instrumental variable methods. *Journal of the American Statistical Association* **116,** 174–191.

Qiu, H. and Luedtke, A. (2020). Leveraging vague prior information in general models via iteratively constructed gamma-minimax estimators. *arXiv preprint arXiv:2012.05465.*

Quinlan, J. A. and Krams, M. (2006). Implementing adaptive designs: Logistical and operational considerations. *Drug Information Journal* **40,** 437–444.

Rabbi, M., Aung, M. H., Zhang, M., and Choudhury, T. (2015). Mybehavior: automatic personalized health feedback from user behaviors and preferences using smartphones. In *Proceedings of the 2015 ACM International Joint Conference on Pervasive and Ubiquitous Computing*, pages 707–718.

Rabbi, M., Klasnja, P., Choudhury, T., Tewari, A., and Murphy, S. (2019). Optimizing mhealth interventions with a bandit. In Baumeister, H. and Montag, C., editors, *Mobile Sensing and Digital Phenotyping: New Developments in Psychoinformatics.* Springer.

Railsback, S. and Grimm, V. (2019). *Agent-based and individual-based modeling: a practical introduction.* Princeton University Press.

Ravanbakhsh, S., Schneider, J., and Poczos, B. (2016). Deep learning with sets and point clouds. *arXiv preprint arXiv:1611.04500.*

Ravanbakhsh, S., Schneider, J., and Poczos, B. (2017). Equivariance through parameter-sharing. In *Proceedings of the 34th International Conference on Machine Learning-Volume 70*, pages 2892–2901. JMLR. org.

Ravi, S. and Larochelle, H. (2017). Optimization as a model for few-shot learning. In *International Conference on Learning Representations (ICLR)*. https://openreview.net/forum?id=rJY0-Kcll.

Renfro, L. A. and Mandrekar, S. J. (2018). Definitions and statistical properties of master protocols for personalized medicine in oncology. *Journal of Biopharmaceutical Statistics* **28,** 217–228.

Restelli, U., Scolari, F., Bonfanti, P., Croce, D., and Rizzardini, G. (2015). New Highly Active Antiretroviral drugs and generic drugs for the treatment of HIV infection: a budget impact analysis on the Italian National Health Service (Lombardy Region, Northern Italy). *BMC Infect. Dis.* **15,** 323.

Richardson, A., Hudgens, M. G., Gilbert, P. B., and Fine, J. P. (2014). Nonparametric bounds and sensitivity analysis of treatment effects. *Statistical Science* **29,** 596.

Riley, W. T., Rivera, D. E., Atienza, A. A., Nilsen, W., Allison, S. M., and Mermelstein, R. (2011). Health behavior models in the age of mobile interventions: are our theories up to the task? *Translational Behavioral Medicine* **1,** 53–71.

Rimfeld, K., Malanchini, M., Spargo, T., Spickernell, G., Selzam, S., McMillan, A., Dale, P. S., Eley, T. C., and Plomin, R. (2019). Twins early development study: A genetically sensitive investigation into behavioral and cognitive development from infancy to emerging adulthood. *Twin Research and Human Genetics* **22,** 508–513.

Rindtorff, N. T., Lu, M., Patel, N. A., Zheng, H., and D'Amour, A. (2019). A biologically plausible benchmark for contextual bandit algorithms in precision oncology using in vitro data. *arXiv preprint arXiv:1911.04389.*

Riviere, M.-K., Dubois, F., and Zohar, S. (2015). Competing designs for drug combination in phase I dose-finding clinical trials. *Statistics in Medicine* **34,** 1–12.

Riviere, M.-K., Yuan, Y., Dubois, F., and Zohar, S. (2014). A Bayesian dose-finding design for drug combination clinical trials based on the logistic model. *Pharmaceutical Statistics* **13,** 247–257.

Riviere, M.-K., Yuan, Y., Jourdan, J.-H., Dubois, F., and Zohar, S. (2018). Phase I/II dose-finding design for molecularly targeted agent: plateau determination using adaptive randomization. *Statistical Methods in Medical Research* **27,** 466–479.

Robbins, H. (1956). A sequential decision problem with a finite memory. *Proceedings of the National Academy of Sciences* **42,** 920–923.

Robbins, H. et al. (1952). Some aspects of the sequential design of experiments. *Bulletin of the American Mathematical Society* **58,** 527–535.

Robert, C. and Casella, G. (2004). *Monte Carlo statistical methods.* Springer Texts in Statistics. Springer-Verlag, New York, second edition.

Robert, C. and Casella, G. (2010). *Introducing Monte Carlo methods with R.* Use R! Springer, New York.

Robertson, D. S., Choodari-Oskooei, B., Dimairo, M., Flight, L., Pallmann, P., and Jaki, T. (2023). Point estimation for adaptive trial designs I: A methodological review. Statistics in Medicine **42**, 122–145.

Robertson, D. S., Lee, K. M., Lopez-Kolkovska, B. C., and Villar, S. S. (2023). Response-adaptive randomization in clinical trials: from myths to practical considerations. *Statistical Science* **38**, 185–208.

Robertson, D. S. and Wason, J. (2019). Familywise error control in multi-armed response-adaptive trials. *Biometrics* **75,** 885–894.

Robins, J., Li, L., Tchetgen, E., and van der Vaart, A. (2008). Higher order influence functions and minimax estimation of nonlinear functionals. In *Probability and Statistics: Essays in Honor of David A. Freedman*, pages 335–421. Institute of Mathematical Statistics.

Robins, J., Orellana, L., and Rotnitzky, A. (2008). Estimation and extrapolation of optimal treatment and testing strategies. *Statistics in Medicine* **27,** 4678–4721.

Robins, J. and Rotnitzky, A. (1995). Semiparametric efficiency in multivariate regression models with missing data. *Journal of the American Statistical Association* **90,** 122–129.

Robins, J. M. (1986). A new approach to causal inference in mortality studies with a sustained exposure period - application to control of the healthy worker survivor effect. *Mathematical Modelling* **7,** 1393–1512.

Robins, J. M. (1989). The analysis of randomized and non-randomized AIDS treatment trials using a new approach to causal inference in longitudinal studies. *Health Service Research Methodology: A Focus on AIDS* pages 113–159.

Robins, J. M. (1994). Correcting for non-compliance in randomized trials using structural nested mean models. *Communications in Statistics – Theory and Methods* **23,** 2379–2412.

Robins, J. M. (1997). Causal inference from complex longitudinal data. In *Latent variable modeling and applications to causality*, pages 69–117. Springer.

Robins, J. M. (1999). Association, causation, and marginal structural models. *Synthese* **121,** 151–179.

Robins, J. M. (2004). Optimal structural nested models for optimal sequential decisions. In *Proceedings of the Second Seattle Symposium in Biostatistics*, pages 189–326. Springer.

Robins, J. M. and Hernán, M. A. (2009). Estimation of the causal effects of time-varying exposures. *Longitudinal Data Analysis* **553,** 599.

Robins, J. M., Li, L., Mukherjee, R., Tchetgen, E. T., and van der Vaart, A. (2017). Minimax estimation of a functional on a structured high-dimensional model. *The Annals of Statistics* pages 1951–1987.

Robins, J. M., Li, L., Tchetgen Tchetgen, E. J., and van der Vaart, A. W. (2009). Quadratic semiparametric von mises calculus. *Metrika* **69,** 227–247.

Robins, J. M. and Rotnitzky, A. (2001). Comments on: Inference for semiparametric models: Some questions and an answer. *Statistica Sinica* **11,** 920–936.

Robinson, M. R., Kleinman, A., Graff, M., Vinkhuyzen, A. A., Couper, D., Miller, M. B., Peyrot, W. J., Abdellaoui, A., Zietsch, B. P., Nolte, I. M., et al. (2017). Genetic evidence of assortative mating in humans. *Nature Human Behaviour* **1,** 1–13.

Robinson, P. M. (1988). Root-n-consistent semiparametric regression. *Econometrica: Journal of the Econometric Society* pages 931–954.

Rodriguez Duque, D., Stephens, D. A., Moodie, E. E. M., and Klein, M. B. (2023). Semiparametric Bayesian inference for dynamic treatment regimes via dynamic regime marginal structural models. *Biostatistics* **24,** 708–727.

Romano, J. P., Shaikh, A., and Wolf, M. (2011). Consonance and the closure method in multiple testing. *The International Journal of Biostatistics* **7.**

Rosenbaum, P. R. and Rubin, D. B. (1983). The central role of the propensity score in observational studies for causal effects. *Biometrika* **70,** 41–55.

Rosenberg, N. A., Edge, M. D., Pritchard, J. K., and Feldman, M. W. (2019). Interpreting polygenic scores, polygenic adaptation, and human phenotypic differences. *Evolution, Medicine, and Public Health* **2019,** 26–34.

Rosenberger, W. F. and Lachin, J. M. (2015). *Randomization in clinical trials: theory and practice.* John Wiley & Sons.

Rosenberger, W. F. and Sverdlov, O. (2008). Handling covariates in the design of clinical trials. *Statistical Science* **23,** 404–419.

Rothman, K. J., Greenland, S., and Lash, T. L. (2008). *Modern Epidemiology.* Philadelphia: Lippincott Williams & Wilkins.

Rothman, K. J., Greenland, S., and Walker, A. M. (1980). Concepts of interaction. *American Journal of Epidemiology* **112,** 467–470.

Rothwell, P. M. (1995). Can overall results of clinical trials be applied to all patients? *The Lancet* **345,** 1616–1619.

Rothwell, P. M. (2005). Subgroup analysis in randomised controlled trials: importance, indications, and interpretation. *The Lancet* **365,** 176–186.

Rotnitzky, A., Smucler, E., and Robins, J. M. (2019). Characterization of parameters with a mixed bias property. *arXiv preprint arXiv:1904.03725.*

Royston, P., Bratton, D., Choodari-Oskooei, B., and Barthel, F. M.-S. (2014). NSTAGE: Stata module for multi-arm, multi-stage (MAMS) trial designs for time-to-event outcomes. Statistical Software Components, Boston College Department of Economics.

Ruan, Y., Lin, Y.-F., Feng, Y.-C. A., Chen, C.-Y., Lam, M., Guo, Z., He, L., Sawa, A., Martin, A. R., Qin, S., et al. (2022). Improving polygenic prediction in ancestrally diverse populations. *Nature Genetics* **54,** 573–580.

Rubin, D. (1980). Discussion of "Randomization analysis of experimental data in the Fisher randomization test" by D. Basu. *Journal of the American Statistical Association* **75,** 591–593.

Rubin, D. B. (1974). Estimating causal effects of treatments in randomized and nonrandomized studies. *Journal of Educational Psychology* **66,** 688.

Rubin, D. B. (1978). Bayesian inference for causal effects: The role of randomization. *The Annals of Statistics* **6,** 34–58.

Rubin, D. B. (1981). The Bayesian bootstrap. *The Annals of Statistics* **9,** 130–134.

Rubin, D. B. and van der Laan, M. J. (2006). Extending marginal structural models through local, penalized, and additive learning. *UC Berkeley Division of Biostatistics Working Paper Series* **212,** 1–20.

Rusmevichientong, P. and Tsitsiklis, J. N. (2010). Linearly parameterized bandits. *Mathematics of Operations Research* **35,** 395–411.

Russo, D., Van Roy, B., Kazerouni, A., Osband, I., and Wen, Z. (2017). A tutorial on Thompson sampling. *arXiv:1707.02038 [cs]* arXiv: 1707.02038.

Ryan, E. G., Drovandi, C. C., McGree, J. M., and Pettitt, A. N. (2016). A review of modern computational algorithms for Bayesian optimal design. *International Statistical Review* **84,** 128–154.

Saarela, O., Arjas, E., Stephens, D. A., and Moodie, E. E. M. (2015). Predictive Bayesian inference and dynamic treatment regimes. *Biometrical Journal* **57,** 941–958.

Saarela, O., Belzile, L. R., and Stephens, D. A. (2016). A Bayesian view of doubly robust causal inference. *Biometrika* **103,** 667–681.

Saarela, O., Stephens, D. A., Moodie, E. E. M., and Klein, M. B. (2015). On Bayesian estimation of marginal structural models. *Biometrics* **71,** 279–288.

Sampson, A. R. and Sill, M. W. (2005). Drop-the-losers design: normal case. *Biometrical Journal* **47,** 257–268.

Sanchez-Kam, M., Gallo, P., Loewy, J., Menon, S., Antonijevic, Z., Christensen, J., Chuang-Stein, C., and Laage, T. (2014). A practical guide to data monitoring committees in adaptive trials. *Therapeutic Innovation & Regulatory Science* **48,** 316–326.

Sanderson, E., Glymour, M. M., Holmes, M. V., Kang, H., Morrison, J., Munafò, M. R., Palmer, T., Schooling, C. M., Wallace, C., Zhao, Q., et al. (2022). Mendelian randomization. *Nature Reviews Methods Primers* **2,** 1–21.

Sanjak, J. S., Long, A. D., and Thornton, K. R. (2017). A model of compound heterozygous, loss-of-function alleles is broadly consistent with observations from complex-disease GWAS datasets. *PLoS Genetics* **13,** e1006573.

Sant'Anna, P. H. and Zhao, J. (2020). Doubly robust difference-in-differences estimators. *Journal of Econometrics* **219,** 101–122.

Sarkar, J. (1991). One-armed bandit problems with covariates. *The Annals of Statistics* **19,** 1978–2002.

Savy, N., Saint-Pierre, P., Savy, S., Julien, S., and Pham, E. (2019). "in silico clinical trials": a way to improve drug development? In *Proceedings of JSM 2019 - Biopharmaceutical Session*.

Savy, N., Savy, S., Andrieu, S., and Marque, S. (2018). *Simulated Clinical Trials: Principle, Good Practices, and focus on Virtual Patients Generation*, chapter 22. Proceeding International Workshop in Simulation 2015. Springer-Verlag.

Schafer, C. M. and Stark, P. B. (2009). Constructing confidence regions of optimal expected size. *Journal of the American Statistical Association* **104,** 1080–1089.

Scharfstein, D. O., Rotnitzky, A., and Robins, J. M. (1999). Adjusting for nonignorable drop-out using semiparametric nonresponse models. *Journal of the American Statistical Association* **94,** 1096–1120.

Schick, A. (1986). On asymptotically efficient estimation in semiparametric models. *The Annals of Statistics* **14,** 1139–1151.

Schmidhuber, J. (1987). *Evolutionary principles in self-referential learning, or on learning how to learn: the meta-meta-... hook*. PhD thesis, Technische Universität München.

Schmidli, H., Bretz, F., Racine, A., and Maurer, W. (2006). Confirmatory seamless phase II/III clinical trials with hypotheses selection at interim: applications and practical considerations. *Biometrical Journal* **48,** 635–643.

Schneider, L. S., Tariot, P. N., Lyketsos, C. G., Dagerman, K. S., Davis, K. L., Davis, S., Hsiao, J. K., Jeste, D. V., Katz, I. R., Olin, J. T., et al. (2001). National institute of mental health clinical antipsychotic trials of intervention effectiveness (CATIE): Alzheimer disease trial methodology. *The American Journal of Geriatric Psychiatry* **9,** 346–360.

Schulte, P. J., Tsiatis, A. A., Laber, E. B., and Davidian, M. (2014). Q-and A-learning methods for estimating optimal dynamic treatment regimes. *Statistical Science: A Review Journal of the Institute of Mathematical Statistics* **29,** 640.

Schulz, J. and Moodie, E. E. M. (2020). Doubly robust estimation of optimal dosing strategies. *Journal of the American Statistical Association* **116(533),** 256–268.

Schumann, C., Lang, Z., Mattei, N., and Dickerson, J. P. (2019). Group fairness in bandit arm selection. *arXiv preprint arXiv:1912.03802*.

Schwarz, G. E. (1978). Estimating the dimension of a model. *The Annals of Statistics* **6,** 461–464.

Semenova, V. and Chernozhukov, V. (2017). Estimation and inference about conditional average treatment effect and other structural functions. *Econometrics Journal*, https://api.semanticscholar.org/CorpusID:221112509.

Sen, R., Shanmugam, K., Dimakis, A. G., and Shakkottai, S. (2017). Identifying best interventions through online importance sampling. In *International Conference on Machine Learning*, pages 3057–3066. PMLR.

Senn, S. (2021). *Statistical Issues in Drug Development.* Statistics in Practice. Wiley.

Shalit, U., Johansson, F. D., and Sontag, D. (2017). Estimating individual treatment effect: generalization bounds and algorithms. In *International Conference on Machine Learning*, pages 3076–3085. PMLR.

Shaw, P. A., Deffner, V., Keogh, R. H., Tooze, J. A., Dodd, K. W., Küchenhoff, H., Kipnis, V., and Freedman, L. S. (2018). Epidemiologic analyses with error-prone exposures: review of current practice and recommendations. *Annals of Epidemiology* **28(11),** 821–828.

Shaw, P. A., Gustafson, P., Carroll, R. J., Deffner, V., Dodd, K. W., Keogh, R. H., Kipnis, V., Tooze, J. A., Wallace, M. P., Küchenhoff, H., and Freedman, L. S. (2020). STRATOS guidance document on measurement error and misclassification of variables in observational epidemiology: Part 2 - sample size, more complex methods of adjustment and advanced topics. *Statistics in Medicine* **39(16),** 2232–2263.

Shen, C., Wang, Z., Villar, S., and van der Schaar, M. (2020). Learning for dose allocation in adaptive clinical trials with safety constraints. In *International Conference on Machine Learning*, pages 8730–8740. PMLR.

Sheppard, A. (2018). Generic medicines: essential contributors to the long-term health of society. Technical report, IMS health. [Cited 2018 April 18].

Shi, C., Fan, A., Song, R., and Lu, W. (2018). High-dimensional A-learning for optimal dynamic treatment regimes. *The Annals of Statistics* **46,** 925–957.

Shi, C., Song, R., and Lu, W. (2016). Robust learning for optimal treatment decision with NP-dimensionality. *Electronic Journal of Statistics* **10,** 2894–2921.

Shi, C., Song, R., and Lu, W. (2021). Concordance and value information criteria for optimal treatment decision. *The Annals of Statistics* **49,** 49–75.

Shi, J., Park, J.-H., Duan, J., Berndt, S. T., Moy, W., Yu, K., Song, L., Wheeler, W., Hua, X., Silverman, D., et al. (2016). Winner's curse correction and variable thresholding improve performance of polygenic risk modeling based on genome-wide association study summary-level data. *PLoS Genetics* **12,** e1006493.

Shortreed, S. M. and Ertefaie, A. (2017). Outcome-adaptive lasso: Variable selection for causal inference. *Biometrics* **73,** 1111–1122.

Shortreed, S. M. and Moodie, E. E. M. (2012). Estimating the optimal dynamic antipsychotic treatment regime: Evidence from the sequential multiple-assignment randomized clinical antipsychotic trials of intervention and effectiveness schizophrenia study. *Journal of the Royal Statistical Society: Series C (Applied Statistics)* **61,** 577–599.

Shrestha, S. and Jain, S. (2021). A Bayesian-bandit adaptive design for n-of-1 clinical trials. *Statistics in Medicine* **40,** 1825–1844.

Siegfried, R. (2014). *Modeling and Simulation of Complex Systems: A Framework for Efficient Agent-Based Modeling and Simulation.* Springer Fachmedien Wiesbaden, Wiesbaden.

Silvapulle, M. J. (2001). Tests against qualitative interaction: exact critical values and robust tests. *Biometrics* **57,** 1157–1165.

Simoneau, G., Moodie, E. E. M., Nijjar, J. S., and W., P. R. (2019). Estimating optimal dynamic treatment regimes with survival outcomes. *Journal of the American Statistical Association* **115(531),** 1531–1539.

Simoneau, G., Moodie, E. E. M., Wallace, M. P., and W., P. R. (2020). Optimal dynamic treatment regimes with survival endpoints: Introducing the DWSurv function in the R package DTRreg. *Journal of Statistical Computation and Simulation* **90(16),** 2991–3008.

Singh, A. and Joachims, T. (2018). Fairness of exposure in rankings. In *Proceedings of the 24th ACM SIGKDD International Conference on Knowledge Discovery & Data Mining*, pages 2219–2228.

Siva, N. (2008). 1000 genomes project. *Nature Biotechnology* **26,** 256–257.

Sklar, A. (1996). Random variables, distribution functions, and copulas: a personal look backward and forward. *Lecture Notes - Monograph Series* pages 1–14.

Slivkins, A. et al. (2019). Introduction to multi-armed bandits. *Foundations and Trends® in Machine Learning* **12,** 1–286.

Smith, C. T., Williamson, P. R., and Beresford, M. W. (2014). Methodology of clinical trials for rare diseases. *Best Practice & Research Clinical Rheumatology* **28,** 247–262.

Sohail, M., Maier, R. M., Ganna, A., Bloemendal, A., Martin, A. R., Turchin, M. C., Chiang, C. W., Hirschhorn, J., Daly, M. J., Patterson, N., et al. (2019). Polygenic adaptation on height is overestimated due to uncorrected stratification in genome-wide association studies. *Elife* **8,** e39702.

Song, J. W. and Chung, K. C. (2010). Observational studies: cohort and case-control studies. *Plastic and Reconstructive Surgery* **126,** 2234.

Song, R., Kosorok, M., Zeng, D., Zhao, Y., Laber, E., and Yuan, M. (2015a). On sparse representation for optimal individualized treatment selection with penalized outcome weighted learning. *Stat* **4,** 59–68.

Song, R., Wang, W., Zeng, D., and Kosorok, M. R. (2015b). Penalized Q-learning for dynamic treatment regimes. *Statistica Sinica* **25,** 901–920.

Song, S., Jiang, W., Hou, L., and Zhao, H. (2020). Leveraging effect size distributions to improve polygenic risk scores derived from summary statistics of genome-wide association studies. *PLoS Computational Biology* **16,** e1007565.

Speed, D. and Balding, D. J. (2019). Sumher better estimates the SNP heritability of complex traits from summary statistics. *Nature Genetics* **51,** 277–284.

Speed, D., Cai, N., Johnson, M. R., Nejentsev, S., and Balding, D. J. (2017). Reevaluation of SNP heritability in complex human traits. *Nature Genetics* **49,** 986–992.

Spicker, D. and Wallace, M. P. (2020). Measurement error and precision medicine: Error-prone tailoring covariates in dynamic treatment regimes. *Statistics in Medicine* **39(26),** 3732–3755.

Spiegelhalter, D. J., Abrams, K. R., and Myles, J. P. (2004). *Bayesian approaches to clinical trials and health-care evaluation.* John Wiley & Sons, Hoboken, NJ.

Splawa-Neyman, J., Dabrowska, D., and Speed, T. (1990). On the application of probability theory to agricultural experiments (English translation by D. M. Dabrowska and T. P. Speed). *Statistical Science* **5,** 465–472.

Stallard, N., Hampson, L., Benda, N., Brannath, W., Burnett, T., Friede, T., Kimani, P. K., Koenig, F., Krisam, J., Mozgunov, P., et al. (2020). Efficient adaptive designs for clinical trials of interventions for COVID-19. *Statistics in Biopharmaceutical Research* **12,** 483–497.

Stallard, N. and Todd, S. (2003). Sequential designs for phase III clinical trials incorporating treatment selection. *Statistics in Medicine* **22,** 689–703.

Stallard, N., Todd, S., Parashar, D., Kimani, P. K., and Renfro, L. A. (2019). On the need to adjust for multiplicity in confirmatory clinical trials with master protocols. *Annals of Oncology* **30,** 506.

Statistica (2018). Penetration rate of generics in units by market size in France 2008-2014. Technical report, Statistica. [Cited 2018 April 18].

Steihaug, T. (1983). The conjugate gradient method and trust regions in large scale optimization. *SIAM Journal on Numerical Analysis* **20,** 626–637.

Stein, C. (1956). Efficient nonparametric testing and estimation. *Proceedings of the Third Berkeley Symposium on Mathematical Statistics and Probability* **1,** 187–195.

Stephens, D. A., Nobre, W. S., Moodie, E. E. M., and Schmidt, A. M. (2023). Causal inference under mis-specification: adjustment based on the propensity score. *Bayesian Analysis* **18(2)**, 639–694.

Stöber, J., Hong, H., Czado, C., and Ghosh, P. (2015). Comorbidity of chronic diseases in the elderly: Patterns identified by a copula design for mixed responses. *Computational Statistics & Data Analysis* **88,** 28–39.

Sun, J., Wang, Y., Folkersen, L., Borné, Y., Amlien, I., Buil, A., Orho-Melander, M., Borglum, A. D., Hougaard, D. M., Melander, O., et al. (2021). Translating polygenic risk scores for clinical use by estimating the confidence bounds of risk prediction. *Nature Communications* **12,** 1–9.

Sun, W., Dey, D., and Kapoor, A. (2017). Safety-aware algorithms for adversarial contextual bandit. In *International Conference on Machine Learning*, pages 3280–3288. PMLR.

Supervie, V. and Ekouevi, D. (2014). Overview of the HIV epidemics in France and worldwide. *La Revue du praticien* **64,** 1060–1066.

Sutton, R. S. (1997). On the significance of Markov decision processes. In *Artificial Neural Networks—ICANN'97: 7th International Conference Lausanne, Switzerland, October 8–10, 1997 Proceeedings 7*, pages 273–282. Springer.

Sutton, R. S. and Barto, A. G. (1998). *Reinforcement learning: An introduction*, volume 1. MIT Press Cambridge.

Sutton, R. S. and Barto, A. G. (2018). *Reinforcement learning: An introduction.* MIT Press.

Sverdlov, O. (2015). *Modern adaptive randomized clinical trials: statistical and practical aspects*, volume 81. CRC Press.

Sverdlov, O. and Rosenberger, W. F. (2013). On recent advances in optimal allocation designs in clinical trials. *Journal of Statistical Theory and Practice* **7,** 753–773.

Sydes, M. R., Parmar, M. K., James, N. D., Clarke, N. W., Dearnaley, D. P., Mason, M. D., Morgan, R. C., Sanders, K., and Royston, P. (2009). Issues in applying multi-arm multi-stage methodology to a clinical trial in prostate cancer: the MRC STAMPEDE trial. *Trials* **10,** 39.

Taliun, D., Harris, D. N., Kessler, M. D., Carlson, J., Szpiech, Z. A., Torres, R., Taliun, S. A. G., Corvelo, A., Gogarten, S. M., Kang, H. M., et al. (2021). Sequencing of 53,831 diverse genomes from the NHLBI TOPMed program. *Nature* **590,** 290–299.

Tamhane, A. C., Hochberg, Y., and Dunnett, C. W. (1996). Multiple test procedures for dose finding. *Biometrics* **52,** 21–37.

Tamura, R. N., Krischer, J. P., Pagnoux, C., Micheletti, R., Grayson, P. C., Chen, Y.-F., and Merkel, P. A. (2016). A small n sequential multiple assignment randomized trial design for use in rare disease research. *Contemporary Clinical Trials* **46,** 48–51.

Tannenbaum, S., Holford, N., Lee, H., Peck, C., and Mould, D. (2006). Simulation of correlated continuous and categorical variables using a single multivariate distribution. *Journal of Pharmacokinetics and Pharmacodynamics* **33,** 773–794.

Taylor, J. and Tibshirani, R. (2018). Post-selection inference for ℓ_1-penalized likelihood models. *Canadian Journal of Statistics* **46,** 41–61.

Tchetgen Tchetgen, E. J. and Shpitser, I. (2012). Semiparametric theory for causal mediation analysis: efficiency bounds, multiple robustness, and sensitivity analysis. *The Annals of Statistics* **40,** 1816.

Tchetgen Tchetgen, E. J. and VanderWeele, T. J. (2012). On causal inference in the presence of interference. *Statistical Methods in Medical Research* **21,** 55–75.

Tchetgen Tchetgen, E. J., Ying, A., Cui, Y., Shi, X., and Miao, W. (2020). An introduction to proximal causal learning. *arXiv preprint arXiv:2009.10982.*

Tehranisa, J. S. and Meurer, W. J. (2014). Can response-adaptive randomization increase participation in acute stroke trials? *Stroke* **45,** 2131–2133.

Tesfatsion, L. and Judd, K. (2006). *Handbook of computational economics: agent-based computational economics.* Elsevier.

Tewari, A. and Murphy, S. A. (2017a). Contextual bandits in mobile health. In Rehg, J. M., Murphy, S. A., and Kumar, S., editors, *Mobile Health Sensors, Analytic Methods, and Applications*, pages 495–518. Springer.

Tewari, A. and Murphy, S. A. (2017b). From ads to interventions: Contextual bandits in mobile health. In Rehg, J., Murphy, S. A., and Kumar, S., editors, *Mobile Health: Sensors, Analytic Methods, and Applications.* Springer.

Thall, P. F. (2020). *Statistical Remedies for Medical Researchers.* Springer Nature.

Thall, P. F. (2021). Adaptive enrichment designs in clinical trials. *Annual Review of Statistics and Its Application* **8,** 393–411.

Thall, P. F., Millikan, R. E., and Sung, H.-G. (2000). Evaluating multiple treatment courses in clinical trials. *Statistics in Medicine* **19,** 1011–1028.

Thall, P. F. and Nguyen, H. Q. (2012). Adaptive randomization to improve utility-based dose-finding with bivariate ordinal outcomes. *Journal of Biopharmaceutical Statistics* **22,** 785–801.

Thall, P. F., Nguyen, H. Q., and Estey, E. H. (2008). Patient-specific dose finding based on bivariate outcomes and covariates. *Biometrics* **64,** 1126–1136.

Thall, P. F., Simon, R., and Ellenberg, S. S. (1988). Two-stage selection and testing designs for comparative clinical trials. *Biometrika* **75,** 303–310.

Thall, P. F., Simon, R., and Ellenberg, S. S. (1989). A two-stage design for choosing among several experimental treatments and a control in clinical trials. *Biometrics* **45,** 537–547.

Thall, P. F. and Wathen, J. K. (2005). Covariate-adjusted adaptive randomization in a sarcoma trial with multi-stage treatments. *Statistics in Medicine* **24,** 1947–1964.

Thall, P. F. and Wathen, J. K. (2007). Practical Bayesian adaptive randomisation in clinical trials. *European Journal of Cancer* **43,** 859–866.

Thall, P. F., Wathen, J. K., Bekele, B. N., Champlin, R. E., Baker, L. H., and Benjamin, R. S. (2003). Hierarchical Bayesian approaches to phase II trials in diseases with multiple subtypes. *Statistics in Medicine* **22,** 763–780.

Thiébaut, A. C. M., Freedman, L. S., Carroll, R. J., and Kpinis, V. (2007). Is it necessary to correct for measurement error in nutritional epidemiology? *Annals of Internal Medicine* **146,** 65.

Thiele, J. C. (2017). *RNetLogo: An Interface to the Agent-Based Modelling Platform 'NetLogo'.* R package version 1.0.4.

Thomas, M., Sakoda, L. C., Hoffmeister, M., Rosenthal, E. A., Lee, J. K., van Duijnhoven, F. J., Platz, E. A., Wu, A. H., Dampier, C. H., de la Chapelle, A., et al. (2020). Genome-wide modeling of polygenic risk score in colorectal cancer risk. *The American Journal of Human Genetics* **107,** 432–444.

Thombs, B. D., De Jonge, P., Coyne, J. C., Whooley, M. A., Frasure-Smith, N., Mitchell, A. J., Zuidersma, M., Eze-Nliam, C., Lima, B. B., Smith, C. G., et al. (2008). Depression screening and patient outcomes in cardiovascular care: a systematic review. *Journal of the American Medical Association* **300,** 2161–2171.

Thompson, W. R. (1933). On the likelihood that one unknown probability exceeds another in view of the evidence of two samples. *Biometrika* **25,** 285–294.

Thrun, S. and Pratt, L. (1998). Learning to learn: Introduction and overview. In *Learning to learn*, pages 3–17. Springer.

Tian, L., Alizadeh, A. A., Gentles, A. J., and Tibshirani, R. (2014). A simple method for estimating interactions between a treatment and a large number of covariates. *Journal of the American Statistical Association* **109,** 1517–1532.

Tian, X. and Taylor, J. (2017). Asymptotics of selective inference. *Scandinavian Journal of Statistics* **44,** 480–499.

Tibshirani, J., Athey, S., Sverdrup, E., and Wager, S. (2022). *grf: Generalized Random Forests.* R package version 2.1.0.

Tibshirani, R. (1996). Regression shrinkage and selection via the lasso. *Journal of the Royal Statistical Society: Series B (Statistical Methodology)* **58,** 267–288.

Tibshirani, R. J., Rinaldo, A., Tibshirani, R., and Wasserman, L. (2018). Uniform asymptotic inference and the bootstrap after model selection. *The Annals of Statistics* **46,** 1255–1287. Publisher: Institute of Mathematical Statistics.

Tighiouart, M. and Rogatko, A. (2010). Dose finding with escalation with overdose control (ewoc) in cancer clinical trials. *Statistical Science* **25,** 217–226.

Tokic, M. (2010). Adaptive ε-greedy exploration in reinforcement learning based on value differences. In *Annual Conference on Artificial Intelligence*, pages 203–210. Springer.

Tomkins, S., Liao, P., Klasnja, P., and Murphy, S. (2021). IntelligentPooling: Practical Thompson sampling for mHealth. *Machine Learning* **110,** 2685–2727.

Torkamani, A., Wineinger, N. E., and Topol, E. J. (2018). The personal and clinical utility of polygenic risk scores. *Nature Reviews Genetics* **19,** 581–590.

Tran-Thanh, L., Chapman, A., De Cote, E. M., Rogers, A., and Jennings, N. R. (2010). Epsilon–first policies for budget–limited multi-armed bandits. In *Proceedings of the AAAI Conference on Artificial Intelligence*, volume 24.

Tran-Thanh, L., Chapman, A., Rogers, A., and Jennings, N. (2012). Knapsack based optimal policies for budget–limited multi–armed bandits. In *Proceedings of the AAAI Conference on Artificial Intelligence*, volume 26.

Trapero-Bertran, M. and Oliva-Moreno, J. (2014). Economic impact of HIV/AIDS: a systematic review in five European countries. *Health Econ Rev* **4,** 15.

Trippa, L., Lee, E. Q., Wen, P. Y., Batchelor, T. T., Cloughesy, T., Parmigiani, G., and Alexander, B. M. (2012). Bayesian adaptive randomized trial design for patients with recurrent glioblastoma. *Journal of Clinical Oncology* **30,** 3258.

Tsiatis, A. A. (2006). *Semiparametric Theory and Missing Data.* New York: Springer.

Tsiatis, A. A., Davidian, M., Holloway, S. T., and Laber, E. B. (2019). *Dynamic treatment regimes: Statistical methods for precision medicine.* CRC press.

Tsuo, K., Zhou, W., Wang, Y., Kanai, M., Namba, S., Gupta, R., Majara, L., Nkambule, L. L., Okada, Y., Morisaki, T., et al. (2022). Multi-ancestry meta-analysis of asthma identifies novel associations and highlights the value of increased power and diversity. *Cell Genomics* **8,** 100212.

Tsybakov, A. B. (2009). *Introduction to Nonparametric Estimation.* New York: Springer.

Urach, S. and Posch, M. (2016). Multi-arm group sequential designs with a simultaneous stopping rule. *Statistics in Medicine* **35,** 5536–5550.

Uricchio, L. H. (2020). Evolutionary perspectives on polygenic selection, missing heritability, and GWAS. *Human Genetics* **139,** 5–21.

US Department of Health and Human Services Food and Drug Administration (2019). Adaptive design clinical trials for drugs and biologics guidance for industry.

Vaish, R., Wyngarden, K., Chen, J., Cheung, B., and Bernstein, M. S. (2014). Twitch crowdsourcing: crowd contributions in short bursts of time. In *Proceedings of the SIGCHI conference on human factors in computing systems*, pages 3645–3654.

van der Laan, M. J. (2013). Targeted learning of an optimal dynamic treatment, and statistical inference for its mean outcome. *UC Berkeley Division of Biostatistics Working Paper Series* **317,** 1–90.

van der Laan, M. J. (2014). Causal inference for a population of causally connected units. *Journal of Causal Inference* **2,** 13–74.

van der Laan, M. J. and Dudoit, S. (2003). Unified cross-validation methodology for selection among estimators and a general cross-validated adaptive epsilon-net estimator: Finite sample oracle inequalities and examples. Technical report, UC Berkeley Division of Biostatistics, Berkeley CA.

van der Laan, M. J. and Luedtke, A. R. (2015). Targeted learning of the mean outcome under an optimal dynamic treatment rule. *Journal of Causal Inference* **3,** 61–95.

van der Laan, M. J. and Petersen, M. L. (2007). Causal effect models for realistic individualized treatment and intention to treat rules. *The International Journal of Biostatistics* **3,** 1–55.

van der Laan, M. J., Polley, E. C., and Hubbard, A. E. (2007). Super learner. *Statistical Applications in Genetics and Molecular Biology* **6,**.

van der Laan, M. J. and Robins, J. M. (2003). *Unified Methods for Censored Longitudinal Data and Causality.* Springer Science & Business Media.

van der Laan, M. J. and Rose, S. (2011). *Targeted Learning: Causal Inference for Observational and Experimental Data.* Springer Science & Business Media.

van der Laan, M. J. and Rubin, D. (2006). Targeted maximum likelihood learning. *The International Journal of Biostatistics* **2,** 1–40.

van der Vaart, A. W. (2000). *Asymptotic statistics*, volume 3. Cambridge University Press.

van der Vaart, A. W. (2002). Semiparametric statistics. *In: Lectures on Probability Theory and Statistics* pages 331–457.

van der Vaart, A. W., Dudoit, S., and van der Laan, M. J. (2006). Oracle inequalities for multi-fold cross validation. *Statistics & Decisions* **24,** 351–371.

van der Vaart, A. W. and Wellner, J. A. (1996). *Weak Convergence and Empirical Processes.* Springer.

van der Wijst, M. G., de Vries, D. H., Groot, H. E., Trynka, G., Hon, C.-C., Bonder, M.-J., Stegle, O., Nawijn, M., Idaghdour, Y., van der Harst, P., et al. (2020). Science forum: The single-cell eQTLGen consortium. *Elife* **9,** e52155.

VanderWeele, T. (2015). *Explanation in causal inference: methods for mediation and interaction.* Oxford University Press.

VanderWeele, T. J. (2009). On the distinction between interaction and effect modification. *Epidemiology* **20,** 863–871.

VanderWeele, T. J. and Knol, M. J. (2011). Interpretation of subgroup analyses in randomized trials: heterogeneity versus secondary interventions. *Annals of Internal Medicine* **154,** 680–683.

VanderWeele, T. J. and Knol, M. J. (2014). A tutorial on interaction. *Epidemiologic Methods* **3,** 33–72.

VanderWeele, T. J. and Robins, J. M. (2007). The identification of synergism in the sufficient-component-cause framework. *Epidemiology* **18,** 329–339.

Vassos, E., Di Forti, M., Coleman, J., Iyegbe, C., Prata, D., Euesden, J., O'Reilly, P., Curtis, C., Kolliakou, A., Patel, H., et al. (2017). An examination of polygenic score risk prediction in individuals with first-episode psychosis. *Biological Psychiatry* **81,** 470–477.

Ventz, S., Barry, W. T., Parmigiani, G., and Trippa, L. (2017). Bayesian response-adaptive designs for basket trials. *Biometrics* **73,** 905–915.

Vickerstaff, V., Omar, R. Z., and Ambler, G. (2019). Methods to adjust for multiple comparisons in the analysis and sample size calculation of randomised controlled trials with multiple primary outcomes. *BMC Medical Research Methodology* **19,** 1–13.

Viele, K., Broglio, K., McGlothlin, A., and Saville, B. R. (2020). Comparison of methods for control allocation in multiple arm studies using response adaptive randomization. *Clinical Trials* **17,** 52–60.

Vilalta, R. and Drissi, Y. (2002). A perspective view and survey of meta-learning. *Artificial Intelligence Review* **18,** 77–95.

Vilhjálmsson, B. J., Yang, J., Finucane, H. K., Gusev, A., Lindström, S., Ripke, S., Genovese, G., Loh, P.-R., Bhatia, G., Do, R., et al. (2015). Modeling linkage disequilibrium increases accuracy of polygenic risk scores. *The American Journal of Human Genetics* **97,** 576–592.

Villar, S. S., Bowden, J., and Wason, J. (2015). Multi-armed bandit models for the optimal design of clinical trials: benefits and challenges. *Statistical Science* **30,** 199.

Villar, S. S., Bowden, J., and Wason, J. (2018). Response-adaptive designs for binary responses: How to offer patient benefit while being robust to time trends? *Pharmaceutical Statistics* **17,** 182–197.

Vinyals, O., Blundell, C., Lillicrap, T., and Wierstra, D. (2016). Matching networks for one shot learning. In *Advances in Neural Information Processing Systems*, pages 3630–3638.

Visscher, P. M., Wray, N. R., Zhang, Q., Sklar, P., McCarthy, M. I., Brown, M. A., and Yang, J. (2017). 10 years of GWAS discovery: biology, function, and translation. *The American Journal of Human Genetics* **101,** 5–22.

von Mises, R. (1947). On the asymptotic distribution of differentiable statistical functions. *The Annals of Mathematical Statistics* **18,** 309–348.

Wager, S. and Xu, K. (2021). Diffusion asymptotics for sequential experiments. *arXiv preprint arXiv:2101.09855*.

Wald, A. (1947). *Sequential analysis*. John Wiley.

Wallace, M. P. and Moodie, E. E. M. (2015). Doubly-robust dynamic treatment regimen estimation via weighted least squares. *Biometrics* **71,** 636–644.

Wallace, M. P., Moodie, E. E. M., and A., S. D. (2017). Dynamic treatment regimen estimation via regression-based techniques: Introducing R package DTRreg. *Journal of Statistical Software* **80(2),** 1–20.

Wang, C.-C., Kulkarni, S. R., and Poor, H. V. (2005). Arbitrary side observations in bandit problems. *Advances in Applied Mathematics* **34,** 903–938.

Wang, L., Bai, Y., Sun, W., and Joachims, T. (2021). Fairness of exposure in stochastic bandits. *arXiv preprint arXiv:2103.02735*.

Wang, L., Laber, E. B., and Witkiewitz, K. (2017). Sufficient Markov decision processes with alternating deep neural networks. *arXiv preprint arXiv:1704.07531*.

Wang, L., Rotnitzky, A., Lin, X., Millikan, R. E., and Thall, P. F. (2012). Evaluation of viable dynamic treatment regimes in a sequentially randomized trial of advanced prostate cancer. *Journal of the American Statistical Association* **107,** 493–508.

Wang, L. and Tchetgen Tchetgen, E. (2018). Bounded, efficient and multiply robust estimation of average treatment effects using instrumental variables. *Journal of the Royal Statistical Society: Series B (Statistical Methodology)* **80,** 531–550.

Wang, L., Zhang, W., He, X., and Zha, H. (2018). Supervised reinforcement learning with recurrent neural network for dynamic treatment recommendation. In *Proceedings of the 24th ACM SIGKDD International Conference on Knowledge Discovery & Data Mining*, pages 2447–2456.

Wang, R., Lagakos, S. W., Ware, J. H., Hunter, D. J., and Drazen, J. M. (2007). Statistics in medicine—reporting of subgroup analyses in clinical trials. *New England Journal of Medicine* **357,** 2189–2194.

Wang, Y.-X., Agarwal, A., and Dudık, M. (2017). Optimal and adaptive off-policy evaluation in contextual bandits. In *International Conference on Machine Learning*, pages 3589–3597. PMLR.

Wason, J., Stallard, N., Bowden, J., and Jennison, C. (2017). A multi-stage drop-the-losers design for multi-arm clinical trials. *Statistical Methods in Medical Research* **26,** 508–524.

Wason, J. M., Brocklehurst, P., and Yap, C. (2019). When to keep it simple–adaptive designs are not always useful. *BMC Medicine* **17,** 1–7.

Wason, J. M. and Robertson, D. S. (2021). Controlling type i error rates in multi-arm clinical trials: a case for the false discovery rate. *Pharmaceutical Statistics* **20,** 109–116.

Wason, J. M. and Trippa, L. (2014). A comparison of Bayesian adaptive randomization and multi-stage designs for multi-arm clinical trials. *Statistics in Medicine* **33,** 2206–2221.

Wassmer, G. and Pahlke, F. (2019). *rpact: Confirmatory Adaptive Clinical Trial Design and Analysis*. R package version 2.0.6.

Watkins, C. J. C. H. (1989). *Learning from Delayed Rewards*. PhD thesis, King's College, Cambridge, UK.

Wei, B., Braun, T. M., Tamura, R. N., and Kidwell, K. (2020). Sample size determination for Bayesian analysis of small n sequential, multiple assignment, randomized trials (snSMARTs) with three agents. *Journal of Biopharmaceutical Statistics* **30,** 1109–1120.

Wei, B., Braun, T. M., Tamura, R. N., and Kidwell, K. M. (2018). A Bayesian analysis of small n sequential multiple assignment randomized trials (snSMARTs). *Statistics in Medicine* **37,** 3723–3732.

Wei, C.-Y. and Luo, H. (2021). Non-stationary reinforcement learning without prior knowledge: An optimal black-box approach. *arXiv preprint arXiv:2102.05406.*

Weiner, D. J., Nadig, A., Jagadeesh, K. A., Dey, K. K., Neale, B. M., Robinson, E. B., Karczewski, K. J., and O'Connor, L. J. (2022). Polygenic architecture of rare coding variation across 400,000 exomes. *medRxiv.*

Weissbrod, O., Hormozdiari, F., Benner, C., Cui, R., Ulirsch, J., Gazal, S., Schoech, A. P., van de Geijn, B., Reshef, Y., Márquez-Luna, C., et al. (2020). Functionally informed fine-mapping and polygenic localization of complex trait heritability. *Nature Genetics* **52,** 1355–1363.

Weissbrod, O., Kanai, M., Shi, H., Gazal, S., Peyrot, W., Khera, A., Okada, Y., Martin, A., Finucane, H., Price, A. L., et al. (2021). Leveraging fine-mapping and non-european training data to improve trans-ethnic polygenic risk scores. *medRxiv.*

Wen, X. and Stephens, M. (2010). Using linear predictors to impute allele frequencies from summary or pooled genotype data. *The Annals of Applied Statistics* **4,** 1158.

Westling, T. and Carone, M. (2020). A unified study of nonparametric inference for monotone functions. *The Annals of Statistics* **48,** 1001.

Wheeler, G. M., Mander, A. P., Bedding, A., Brock, K., Cornelius, V., Grieve, A. P., Jaki, T., Love, S. B., Weir, C. J., Yap, C., et al. (2019). How to design a dose-finding study using the continual reassessment method. *BMC Medical Research Methodology* **19,** 1–15.

Wheeler, G. M., Sweeting, M. J., and Mander, A. P. (2017). Toxicity-dependent feasibility bounds for the escalation with overdose control approach in phase I cancer trials. *Statistics in Medicine* **36,** 2499–2513.

Whitehead, J., Zhou, Y., Stevens, J., Blakey, G., Price, J., and Leadbetter, J. (2006). Bayesian decision procedures for dose-escalation based on evidence of undesirable events and therapeutic benefit. *Statistics in Medicine* **25,** 37–53.

Wilkins, M. R., Mckie, M. A., Law, M., Roussakis, A. A., Harbaum, L., Church, C., Coghlan, J. G., Condliffe, R., Howard, L. S., Kiely, D. G., et al. (2021). Positioning imatinib for pulmonary arterial hypertension: A phase I/II design comprising dose finding and single-arm efficacy. *Pulmonary Circulation* **11,** 20458940211052823.

Williamson, T., Eliasziw, M., and Fick, G. H. (2013). Log-binomial models: exploring failed convergence. *Emerging Themes in Epidemiology* **10,** 1–10.

Wing, C., Simon, K., and Bello-Gomez, R. A. (2018). Designing difference in difference studies: best practices for public health policy research. *Annual Review of Public Health* **39,** 453–469.

Witte, J. S., Visscher, P. M., and Wray, N. R. (2014). The contribution of genetic variants to disease depends on the ruler. *Nature Reviews Genetics* **15,** 765–776.

Wojcik, G. L., Graff, M., Nishimura, K. K., Tao, R., Haessler, J., Gignoux, C. R., Highland, H. M., Patel, Y. M., Sorokin, E. P., Avery, C. L., et al. (2019). Genetic analyses of diverse populations improves discovery for complex traits. *Nature* **570,** 514–518.

Woodcock, J. and LaVange, L. M. (2017). Master protocols to study multiple therapies, multiple diseases, or both. *New England Journal of Medicine* **377,** 62–70.

Woodroofe, M. (1979). A one-armed bandit problem with a concomitant variable. *Journal of the American Statistical Association* **74,** 799–806.

Wu, H., Srikant, R., Liu, X., and Jiang, C. (2015). Algorithms with logarithmic or sublinear regret for constrained contextual bandits. *arXiv preprint arXiv:1504.06937.*

Wu, J. et al. (2021). Ranking tailoring variables for constructing individualized treatment rules: an application to schizophrenia. *Journal of the Royal Statistical Society, Series C* **23,** 96–97.

Wu, K.-H. H., Douville, N. J., Konerman, M. C., Mathis, M. R., Scott, H. L., Wolford, B. N., Surakka, I., Sarah, G. E., Hyeon, J., Hirbo, J., et al. (2021). Polygenic risk score from a multi-ancestry GWAS uncovers susceptibility of heart failure. *medRxiv.*

Wu, P., Zeng, D., Fu, H., and Wang, Y. (2020). On using electronic health records to improve optimal treatment rules in randomized trials. *Biometrics* **76,** 1075–1086.

Wu, Y., Shariff, R., Lattimore, T., and Szepesvári, C. (2016). Conservative bandits. In *International Conference on Machine Learning*, pages 1254–1262. PMLR.

Xia, Y., Li, H., Qin, T., Yu, N., and Liu, T.-Y. (2015). Thompson sampling for budgeted multi-armed bandits. In *Proceedings of the 24th International Conference on Artificial Intelligence*, pages 3960–3966.

Xiaohong Chen and White, H. (1999). Improved rates and asymptotic normality for nonparametric neural network estimators. *IEEE Transactions on Information Theory* **45,** 682–691. Conference Name: IEEE Transactions on Information Theory.

Xu, Y. (2017). Generalized synthetic control method: Causal inference with interactive fixed effects models. *Political Analysis* **25,** 57–76.

Xub, X. and Bretz, F. (2017). The MCP-Mod methodology: Practical considerations and the dosefinding R package. In O'Quigley, J., Iasonos, A., and Bornkamp, B., editors, *Handbook of Methods for Designing, Monitoring, and Analyzing Dose-Finding Trials*, chapter 12, pages 205–227. CRC Press, Taylor and Francis Group.

Yan, F., Thall, P., Lu, K., Gilbert, M., and Yuan, Y. (2018). Phase I-II clinical trial design: a state-of-the-art paradigm for dose finding. *Annals of Oncology* **29,** 694–699.

Yang, J., Benyamin, B., McEvoy, B. P., Gordon, S., Henders, A. K., Nyholt, D. R., Madden, P. A., Heath, A. C., Martin, N. G., Montgomery, G. W., et al. (2010). Common SNPs explain a large proportion of the heritability for human height. *Nature Genetics* **42,** 565–569.

Yang, J., Ferreira, T., Morris, A. P., Medland, S. E., Madden, P. A., Heath, A. C., Martin, N. G., Montgomery, G. W., Weedon, M. N., Loos, R. J., et al. (2012). Conditional and joint multiple-SNP analysis of GWAS summary statistics identifies additional variants influencing complex traits. *Nature Genetics* **44,** 369–375.

Yang, J., Zeng, J., Goddard, M. E., Wray, N. R., and Visscher, P. M. (2017). Concepts, estimation and interpretation of SNP-based heritability. *Nature Genetics* **49,** 1304–1310.

Yang, S. and Zhou, X. (2020). Accurate and scalable construction of polygenic scores in large biobank data sets. *The American Journal of Human Genetics* **106,** 679–693.

Yang, Y., Zhu, D., et al. (2002). Randomized allocation with nonparametric estimation for a multi-armed bandit problem with covariates. *The Annals of Statistics* **30,** 100–121.

Yao, J., Brunskill, E., Pan, W., Murphy, S., and Doshi-Velez, F. (2020). Power-constrained bandits. *arXiv preprint arXiv:2004.06230.*

Yi, G. (2017). *Statistical Analysis with Measurement Error or Misclassification.* Springer; New York, NY.

Yin, G. (2012). *Clinical trial design: Bayesian and frequentist adaptive methods*, volume 876. John Wiley & Sons.

Yin, G., Li, Y., and Ji, Y. (2006). Bayesian dose-finding in phase I/II clinical trials using toxicity and efficacy odds ratios. *Biometrics* **62,** 777–787.

Yom-Tov, E., Feraru, G., Kozdoba, M., Mannor, S., Tennenholtz, M., and Hochberg, I. (2017). Encouraging physical activity in patients with diabetes: intervention using a reinforcement learning system. *Journal of Medical Internet Research* **19,** e338.

Young, J. G., Hernán, M. A., and Robins, J. M. (2014). Identification, estimation and approximation of risk under interventions that depend on the natural value of treatment using observational data. *Epidemiologic Methods* **3,** 1–19.

Yu, Z., Jin, J., Tin, A., Köttgen, A., Yu, B., Chen, J., Surapaneni, A., Zhou, L., Ballantyne, C. M., Hoogeveen, R. C., et al. (2021). Polygenic risk scores for kidney function and their associations with circulating proteome, and incident kidney diseases. *Journal of the American Society of Nephrology* **32,** 3161–3173.

Yuan, M. and Lin, Y. (2006). Model selection and estimation in regression with grouped variables. *Journal of The Royal Statistical Society, Series B (Statistical Methodology)* **68,** 49–67.

Yuan, Y., Hess, K. R., Hilsenbeck, S. G., and Gilbert, M. R. (2016). Bayesian optimal interval design: a simple and well-performing design for phase I oncology trials. *Clinical Cancer Research* **22,** 4291–4301.

Yusuf, S., Wittes, J., Probstfield, J., and Tyroler, H. A. (1991). Analysis and interpretation of treatment effects in subgroups of patients in randomized clinical trials. *Journal of the American Medical Association* **266,** 93–98.

Zagoraiou, M. (2017). Choosing a covariate-adaptive randomization procedure in practice. *Journal of Biopharmaceutical Statistics* **27,** 845–857.

Zaheer, M., Kottur, S., Ravanbakhsh, S., Poczos, B., Salakhutdinov, R. R., and Smola, A. J. (2017). Deep sets. In *Advances in Neural Information Processing Systems*, pages 3391–3401.

Zeger, S. L., Thomas, D., Dominici, F., Samet, J. M., Schwartz, J., Dockery, D., and Cohen, A. (2000). Exposure measurement error in time-series studies of air pollution: concepts and consequences. *Environmental Health Perspectives* **108(5),** 419–426.

Zeng, P., Hao, X., and Zhou, X. (2018). Pleiotropic mapping and annotation selection in genome-wide association studies with penalized gaussian mixture models. *Bioinformatics* **34,** 2797–2807.

Zhan, R., Hadad, V., Hirshberg, D. A., and Athey, S. (2021). Off-policy evaluation via adaptive weighting with data from contextual bandits. In *Proceedings of the 27th ACM SIGKDD Conference on Knowledge Discovery & Data Mining*, pages 2125–2135.

Zhang, B., Tsiatis, A. A., Davidian, M., Zhang, M., and Laber, E. (2012). Estimating optimal treatment regimes from a classification perspective. *Stat* **1,** 103–114.

Zhang, B., Tsiatis, A. A., Laber, E. B., and Davidian, M. (2012). A robust method for estimating optimal treatment regimes. *Biometrics* **68,** 1010–1018.

Zhang, B., Tsiatis, A. A., Laber, E. B., and Davidian, M. (2013). Robust estimation of optimal dynamic treatment regimes for sequential treatment decisions. *Biometrika* **100,** 681–694.

Zhang, C.-H. (2010). Nearly unbiased variable selection under minimax concave penalty. *The Annals of Statistics* **38,** 894 – 942.

Zhang, C.-H. and Zhang, S. S. (2014). Confidence intervals for low dimensional parameters in high dimensional linear models. *Journal of the Royal Statistical Society: Series B (Statistical Methodology)* **76,** 217–242.

Zhang, H., Zhan, J., Jin, J., Zhang, J., Ahearn, T. U., Yu, Z., O'Connell, J., Jiang, Y., Chen, T., Garcia-Closas, M., et al. (2022). Novel methods for multi-ancestry polygenic prediction and their evaluations in 3.7 million individuals of diverse ancestry. *bioRxiv.*

Zhang, J. and Braun, T. M. (2013). A phase I Bayesian adaptive design to simultaneously optimize dose and schedule assignments both between and within patients. *Journal of the American Statistical Association* **108,** 892–901.

Zhang, K., Janson, L., and Murphy, S. (2020). Inference for batched bandits. *Advances in Neural Information Processing Systems* **33,** 9818–9829.

Zhang, K. W., Janson, L., and Murphy, S. A. (2021). Statistical inference with m-estimators on bandit data. *arXiv preprint arXiv:2104.14074.*

Zhang, K. W., Janson, L., and Murphy, S. A. (2022). Statistical inference after adaptive sampling in non-Markovian environments. *arXiv preprint arXiv:2202.07098.*

Zhang, Y. and Yang, Q. (2021). A survey on multi-task learning. *IEEE Transactions on Knowledge and Data Engineering.*

Zhao, L., Tian, L., Cai, T., Claggett, B., and Wei, L.-J. (2013). Effectively selecting a target population for a future comparative study. *Journal of the American Statistical Association* **108,** 527–539.

Zhao, P. and Yu, B. (2006). On Model Selection Consistency of Lasso. *Journal of Machine Learning Research* **7,** 23.

Zhao, Q., Small, D. S., and Ertefaie, A. (2017). Selective inference for effect modification via the lasso. *arXiv preprint arXiv:1705.08020.*

Zhao, Y., Zeng, D., Rush, A. J., and Kosorok, M. R. (2012). Estimating individualized treatment rules using outcome weighted learning. *Journal of the American Statistical Association* **107,** 1106–1118.

Zhao, Y., Zeng, D., Socinski, M. A., and Kosorok, M. R. (2011). Reinforcement learning strategies for clinical trials in nonsmall cell lung cancer. *Biometrics* **67,** 1422–1433.

Zhao, Y.-Q., Laber, E. B., Ning, Y., Saha, S., and Sands, B. E. (2019). Efficient augmentation and relaxation learning for individualized treatment rules using observational data. *The Journal of Machine Learning Research* **20,** 1821–1843.

Zhao, Y.-Q., Zeng, D., Laber, E. B., and Kosorok, M. R. (2015). New statistical learning methods for estimating optimal dynamic treatment regimes. *Journal of the American Statistical Association* **110,** 583–598.

Zheng, J., Erzurumluoglu, A. M., Elsworth, B. L., Kemp, J. P., Howe, L., Haycock, P. C., Hemani, G., Tansey, K., Laurin, C., Pourcain, B. S., et al. (2017). LD hub: a centralized database and web interface to perform LD score regression that maximizes the potential of summary level GWAS data for SNP heritability and genetic correlation analysis. *Bioinformatics* **33,** 272–279.

Zheng, W. and van der Laan, M. J. (2010). Asymptotic theory for cross-validated targeted maximum likelihood estimation. *UC Berkeley Division of Biostatistics Working Paper Series* **Paper 273,** 1–58.

Zheng, W. and van der Laan, M. J. (2011). Cross-Validated Targeted Minimum-Loss-Based Estimation. In *Targeted Learning: Causal Inference for Observational and Experimental Data,* pages 459–474. Springer New York, New York, NY.

Zhong, X., Cheng, B., Qian, M., and Cheung, Y. K. (2019). A gate-keeping test for selecting adaptive interventions under general designs of sequential multiple assignment randomized trials. *Contemporary Clinical Trials* **85,** 105830.

Zhou, D. and Tomlin, C. (2018). Budget-constrained multi-armed bandits with multiple plays. In *Proceedings of the AAAI Conference on Artificial Intelligence*, volume 32.

Zhou, X., Mayer-Hamblett, N., Khan, U., and Kosorok, M. R. (2017). Residual weighted learning for estimating individualized treatment rules. *Journal of the American Statistical Association* **112,** 169–187.

Zhou, Z., Wang, Y., Mamani, H., and Coffey, D. G. (2019). How do tumor cytogenetics inform cancer treatments? dynamic risk stratification and precision medicine using multi-armed bandits. *Dynamic Risk Stratification and Precision Medicine Using Multi-armed Bandits (June 17, 2019).*

Zhu, H. and Zhou, X. (2020). Statistical methods for SNP heritability estimation and partition: a review. *Computational and Structural Biotechnology Journal* **18,** 1557–1568.

Zhu, W., Zeng, D., and Song, R. (2019). Proper inference for value function in high-dimensional Q-learning for dynamic treatment regimes. *Journal of the American Statistical Association* **114,** 1404–1417.

Zigler, C. M. and Dominici, F. (2014). Uncertainty in propensity score estimation: Bayesian methods for variable selection and model-averaged causal effects. *Journal of the American Statistical Association* **109,** 95–107.

Zimmert, M. (2018). Efficient difference-in-differences estimation with high-dimensional common trend confounding. *arXiv preprint arXiv:1809.01643.*

Zohar, S. and Chevret, S. (2007). Recent developments in adaptive designs for phase I/II dose-finding studies. *Journal of Biopharmaceutical Statistics* **17,** 1071–1083.

Zou, H. (2006). The adaptive lasso and its oracle properties. *Journal of the American Statistical Association* **101,** 1418–1429.

Zou, H. and Hastie, T. (2005). Regularization and variable selection via the elastic net. *Journal of the Royal Statistical Society: Series B (Statistical Methodology)* **67,** 301–320.

Zucker, D. R., Ruthazer, R., and Schmid, C. H. (2010). Individual (n-of-1) trials can be combined to give population comparative treatment effect estimates: methodologic considerations. *Journal of Clinical Epidemiology* **63,** 1312–1323.

Index

Note: Page numbers in **bold** and *italic* refer to tables and figures, respectively.